DELAWARE ACADEMY OF MEDICINE
LEWIS B. FLINN LIBRARY
1925 LOVERING AVE.
WILMINGTON, DEL. 19806

SURGICAL PROBLEMS AFFECTING THE PATIENT WITH CANCER: INTERDISCIPLINARY MANAGEMENT

Surgical Problems Affecting the Patient with Cancer: Interdisciplinary Management

Alan T. Lefor, M.D.
Associate Professor of Surgery and Oncology
Department of Surgery and the
University of Maryland Cancer Center
University of Maryland at Baltimore
Baltimore, Maryland

With 24 Contributors

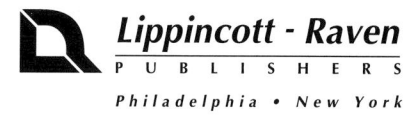

Lippincott - Raven
PUBLISHERS
Philadelphia • New York

Assistant Editor: Eileen Wolfberg
Production Editor: Virginia Barishek
Production: Textbook Writers Associates
Interior Designer: Martha White Tenney
Cover Designer: Thomas M. Jackson
Indexer: Alphabyte, Inc.
Compositor: The Composing Room of Michigan, Inc.
Printer/Binder: Quebecor/Kingsport

Copyright © 1996, by Lippincott–Raven Publishers. All rights reserved. This book is protected by copyright. No part of it may be reproduced, stored in a retrieval system, or transmitted, in any form or by any means—electronic, mechanical, photocopy, recording, or otherwise—without the prior written permission of the publisher, except for brief quotations embodied in critical articles and reviews. Printed in the United States of America. For information write Lippincott–Raven Publishers, 227 East Washington Square, Philadelphia, PA 19106.

Library of Congress Cataloging-in-Publication Data

Surgical problems affecting th patient with cancer :
 interdisciplinary management / [edited by] Alan T. Lefor.
   p. cm.
 Includes bibliographical references and index.
 ISBN 0-397-51402-6 (alk. paper)
  1. Cancer—Complications—Surgery. 2. Cancer—Complications—Treatment. I. Lefor, Alan T.
  [DNLM: 1. Neoplasms—complications.
  2. Neoplasms—surgery. QZ 200 S9615 1996]
RD651.S886 1996
616.99'4059—dc20
DNLM/DLC
for Library of Congress   95-41063
                                                CIP

The material contained in this volume was submitted as previously unpublished material, except in the instances in which credit has been given to the source from which some of the illustrative material was derived.

Great care has been taken to maintain the accuracy of the information contained in the volume. However, neither Lippincott–Raven Publishers nor the editors can be held responsible for errors or for any consequences arising from the use of the information herein.

The authors and publisher have exerted every effort to ensure that drug selection and dosage set forth in this text are in accord with current recommendations and practice at the time of publication. However, in view of ongoing research, changes in government regulations, and the constant flow of information relating to drug therapy and drug reactions, the reader is urged to check the package insert for each drug for any change in indications and dosage and for added warnings and precautions. This is particularly important when the recommended agent is a new or infrequently employed drug.

Materials appearing in this book prepared by individuals as part of their official duties as U.S. Government employees are not covered by the above-mentioned copyright.

9 8 7 6 5 4 3 2 1

To Mom and Dad for the beginning,
to Sheila for the present,
to Maarten for the promise of the future

Contributors

Adrian Barbul, M.D.
Department of Surgery
Sinai Hospital of Baltimore and Johns Hopkins University
Baltimore, Maryland

David L. Bogdonoff, M.D.
Associate Professor of Anesthesiology and Surgery
Departments of Anesthesiology and Surgery
University of Virginia School of Medicine
Charlottesville, Virginia

William E. Burak, Jr, M.D.
Clinical Assistant Professor
Division of Surgical Oncology
Ohio State University College of Medicine
Columbus, Ohio

Pauline W. Chen, M.D.
Resident, Department of Surgery
Yale University
New Haven, Connecticut

Brian J. Eastridge, M.D.
Administrative Chief Resident
Department of Surgery
University of Maryland Medical Center
Baltimore, Maryland

Stephen E. Ettinghausen, M.D.
Division of Surgical Oncology
Washington Cancer Institute
Washington Hospital Center
Washington, D.C.

William B. Farrar, M.D.
Director, Division of Surgical Oncology
Department of Surgery
Arthur G. James Cancer Hospital and Research Institute
Ohio State University College of Medicine
Columbus, Ohio

Michael Fiocco, M.D.
Assistant Professor of Surgery
Division of Cardiothoracic Surgery
Department of Surgery
University of Maryland School of Medicine
Baltimore, Maryland

William E. Fisher, M.D.
Division of Surgical Oncology
Department of Surgery
Ohio State University School of Medicine
Columbus, Ohio

Meyer R. Heyman, M.D.
Associate Professor of Medicine and Oncology
Division of Hematology/Medical Oncology
University of Maryland Cancer Center
University of Maryland School of Medicine
Baltimore, Maryland

Mark J. Krasna, M.D.
Assistant Professor of Surgery
Chief, General Thoracic Surgery
Division of Cardiothoracic Surgery
Department of Surgery
University of Maryland School of Medicine
Baltimore, Maryland

Alan T. Lefor, M.D.
Associate Professor of Surgery and Oncology
Department of Surgery and the University
  of Maryland Cancer Center
University of Maryland School of
  Medicine
Baltimore, Maryland

Michael P. Lilly, M.D.
Associate Professor of Surgery
Division of Vascular Surgery
Department of Surgery
University of Maryland School of
  Medicine
Baltimore, Maryland

Donald D. Mathes, M.D.
Assistant Professor of Anesthesiology
Department of Anesthesiology
The Bowman Gray School of Medicine
  of Wake Forest University
Winston-Salem, North Carolina

Gregory P. Midis, M.D.
Fellow, Department of Surgical Oncology
M.D. Anderson Cancer Center
Houston, Texas

James L. Peacock, M.D.
Assistant Professor of Surgery and
  Oncology
University of Rochester School of Medicine
  & Dentistry
Rochester, New York

Michael R. Schäffer, M.D.
Department of Surgery
Chirurgische Klinik
Eberhard-Karls-Universität Tübingen
Tübingen, Germany

Hank J. Schneider, M.D.
Department of Surgery
Oregon Health Sciences University
Portland, Oregon

Carl Shanholtz, M.D.
Assistant Professor of Medicine
  and Member, Program in Oncology
Director of Critical Care
University of Maryland Cancer Center
Baltimore, Maryland

William F. Sindelar, M.D., Ph.D.
Senior Investigator
Surgery Branch, National Cancer
  Institute
Bethesda, Maryland

James V. Sitzmann, M.D.
Professor and Robert J. Coffey Chair
Department of Surgery
Georgetown University
Washington, D.C.

John Skibber, M.D.
Assistant Professor of Surgery
Department of Surgical Oncology
M.D. Anderson Cancer Center
Houston, Texas

Irene Perez Vetto, B.S.N., R.N., O.C.N.
Department of Surgery
Oregon Health Sciences University
Portland, Oregon

John T. Vetto, M.D.
Assistant Professor of Surgery
Section of Surgical Oncology
Department of Surgery
Oregon Health Sciences University
Portland, Oregon

Eric A. Wiebke, M.D.
Assistant Professor of Surgery
Department of Surgery
Indiana University School of Medicine
Indianapolis, Indiana

Foreword

Surgery remains the mainstay of treatment for patients with cancer. Of the 50% of patients with cancer who will be cured by appropriate modern treatment, surgery is estimated to play a role in more than two-thirds of these curative treatments. The role of surgery as a primary treatment or its integration as part of the multimodality treatment of cancer patients is constantly being refined and is described in standard texts of cancer treatment.

The surgeon, however, plays a major additional role in the management of diverse problems that arise in the cancer patient and this text deals, in detail, with these issues. Either as a result of the local effects caused by growing cancer nodules or consequences that arise from the aggressive application of cancer treatments, the surgeon often is called on to deal with difficult problems in this challenging patient population.

The aggressive use of modern chemotherapy has dramatically increased the need for vascular access and this book deals with the problems of gaining vascular access and the management of problems resulting from extravasation of chemotherapeutic agents. The hematopoietic suppression resulting from chemotherapy leads to unique problems such as the management of abdominal pain in neutropenic patients, the management of gastrointestinal bleeding in patients with thrombocytopenia, or the inhibition of wound healing resulting from the administration of chemotherapy and radiation therapy. Separate chapters deal with these issues. The application of radiation therapy can lead to problems with intestinal motility, perforation, and fibrosis; the difficult problems that arise in these clinical situations often require surgical intervention.

Surgery continues to play a major role in primary cancer treatment but the surgeon does much more as well. This text delineates many of the important roles of the surgeon as the natural history of the disease evolves in the cancer patient.

Steven A. Rosenberg, M.D., Ph.D.

Preface

Although there are a number of excellent surgical oncology textbooks available that discuss the surgical treatment of cancer, many conditions arise in the course of cancer therapy for which surgeons are asked to serve as consultants. This often occurs while the patient is treated by other oncology caregivers and does not fall into discussions contained in textbooks of surgical oncology. This volume brings together a single reference source for the oncology professional that provides information on dealing with a variety of surgical conditions encountered in the cancer patient. Some management problems discussed in this book also are seen in patients without malignancy. In those cases, aspects of diagnosis or treatment that are affected by coexisting malignancy are amplified.

This book is presented in three parts:

- Part I deals specifically with gastrointestinal and abdominal problems often seen in the oncology patient. Chapter 1 gives an excellent overview of abdominal problems in patients with cancer. Chapters 2 through 8 each focuses on specific gastrointestinal and abdominal problems often confronted by the general surgeon as a consultant.
- Part II focuses on extra-abdominal surgical problems of interest to the consulting surgeon, including chapters on venous access, chemotherapy extravasation, vascular problems, and thoracic problems.
- Part III contains five chapters that provide information regarding systemic issues that is specifically useful to the surgeon caring for the cancer patient. Chapters include: *Preoperative Evaluation of the Cancer Patient, Chemotherapy and Wound Healing, Nutritional Support in the Cancer Patient, Infections in the Immunocompromised Patient,* and *Cancer-Related Hematologic Abnormalities in Surgical Patients.*

This information has been compiled to make the surgical decision-making process easier and, ultimately, to improve the care of the cancer patient by surgeons. Because much of cancer care is multidisciplinary, this information will also be of interest to non-surgeons involved in the care of the cancer patient. Although the resulting volume is an effort of many, I alone am responsible for any errors in content.

Alan T. Lefor, M.D.

Acknowledgments

I am deeply grateful to each of the contributors for their significant efforts despite the rigors of busy clinical practices and academic responsibilities. Each of them is actively engaged in the practice of caring for cancer patients. I am also deeply indebted to the staff at Lippincott–Raven Publishers, particularly Mr. J. Stuart Freeman, without whose support from its inception, this project would have never come to fruition, and to Ms. Eileen Wolfberg whose support has been unflagging and essential. The extraordinary patience and fortitude shown by Ms. Geraldine McGowan of Textbook Writers Associates in the production of this work is acknowledged.

I also wish to acknowledge the constant support of my department chairman, Dr. Anthony L. Imbembo, who has enabled me to continue my pursuits in an outstanding academic environment.

Most importantly, I express my deepest gratitude to the families and friends of my contributors, who understand one of the paradoxes of an academic career. For it is from them that academic pursuits ultimately take valuable time, whereas it is also our families and friends who make much of life worthwhile.

A. T. L.

Contents

Contributors   vii

Foreword   ix
Steven A. Rosenberg, M.D., Ph.D.

Preface   xi

I. Abdominal Surgical Problems   1

1. **Abdominal Pain in the Neutropenic Cancer Patient**   3
   Gregory P. Midis and John Skibber

2. **Malignant Gastrointestinal Obstruction**   25
   Eric A. Wiebke

3. **Gastrointestinal Bleeding and Perforation in the Cancer Patient**   61
   William E. Burak, Jr. and William B. Farrar

4. **Inflammatory Lesions of the Gastrointestinal Tract**   97
   William E. Fisher, William E. Burak, Jr., and William B. Farrar

5. **Hepatobiliary Disease in the Cancer Patient**   111
   James V. Sitzmann

6. **Management of Malignant Ascites**   125
   Eric A. Wiebke

7. Intestinal Complications of Radiation Therapy   143
   Pauline W. Chen and William F. Sindelar

8. Constipation and Chemotherapy-Induced Emesis   161
   John T. Vetto, Hank J. Schneider, and Irene Perez Vetto

II. Extra-Abdominal Surgical Problems   181

9. Chronic Venous Access in the Cancer Patient   183
   Brian J. Eastridge and Alan T. Lefor

10. Management of Chemotherapy Extravasation   211
    Stephen E. Ettinghausen

11. Vascular Problems in the Cancer Patient   223
    Michael P. Lilly

12. Thoracic Problems in the Cancer Patient   249
    Michael Fiocco and Mark J. Krasna

III. Systemic Considerations in the Surgical Treatment of the Cancer Patient   271

13. Preoperative Evaluation of the Cancer Patient   273
    Donald D. Mathes and David L. Bogdonoff

14. Chemotherapy and Wound Healing   305
    Michael R. Schäffer and Adrian Barbul

15. Nutritional Support in the Cancer Patient   321
    James L. Peacock

16. Infections in the Immunocompromised Patient   343
    Carl Shanholtz

17. Cancer and Therapy-Related Hematolgic Abnormalities   373
    Meyer R. Heyman

Index   393

ABDOMINAL SURGICAL PROBLEMS

I

Abdominal Pain in the Neutropenic Cancer Patient

GREGORY P. MIDIS
JOHN SKIBBER

Most general surgeons practicing outside of major cancer centers dread the consultation for abdominal pain in the cancer patient. Other than gastrointestinal bleeding, nearly all consultations for evaluation of abdominal visceral disease center around the symptom of pain. The cancer patient should be evaluated and treated as any other patient with the same symptomatology. Most abdominal pain will resolve without aggressive intervention. Problems commonly seen in noncancer patients are also common in cancer patients and may occur with increased frequency as a result of decreased immunocompetence. Both this altered immunity and medications such as steroids may mask the signs and symptoms of a gastrointestinal catastrophe. Abdominal pain, therefore, is more of a diagnostic challenge in this patient population. A thorough, methodical approach is warranted in evaluating these patients. It is also important for the general surgeon to be familiar with the causes of abdominal pain that are unique to the cancer patient.

This chapter focuses on select abdominal problems likely to be seen in cancer patients by a consulting surgeon. A separate section is included on abdominal pain in the bone marrow transplant patient. This organization was chosen because certain causes of abdominal pain apply only to the cancer patient population.

The algorithm in Figure 1-1 will serve as a useful guide to the organization of both this chapter and to this section of the book focusing on gastrointestinal disease. If one is consulted for gastrointestinal bleeding, appropriate resuscitation and evaluation initially have been performed. (This is more fully discussed in Chapter 3.) Most other consultations for abdominal problems will usually be for pain. After a thorough evaluation including history, physical examination, and appropriate radiologic studies, a clinical picture will emerge. If the pain is not extra-abdominal (referred), it can be classified under the headings of *obstruction*, *inflammatory* (including infection or sepsis), *vascular* or *ischemic*, or *other* to include pain from drug reactions, organomegaly, retroperitoneal hemorrhage, tumor, or metabolic derangements. Each section in this chapter focuses on select topics from some of these categories.

Although this chapter serves as an overview, other chapters of this book focus in detail on some of the problems causing abdominal pain in the cancer patient. In order that each chapter may be useful alone, there is some overlap found particularly between this chapter and those that follow it. Gastrointestinal obstruction is discussed in Chapter 2. Gastrointestinal bleeding and perforation are thoroughly discussed in Chapter 3. Inflammatory conditions of the gastroin-

```
                          Initial Consultation
                         /                    \
                        /                      \
                       /                        Gastrointestinal Bleeding
                      ↓                                  ↓
              Abdominal Pain                          Therapy
             /            \
            ↓              ↓
    Extra-abdominal    Intra-abdominal
    Source (Referred)     Source
                            ↓
                        Evaluation
                      ("Clinical Picture")
```

Obstruction		Vascular/Ischemic	Inflammation/Infection	Other
Ileus	**Mechanical Obstruction**	Mesenteric infarct (arterial/venous)		Drug reaction
Medications	Adhesions	Hepatic infarct		Retroperitoneal hemorrhage
Metabolic	Tumor	Splenic infarct		Hepatomegaly
Infection	Hernia	Renal infarct		Splenomegaly
Neurologic	Radiation enteritis	Ruptured aneurysm		Tumor (mass)
	Volvulus			Metabolic
	Intussusception			

Inflammation/Infection:

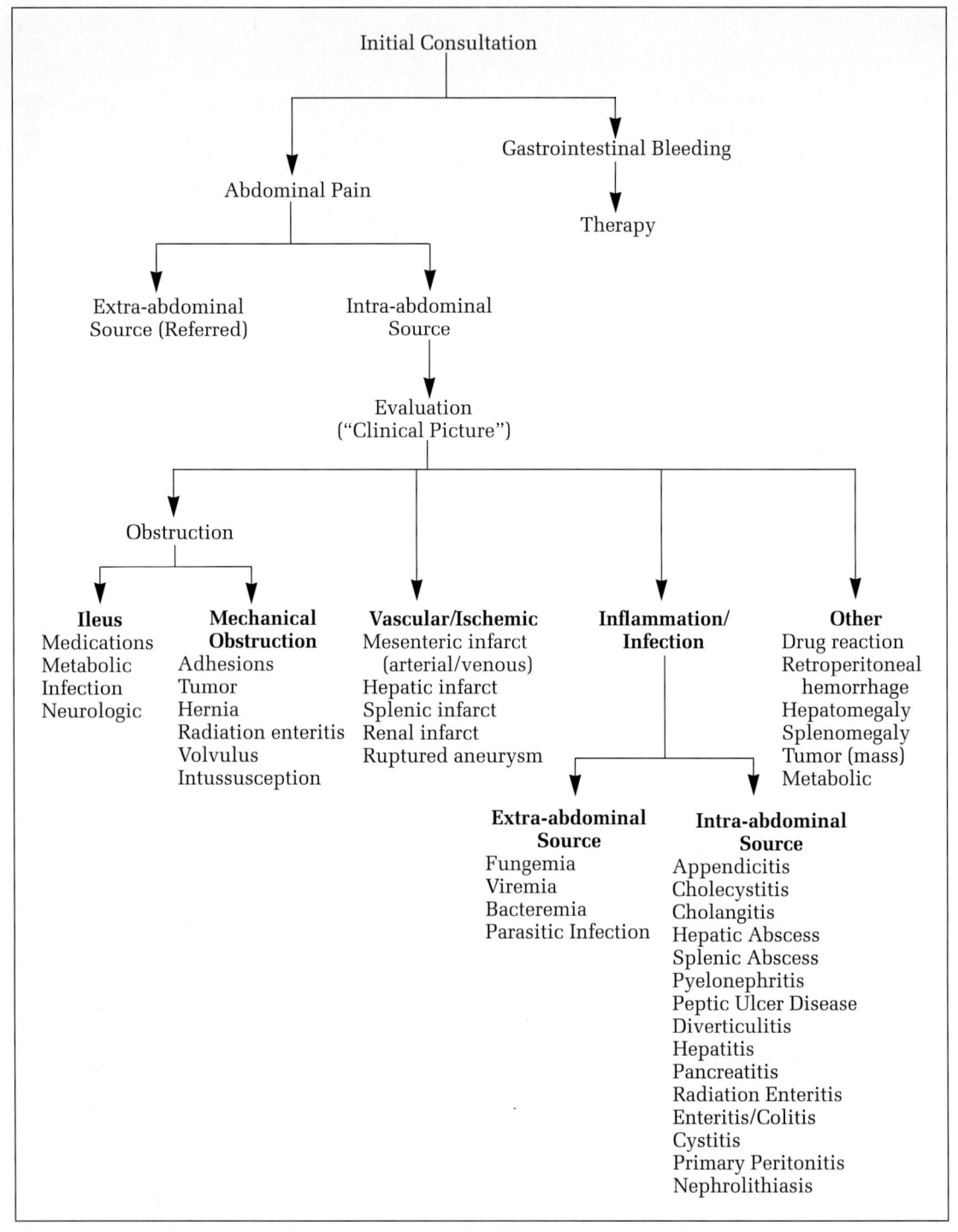

Extra-abdominal Source	Intra-abdominal Source
Fungemia	Appendicitis
Viremia	Cholecystitis
Bacteremia	Cholangitis
Parasitic Infection	Hepatic Abscess
	Splenic Abscess
	Pyelonephritis
	Peptic Ulcer Disease
	Diverticulitis
	Hepatitis
	Pancreatitis
	Radiation Enteritis
	Enteritis/Colitis
	Cystitis
	Primary Peritonitis
	Nephrolithiasis

Figure 1-1. Consultant approach to gastrointestinal problems in cancer patients.

testinal tract are covered in Chapter 4. Hepatobiliary disease is the focus of Chapter 5. The management of malignant ascites is discussed in Chapter 6. The effects of radiation therapy on the intestinal tract are fully covered in Chapter 7. Problems with constipation and chemotherapy-induced emesis are further discussed in Chapter 8. Thus, the chapters in the first section of the book comprise a complete discussion of abdominal problems in the cancer patient.

INFLAMMATORY/INFECTIOUS DISEASES

The algorithm in Figure 1-1 shows both the common and unique causes of abdominal pain that initially result from localized inflammatory or infectious processes. These diseases have been divided into those originating extra-abdominally where the abdominal viscera are target organs and those that originate within the abdominal viscera. Although the majority of these conditions may remain as locoregional disease, many have the potential to cause sepsis, particularly in the neutropenic cancer patient.

This section will focus on aspects of inflammatory and infectious conditions unique to the cancer patient: neutropenic enterocolitis, pancreatitis, perforation, and abdominal manifestations of disseminated infectious diseases. Other inflammatory conditions of the gastrointestinal tract are fully discussed in Chapter 4.

Neutropenic Enterocolitis

The most common cause of abdominal pain in the neutropenic patient is neutropenic enterocolitis (NE). It is also referred to as *typhlitis*, *ileocecal syndrome*, and *neutropenic enteropathy*. Neutropenic enterocolitis is characterized by fever, abdominal pain, nausea, vomiting, diarrhea (often bloody), and depending on the severity, sepsis. It should not be confused with "necrotic enterocolitis," which can occur in the terminal phases of other types of colitis such as pseudomembranous colitis and ischemic colitis. Infectious colitis is not covered in this chapter; it is fully discussed in Chapter 16.

The incidence of neutropenic enterocolitis varies with study type and the patient population examined. It occurs in 2.6% of adults with leukemia, according to one clinical study,[1] and in 12% of patients with leukemia at autopsy.[2] If NE is studied in the context of gastrointestinal (GI) complications or abdominal pain developing in leukemic patients, the incidence is 35% to 62%.[3–5] Neutropenic enterocolitis was the cause of 61% to 100% of acute abdominal conditions requiring surgery in two neutropenic patient populations.[6,7] When the occurrence of NE is sought in patients receiving cytosine arabinoside (Ara-C), it is found to occur in 8.6% of Ara-C administrations, or in 17% of patients treated.[8] This latter figure has varied depending on the dosing of Ara-C, but the range is 2.6% to 32.4% of patients.[8] The incidence in the pediatric population may be different, as neutropenic enterocolitis was found in only 4% of cases of abdominal pain documented in young leukemic patients.[9] In summary, the various incidences may depend on population selection and the problematic nature of documenting this disease given the various degrees of its presentation and the lack of sufficient confirmation through pathology or autopsy examination.

Neutropenic enterocolitis occurs most commonly in leukemic patients after therapy-induced neutropenia. The peak incidence is 7 to 14 days after the initiation of therapy, which usually coincides with the neutrophil count nadir. It also has been documented in patients with other conditions such as aplastic anemia,[10,11] cyclic neutropenia,[11,12] solid tumors,[11,13] myeloma,[11] and in therapy associated with bone-marrow transplantation.[14,15]

Although many chemotherapeutic agents have been associated with neutropenic enterocolitis, the most commonly implicated is Ara-C alone or in combination with other agents.[7,8,16–21] It is not surprising that this is one of the most effective agents in treating leukemia. Despite the common use of Ara-C in multiagent regimens with daunorubicin, neutropenic enterocolitis does not occur with daunorubicin alone.[22] Ara-C precipitates NE by initially causing physical damage to the GI tract.

Although the entire GI tract can be affected, there is a predilection for the right colon and cecum for unknown reasons.[8,20,22] The progression of the disease after this initial insult explains the protean clinical manifestations as the disease advances from mild to severe.

Chemical damage to the colon rather than leukemic infiltration is felt to be the initiating event, given the absence of neoplastic cells in colonic specimens.[2,19] Once the mucosa is violated, ulcerations form which lead to focal ischemia and possibly necrosis with no immediate regeneration of cells seen.[22,23] On gross examination, the bowel has transmural edema with patchy areas of ulceration and necrosis, which is worse in the mucosa and submucosal areas compared with the serosa.[23] Less severe cases eventually show microscopic evidence of epithelial regeneration at the crypts.[22] The pathology can also include telangiectasias and intramural hemorrhage associated with either vascular malformation or associated thrombocytopenia.[22] More importantly, these areas of ulceration and necrosis are felt to be portals by which a host of microorganisms gain entry into the circulation. This causes further colonic disease and can lead to sepsis.[20,23,24]

The association of ileus and subsequent stasis with neutropenic enterocolitis is not clearly defined.[13,25] Ischemia is not felt to be a primary etiology in the pathogenesis of neutropenic enterocolitis as it is in ischemic colitis, because the mesenteric vessels in resected colonic specimens are patent.[2] The presence of these macroscopic and microscopic findings varies greatly with the severity of the disease.[25]

Because the colonic mucosal barrier is destroyed, it is not surprising that indigenous flora are the major organisms isolated from pathologic sections of the colon and the blood of patients with neutropenic enterocolitis. These organisms include *Pseudomonas Aeruginosa, Klebsiella Pneumoniae, Escherichia Coli, Enterobacteriaceae*, and *Candida*.[2,19–22,24] Recently the *Clostridia* species, such as *C. septicum*,[20,26] and *C. tertium*,[23] have been implicated as causal agents, which may reflect the altered gastrointestinal flora due to broad-spectrum antibiotic use for long periods of time.

The clinical features of neutropenic enterocolitis include fever, abdominal pain, nausea, and vomiting in a neutropenic patient, usually 7 to 14 days after the initiation of chemotherapy. The presence and severity of symptoms depends on the extent of disease; this can be a spectrum from mild and self-limiting to septic and life-threatening. Because these patients are immunosuppressed, it is generally believed that the physical examination is less useful than normal. In fact, however, most series demonstrated the presence of abdominal pain in neutropenic enterocolitis, a significant percent of which localized to the right lower quadrant.[1,4–6,9,18] Diarrhea, whether bloody or not, can be caused by antibiotics, chemotherapy, or other gastrointestinal conditions such as colitis.

In many cases, neutropenic enterocolitis is associated with sepsis and in 40% to 74% of these patients, bacteria are isolated from the blood.[3,5,7,8,24,25] These organisms are similar to the organisms isolated from the resected segments of the colon in patients with severe neutropenic enterocolitis. Unfortunately, the bacterial isolates are not specific for neutropenic enterocolitis as these are the most common organisms isolated in neutropenic infections.[27] The clinical and laboratory findings, therefore, are nonspecific, and a high index of suspicion is certainly warranted to make the diagnosis.

Plain radiographic evaluation is also nonspecific for neutropenic enterocolitis. Abdominal radiographs usually show mild ileus, focal dilatation of scattered small bowel loops, occasional fluid-filled ascending colon, and sometimes obstruction at the ileocecal junction.[28] If perforation occurs in neutropenic enterocolitis, pneumoperitoneum or pneumatosis intestinalis sometimes can be seen.

Although sonography can be used, computed tomography (CT) scan has become more common for the evaluation of abdominal pain in neutropenic patients. The abdominal computed tomography scan findings in neutropenic enterocolitis are diffuse bowel wall thickening, occasional low attenuation areas consistent with edema or necrosis, pneumatosis, pericolonic fluid, and thickening of fascial planes.[28–30] An example of this is shown in Figure 1-2.

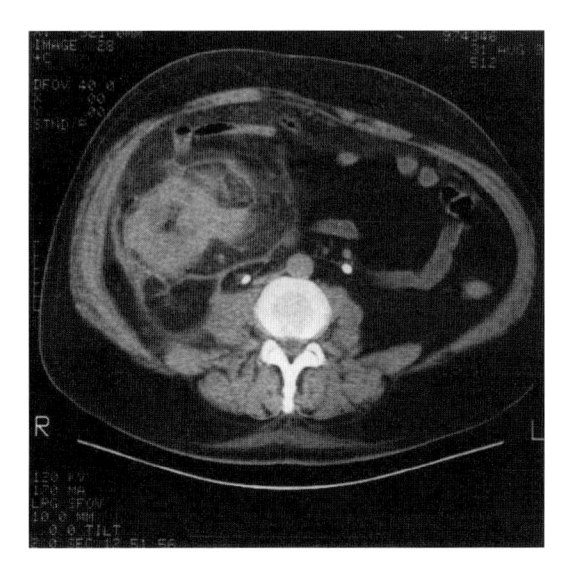

The differential diagnosis of suspected neutropenic enterocolitis includes the conditions listed in Table 1-1. Most of these conditions are commonly found in patients seen in any general surgery practice.

The diagnosis of neutropenic enterocolitis is generally one of exclusion.[18] Careful initial evaluation including history, physical

Table 1-1. Differential Diagnosis of Neutropenic Enterocolitis

Ischemic colitis
Infectious colitis
Mesenteric lymphadenitis
Retroperitoneal hemorrhage
Liver abscess
Nephrolithiasis
Appendicitis
Cholecystitis
Pancreatitis
Radiation enteritis

examination, and plain radiographs will help exclude more common conditions (Table 1-1). Stool evaluation with flexible sigmoidoscopy can help rule out pancolonic infections such as pseudomembranous colitis. Recently, peritoneal lavage has been suggested as a way to distinguish operable and nonoperable neutropenic enterocolitis presentations.[16]

Before discussing therapy, it is useful to put neutropenic enterocolitis in clinical perspective. Most cases of abdominal pain in the neutropenic patient, specifically NE, will resolve with conservative (*i.e.*, nonoperative) therapy.[8,9] In fact, it is in these cases that the diagnosis is questioned. The outcome evaluation of neutropenic enterocolitis patients, whether treated primarily by medical or surgical means, is complicated by selection bias, small numbers of patients in most series, and the poor outcome in general for neutropenic patients with infectious complications. Furthermore, autopsy studies in patients with the clinical diagnosis of NE have not always demonstrated histologic evidence of the disease but rather findings associated with various leukemic complications.[1,4,30]

There are no prospective trials to guide clinicians in choosing medical or surgical therapy. Despite this, some authors support surgical therapy,[1,7,25] whereas others favor conservative (*i.e.*, nonoperative) or medical therapy.[5] Most, however, recommend individualized management, which incorporates both types of therapy.[4,9,19,24,31]

Figure 1-2. This CT scan image was obtained from a 55-year-old man with acute monocytic leukemia receiving chemotherapy who presented with sepsis and right lower quadrant pain. It demonstrates a large right lower quadrant inflammatory process, consistent with necrotizing enterocolitis. At operation he had an ischemic right colon and underwent resection with creation of an ileostomy and mucous fistula.

Initial management should include careful observation, nasogastric decompression, nutritional support, blood products, and broad-spectrum antibiotics. Appropriate radiographs are obtained as needed and include plain radiographs, sonograms, and CT scans; contrast studies are not encouraged given the possibility of severely diseased and possibly perforated bowel. Surgery is reserved for perforation, hemorrhage, abscess, obstruction, or failure to progress with nonoperative management.[24,25]

The appropriate surgical procedure in neutropenic enterocolitis has varied from resection of involved colon with either anastomosis or endostomy and mucous fistula to diversion only. Neither appendectomy with drainage nor diversion alone is useful as the focus of infection remains *in situ*. The success of these procedures has varied from study to study.[3,25,32] In a recent review of combined neutropenic enterocolitis studies from 1973 to 1992, Ettinghausen[24] reported a surgical mortality of 21% and a medical mortality of 48%. Complications in these surgical procedures included wound infection, intra-abdominal sepsis, respiratory failure, and wound dehiscence.

Survival depends on the return of leukocyte counts[4,19,20,24] and improvement in overall condition. Granulocytes and growth factors (G-CSF (granulocyte colony-stimulating factor) and GM-CSF (granulocyte-macrophage)) have been used to hasten immunologic recovery. As discussed in Chapter 17, the period of severe neutropenia may be shortened if these agents are administered shortly after completion of chemotherapy, but their role in the management of neutropenic enterocolitis is unclear.[7]

RECOMMENDED APPROACH TO THE PATIENT WITH NEUTROPENIC ENTEROCOLITIS

Most likely the surgical consultant will be involved in the more complicated cases of neutropenic enterocolitis (*i.e.*, when conservative [nonoperative] therapy has failed or there is high suspicion that the GI tract is the source of sepsis in a neutropenic patient). The algorithm in Figure 1-3 was made to guide the surgeon in the care of these patients. Obviously, superior judgement is needed to know when to abandon this approach and individualize therapy, especially in a disease such as neutropenic enterocolitis with such varied manifestations and outcomes given concurrent medical problems.

The initial evaluation of these patients follows the same guidelines used for any patient with an abdominal problem for which surgical intervention is contemplated. Patients, who on initial evaluation have peritonitis or pneumoperitoneum, are quickly prepared and taken to the operating room. If neutropenic enterocolitis is suspected and the patient has either generalized, or more commonly, right lower quadrant symptoms and signs, the disease processes in Table 1-1 must be considered in the differential diagnosis. The likelihood of *Clostridium difficile* colitis decreases if stool evaluation for toxin and flexible sigmoidoscopy are negative. Often, the differential diagnosis consists of neutropenic enterocolitis and appendicitis. We believe that CT scan is helpful at this point to differentiate these two diagnoses and to evaluate the severity of neutropenic enterocolitis if it is present. If the CT scan demonstrates an abscess, CT-directed or open drainage can be performed; which of these two should be used depends on the judgement of the surgeon and the availability of radiologic expertise.

The CT scan could also identify localized perforation or pneumatosis intestinalis, both of which mandate urgent exploration. If the scan suggests neutropenic enterocolitis without the complications mentioned and the patient is stable, the conservative (nonoperative) management as outlined above can be instituted. If uncertainty exists given all the data, diagnostic laparoscopy should be considered to differentiate appendicitis if possible, and to evaluate the extent of colonic disease.

Recent data on the evaluation of gastrointestinal problems in critically ill patients using laparoscopy has been promising.[33] If managed nonoperatively, the patient should

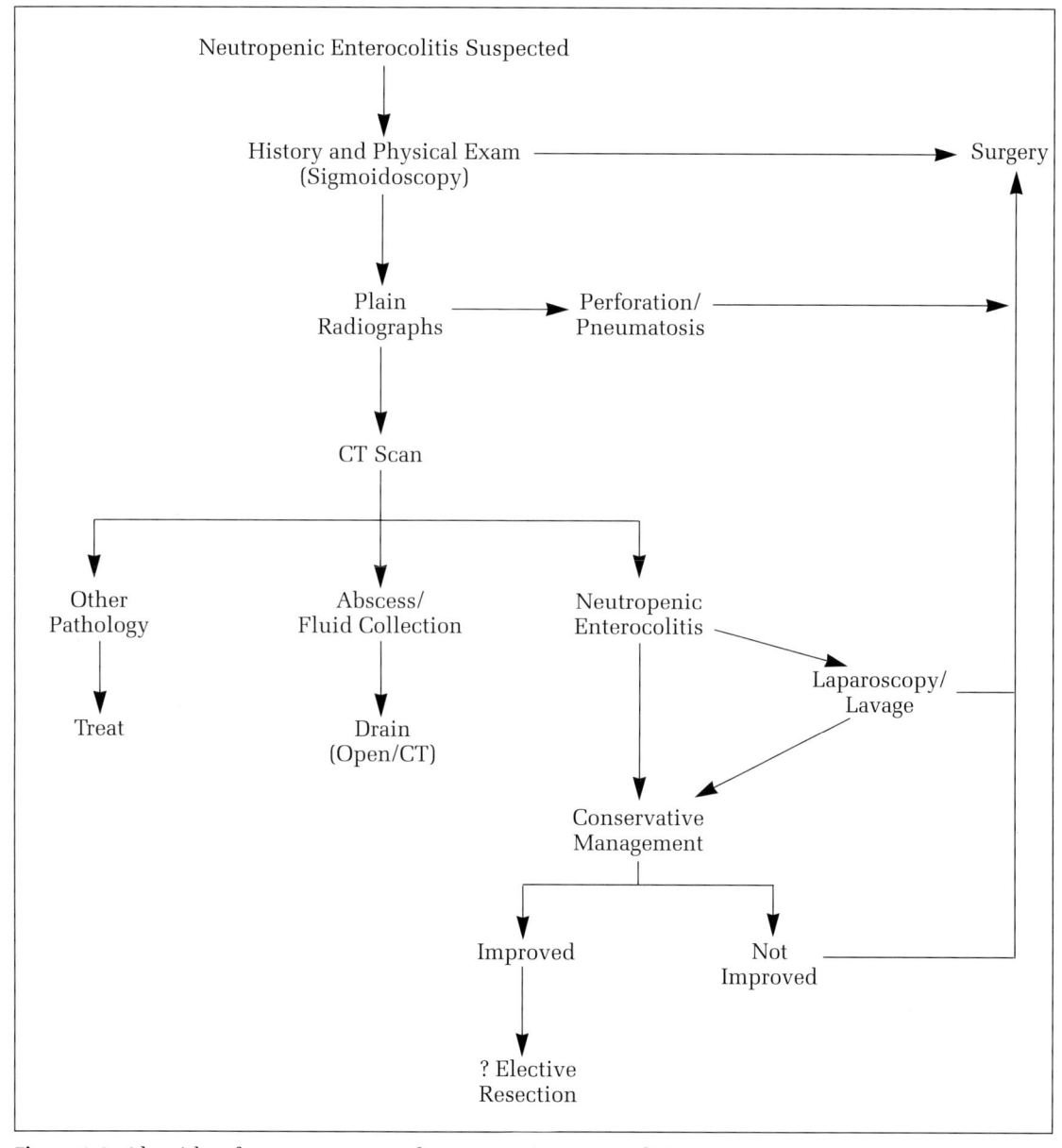

Abdominal Pain in the Neutropenic Cancer Patient

Figure 1-3. Algorithm for management of neutropenic enterocolitis.

be closely monitored with repeat investigations as needed. Any deterioration or failure to improve in a 24- to 48-hour period is justification for exploration. The surgeon will find the evaluation and management of neutropenic enterocolitis to be very similar to ischemic colitis, along with all of the dilemmas associated with the care of these patients.

Once the patient recovers, consideration must be given to recurrence of neutropenic enterocolitis with subsequent courses of therapy. This has been found to occur in a significant number of patients followed after initial neutropenic enterocolitis.[8,19,31] Elective resection has been considered by some of these authors.[8,19,31]

The proper operation to perform is a matter of judgement. As mentioned, simple drainage of the affected area or appendectomy only should not be done. Very careful evaluation of the bowel should be performed prior to resection because areas of normal-appearing serosa could have involved mucosa or submucosa. Once resection is performed, a decision must be made concerning anastomosis in these patients. In the face of no soilage and increased neutrophil counts, anastomosis can be considered, but leakage results in a high morbidity and mortality.

The most conservative surgical treatment and the one recommended would involve a proximal ostomy and distal mucous fistula. Proximal diversion without resection in cases of near obstruction without necrosis has been advocated but its use has been limited.

SUMMARY: NEUTROPENIC ENTEROCOLITIS

1. The peak incidence of neutropenic enterocolitis is 7 to 14 days after therapy begins, and is associated with Ara-C administration. Neutropenic enterocolitis is caused by chemical damage to the colon.
2. Clinical features include fever, abdominal pain, nausea and vomiting with a wide range of severity. Many patients do have pain localized to the right lower quadrant.
3. Initial management includes nasogastric decompression, nutritional support, and antibiotics. Surgery is reserved for perforation, hemorrhage, abscess, obstruction or failure to improve with nonoperative management. Those patients needing bowel resection usually should undergo an ileostomy and mucous fistula rather than primary anastomosis.

Pancreatitis

Pancreatitis is a rare cause of abdominal pain in cancer patients. It has been associated

Table 1-2. Factors Associated With Pancreatitis in the Cancer Patient

Single and multiagent chemotherapy
Tumor lysis
Hepatic intra-arterial chemotherapy
Intraperitoneal chemotherapy
Pancreatic carcinoma
Pancreatic metastatic disease
Bone marrow transplantation

with the entities listed in Table 1-2. Hepatobiliary diseases common in cancer patients are further discussed in Chapter 5.

The most common single chemotherapeutic agent associated with pancreatitis is L-asparaginase, a protein synthesis inhibitor used mainly in the treatment of acute lymphoblastic leukemia. Pancreatitis is the least common toxicity of this drug.[34] In a study of 43 pediatric leukemic patients treated with L-asparaginase, 16% developed pancreatitis; of these 43% occurred during administration of the drug.[34] The incidence of pancreatitis is 0% to 16% in clinical studies,[34] and 0% to 25% in combined autopsy and clinical studies.[35,36]

The clinical presentation in oncology patients does not differ from that seen in other settings. However, it can occur 2 days to 10 weeks after the initiation of therapy, with a median occurrence at 6 days.[36] Although not indicated in all of the studies reviewed, conservative (i.e., nonoperative) therapy was uniformly successful. The role of concomitant steroid administration in potentiating L-aspariase–induced pancreatitis is controversial.[34,36,37]

Another agent implicated in chemotherapy-induced pancreatitis is Ara-C, which was reported in one patient on two administrations of this agent. A review of the literature revealed two additional cases.[38]

Pancreatitis also has been infrequently reported with the use of multi-agent chemotherapy. All cases were mild, and conservative (i.e. nonoperative) therapy resulted in rapid resolution without interference in the treatment regimen.[39–41]

Pancreatitis also can be caused by tumor infiltration of the pancreatic parenchyma. Although it is an uncommon presentation of pancreatic carcinoma,[42] it has been reported as a presentation of metastatic disease to the pancreas. The most common cancer associated with metastasis-induced pancreatitis is bronchogenic carcinoma, the majority of which are small cell carcinomas. The incidence of pancreatitis in small cell lung cancer from an autopsy series was 20% to 40%, whereas the clinical incidence in this same population was 3.3% to 7.5%.[43–45] The diagnosis was made by typical physical examination findings, increased amylase and lipase, with confirmation by computed tomography or sonography. Although it is difficult to derive a treatment plan based on few cases, it appears that in severe cases of pancreatitis, patients do not tolerate chemotherapy well. However, patients who can tolerate chemotherapy when indicated do benefit from treatment.[45,46] These are patients who demonstrate few negative prognostic indicators of pancreatitis.

Tumor lysis is a rare cause of pancreatitis. It has been reported in two cases of lymphoma where exquisite tumor sensitivity to chemotherapy with rapid lysis was thought to have caused pancreatitis. These patients presented with abdominal pain and increased amylase levels; both responded to conservative therapy.[37]

Pancreatitis was a rare complication of intraperitoneal chemotherapy seen in 1 of 43 patients treated with cytoreductive therapy and chemotherapy.[47]

The satisfactory response rates in treating hepatic tumors with intra-arterial chemotherapy has increased the number of patients treated with either pumps or transcatheter interventional techniques. Increases in amylase were seen in patients treated with transcatheter intra-arterial chemotherapy using either gelatin sponges or gelfoam powder embolization. It was not seen in patients given intra-arterial chemotherapy alone. Because prior coil occlusion of the gastroduodenal artery prevented increases in amylase after chemotherapy and embolization, the authors concluded that reflux of embolic materials into the gastroduodenal artery probably causes pancreatitis. Unfortunately, the authors documented increased amylase levels and not clinical pancreatitis.[48] Pancreatitis was also seen in 7% of patients with hepatocellular carcinoma treated with intra-arterial cisplatin. All cases were mild, and the patients recovered with conservative measures.[49] Only 1 of 85 patients treated with continuous hepatic arterial chemotherapy developed pancreatitis in a single institution.[50]

Abdominal pain, nausea, and vomiting are common in patients after bone marrow transplantation. These symptoms are usually associated with the administration of multiple chemotherapeutic agents and radiation or complications such as infection and graft-versus-host disease. Pancreatitis is a possible cause of this abdominal pain. It was found in 7 of 202 (3.5%) bone marrow transplantations at a single institution.[51] Although 4 of these incidents occurred in the peritransplant period, the remainder were diagnosed up to 2 years after transplantation. It is unclear whether pancreatitis in this situation is due to chemotherapy, bone marrow transplantation, graft-versus-host disease, or a combination of all these factors.

In summary, pancreatitis from a variety of causes can be seen in the oncology patient. Fortunately, it is a rare occurrence and most patients recover rapidly with nonoperative measures. As with pancreatitis in any patient, the treatment of necrotizing pancreatitis often requires aggressive surgical therapy to improve overall outcome. Pancreatitis, however, should be included in the differential diagnosis of abdominal pain in the neutropenic cancer patient.

SUMMARY: PANCREATITIS

1. Pancreatitis has been associated with L-asparaginase and Ara-C administration. It can also be caused by direct invasion of the pancreas by tumor.
2. Therapy is usually nonoperative with supportive care only. Patients with necrotizing pancreatitis may require surgical debridement.

Perforation

Gastrointestinal perforation in the neutropenic cancer patient usually is encountered under the following circumstances: as a presentation of cancer, as a benign condition occurring in a cancer patient, or as a result of tumor lysis from therapy. The latter two conditions are the ones most often seen in the neutropenic patient presenting with abdominal pain. A further discussion of gastrointestinal perforation, including other causes not seen primarily in neutropenic cancer patients, is found in Chapter 3.

Perforation should always be included in the differential diagnosis of cancer patients who present with abdominal pain, regardless of the paucity of clinical findings to support the diagnosis. In a review of 272 emergency procedures in 266 adults with cancer, Turnbull[52] found 41 perforations; 31 were considered disease- or treatment-related, and included gastric, small bowel, and colonic perforations. It is not specifically stated which were caused by benign conditions and which were caused directly by the malignancy. In a study of right lower quadrant pain in 129 leukemic patients, 10 perforated viscera were found (excluding the cecum).[9] Of 50 neutropenic patients with abdominal pain seen at Roswell Park Cancer Center (Buffalo, NY) by the surgical service, one perforation was found from gastric lymphoma.[4] In a review of 14 emergency abdominal operations in neutropenic cancer patients at the National Institutes of Health (Bethesda, MD), six perforations were found.[6] Two perforations were seen in 58 neutropenic cancer patients who required surgical consultation for acute abdominal pain.[5] Gastrointestinal perforation is the cause of abdominal pain in a small number of neutropenic cancer patients, and can be spontaneous (no pathology associated) or disease related.

Perforation not localized to an area of cancer is called *spontaneous perforation* and is seen in patients receiving chemotherapy with and without steroids. Twelve cases of spontaneous gastroduodenal perforation were seen at the Memorial Sloan-Kettering Cancer Center (New York, NY) between 1974 and 1987. There was no history of prior ulcer disease, and all patients were receiving chemotherapy or steroids.[53] Also, 21 emergency operations were reviewed in patients with metastatic cancer receiving chemotherapy. Fifteen perforations were found, 10 were in a viscus not involved with cancer (67%).[54] Of 30 perforations in cancer patients receiving chemotherapy and steroids, approximately 50% occurred in areas not involved with tumor.[55] These studies indicate that gastrointestinal perforation in the cancer patient can occur in areas not involved with tumor and usually in the setting of steroids with and without cytotoxic chemotherapy.

Perforation in an area of bowel involved with cancer usually occurs with lymphoma either at the time of presentation or during therapy. It can occur with any primary malignancy or metastatic disease to the bowel, but this is rare.[50,55] It is seen at the time of presentation in 15% to 31% of primary GI tract lymphomas.[56–60] The perforation rate without therapy depends greatly on the stage of disease, as series with higher stage disease (stage III or IV) tend to have higher perforation rates. Because they have not received therapy, these patients are not neutropenic. Therapy is based on standard general surgical principles.

More importantly, perforation is sometimes seen after initiation of therapy for lymphoma. These patients are usually neutropenic, and if receiving steroids, typical presenting signs and symptoms of perforation may be absent.

In a study of patients with non-Hodgkin's lymphoma of the GI tract, 23 initially had surgery and 14 did not; 43% of these nonoperated patients subsequently developed hemorrhage or perforation.[61] In another review of patients with localized and disseminated lymphoma, 24 patients were not initially treated with surgery, and 2 had perforations (8%).[62] In 18 patients receiving therapy for diffuse histiocytic lymphoma most of whom were stage III or IV, 3 had perforations during therapy (19%), and 3 prior to therapy.[59]

In a review of 104 cases of lymphoma,

mostly early stage, 13% experienced hemorrhage or perforation during therapy.[63] In another 20 patients with stage III or IV lymphoma, two perforations were seen (10%).[64] More recently, 70 patients with primarily stage I or II lymphoma were reviewed at the MD Anderson Cancer Center (Houston, TX). Fifty-five received primary chemotherapy with or without radiotherapy; no perforations occurred.[65]

Perforation during therapy of GI tract lymphoma does occur, but the incidence depends on the stage of disease. The greater perforation rate with later stage disease may also reflect a higher overall perforation rate regardless of therapy as indicated previously in patients presenting with perforation. Therapy of GI tract lymphomas in the pediatric population with non-Hodgkin's lymphoma also reveals a 6% to 7% perforation rate.[66,67]

The neutropenic patient may present with some or all of the signs and symptoms of perforation. It is important to remember that this patient population, particularly if receiving steroids, may mask the typical presentation which could have devastating consequences. Although pneumoperitoneum is commonly seen, it may be absent in 51% to 67% of immunocompromised or neutropenic patients.[52]

Perforation of a gastric ulcer is treated with simple closure unless chronicity is seen and malignancy is suspected; simple closure is also recommended for duodenal perforation.[52,53] Small bowel perforation is treated by resection and primary anastomosis unless peritonitis is found or the perforation occurs in conjunction with steroid therapy or neutropenia.[50,52] Colonic perforations are treated with resection and diversion.

SUMMARY: PERFORATION

1. Perforation may be the initial presentation of a malignancy or be a result of tumor lysis caused by therapy. It is found in a small number of neutropenic cancer patients and can be spontaneous or disease related (often in patients with lymphoma).
2. Higher rates of perforation are seen after therapy for lymphoma in patients with more advanced disease.
3. Therapy is based on basic surgical principles. Caution should be exercised in the repair of small bowel perforations in neutropenic patients or in those receiving steroids.

Disseminated Infection

Fungal organisms are second only to bacteria as the cause of infection in neutropenic cancer patients. *Candida* species and *Aspergillus* species are responsible for about 90% of fungal infections in adult neutropenic patients with acute lymphocytic leukemia (ALL).[68] In neutropenic children with cancer, the most common organisms are *Candida*, *Aspergillus*, *Mucor*, and *Phycomycetes*.[69,70] Invasive candidal infection was found in 11% of 1500 bone marrow transplant patients, and invasive *Aspergillus* was found in 4.5 % of patients.[71,72] The most commonly involved sites of infection are the oral cavity, esophagus, GI tract, and lung, with other viscera involved less often.[27,70] Intra-abdominal infections are further discussed in Chapter 16.

Risk factors for candidemia include prolonged bacteremia, neutropenia, fever, administration of antimicrobial agents, multiple antibiotics, and *Candida* organisms in the stool.[68] An additional risk factor in bone marrow transplant patients is donor cell depletion of lymphocytes; in fact, it is the most powerful predictor of fungemia in these patients.[73] Colonization with *Candida* organisms also increases the risk for disseminated infection. It is thought that dissemination occurs from the colonization sites.[27] It was found that 2% to 11% of immunocompromised children colonized with *C. tropicalis* and *C. albicans* developed disseminated fungal infections, whereas none without colonization developed fungemia.[69] The therapy for these infections has traditionally been amphotericin B alone. However, the roles of fluconazole, itraconazole, and other agents as adjuncts or alternative therapy are still investigational.[27]

Abdominal pain is most commonly seen when disseminated fungal infection involves the liver or spleen. This is called *focal hepatic candidiasis, hepatosplenic candidiasis,* or *hepatic candidiasis.* This is a distinct clinical syndrome that differs from disseminated fungal infection by the involvement of only the liver and spleen.[74] Almost every case is seen in granulocytopenic patients post-therapy and is characterized by fever, abdominal pain (diffuse or localized to the right upper quadrant), anorexia, nausea, and vomiting.[74–77] It is caused by focally persistent abscesses in the liver, spleen, and, rarely, the kidneys. It often presents as an increase in liver enzymes in a patient suspected of having fungemia. In addition, an increase in candidal IgM and leukocytosis is sometimes seen.[74,75] The diagnosis is made by CT scan or sonography with the characteristic "bull's eye" lesions seen only when granulocyte counts are recovering. Confirmation is made by biopsy if needed.[74,78] The diagnosis is sometimes difficult to confirm without biopsy as positive blood cultures occur in less than 50% of patients with candidemia.[75] The presentation of hepatosplenic candidiasis is the same in children.[70] As in other forms of *Candida* infection, the treatment is amphotericin B, which can be given systemically or locally by hepatic infusion.[70,74–77] The addition of flucytosine is controversial.[75] Recently, satisfactory results have been seen with fluconazole if amphotericin B fails.[79]

Surgeons should also be aware of other manifestations of candidemia as the presentations are similar to many other common diseases of the abdominal viscera usually treated by surgical means. Biliary tract candidiasis was identified in nine patients: six had disease confined to the gallbladder, and three had disease only in the biliary tree. Therapy was successful with cholecystectomy and antifungal therapy.[80] A case of gangrenous cholecystitis from *C. tropicalis* presenting as acute acalculous cholecystitis was found in a neutropenic cancer patient.[81] These cases demonstrate the myriad presentations of abdominal fungal infections in neutropenic patients.

In addition to hepatoslenic candidiasis, the spleen can be involved as the only manifestation of disseminated fungal infection. Seven immunocompromised cancer patients have been identified with focal splenic abscesses from *Candida* species.[82,83] They presented with fever, no response to antibiotics, and left upper quadrant pain. Their therapy consisted of splenectomy in all cases.

Viral infections are also very common in neutropenic cancer patients. Abdominal involvement is not the rule, but it can be a part of disseminated infections from viruses such as herpes simplex virus (HSV), herpes zoster, varicella zoster virus (VZV), or cytomegalovirus (CMV). The surgical consultant should know that the clinical manifestations of these infections as abdominal involvement is rarely seen without other organ involvement. Viral infections are discussed further in Chapter 16.

HSV occurs in neutropenic cancer patients usually as a reaction to latent virus.[84] It most commonly presents as oral, genital, or mucocutaneous disease.[27,85] It can spread directly or by the hematogenous route to involve the stomach, colon, adrenal glands, liver, or central nervous system.[27,85] Bacterial suprainfection can occur in more severe cases. HSV hepatitis has been identified in bone marrow transplant patients. It presents with fever and abdominal pain; other viscera are commonly involved, but skin lesions are not usually seen.[86] The treatment involves acyclovir and observation; surgical intervention is needed only for complications from severe GI tract disease.

VZV infection in the neutropenic patient usually presents as reactivation of latent virus. Patients more commonly have VZV with disease confined to distinct dermatomal areas, and less commonly varicella-like infection with nonlocalized cutaneous disease.[27,87] Dissemination of VZV is seen in

11% of cancer patients: of these, 75% have cutaneous dissemination, 7% have visceral, and 18% have both cutaneous and visceral dissemination.[27] The most common noncutaneous sites of disease are the lung, followed by the liver, then the central nervous system.[27] Abdominal pain occurs mainly when the liver is involved in this dissemination process. The surgical consultant should remember that visceral involvement without skin disease is rare, and that abdominal symptoms indicative of visceral involvement may precede skin involvement.[88,89] In a study of varicella infection in 31 immunocompromised children, 15 were found to have visceral involvement, and 11 of these 15 complained of abdominal pain from hepatitis. In most cases, pneumonitis, encephalopathy, and coagulopathy were present in addition to liver disease.[88] The mortality from disseminated disease is 7% to 50%.[88,89]

VZV infections occur in 17% to 50% of patients after allogeneic bone marrow transplant.[27,87] In patients with these infections, 75% to 85% present as herpes zoster, and 15% to 25 % present as a varicella-like syndrome.[27] Unlike VZV in bone marrow transplant patients, HSV occurs during the reappearance of immune function, which is 2 to 6 months after bone marrow transplant.[87] Skin lesions typically appear for 5 to 7 days; dissemination is seen in 5 % of cases and occurs during this period of skin disease. Abdominal pain can occur at this time if there is VZV hepatitis, which is characterized by an increase in liver enzymes with a mild increase in bilirubin. The hepatitis is usually self-limited.[87] The diagnosis is made by physical examination and routine laboratory findings supplemented when needed with cultures and immunofluorescence testing.[27,87–89] The treatment for VZV as with HSV is acyclovir.

CMV is also commonly seen in the immunocompromised host. It is the most common viral infection in the period after bone marrow transplant with an incidence of 50% in these patients.[27] As with HSV and VZV, CMV is usually the result of reactivation of latent virus. Most cases involve mild disease with fever, abdominal pain, hepatitis, leukopenia, and thrombocytopenia. Abdominal involvement in more severe cases includes gastritis, esophagitis, and enterocolitis. The most life-threatening CMV infection, however, is pneumonitis.[27] Surgeons will usually be consulted for abdominal pain in more advanced cases where necrosis, obstruction, or perforation may arise in CMV-infected viscera.

SUMMARY: DISSEMINATED INFECTION

1. Disseminated fungal infection involving the liver or spleen may cause abdominal pain. Biliary tract candidiasis also has been described and treated with cholecystectomy and antifungal therapy.
2. Viral infections also are common in neutropenic cancer patients. HSV hepatitis has been described in bone marrow transplant patients. Treatment is with acyclovir. CMV is the most common viral infection in the bone marrow transplant patient and is usually a result of reactivation of latent virus. Abdominal involvement can lead to necrosis, obstruction, or perforation.

OBSTRUCTION

If abdominal pain in the neutropenic cancer patient is associated with the clinical picture of obstruction, a decision is made whether or not the obstruction is mechanical. In the cancer patient, this decision can be difficult. (Gastrointestinal obstruction in the cancer patient is fully discussed in Chapter 2.) This chapter considers only adynamic ileus secondary to chemotherapeutic agents as this is an important cause of obstructive symptoms in the cancer patient.

The use of chemotherapeutic agents to

treat malignant disease can result in profound gastrointestinal adverse effects. Nausea, vomiting, and diarrhea are commonly reported by cancer patients receiving therapy. Most of these toxicities are not associated with abdominal pain. (A complete discussion of nausea in the cancer patient is found in Chapter 8.) However, a less common toxicity, ileus from chemotherapeutic agents, is associated with abdominal pain and must be included in the differential diagnosis of abdominal pain in the neutropenic patient.

The agent most commonly associated with ileus is vincristine (Oncovin), a plant alkaloid. Ileus, constipation, and associated abdominal pain of varying degrees occur from autonomic nerve dysfunction.[90–92] Neurotoxicity in general is the major dose-limiting factor for this drug and its frequency is directly proportional to dose.[91] Acute gastrointestinal symptoms usually occur within a few days of drug administration, and they usually precede other manifestations of neurotoxicity.[90,93] In a study of 392 cases of vincristine therapy, constipation was reported in one third, and decompression of the GI tract was needed in three patients.[93] Abdominal pain was usually seen after the first or second dose, and preceded the discomfort associated with constipation. All gastrointestinal symptoms were dose related. Similar results were identified in a group of 50 leukemic patients treated with vincristine. Of those, 46% experienced abdominal pain and constipation within 3 days of therapy and one fourth had radiologic evidence of adynamic ileus.[94] Vinblastine produces similar gastrointestinal findings, but bone-marrow toxicity usually precedes neurotoxicity and therefore the incidence is usually less as dose adjustments are made earlier.[91]

Therapy is nonoperative with bowel rest, possible nasogastric suction, and frequent monitoring and serial examinations. Colonic ileus (pseudo-obstruction) is dealt with in the usual fashion; colonoscopic decompression is sometimes needed.[50] The manifestations are partially or completely reversible with decreased dosing or drug withdrawal.[91] Operative intervention is rare in the patient with cancer, as is usually the case with adynamic ileus. It is of paramount importance for the surgical consultant to consider other potentially harmful causes of abdominal pain in these patients.

SUMMARY: OBSTRUCTION AND ILEUS

1. Ileus as a result of chemotherapy administration is commonly associated with abdominal pain. Vincristine is commonly associated with ileus as a result of autonomic nerve dysfunction.
2. Therapy is usually nonoperative with bowel rest, nasogastric suction if indicated, and frequent monitoring. Other causes of abdominal pain must be considered.

VASCULAR/ISCHEMIC

Abdominal pain associated with vascular events in the cancer patient is mentioned here for completeness, but will not be discussed further in this chapter. (A discussion of vascular problems in the cancer patient is found in Chapter 11.) There are no specific vascular causes of abdominal pain in the cancer patient that are not also found in the general population and, therefore, one is referred to other sources for discussions of vascular problems that cause abdominal pain. The surgical consultant must review the types of vascular or ischemic events that can occur and keep them in the differential diagnosis of abdominal pain in the cancer patient.

In particular, one must keep in mind the effects of various therapeutic modalities on the vascular system, such as the acceleration of atherosclerotic disease caused by radiation therapy (refer to Chapters 7 and 11 for further discussion of these interactions). Although this may be an unusual effect on the mesenteric vasculature, the effects of radiation on the more commonly involved iliac vessels may complicate vascular reconstruction procedures. In general, there are no other specific considerations in the cancer patient when evaluating and treating abdominal pain of vascular origin compared to the patient without a malignancy.

ABDOMINAL PAIN IN THE BONE MARROW TRANSPLANT PATIENT

This section has been included because abdominal pain in the recent bone marrow transplant (BMT) patient has several unique causes. It is useful to consider these disease processes together because of their often similar presentations.

Bone marrow transplantation has been used successfully to treat hematologic malignancies, severe aplastic anemia, immunodeficiency states, and congenital disorders. More recently, BMT has become part of the armamentarium in treating solid tumors such as breast and ovarian cancer.[95] Abdominal pain, along with nausea and diarrhea, is common in patients after transplantation. In a retrospective study of 45 autologous BMT patients followed to 100 days post-transplant, abdominal pain was documented in 51%. Surgical consultation was obtained in 22% of the patients with pain, and 40% of the consulted patients required laparotomy.[96] Given this frequency of abdominal pain, it is important for the consulting surgeon to be aware of the unique causes of abdominal pain in this increasing patient population while still considering the more common causes of abdominal pain. This section will review the more common causes of abdominal pain in bone marrow transplant patients.

Table 1-3 gives the differential diagnosis of common causes of abdominal pain in BMT patients. In most cases, a combination of these causes exists and some, such as graft-versus-host disease (GVHD), can have a wide range of severity. As the bone marrow transplant patient progresses through different phases of the transplantation process, certain causes

Table 1-3. Common Causes of Abdominal Pain in Bone Marrow Transplant Patients

Chemoradiation
GVHD (single or multiorgan; acute and chronic)
Disseminated infection
Veno-occlusive disease of the liver
Enterocolitis
Pancreatitis
Adverse drug reactions
Cholecystitis
Gastroduodenal erosions and ulcerations
Hepatitis

of abdominal pain become more common. This chronology is of paramount importance in the evaluation of these patients. It is also important to remember that despite resolution of their neutropenia after successful bone marrow engraftment, the host remains immunodeficient for about 2 months.[27]

Crampy abdominal pain and diarrhea are common immediately after bone marrow transplant. This is usually due to the intense chemoradiation given as preparative treatment for transplantation. This consists of total body irradiation and chemotherapy, which causes intestinal epithelial damage. It develops by 10 days post-transplant and is usually resolved by day 20 unless GVHD intercedes.[97] Although most cases are mild, surgical intervention occasionally is required because of perforation or bleeding.[97]

These clinical findings must be differentiated from infection and GVHD, which have identical presentations. Infectious enteritis in BMT patients can be bacterial, viral, fungal, or parasitic and can vary greatly in severity. The diagnosis consists of a combination of biopsy, stool culture, and serology where appropriate. Occasionally, surgery is required for complications in severe cases.[97]

Gastrointestinal manifestations of GVHD include crampy abdominal pain, anorexia, diarrhea, nausea, and vomiting. It is a disease complex caused by donor T-cell–mediated destruction of normal host cells after activation by minor histocompatibility antigenic differences.[98,99] Both acute and chronic forms of GVHD exist, and they differ in onset and sites of organ involvement. It is a significant problem that occurs in 50% to 80% of allogeneic bone marrow transplants and is responsible for 12% to 20% of the post-transplant mortality.[99–101] Acute GVHD usually develops between 7 to 21 days post-transplant, and the major organs involved include skin, liver, and the GI tract.[102]

The gastrointestinal symptoms of GVHD can vary from mild and self-limiting to severe and life-threatening. Hepatic and gastrointestinal manifestations usually follow skin involvement that is characterized by a maculopapular rash.[101] The liver is the second most common organ involved, and hepatic disease manifests as an increase in liver function tests with a cholestatic picture.[101] The third most commonly involved organ is the GI tract. This includes focal or diffuse disease from the stomach to the colon and myriad clinical presentations depending on severity. Gastrointestinal involvement may be complicated by subsequent infection at damaged mucosal sites. This makes differentiating GVHD from enteritis difficult in certain cases. Most patients have cutaneous disease, and some have hepatic involvement when gastrointestinal symptoms appear; however, it is important to note that for some patients, gastrointestinal manifestations are the only evidence of GVHD.[97,100,101] Once the diagnosis is suspected clinically, biopsy of affected areas is used to establish the diagnosis.

Acute GVHD can also affect focal areas of the GI tract.[100] Upper gastrointestinal GVHD was identified as a distinct clinical entity in 62 of 469 allogeneic BMT patients in a study from one institution. In 25 of these patients, the skin and upper GI tract were the only sites involved, whereas the other 37 had diffuse organ involvement.[103] Whether focal or diffuse, acute GVHD can follow an indolent course or progress to greater severity with complications such as perforation, bleeding, or infection. Once acute GVHD has resolved, abdominal pain and diarrhea can persist for weeks.[97]

Chronic GVHD usually occurs 80 to 400 days post-transplant, and in 70% to 80% cases, it is preceded by acute GVHD.[97,101,102] It is the most common late complication of allogeneic bone marrow transplant, with an incidence of 20% to 40% in patients surviving the first 100 days post-transplant.[101] It is characterized by increased collagen deposition in the dermis and mucosal surfaces, as well as autoantibody production.[101,102] This leads to a clinical picture of cutaneous disease, esophagitis, oral lesions, hepatic and gastrointestinal involvement, and immunosuppression.[101] The most common cause of death in these patients is infection secondary to immunosuppression.[97]

Abdominal manifestations include both hepatic and diffuse GI disease, but the extent of organ involvement is highly variable. Hepatic disease is seen in 90% of patients and is characterized by right upper quadrant pain, jaundice, and elevation of liver function tests. At this period of post bone marrow transplant, the differential diagnosis for these symptoms is chronic viral infection, adverse drug reactions, and cholecystitis.[97,101] Gastrointestinal involvement in chronic GVHD is a result of collagen deposition in the bowel wall. This causes decreased gut motility and malabsorption, which consequently causes colicky abdominal pain, diarrhea, and malnutrition.[97,100,102]

The cause of right upper quadrant pain in the bone marrow transplant patient may be difficult to determine because of the similar presentation of many diseases and the frequency of this clinical finding. Important causes include adverse drug reactions, infection, cholecystitis, hepatic veno-occlusive disease (VOD), hepatic GVHD, and gastroduodenal ulcerations or erosions.

Hepatic VOD is a common complication of bone marrow transplant that occurs within 2 to 3 weeks of transplantation in 20% to 30% of patients. (Further discussion of hepatic vascular occlusive disease can be found in Chapter 5.) It is caused by the intensive chemotherapy or combined chemoradiation treatment that is given as a preparative regimen before marrow transplantation.[97,104,105] Clinically, a characteristic chronology is seen that begins with weight gain and jaundice. This can progress to abdominal pain, ascites, and encephalopathy. These findings in this post-transplant period can be used to differentiate VOD from GVHD, which almost always begins after day 20.[97] Other causes of right upper quadrant pain can be ruled out with standard imaging modalities. Ultimately, the diagnosis is made by liver biopsy, which in VOD shows centrilobar hemorrhagic necrosis causing obliteration of sinusoids and terminal hepatic venules.[104] This results clinically in hepatomegaly, ascites, and an elevation in liver function tests.[97] Although in the past, therapy was only supportive in nature, recent use of thrombolytic therapy has shown promise in select patients.[105] VOD resolves in 55% of patients, persists in 13%, and contributes to death in 32%, usually from multiorgan failure.[97,105] In general, there is no role for surgical therapy in this disease. Patients with ascites from chronic venous obstruction may benefit from peritoneovenous shunting, which is further discussed in Chapter 6. However, surgeons should be aware of this common cause of right upper quadrant pain in order to avoid unnecessary laparotomy.

Cholecystitis has been reported after bone marrow transplant. However, the signs and symptoms may be masked because of immune suppression and frequency of pain in the right upper quadrant post-transplantation. Cholecystitis occurred in 8 of 770 recipients of both allogeneic and autologous bone marrow transplants. Sixty-three percent of cases were acalculous.[106] The diagnosis was often difficult using standard laboratory and radiographic evaluations. Another institution recorded only two cases of acute acalculous cholecystitis after bone marrow transplant; both were treated successfully with cholecystectomy.[107] Given the small number of reports in this patient population, it is possible that the incidence of cholecystitis is the same post-transplant as in any other critically ill patient population. The surgical consultant should also be aware that the gallbladder can also rarely be involved by leukemic infiltrates that may present as cholecystitis.[109]

Abdominal pain, particularly right upper quadrant pain after bone marrow transplant may also be caused by a variety of infectious diseases originating in the abdomen, such as hepatitis, visceral abscess, or enteritis. Abdominal symptoms may also be the result of disseminated bacterial, fungal, viral, or parasitic disease such as discussed in a previous section.[97]

SUMMARY: ABDOMINAL PAIN IN THE BONE MARROW TRANSPLANT PATIENT

1. Crampy abdominal pain and diarrhea are common after bone marrow transplantation. They usually develop by 10 days post-transplant and resolve by 20 days post-transplant as a result of intestinal epithelial damage. Infection and GVHD have identical presentations.
2. Gastrointestinal manifestations of GVHD include crampy abdominal pain, anorexia, diarrhea, nausea, and vomiting. GVHD occurs in 50% to 80% of patients receiving allogeneic bone marrow transplant and is responsible for 12% to 20% of post-transplant mortality. Gastrointestinal manifestations usually follow skin involvement and can include focal or diffuse disease from stomach to colon. Furthermore, chronic GVHD can occur 80 to 400 days post-transplant, and is usually preceded by acute GVHD.
3. Vascular occlusive disease is also seen in the bone marrow transplant population and usually presents with abdominal pain, jaundice, ascites, and encephalopathy. Thrombolytic therapy may have a role, but therapy is usually limited to supportive care.
4. Acalculous cholecystitis has also been reported post bone marrow transplant.

The typical clinical findings may be masked because of immunosuppression.

∎

SUMMARY

The surgical consultant will be called to see gastrointestinal problems in cancer patients caused directly by tumors and the intensive therapies used to treat them. As the number of cytotoxic agents increases and the doses intensify, the abdominal complications will certainly increase. Cancer patients should be treated aggressively if ethically appropriate. Reluctance to offer adequate and timely surgical therapy to these patients because of their "cancer" diagnosis is not justified. This chapter has emphasized that the general surgeon—not just the surgical oncologist—can manage the majority of these problems using standard surgical therapy. No surgeon should be intimidated because of the often complex nature of these patients' illnesses. To treat these patients adequately, however, it is important to be aware of the unique causes of abdominal pain in the cancer patient. Finally, it is also important to remember that the successful treatment of cancer patients involves close cooperation between surgeons and other members of the multidisciplinary team.

REFERENCES

1. Mower W, Hawkins J, Nelson E. Neutropenic enterocolitis in adults with acute leukemia. Arch Surg 1986;121:571.
2. Steinberg D, Gold J, Brodin A. Necrotizing enterocolitis in leukemia. Arch Intern Med 1973;131:538.
3. Villar H, Warneke J, Peck M, et al. Role of surgical treatment in the management of complications of the gastrointestinal tract in patients with leukemia. Surg Gynecol Obstet 1987;165:217.
4. Wade D, Douglass H, Nava H, et al. Abdominal pain in neutropenic patients. Arch Surg 1990;125:1119.
5. Starnes H, Moore F, Mentzer S, et al. Abdominal pain in neutropenic cancer patients. Cancer 1986;57:616.
6. Glenn J, Funkhouser W, Schneider P. Acute illnesses necessitating urgent abdominal surgery in neutropenic cancer patients: description of 14 cases and review of the literature. Surgery 1989;105:778.
7. Martell R, Jacobs P. Surgery for the acute abdomen in adults with leukemia. Postgrad Med J 1986;62:915.
8. Vlasveld L, Zwaan F, Fibbe R, et al. Neutropenic enterocolitis following treatment with cytosine arabinoside-containing regimens for hematological malignancies: a potentiating role for amsacrine. Ann Hematol 1991;62:129.
9. Skibber J, Matter G, Pizzo P, et al. Right lower quadrant pain in young patients with leukemia. Ann Surg 1987;206:711.
10. Weinberger M, Hollingsworth H, Feuerstein I, et al. Successful surgical management of neutropenic enterocolitis in two patients with severe aplastic anemia. Arch Intern Med 1993;153:107.
11. Abbasoglu O, Cakmakci M. Neutropenic enterocolitis in patients without leukemia. Surgery 1993;113:113.
12. Geelhoed G, Kane M, Dale D, et al. Colon ulceration and perforation in cyclic neutropenia. J Pediatr Surg 1973;8:379.
13. Kingry R, Hobson R, Muir R. Cecal necrosis and perforation with systemic chemotherapy. Am Surg 1973;39:129.
14. Mehta J, Nagler A, Or R, et al. Neutropenic enterocolitis and intestinal perforation associated with carboplatin-containing conditioning regimen for autologous bone marrow transplantation. Acta Oncol 1992;31:591.
15. Or R, Mehta O, Nagler A, et al. Neutropenic enterocolitis associated with autologous bone marrow transplantation. Bone Marrow Transplant 1992;9:383.
16. Sauter E, Vauthey J, Bolton J, et al. Selective management of patients with neutropenic enterocolitis using peritoneal lavage. J Surg Oncol 1990;45:63.
17. Anderson P. Neutropenic enterocolitis treated by primary resection with anastomosis in a leukemic patient receiving chemotherapy. Aust N Z J Surg 1993;63:74.
18. Wade D, Nava H, Douglass H. Neutropenic enterocolitis: clinical diagnosis and treatment. Cancer 1992;69:17.
19. Moir C, Scudamore C, Benny W. Typhlitis: selective surgical management. Am J Surg 1986;151:563.
20. Newbold K. Neutropenic enterocolitis: clinical and pathological review. Dig Dis 1989;7:281.
21. Dosik G, Luna M, Valdivieso M, et al. Necrotizing colitis in patients with cancer. Am J Med 1979;67:646.

22. Slavin R, Dias M, Saral R. Cytosine-arabinoside induced gastrointestinal toxic alterations in sequential chemotherapeutic protocols. Cancer 1978;42:1747.
23. Coleman N, Speirs G, Khan J, et al. Neutropenic enterocolitis associated with Clostridium tertium. J Clin Pathol 1993;46:180.
24. Ettinghausen S. Collagenous colitis, eosinophilic colitis, and neutropenic colitis. Surg Clin North Am 1993;73:993.
25. Alt B, Glass N, Sollinger H. Neutropenic enterocolitis in adults: review of the literature and assessment of surgical intervention. Am J Surg 1985;149:405.
26. King A, Rampling A, Wight D, Warren R. Neutropenic enterocolitis due to Clostridium septicum infection. J Clin Pathol 1984;37:335.
27. Rosenberg A, Brown A. Infection in the cancer patient. Dis Mon 1993;39:507.
28. Adams G, Rauch R, Kelvin F, et al. CT detection of typhlitis. J Comput Assist Tomogr 1985;9:363.
29. Jones B, Fishman E. CT of the gut in the immunocompromised host. Radiol Clin North Am 1989;27:763.
30. Frick M, Maile C, Crass J, et al. Computed tomography of neutropenic colitis. AJR 1984;143:763.
31. Keidan R, Fanning J, Gatenby R, et al. Recurrent typhlitis: a disease resulting from aggressive chemotherapy. Dis Colon Rectum 1989;32:206.
32. Koea J, Shaw J. Surgical management of neutropenic enterocolitis. Br J Surg 1989;76:821.
33. Bender J, Talamini M. Diagnostic laparoscopy in critically ill intensive-care-unit patients. Surg Endosc 1992;6:302.
34. Weetman R, Baehner R. Latent onset of clinical pancreatitis in children receiving L-asparaginase therapy. Cancer 1974;34:780.
35. Whitecar J, Bodey G, Harris J, et al. Current concepts: L-asparaginase. N Engl J Med 1970;282:732.
36. Mallory A, Kern F. Drug-induced pancreatitis: a critical review. Gastroenterology 1980;78:813.
37. Spiegel R, Magrath I. Tumor lysis pancreatitis. Med Pediatr Oncol 1979;7:169.
38. Altman A, Dinndorf P, Quinn J. Acute pancreatitis in association with cytosine arabinoside therapy. Cancer 1982;49:1384.
39. Socinski M, Garnick M. Acute pancreatitis associated with chemotherapy for germ cell tumors in two patients. Ann Intern Med 1988;108:567.
40. Batson O, Branda R. Acute pancreatitis complicating therapy of Hodgkins disease. Am J Hematol 1990;33:78.
41. Newman C, Ellis D. Pancreatitis during combination chemotherapy. Clin Oncol 1979;5:83.
42. Warshaw A, Castillo C. Medical progress: pancreatic carcinoma. N Engl J Med 1992;326:455.
43. Gutman M, Inbar M, Klausner J. Metastases-induced acute pancreatitis: a rare presentation of cancer. Eur J Surg Oncol 1993;19:302.
44. Chowhan N, Madajewicz S. Management of metastases-induced acute pancreatitis in small cell carcinoma of the lung. Cancer 1990;65:1445.
45. Yeung K, Haidak D, Brown J, et al. Metastses-induced acute pancreatitis in small cell bronchogenic carcinoma. Arch Intern Med 1979;139:552.
46. Stewart K, Dickout W, Urschel J. Metastasis-induced acute pancreatitis as the initial manifestation of bronchogenic carcinoma. Chest 1993;104:98.
47. Esquivel J, Vidal-Jove J, Steves M, et al. Morbidity and mortality of cytoreductive surgery and intraperitoneal chemotherapy. Surgery 1993;113:631.
48. Kishimoto W, Nakao A, Takagi H, et al. Acute pancreatitis after transcatheter arterial embolization (TAE) for hepatocellular carcinoma. Am J Gastroenterol 1989;84:1396.
49. Shibata J, Fujiyama S, Sato T, et al. Hepatic arterial injection chemotherapy with cisplatin suspended in an oily lymphographic agent for hepatocellular carcinoma. Cancer 1989;64:1586.
50. Kemeny M, Brennan M. The surgical complications of chemotherapy in the cancer patient. Curr Probl Surg 1987;24:609.
51. Werlin S, Casper J, Antonson D, et al. Pancreatitis associated with bone marrow transplantation in children. Bone Marrow Transplant 1992;10:65.
52. Turnbull A. Abdominal and upper gastrointestinal emergencies. In Turnbull A, (ed). Surgical emergencies in the cancer patient. Chicago: Year Book Medical Publishers, 1987:152.
53. Ricci J, Turnbull A. Spontaneous gastroduodenal perforation in cancer patients receiving cytotoxic therapy. J Surg Oncol 1989;41:219.
54. Ferrara J, Martin E, Carey L. Morbidity of emergency operations in patients with metastatic cancer receiving chemotherapy. Surgery 1982;92:605.
55. Torosian M, Turnbull D. Emergency laparotomy for spontaneous intestinal and colon perforations in cancer patients receiving corticosteroids and chemotherapy. J Clin Oncol 1988;6:291.
56. Domizio P, Owen R, Sheperd N, et al. Primary lymphoma of the small intestine. Am J Surg Pathol 1993;17:429.
57. Serour F, Dona G, Birkenfeld S, et al. Primary neoplasms of small bowel. J Surg Oncol 1992;49:29.

58. Desa L, Bridger J, Grace P, et al. Primary jejunoileal tumors: review of 45 cases. World J Surg 1991;15:81.
59. Hande K, Fisher R, DeVita V, et al. Diffuse histiocytic lymphoma involving the gastrointestinal tract. Cancer 1978;41:1984.
60. Roxenfelt F, Rosenberg S. Diffuse histiocytic lymphoma presenting with gastrointestinal tract lesions. Cancer 1980;45:2188.
61. List A, Greer J, Cousar J, et al. Non-Hodgkin's lymphoma of the gastrointestinal tract: an analysis of clinical and pathologic features affecting outcome. J Clin Oncol 1988;6:1125.
62. Talamonti M, Dawes C, Joehl R, et al. Gastrointestinal lymphoma. Arch Surg 1990;125:972.
63. Weingard D, Decosse J, Sherlock P, et al. Gastrointestinal Lymphoma: a 30-year review. Cancer 1982;49:1258.
64. Randall J, Obeid M, Blackledge G. Hemorrhage and perforation of gastrointestinal neoplasms during chemotherapy. Ann R Coll Surg Engl 1986;68:286.
65. Yahanda A, Mansfield P. The role of locoregional therapy in the treatment of stage IE and IIE gastric lymphoma. Presented at the 47th Scientific Program of the Society of Surgical Oncology, Houston, Texas, 1994.
66. Rivera-Luna R, Guerra G. Abdominal lymphoma and intestinal perforation. J Clin Oncol 1989;7:285.
67. Meyers P, Potter V, Wollner N, et al. Bowel perforation during initial treatment for childhood non-Hodgkin's lymphoma. Cancer 1985;56:259.
68. Richet H, Andremont A, Tancrede C, et al. Risk factors for candidemia in patients with acute lymphoblastic leukemia. Rev Infect Dis 1991;13:211.
69. Marina N, Flynn P, Rivera G, et al. Candida tropicalis and candida albicans fungemia in children with leukemia. Cancer 1991;68:594.
70. Pizzo P, Walsh T. Fungal infections in the pediatric cancer patient. Semin Oncol 1990;17:6.
71. Goodrich J, Reed E, Mori M, et al. Clinical features and analysis of risk factors for invasive candidal infection after marrow transplantation. J Infect Dis 1991;164:731.
72. Meyers J. Fungal infections in bone marrow transplant patients. Semin Oncol 1990;17:10.
73. Pirsch J, Maki D. Infectious complications in adults with bone marrow transplantation and T-cell depletion of donor marrow. Ann Intern Med 1986;104:619.
74. von Eiff M, Essink M, Roos N, et al. Hepatosplenic candidiasis, a late manifestation of Candida septicaemia in neutropenic patients with haematologic malignancies. Blutalkohol 1990;60:242.
75. Tashjian L, Abramson J, Peacock J. Focal hepatic candidiasis: a distinct variant of candidiasis in immunocompromised patients. Rev Infect Dis 1984;6:689.
76. Haron J, Feld R, Tuffnell P, et al. Hepatic candidiasis: an increasing problem in immunocompromised patients. Am J Med 1987;83:17.
77. Blade J, Lopez-Guillermo A, Rozman C, et al. Chronic systemic candidiasis in acute leukemia. Ann Hematol 1992;64:240.
78. Thaler M, Pastakia B, Shawker T, et al. Hepatic candidiasis in cancer patients: the evolving picture of the syndrome. Ann Intern Med 1988;108:88.
79. Kauffman C, Bradley S, Ross S, et al. Hepatosplenic candidiasis: successful treatment with Fluconazole. Am J Med 1991;91:137.
80. Morris A, Sands M, Shiraki M, et al. Gallbladder and biliary tract candidiasis: nine cases and review. Rev Infect Dis 1990;12:483.
81. McGuire N, Hutson J, Hueble H. Gangrenous cholecystitis secondary to Candida tropicalis infection in a patient with leukemia. Clin Infect Dis 1992;14:367.
82. Hatley R, Donaldson J, Raffensperger J, et al. Splenic microabscesses in the immune-compromised patient. J Pediatr Surg 1989;24:697.
83. Page C, Coltman C, Robertson H, et al. Candidal abscess of the spleen in patients with acute leukemia. Surg Gynecol Obstet 1980;151:604.
84. Lazarus H, Cregar R, Gerson S. Infectious emergencies in oncology patients. Semin Oncol 1989;16:543.
85. Bustamante C, Wade J. Herpes simplex virus infection in the immunocompromised cancer patient. J Clin Oncol 1991;9:1903.
86. Johnson J, Egaas S, Gleaves C, et al. Hepatitis due to herpes simplex virus in marrow-transplant recipients. Clin Infect Dis 1992;14:38.
87. Feldman S. Varicella zoster infections in bone marrow transplantations. Recent Results Cancer Res 1993;132:175.
88. Morgan E, Smalley L. Varicella in immunocompromised children. Am J Dis Child 1983;137:883.
89. Stemmer S, Kinsman K, Tellschow S, et al. Fatal noncutaneous visceral infection with Varicella-Zoster virus in a patient with lymphoma after autologous bone marrow transplantation. Clin Infect Dis 1993;16:497.
90. Mitchell E, Schein P. Gastrointestinal toxicity of chemotherapeutic agents. In: Perry M, ed. The chemotherapy sourcebook. Baltimore: Williams and Wilkins, 1992:620.
91. Weiss H, Walker M, Wiernik P. Neurotoxicity

of commonly used antineoplastic agents. N Engl J Med 1974;291:127.
92. Rosenthal S, Kaufman S. Vincristine neurotoxicity. Ann Intern Med 1974;80:733.
93. Holland J, Scharlau C, Gailani S, et al. Vincristine treatment of advanced cancer: a cooperative study of 392 cases. Cancer Res 1973;33:1258.
94. Sandler S, Tobin W, Henderson E. Vincristine-induced neuropathy. Neurology 1969;19:367.
95. Hurd D. Bone marrow transplantation for cancer: an overview. Recent Results Cancer Res 1993;132:1.
96. Morton B, Wagman L, O'Donnell M. Significance and implications of abdominal pain in autologous bone marrow transplant patients. Presented at the 42nd Annual Cancer Symposium of the Society of Surgical Oncology, May 21-4, 1989, San Francisco, CA.
97. McDonald G, Shulman H, Sullivan K, et al. Intestinal and hepatic complications of human bone marrow transplantation. Parts I and II. Gastroenterology 1986;90:460,770.
98. Vogelsang G. Acute and chronic graft-versus-host disease. Curr Opin Oncol 1993;5:276.
99. Korngold R. Biology of graft-versus-host disease. Am J Pediatr Hematol Oncol 1993;15:18.
100. Barrett A. Graft-versus-host disease: basic considerations. Recent Results Cancer Res 1993;132:185.
101. Vogelsang G, Wagner J. Graft-versus-host disease. Hematol Oncol Clin North Am 1990;4:625.
102. Parkman R. Graft-versus-host disease. Annu Rev Med 1991;42:189.
103. Weisdorf D, Snover D, Haake R, et al. Acute upper gastrointestinal graft-versus-host disease: clinical significance and response to immunosuppressive therapy. Blood 1990;76:624.
104. Gottesman L, Turnbull A, O'Reilly R. Surgical implications of hepatic venocclusive disease following bone marrow transplantation. J Surg Oncol 1988;37:113.
105. Bearman S, Shuhart M, Hinds M, et al. Recombinant human tissue plasminogen activator for the treatment of established severe venocclusive disease of the liver after bone marrow transplantation. Blood 1992;80:2458.
106. Jardines L, O'Donnell M, Johnson D, et al. Acalculous cholecystitis in bone marrow transplant patients. Cancer 1993;71:354.
107. Pitkaranta P, Haapiainen R, Taavitsainen M, et al. Acalculous cholecystitis after bone marrow transplantation in adults with acute leukemia. Eur J Surg 1991;157:361.
108. Hurley R, Weisdorf D, Jessurun J, et al. Relapse of acute leukemia presenting as acute cholecystitis following bone marrow transplantation. Bone Marrow Transplant 1992;10:387.

2

Malignant Gastrointestinal Obstruction

ERIC A. WIEBKE

Malignant obstruction of the gastrointestinal tract is common. From the esophagus to the anus, malignancies often present with signs and symptoms of obstruction. The diagnosis, evaluation, and treatment of primary gastrointestinal cancers are usually straightforward. Recurrent or metastatic cancer causing bowel obstruction, on the other hand, can be therapeutically challenging. The degree of surgical intervention necessary, if indicated, must be carefully considered and the therapy for these patients must be individualized.

In this chapter, the evaluation and treatment of primary and recurrent malignancies of the gastrointestinal tract that cause obstruction are discussed. The approach to patients with recurrent disease or peritoneal carcinomatosis causing obstruction is formidable and the possible interventions more varied and less standardized.

ESOPHAGEAL CANCER INCLUDING THE GASTRIC CARDIA

Carcinoma of the esophagus often presents with locally advanced disease and evidence of partial esophageal occlusion. The clinical presentation is one of weight loss, inability to swallow solids initially, progressing to difficulty with liquids and odynophagia (pain with swallowing). The tumors are often bulky with regional lymph node and adjacent organ involvement, and usually cannot be resected for cure. Many, however, are resected for palliation. Palliative procedures other than resection include stenting, laser ablation, and radiation therapy. Each approach has been associated with a wide range of clinical outcomes.

Resection of esophageal cancer is attempted in approximately one third of cases, and survival in resected patients averages many months. Local recurrence rates of up to 50% have been reported despite resectional therapy. Attempts to improve resectability rates and decrease local recurrence rates by providing patients with preoperative radiation and chemotherapy have been successful in certain circumstances, yet the survival data overall does not seem significantly altered.[1,2] The Vanderbilt group[2] most recently reported on 58 patients with adenocarcinoma of the esophagus treated with preoperative radiation and chemotherapy (3000 cGy and cisplatin/5-Fluorouracil/leucovorin) and resection, or resection alone in a nonrandomized study.[3] Toxicity of the neoadjuvant therapy was minimal.

Sixteen patients treated with resection had a mean survival time of 8 months; 23 patients treated with preoperative chemoradiation therapy had average survival times of greater than 26 months. The 24 month actuarial survival was 15% for those treated with resection alone and 76% for those treated with multimodality therapy. A randomized trial of preoperative chemotherapy (5-FU and cisplatin-based) for patients with squamous cell carcinoma of the esophagus revealed similar resectability rates for both the treated and resection alone groups, higher postoperative complication and death rates for the treated group, and similar survival rates (median survival for both groups was 10 months).[1] These authors concluded that preoperative chemotherapy for squamous cell cancers was of no benefit, and actually increased operative morbidity and mortality. Next, 68 patients with biopsy-proved cancer of the esophagus were treated with preoperative radiation therapy (3000 cGy over 3 weeks).[4] Forty-three patients had squamous cell carcinoma, 22 had adenocarcinoma, and 3 had other malignancies. Eleven patients developed local recurrence and 30 developed metastases. Mean survival time was 39.7 months for squamous cell tumors and 23.9 months for adenocarcinomas; overall mean survival time was 32.5 months.

The surgical approaches to thoracic esophageal cancers are limited to two general categories: resection including aggressive mediastinal dissection via a thoracotomy and transhiatal esophagectomy. Survival seems comparable between the two groups, although this is somewhat controversial. Skinner et al[5] have been advocates of radical *en bloc* esophagectomy in selected patients, and others also conclude that radical lymphadenectomy improves survival.[6] Orringer[7] and Gadacz[8] have pointed out that transhiatal esophagectomy results in similar survival rates, stage for stage, as the more radical operations, with less operative morbidity and mortality. Figure 2-1 shows a barium esophagogram of a dysphagic 65-year-old man who had an endoscopically confirmed adenocarcinoma of the distal esophagus. His evaluation included abdominal and chest computed tomography (CT) scans which did not reveal metastatic disease, lymphadenopathy, or local invasion by the tumor. He underwent a successful transhiatal esophagectomy with

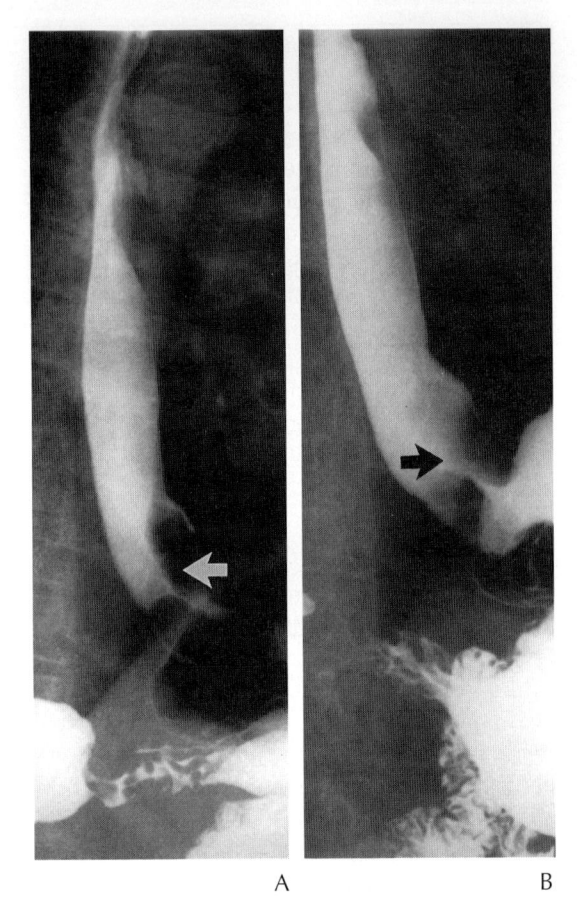

Figure 2-1. A 65-year-old man was evaluated for progressive dysphagia for solids and liquids and a 35-pound weight loss. Barium swallow (*arrows*) revealed a near-obstructing lesion at the gastroesophageal junction. Endoscopy confirmed the lesion, and biopsy showed it to be an adenocarcinoma of the distal esophagus. Transhiatal esophagectomy was performed with excellent relief of symptoms; however the patient succumbed to metastatic disease 1 year later.

excellent relief of the dysphagia. The patient succumbed to metastatic disease 1 year later but was free from locally recurrent disease.

Surgical palliation consists of esophagectomy, more commonly transhiatal than transthoracic, and should not include mediastinal dissection. Because the involvement of regional lymph nodes is so common with midesophageal lesions and portends poor survival even when the resection is accompanied by lymph node dissection, many surgeons approach all cancers of this location with the transhiatal approach. Palliative surgery in the hands of experienced surgeons is very good. Palliation with a bypass, for example, using a retrosternal colonic or gastric tube, leaving the cancer *in situ*, cannot be recommended. Although some investigators claim that a small group of patients who cannot be palliated by other means will benefit from bypass surgery,[9] Orringer and colleagues[10] point out that these patients have survival times of less than 6 months when the tumor cannot be resected, and that a procedure with a 20% to 30% mortality rate cannot be justified. Combinations of the nonoperative therapies described below are more reasonable for this group of patients.

Nonoperative palliation seems to be reasonable in those patients who are medically and nutritionally unfit for large resections, but the long-term results are poor. The options include stenting, laser tumor ablation with or without dilatation, and radiation therapy. Recurrent esophageal cancer can occur at the suture line, causing malignant stricture and obstruction, or when present in mediastinal lymph nodes, cause obstruction by extrinsic compression of the esophagus. Neither type of recurrence is amenable to further surgical therapy. Palliative options are the same as above.

Results of Stenting

Stenting of obstructing, unresectable esophageal lesions or recurrent tumors with Celestin™ or Atkinson™ tubes has been performed for many years. The results in general are poor, and the mortality and complication rates, including esophageal perforation, can be high (each greater than 10%). Operative placement of rigid stents carries the highest morbidity and mortality and should be avoided at all costs. In a report of 33 patients who underwent operative esophageal intubation, the mortality rate was 27% and mean survival time was 3.7 months.[11] Stenting is, however, the palliative procedure of choice for malignant tracheoesophageal fistula. Expandable stents, first used for malignant biliary obstruction,[12,13] are now being used for malignant esophageal obstruction.[14] Their palliative effectiveness is unknown at this time. A report of six patients treated with endoscopically placed self-expanding silicone-coated stents revealed excellent palliation in all, which was reportedly sustained.[14] Complications included stent migration, food impaction, and perforation. Theoretical advantages over standard stenting and laser therapy were discussed; advantages included lower cost, one-time application, lower risk of recurrent obstruction, ability to treat submucosal lesions not accessible to laser therapy, and lower complication rates compared with standard stents.

Figure 2-2 shows an endoscopically placed stent used for recurrent dysphagia after resection of a gastroesophageal junction adenocarcinoma. Because positive lymph nodes were found at the time of the original resection, this 51-year-old man underwent postoperative chemoradiation therapy. When an anastomotic recurrence developed, he was not a candidate for further radiation therapy. He was initially treated with continued chemotherapy and dilatations. He had progressive mediastinal node involvement causing obstruction at multiple levels of the esophagus, however, and was palliated with an endoscopically placed stent. Although survival was short, he was able to swallow liquids and his own secretions.

RESULTS OF ENDOSCOPIC LASER TUMOR ABLATION

Endoscopic tumor ablation using the laser has been relatively successful, but its use is limited to a few centers experienced with the technique. Currently, endoscopic laser therapy is performed with a neodymium: yttrium-aluminum-garnet (Nd:YAG) laser. A single session, retrograde technique as described by Pietrafitta and Dwyer[15] is typically used. Palliation can be achieved in up to 85% of individuals.[16,17] Adenocarcinomas are treated more effectively.[18] The main drawbacks in-

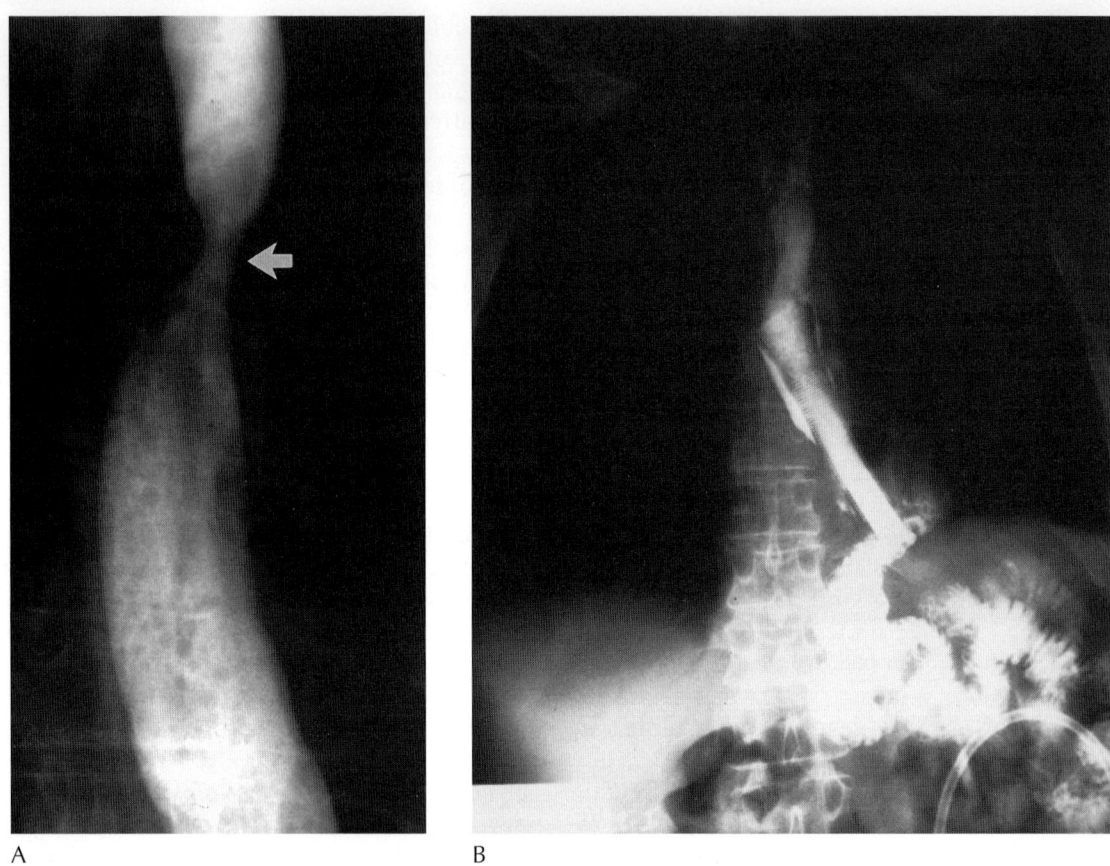

Figure 2-2. A 51-year-old man with biopsy-proved adenocarcinoma of the GE junction involving the distal esophagus and proximal stomach. The patient underwent total gastrectomy and distal esophagectomy. He received postoperative chemoradiation therapy for positive lymph nodes, but developed recurrent dysphagia. Evaluation revealed anastomotic recurrence secondary to extrinsic compression by involved lymph nodes. **A.** Progressive mediastinal nodal involvement (*arrow*) and dysphagia necessitated placement of a stent (**B**), which allowed for swallowing of saliva and liquids.

clude the need for repeat treatments and the risk of perforation.

Ferraro et al[19] used laser therapy to treat 41 patients with advanced esophageal cancers. The average number of treatments per patient was 2.7. One major complication and death occurred with a total of 112 treatments and survival from date of diagnosis averaged just under 5 months. The results, in general, were good, with an 86% initial success rate.

Sankar and Joffe[20] described Nd:YAG laser therapy combined with esophageal dilatation in 20 consecutive patients. In their patients, 11 had squamous cell and 9 had adenocarcinoma. Total obstruction was found in 10 patients. Three complications occurred, all in patients previously treated with combined chemoradiation therapy; nine were treated twice and two were treated more than two times. All patients were relieved of dysphagia. Mean survival of the group was 18.5 weeks.

These and other studies confirm the safety and efficacy of endoscopic Nd:YAG laser therapy for palliation of obstructing esophageal cancers.[15] The role of additional dilatation is not clear. The results are comparable to those of radiation therapy, which is currently the most widely used palliative treatment modality for esophageal cancer.

RESULTS OF RADIATION THERAPY

Radiation therapy has been the mainstay for the palliative treatment of unresectable esophageal cancer. The results in general have been discouraging, although recent reports have been more favorable. Palliation is often rapid, rendering patients able to eat for much of their remaining life. The morbidity is minimal and, unlike surgery, there is virtually no mortality associated with the treatment. As an example of the effectiveness of radiation in the treatment of esophageal cancer, a review by Caspers et al[21] showed that of patients with obstructions, 71% responded to radiation and 76% were able to eat. The palliation lasted an average of 7.5 months. Palliation typically lasts 5 to 10 months with up to 85% of patients receiving symptomatic benefit. High dose regimens (>6000 cGy) seem to be most effective.[22,23]

Treatment of esophageal cancer by chemotherapy alone is not effective, and there is no good data on the use of chemotherapy combined with radiation for palliation of advanced, unresectable esophageal cancers. Given the added toxicity of cytotoxic agents and the good results of radiation alone, this approach does not seem warranted.

SUMMARY: ESOPHAGEAL CANCER

1. Esophageal malignancies often present with advanced disease. Resection for cure or palliation would be undertaken in the medically and nutritionally fit patient. Results are good in experienced hands.
2. There are some data to indicate that preoperative chemoradiation therapy may improve both resectability and local control rates. It is not clear that survival is improved.
3. Palliation for unresectable esophageal malignancies includes radiation therapy and laser ablation therapy; each of these is particularly well suited for obstructing cancers. Stenting is another, albeit less attractive, option. There is currently no place for bypass procedures in the palliation of advanced or recurrent esophageal cancer.

CANCER OF THE STOMACH

Unlike cancers of the gastroesophageal junction, cancers of the body and antrum of the stomach rarely present with obstruction and more often are associated with early satiety, pain, and weight loss. Large antral lesions may present with gastric outlet obstruction, but the diagnosis is usually made before this late stage. Diffuse involvement of the stomach by tumor can result in abnormal gastric emptying in the absence of true obstruction. In the past, gastric outlet obstruction was typically a complication of advanced peptic ulcer disease.[24] Johnson and Ellis[25] have reported that the ratio of benign to malignant causes of gastric outlet obstruction, once 2:1, is now reversed, and they found a ratio of 3.5:1 for malignant to benign causes. They suggested that gastric outlet obstruction now predicts malignancy, and that this should be confirmed with endoscopic biopsy.

An attempt at curative resection of these cancers should be undertaken in the absence of evidence of distant metastases. The optimal procedure to be performed depends on tumor size and location. In general, lesions of the proximal stomach and body are treated with total gastrectomy, and antral lesions by distal gastrectomy. Gastrectomy for palliation of these cancers is commonly performed and is indicated in individuals otherwise medically and nutritionally fit. The goal is to provide prolonged symptomatic relief. In experienced hands, the operative mortality and morbidity are relatively low, and patients can obtain significant symptomatic relief.

The exception to this recommendation

may be the patient with linitis plastica. A report of 26 patients with linitis plastica revealed very poor results in patients undergoing palliative resections.[26] Survival comparisons showed mean survival of 6.6 months in the nonresection group and 7.2 months in the resection group. Patients who underwent palliative gastrectomy in the presence of peritoneal, hepatic, or pancreatic involvement had a mean survival time of 4 months. These authors concluded that linitis plastica in general was not a surgical disease and that palliative resections were not warranted.

Other comparisons of patients undergoing exploration only, gastrojejunostomy bypass, and palliative resection consistently show a trend toward better palliation and improved survival for the resection groups in the many retrospective series reported.[27-30] Although none of these studies controlled for patient selection for resection or bypass, the data overall is compelling. Patients who underwent curative or palliative total gastrectomy for gastric cancer were evaluated at the MD Anderson Hospital (Houston, TX).[28] Of the 219 patients studied, 151 had potentially curative procedures, 45 had palliative procedures, 21 had exploration or bypass, and 2 had other procedures. Complication and operative mortality rates were comparable between the resection groups; however, operative mortality was highest in the exploration or bypass group. Overall survival was poorest in the exploration or bypass group. An analysis of 144 patients with gastric cancer who underwent curative resection (69 patients), palliative resection (55 patients), or gastrojejunostomy (20 patients) revealed similar findings; however, the analysis also included the effectiveness of palliation.[30] There were 105 patients available for follow-up. Complication rates and operative mortality were comparable between all three groups. The bypass procedure provided short-lived palliation (mean 5.9 months) in 80% of survivors. Palliative resection, on the other hand, provided longer palliation (mean 14.6 months) in more patients. Resection was therefore felt to be preferable to bypass for palliation given the nearly identical morbidity and mortality rates.

Nonresectional operative palliation by placement of gastrostomy or jejunostomy tubes is usually not warranted if preoperative evaluation determines that the cancer is unresectable. If a gastric cancer is found to be unresectable during exploration, gastrojejunostomy has been the most commonly performed palliative procedure, although the results are poor enough to question its use. As noted above, palliation is typically very short-lived. In another study of 51 patients with gastric cancer who underwent palliative procedures, 25 had gastrojejunostomy.[29] Some benefit was seen in only 8 (30%) of these patients.

Nonoperative palliation includes chemoradiation therapy, percutaneous gastrostomy (endoscopic [PEG] or radiologic), and placement of self-expanding stents.

RESULTS WITH PALLIATIVE CHEMORADIATION THERAPY

Single agent chemotherapy produces response rates between 15% and 20%.[31] Responses are short-lived and do not impact on survival. Combination chemotherapy produces response rates of 30% to 40%.[32-34] The most commonly used regimen in the past has been the combination 5-Fluorouracil, adriamycin, and mitomycin-C (FAM). Although the response rates are higher, survival is no different than with a single agent.

Palliation of pain and bleeding from unresectable gastric cancer by radiation therapy is occasionally seen, although relief of obstruction is not. Therefore, radiation therapy cannot be recommended for palliation of obstruction.

PALLIATIVE PERCUTANEOUS GASTROSTOMY TUBE PLACEMENT

PEG tubes, or percutaneous gastrostomy tubes, may be placed for palliation, although there are no data to support or refute this recommendation. These gastrostomy tubes allow for decompression, if needed. Jejunostomy tubes may be placed through the gastrostomy tubes under endoscopic or radiologic guidance, and these can help with nutritional support through jejunal feedings. In general, these procedures are very safe with low complication rates, do not require general anesthetics for placement, and are very comfortable for the patients.

RESULTS OF STENT PLACEMENT

Self-expanding stents have been used in vascular surgery and for malignant biliary obstruction. Their use is described in case reports of patients with gastric outlet obstruction.[35] Stents may be most suitable for patients with extrinsic obstruction. It is not clear that long-term palliation can be obtained with primary malignancies using these devices because of the risk of tumor ingrowth into the mesh stent. Large groups of patients have not been reported. Laser ablation, successful in malignant esophageal and rectal obstruction, has had limited use in malignant gastric outlet obstruction.

SUMMARY: CANCER OF THE STOMACH

1. Obstructing gastric cancers should be resected when possible: antrectomy for distal lesions and total gastrectomy for proximal lesions. Palliative resection procedures are effective in experienced hands. One of the most common palliative surgical procedures performed for unresectable gastric cancer is gastrojejunostomy. Published reports indicate short survival times and ineffective palliation in patients undergoing bypass procedures and their use cannot be recommended.
2. There does not appear to be a role for chemotherapy or radiation therapy in the palliation of obstructing gastric cancer.
3. The results of other nonoperative palliative procedures for gastric cancer are not known. The techniques include percutaneous gastrostomy and placement of self-expanding stents. The benefits of these procedures seem to be their safety and high level of patient comfort.

CANCER OF THE PERIAMPULLARY REGION

Periampullary (distal common bile duct, duodenal, and ampullary) and pancreatic malignancies are rarely curable. The most common malignancy in this group is adenocarcinoma of the head of the pancreas. By the time these malignancies present with duodenal obstruction, they are usually unresectable. Obstruction of the biliary tree due to more proximal lesions (cholangiocarcinomas) is fully discussed in Chapter 5.

Patients with periampullary cancers should undergo careful evaluation for evidence of metastases and local extension into adjacent blood vessels. The work-up may include an abdominal CT scan, cholangiogram, and mesenteric arteriogram with venous phase. The role of endoscopic ultrasound as a staging tool has yet to be determined. If there is no evidence of unresectability on these studies, and the patient is medically fit, resection should be attempted. Resection represents the best intervention for relief and prevention of biliary and duodenal obstruction. If the tumor is unresectable or metastases to regional lymph nodes or the liver are present, surgical palliation of biliary and duodenal obstruction should be performed.

Approximately 25% of patients with unresectable pancreatic head malignancies will go on to develop duodenal obstruction, whereas 75% present with biliary obstruction and jaundice. Although biliary obstruction can be successfully relieved with endoscopically placed stents, gastrointestinal obstruction can be relieved only surgically. In the past, high morbidity and mortality rates were associated with surgical bypass procedures for unresectable periampullary malignancies. Recently, with reports of low complication and mortality rates for pancreaticoduodenectomy, the role of combined palliative surgical bypass for biliary and duodenal obstruction by these tumors has been reexamined.

Careful selection of bypass candidates is important. Meinke et al[36] compared 105 patients with cancer of the head of the pancreas who underwent biliary bypass only with 111 who underwent combined biliary and duodenal bypass (double bypass). The 30-day operative mortality was 14% for both groups. In the biliary bypass only group, 31 patients (30%) subsequently developed gastric outlet obstruction. The number of patients who developed duodenal obstruction after the double bypass procedure was unfortunately not reported, although a 15% rate of gastric outlet obstruction was reported. They concluded that many patients were at risk of developing gastric outlet obstruction and that this high number justified the performance of gastrojejunostomy.

More recently, Lillemoe et al[37] published a report of 118 consecutive patients who underwent palliative bypass procedures for unresectable periampullary malignancies. The most common procedure performed was a double bypass (75%). Gastrojejunostomy, alone or combined with biliary bypass, was performed in 107 of 118 patients (91%), and 3 additional patients had a gastrojejunostomy performed at the time of a previous operation. The 30-day mortality rate was 3.3% and the complication rate 37%, including delayed gastric emptying in 8%. The mean survival time was 7.7 months. At follow-up, only 4% of the patients developed gastric outlet obstruction. Despite support for nonoperative palliation of biliary obstruction in these patients as described in randomized trials,[37] data from The Johns Hopkins Hospital (Baltimore, MD) supports selective use of combined duodenal and biliary bypass procedures in patients who have unresectable periampullary malignancies at the time of exploration.[37] These patients, in general, had aggressive preoperative evaluation for evidence of local unresectability or metastatic spread and were thus candidates for aggressive resection at the time of their exploration. They recommended retrocolic loop gastrojejunostomy as the gastrointestinal bypass procedure of choice, as lower incidences of delayed gastric emptying (6% versus 17%) and late gastric outlet obstruction (2% versus 9%) were noted when compared to the antecolic bypass.

Successful palliation and prevention of duodenal obstruction as described requires careful patient selection. Those who have no or minimal symptoms fare well. The palliation and relief of gastric outlet obstruction in patients with long-standing, advanced obstruction is much more difficult, and in this group of patients with advanced cancer, malnutrition, and chronic gastric distension, the morbidity and mortality from surgical intervention are high. Weaver et al[38] looked specifically at the benefit of gastrojejunostomy in pancreatic cancer patients. They divided patients into two groups: 45 patients without duodenal obstruction and 36 patients with duodenal obstruction. Thirty day mortalities after gastrojejunostomy were 40% and 70%, respectively. In a subset of 21 patients who had nausea and vomiting, 90% died within 30 days of gastric bypass. They concluded that gastric outlet obstruction was a terminal event and that intervention was not justified. No explanation was given for the 40% mortality rate of the unobstructed patients, which is very high and has not been observed in other studies.

Doberneck and Berndt[39] showed that delayed gastric emptying complicated gastrojejunostomy for pancreatic cancer. Delayed gastric emptying complicated 26% of their patients after gastrojejunostomy. The study was small, thus conclusions could not be specifically made. They confirmed, however, that delayed gastric emptying occurred more frequently in those patients undergoing bypass who had duodenal obstruction by cancer.

The UCLA group described their experience with palliative procedures for pancreatic cancer.[40] Looking specifically at the palliation for duodenal obstruction, they described 50 patients who underwent bypass for evidence of obstruction, albeit early obstruction, and 20 bypasses performed prophylactically, with mortality rates of 12% and 5%, respectively. Only two failed completely, and overall, 20% had some problem with the gastrojejunostomy. Of 80 patients who underwent biliary bypass alone, 20 (25%) required subsequent gastrojejunostomy, and all functioned within 10 days. An additional 19 patients (24%) developed marked nausea and vomiting in the terminal stages of their disease and were not subjected to surgical bypass. Because of the high rate of development of duodenal obstruction, and the low mortality rates associated with bypass, gastrojejunostomy was recommended for all patients undergoing operative biliary bypass.

A completely different approach to these patients has been described in 19 patients from Wayne State University (Detroit, MI), all of whom underwent antrectomy and gastrojejunostomy for malignant duodenal obstruction.[41] Twelve patients were tolerating regular food at the time of their deaths (4 to 21 months after resection), and the remaining 9 survivors were tolerating a regular diet 9 to 29 months after resection. Biliary bypass was mandatory. This same institution, however, previously reported mortality rates of 40% to 90% after gastrojejunostomy alone.[38] The finding of improved operative morbidity and mortality after the more aggressive procedure was not addressed. The procedure has not gained wide acceptance.

In a report of 51 patients who underwent palliative surgery for unresectable pancreatic cancer, four patients with duodenal obstruction underwent gastrojejunostomy.[42] Three of these subsequently experienced impaired gastric emptying. This illustrates the problem facing patients with established gastric outlet obstruction: the results of bypass surgery are very poor. Because of this, and encouraged by the results of self-expanding stent placement for esophageal and biliary malignancies, some have applied this technique to the obstructed duodenum. A report of three patients showed this method provided ease of insertion and good palliation with no morbidity.[43] The stents were passed through a PEG tube under direct peroral endoscopic visualization.

To summarize, patients explored for potential resection of periampullary cancers should undergo double bypass if they are found to be unresectable. The loop gastrojejunostomy should be performed in a retrocolic fashion. For those patients who present with unresectable cancer and no duodenal obstruction, exploration and bypass can be safely performed but is probably not justified: biliary decompression can be achieved successfully with endoscopic stents and the rate of development of duodenal obstruction is less than 25%. For those patients who present with advanced malignancy and evidence of gastric outlet obstruction due to duodenal invasion, operation results in high morbidity and mortality rates because this represents end-stage disease and life expectancy is very limited. Palliation of nausea and vomiting may be obtained by nasogastric decompression and by the use of antiemetic medications, although newer techniques such as self-expanding stent placement may be a safe alternative.

SUMMARY: CANCER OF THE PERIAMPULLARY REGION

1. Patients found to be unresectable at the time of exploration for periampullary malignancies should undergo palliative combined biliary and gastric bypass procedures. Although duodenal obstruction will occur less than 25% of the time, there is essentially no added morbidity to gastrojejunostomy when done at the time of biliary bypass.
2. The results of gastrojejunostomy performed for established gastric outlet ob-

struction are poor and the procedure should probably be avoided in this group of patients. If expected survival is short, antiemetics and nasogastric tube decompression should be used.

CANCER OF THE MESENTERIC SMALL BOWEL

Primary Malignancies

Small bowel malignancies account for 1% to 3% of gastrointestinal malignancies.[44,45] The most common malignancy is adenocarcinoma, followed by carcinoid tumors, although a recent report revealed lymphoma to be the second most common small bowel malignancy.[46] Surprisingly, pain is the predominant presenting complaint of patients with small bowel cancers. The course is often indolent, with delays in diagnosis being typical, and the diagnosis is usually made at the time of exploration. Obstruction is a common problem in patients with these lesions.

Adenocarcinomas of the jejunum and ileum together represent approximately 50% of small intestinal adenocarcinomas, with the remaining being duodenal lesions. Most of the patients present with evidence of partial or complete obstruction. Although resection is often possible, lymph node metastases are common, adversely affecting survival. There are no data regarding the use of adjuvant chemotherapy in these patients because patient numbers are very small. Carcinoid tumors, on the other hand, are more common in the ileum. Their presentation is indolent and a long history of vague complaints is common. Carcinoid syndrome is unusual at the time of diagnosis and thus does not aid in the

Figure 2-3. A 69-year-old man presented with 3 days of distension, nausea, and vomiting preceded by 2 weeks of intermittent crampy abdominal pain. Examination revealed a palpable mass in the lower abdomen. **A.** Supine abdominal radiograph revealing multiple loops of dilated small bowel and no gas in colon or rectum, compatible with a small bowel obstruction. **B.** Palpable mass on examination evaluated with abdominal and pelvic CT scan. This study revealed a 10 cm x 8 cm mass (*arrow*) involving the small bowel mesentery. At exploration, a large mass involving the jejunum was found and resected. Pathology revealed malignant stromal cell tumor.

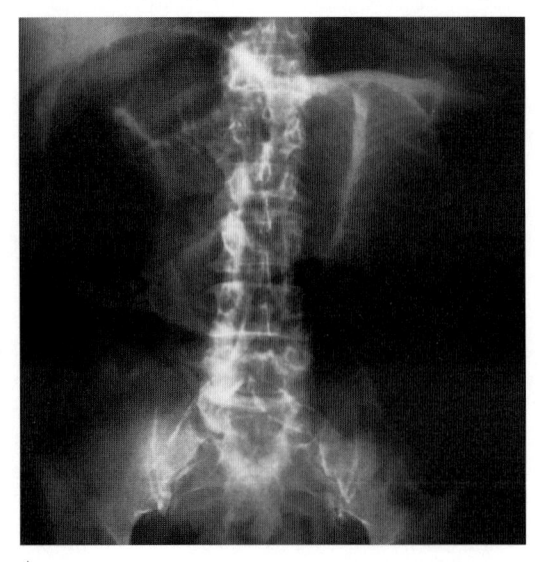

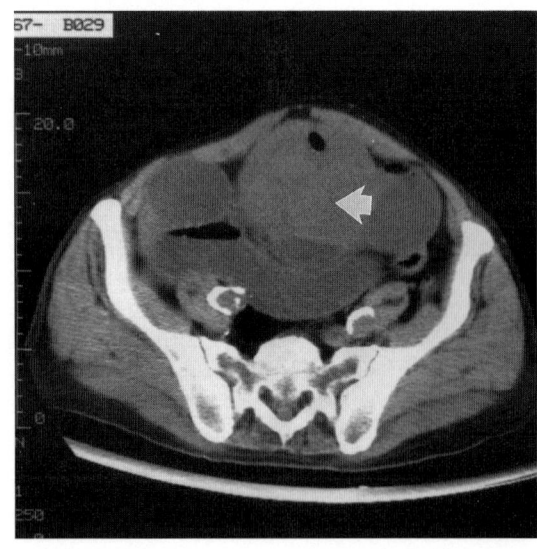

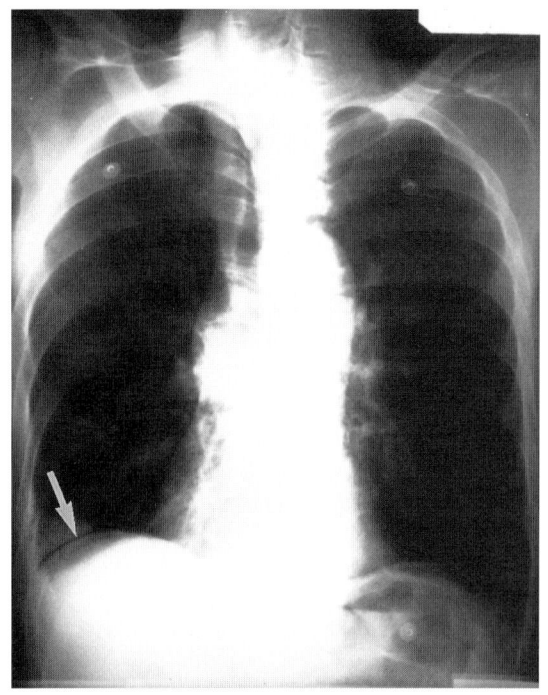

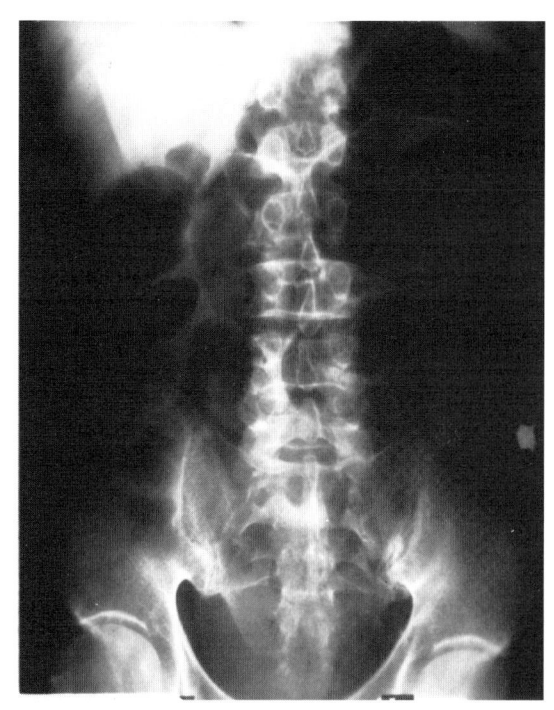

Figure 2-4. A 70-year old man developed severe abdominal pain after a 5-day history of progressive distension, crampy pain, nausea, and vomiting. **A.** Upright chest film revealed free intraperitoneal air (*arrow*). **B.** Abdominal film revealed dilated small bowel loops and some colonic gas. At exploration, a large mass involving two segments of small intestine and the dome of the bladder mass resected. Pathology revealed a large cell lymphoma with nodal involvement for which the patient received postoperative chemotherapy.

preoperative diagnosis of these unusual tumors. Lymph node metastases are common. Resection of involved bowel and mesentery and associated lymph nodes is indicated, and careful exploration for second primary sites and liver metastases is important.

Lymphoma involving the small bowel is uncommon; it is usually diagnosed at exploration for a bowel obstruction. The lesion is resected along with the adjacent mesentery. Patients with evidence of lymph node involvement by lymphoma, or who have not been completely resected, should undergo postoperative chemotherapy. For lymphoma isolated to the bowel wall, resection alone may be sufficient,[44] although this is controversial.[47]

Figures 2-3 and 2-4 show primary small bowel malignancies causing small intestinal obstruction. Figure 2-3 is an abdominal radiograph of a 69-year-old man with a long history of intermittent crampy abdominal pain. He finally sought medical attention when he developed progressive abdominal distension, nausea, and vomiting. Physical examination revealed abdominal distension and tympany, as well as a large mass in the lower abdomen. His plain radiographs revealed dilated small intestinal loops and no colonic gas. The mass was evaluated with a CT scan of the abdomen and pelvis. This revealed a large lesion that seemed to involve the small bowel mesentery. This was confirmed at operation where a large mass involving the jejunum was resected. Pathology revealed a malignant stromal cell tumor.

A 70-year-old man presented with 5 days of worsening crampy abdominal pain, distension, and vomiting. On examination, he had evidence of peritonitis. His admission chest and abdominal radiographs are shown in Figure 2-4. These showed free intraperitoneal air, consistent with a perforated viscus, and dilated small bowel loops. At exploration, an infiltrating mass was resected along with two segments of small bowel and the dome of the bladder. Microscopic examination of the specimen revealed a large cell lymphoma with positive lymph nodes. The patient received postoperative chemotherapy.

Metastatic Lesions to the Small Bowel

The small bowel is a common site for metastatic spread of many cancers, with melanoma being the most common extra-abdominal cancer metastasizing to the small bowel. A report from the Mayo Clinic of 41 patients with melanoma metastatic to the gastrointestinal tract[48] revealed the small intestine as the most common site, representing 71% of cases. Although mean survival was less than 1 year for the entire group, small bowel metastases had a significantly worse prognosis. Despite this poor survival, exploration and attempted resection of disease was felt to provide effective palliation. Intra-abdominal cancers, such as ovarian, gastric, and colorectal, frequently result in carcinomatosis involving the small intestine. Bleeding and obstruction are frequent presenting signs. Management of these difficult problems is addressed in more detail below.

SUMMARY: CANCER OF THE MESENTERIC SMALL BOWEL

1. Primary small bowel malignancies are rare and include adenocarcinoma, carcinoid, and lymphoma. Although abdominal pain is the most common presenting complaint, small bowel obstruction is common. Resection is the initial treatment of choice for all of these neoplasms, including lymphoma, where the risk of perforation and hemorrhage while on chemotherapy is high.
2. The role of adjuvant chemotherapy in the treatment of stage I and II small bowel lymphoma is controversial; however, most clinicians now recommend additional chemotherapy for this group of patients.

MALIGNANT OBSTRUCTION AND CARCINOMA OF THE COLON AND RECTUM

Colon and rectal cancer together are the second most common cause of cancer mortality in the United States. The American Cancer Society estimates that 149,000 new cases will be diagnosed and 56,000 people will die of colorectal cancer in the United States in 1995.[49] Over the past decade, there has been a trend toward decreasing mortality rates, and current overall 5-year survival rates are approximately 55%. Despite these small but welcome improvements in survival, colorectal cancer remains a significant public health problem. It is hoped that continued efforts in screening for occult disease, colonoscopic polypectomy, and improvements in adjuvant therapy will improve survival further.

Colorectal cancers often present in an indolent fashion. Whereas one might expect obstruction to be common, colorectal cancer patients present with obstruction only 8% to 16% of the time. Obstruction is more common at the hepatic and splenic flexures and in the descending colon; obstruction is less common for cecal and rectal neoplasms. The management of obstructing colorectal cancers has undergone an interesting evolution over the past two decades, especially when considering left-sided lesions. In general, obstruction is felt to be a poor prognostic sign. When survival between patients with and without obstruction are compared, controlling for stage of disease, obstructed patients consistently have worse survival rates.[50] The National Surgical Adjuvant Breast and Bowel Project (NSABP) analyzed 1021 patients with stage B and C cancers enrolled in two studies, specifically looking at location of the primary tumor and presence of obstruction as prognostic determinants.[51]

In this study, 140 patients (14%) presented with acute obstruction. There was a surprisingly even distribution of obstructing lesions throughout the colon and rectum, but the descending colon accounted for 21% of all obstructing lesions. The proportion of lesions presenting with obstruction was highest for the splenic flexure (37%); this finding has been noted in other studies. Only 16% of obstructing lesions were located in the sigmoid colon, and 4% of obstructing lesions were rectal cancers. The data were first examined without regard to nodal status: for all patients, there was a significant decrease in disease-free survival for those with obstruction. Looking specifically at location of primary, right-sided lesions revealed significantly worse disease-free survival when obstructed (53% versus 20% treatment failure rate). Lesions in the descending and sigmoid colon had the same outcome whether or not obstruction was present. When controlling for lymph node status, disease-free survival was significantly worse for obstructed patients with either negative or positive nodes.

After publication of the NSABP data, the Gastrointestinal Tumor Study Group (GITSG) examined its data on colon cancer patients in an effort to define prognostic factors affecting overall and disease-free survival.[52] This group evaluated 572 patients with stage B2 and C colon lesions. Unlike the NSABP report, rectal cancers were not included in the analysis. Tumor location had no effect on survival. There was no relation identified between primary location and obstruction. Eighty patients had obstructions. Survival was adversely affected by the presence of obstruction, independent of stage. For all patients, 5-year survival was approximately 45% in those patients with obstructions and 60% in patients with no obstruction, the difference being statistically significant ($p<0.003$).

A review of 77 patients with obstructing colon cancer treated at the Massachusetts General Hospital (Boston, MA) confirmed the NSABP and GITSG findings.[53] Actuarial survival was worse for patients with obstructions compared with those with no obstruction (31% versus 59%) as was disease-free survival (44% versus 75%). Failure rates were much higher: 42% versus 14% for local failure and 44% versus 21% for distant metastases. The findings of worse survival and higher local and distant failure rates held, in general, stage for stage when compared with patients with no obstruction. These researchers could not identify survival differences based on primary location, with obstructing left-sided lesions resulting in 5-year disease-free survival of 44% and right-sided lesions 47% (versus 67% and 74% for those patients with no obstruction, respectively).

In another analysis of clinical and pathologic variables of potential prognostic importance in patients with colorectal cancer, 709 patients were reviewed.[54] The analysis revealed stage of disease to have the strongest association with survival. Independent of stage, the following variables (ranked according to their relative importance to patient survival) showed an association: tumor grade, level of direct spread, presence of venous invasion, age, sex, and presence of obstruction. Obstruction was associated with a worse 5-year survival (19% versus 38%; $p=0.001$) in the univariate analysis. In the multivariate analysis, obstruction lost much of its importance ($p=0.018$), with stage, patient age, and tumor grade being by far the most important variables. Obstruction was, however, the only symptom or sign that maintained some independent prognostic importance (abdominal pain, anemia, altered bowel habits, abnormal abdominal examination, and duration of symptoms did not).

In a Danish series of 156 patients with malignant obstruction of the colon and rectum, 29% had disseminated disease, and in more than 20% palliative treatment only was given (diversion or bypass) with a 49% operative mortality rate.[55] For the remaining patients undergoing primary or staged resection of the tumor, the mortality rate was 5%. The majority of patients with right-sided lesions underwent right hemicolectomy and anastomosis. Patients with left-sided lesions were subjected to a variety of procedures: the most common was decompressing transverse colostomy followed by staged resection, and the least common was primary resection with anastomosis.

The management of obstructing colon cancer is straight forward with regard to right-sided lesions: most can be safely managed by right hemicolectomy and primary anastomosis. Operative mortality rates of less than 10% can be expected. An example of this approach is shown in Figure 2-5. This 67-year old man presented with hemooccult positive stools and intermittent crampy abdominal pain. A barium enema showed a large cecal lesion only. He underwent an uncomplicated right hemicolectomy with primary anastomosis. Examination of the specimen revealed a moderately differentiated adenocarcinoma of the cecum, and no nodes were involved.

For left-sided lesions, optimal management is less clear, and surgical approaches are evolving. The left colon is defined as including the descending and sigmoid colon. Patients who present with evidence of colonic obstruction should undergo sigmoidoscopy to determine the presence or absence of a rectal lesion, and probably should have a gentle water-soluble contrast enema to define the level of obstruction and to rule out pseudo-obstruction. The surgical intervention for obstructing left-sided lesions must be individualized. The options include: (1) initial decompressing colostomy possibly followed by resection at a later date; (2) resection with colostomy (Hartmann's procedure) possibly followed by colostomy reversal at a later date; and (3) resection with primary anastomosis.

Many of the management decisions regarding obstructing colon cancers have been based on the assumption that primary anastomosis of unprepared colon was unsafe and had a high rate of anastomotic failure. Because of this fear, operative management was formerly based on a three-stage procedure: initial colostomy, resection, and colostomy reversal. This approach is no longer used because each subsequent operation carries its own defined morbidity and mortality. Decompressing colostomy alone can be used in certain situations, such as in the patient with severe underlying medical problems, or in those with disseminated disease whose expected survival time is short. For the most part, however, patients should undergo resection of the cancer. The current controversy lies in whether to perform an end colostomy or primary anastomosis under these circumstances.

Historically, diverting colostomy was recommended as the initial intervention in colorectal cancer patients presenting with obstruction. In 1974, Welch and Donaldson[56]

Figure 2-5. This 67-year-old man presented with hemooccult positive stools and mild crampy abdominal pain. A barium enema showed a large cecal lesion only (*arrow*). The patient underwent a right hemicolectomy with anastomosis. Pathology revealed a moderately differentiated adenocarcinoma and no lymph nodes were involved.

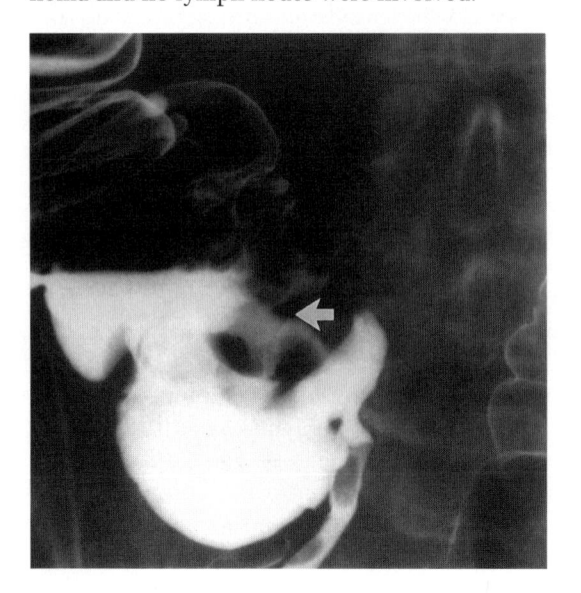

reported on 124 colorectal cancer patients who presented with obstruction. Of these, 85 (69%) underwent diversion as their initial procedure. This represented their preferred approach to obstructing left-sided lesions: 81 of 87 patients (93%) with left-sided lesions initially received diverting colostomies. For left-sided cancers, the data revealed 2% mortality after preliminary diverting colostomy (usually loop transverse colostomy) followed by resection, 60% mortality after primary resection, and 17% mortality after cecostomy. The rationale for initially performing a diverting colostomy was that it allowed for decompression with very low mortality, elective bowel preparation, and subsequent safe resection.

Follow-up data looking at long-term survival, selection of diverted patients who ultimately underwent resection, and explanations for the high mortality of the group who underwent initial diverting cecostomy compared to colostomy were not reported. It appears that many patients who underwent diverting transverse loop colostomy never had a curative resection; this group had a high (47%) mortality rate. In this group of patients, the data are thus not convincing that all patients treated by initial diverting colostomy have lower mortality rates than those undergoing initial resection.

The staged procedure, based on initial decompressing colostomy, has been criticized more recently. Concerns about subsequent general anesthetics and colonic procedures, including colostomy reversals, have in fact revealed real morbidity and mortality associated with each subsequent procedure. There is also conflicting data regarding survival in patients undergoing initial decompression as opposed to initial resection. Initial reports seemed to indicate that survival overall was improved if the lesion could be extirpated at the time of the initial exploration.[57] Others have found no difference in survival between initial resection compared with resection delayed for 2 weeks after diversion.[58] Irvin and Greaney[59] hypothesized that the improved survival noted with immediate tumor resection may have been an artifact due to a high number of right-sided lesions reported. There seems to be uniform agreement, however, that limiting the number of operations to one or two greatly shortens length of hospitalization and limits complications. For example, in a recent report of 115 patients who presented with malignant colorectal obstruction,[60] hospital stay was significantly shorter if the tumor was resected initially, whether or not a diverting stoma was performed. There was no significant difference in operative mortality or survival between the two groups. These findings have led to the more recent push toward one or two-staged procedures for obstructing left-sided colon cancers.

MANAGEMENT OF OBSTRUCTING LEFT-SIDED COLORECTAL CANCERS

Current surgical dogma states that patients with obstructing left-sided cancers should, in general, undergo resection of the tumor and end colostomy (Hartmann's procedure). Intestinal continuity should then be reestablished within 6 to 8 weeks, after colonoscopic evaluation of the remaining colon. Early colostomy reversal should be the goal in order to minimize complications and problems associated with long-term diversion.

Another attractive option for treating these patients is extended right hemicolectomy or subtotal colectomy with primary ileocolic or ileorectal anastomosis. The major drawback to this operation may be the risk of diarrhea, especially in the elderly or debilitated patient. Morgan et al[61] reported from Wales in 1985 on 16 patients treated by extended right hemicolectomy with no perforations had synchronous neoplasms in the right colon. The results of resection were excellent: no anastomotic leaks, and patients averaged one to three bowel movements daily. The operative mortality rate was 12.5%. A subsequent report of 22 patients who underwent subtotal colectomy with primary anastomosis provided similar results.[62] The operative mortality rate was 4.5%. There was one anastomotic leak. Patients ultimately averaged two to three bowel movements per day on a normal diet. Finally, a group of 72 patients who underwent subtotal colectomy for left-sided colorectal cancers included 23 obstructed patients.[63] One death occurred in the elective group and one death in the emergency obstructed group. There were no anastomotic leaks and diarrhea was not a problem. These authors also suggested that even though the quoted risk of synchronous colonic cancers is small (3% to 4%), many of their patients had synchronous cancers and adenomas, and thus resection of proximal colon that has not been colonoscopically or radiologically evaluated was reasonable.

An interesting approach to obstructed patients with colorectal cancer has been reported.[64] Three patients with obstructing sigmoid colon or rectal cancers were treated with endoscopic balloon dilatation of the lesion. This allowed for elective bowel preparation and fluid and electrolyte resuscitation in all patients. Curative resection was then performed in one patient. Another patient with a large rectal cancer refused surgery and colostomy and was successfully palliated with Nd:YAG laser ablation. The third patient presented with obstruction and malignant ascites and achieved good palliation after balloon dilatation and laser ablation.

An approach that has not gained widespread acceptance among surgeons in the United States is the use of primary anastomosis after resection of an unprepared colon. Standard surgical teaching has been that colostomy should be performed in these instances because the risk of anastomotic disruption in a loaded colon is too great. Experimental data have resulted in mixed reports about the necessity of clearing the colon of feces to maintain anastomotic integrity. A rat model revealed high anastomotic leak rates in animals with loaded colons compared with those without fecal material.[65] The many criticisms of this study include the very high leak rates overall when compared with other studies, the lack of strict bowel preparation and the methods to determine level of fecal loading, the absence of antibiotic use, and the concomitant study of materials to drain colonic anastomoses, something that is not done in the United States.

A recent study looked at the role of fecal material as a colonic mucosa-trophic agent.[66] Rats underwent diverting colostomy or sham operation. After sacrifice, colonic segments were analyzed for collagen content and proline incorporation. In the defunctionalized colon and rectum, collagen content was markedly lower and evidence of protein synthesis decreased compared with proximal bowel, which was the same as control animals. Effects on colonic healing were not addressed. Some British surgeons have espoused on-table colonic lavage of the proximal unprepared colon to decrease fecal loading and thus increase the likelihood of primary anastomotic healing. This approach is messy and time consuming and has not gained acceptance in the United States.

In questioning whether or not fecal loading of the colon is a contraindication to primary anastomosis, some investigators have begun to look at the results of left colon resection and primary anastomosis in unprepared bowel.[67] All maintain that the decision to perform an anastomosis under these circumstances should not be based on the presence of stool in the colon, but on other principles including the construction of a tension-free anastomosis, the maintenance of an adequate blood supply to the colonic segments, and the absence of gross peritoneal contamination. Under these conditions, with adequate colonic decompression, all maintain that primary anastomosis can be safely performed. Although current experience with primary repair of traumatic colorectal injuries has been convincing and encouraging, such that it is now the accepted approach to the majority of these injuries, it is not clear that results from this population of healthy individuals without obstructions can be applied to elderly individuals with obstructions who typically have many concurrent medical problems.

Four British reports,[68-71] however, describe the use of this technique in elderly patients with obstructions undergoing emergency colon surgery. A total of 81 patients underwent partial colectomy for obstruction with primary colocolonic or colorectal anastomosis. White and Macfie[68] reported on 35 patients with obstructing left-sided colorectal cancers who underwent resection and primary anastomosis. Twenty-nine patients underwent partial colectomies and anastomosis and the remaining six had subtotal colectomies with ileocolic anastomosis, abdominoperineal resection, or a Hartmann's procedure. Four anastomotic leaks were reported, and one was lethal. These authors felt that the overall length of hospitalization was shorter than could be obtained with staged procedures, and that overall morbidity and mortality were similar.

Irving and Scrimgeour[69] reported on 72 consecutive patients who underwent elective (53) or emergency (19) colectomy with primary anastomosis without bowel preparation. In this group, there were 12 emergency left-sided resections (not necessarily for obstruction). No anastomotic leaks were reported for the entire series, and the mean length of hospitalization for the entire group was 12 days. These authors concluded that mechanical bowel preparation was not needed for colorectal surgery provided appropriate intravenous antibiotics were given preoperatively. A report of 126 emergency colorectal procedures concluded that morbidity and mortality were acceptable for resection and primary anastomosis.[70] Specifically, 22 patients with obstruction underwent left-sided resections with primary anastomosis and no colostomy.

Also of interest, 27 patients underwent the same procedure in the face of peritonitis secondary to acute diverticulitis, ischemia, malignancy, or inflammatory bowel disease. Although not specifically assigned to groups, a total of seven anastomotic leaks developed: six in the groups undergoing primary anastomosis, of which three were in the left-sided groups. Two were converted to end colostomies. There were no deaths attributable to anastomotic leak.

Finally, Dorudi et al[71] reported on 18 consecutive patients who underwent resection and primary anastomosis for obstructing left-sided colorectal cancers. There were no anastomotic leaks and the average length of hospitalization was 11 days. All of these reports describe safe primary anastomosis of unprepared colon in an elderly population undergoing emergency colorectal surgery.

Figure 2-6 illustrates a near-obstructing descending colon adenocarcinoma on barium enema. Colonoscopic examination could not be performed proximal to the tight lesion, and the barium study was ordered. The patient had a gentle bowel preparation and underwent a successful left hemicolectomy with primary anastomosis. A partial small bowel resection of an involved segment was also performed. Liver metastases were also found.

Figure 2-6. A 66-year-old man with a biopsy-proved adenocarcinoma of the descending colon. Gastroenterologists were unable to colonoscopically evaluate the colon proximal to lesion. Barium enema confirmed near-obstructing lesion (*arrow*). Left hemicolectomy with anastomosis and partial enterectomy for involved small bowel were performed. Liver metastases were also found.

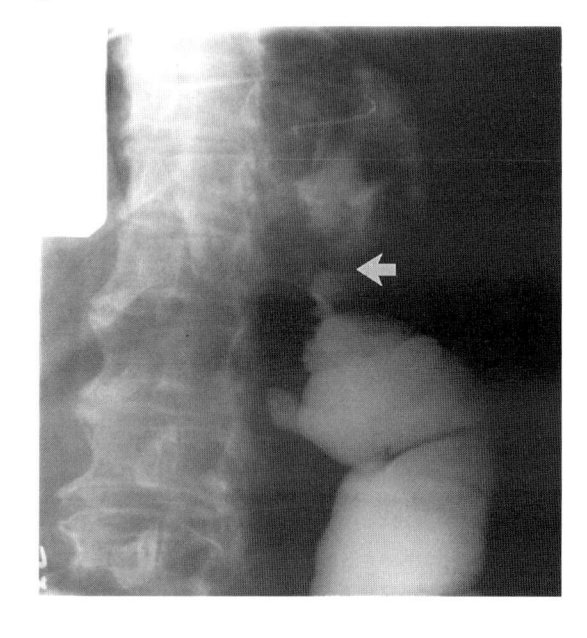

MANAGEMENT OF OBSTRUCTING RECTOSIGMOID AND RECTAL CANCER

Cancers of the low sigmoid colon and upper rectum are treated in general by resection and primary anastomosis. Low-lying rectal cancers in general are treated by abdominoperineal resection. In the face of acute obstruction, however, abdominoperineal resection may not be appropriate. Sigmoid colostomy and mucous fistula with intraoperative evaluation of the extent of pelvic disease and extrapelvic metastases allow for careful planning of the most effective treatment approach. Patients without significant pelvic disease can undergo bowel preparation along with fluid, electrolyte imbalance, and nutritional resuscitation followed by resection. Patients with more extensive pelvic spread can be considered for pre-resectional chemoradiation therapy. Radiation therapy alone often downstages both T and N tumor classifications, and renders many unresectable patients resectable.[72]

Studies have shown that for preoperative radiation therapy to be effective, full doses must be used (>4500 cGy). This results in resectability rates of 50% to 60%.[73] Nonrandomized studies have shown significant improvements in 5-year survival rates and local failure rates.[74–76] Randomized studies have not confirmed these differences, although none used adequate doses of radiation.[72] Although there are few studies that specifically address these issues regarding the addition of chemotherapy to radiation therapy, Frykolm et al[77] showed a doubling of resectability rates with chemoradiation therapy, from 34% to 71%, compared to radiation therapy alone. Local failure rates may also be improved with radiation or chemoradiation therapy. Local failure rates after resection of locally advanced lesions are more than 50%; preoperative radiation reduces this to 24% to 50%; and combination chemoradiation therapy may reduce this further to 13% to 20%. Patients with metastatic rectal cancer can undergo palliative abdominoperineal resection or chemoradiation therapy if the disease is locally advanced.

The patient who presents with an obstructing and presumably resectable cancer of the rectum or rectosigmoid colon often requires relief of the obstruction before resection can be carried out. An alternative to initial diverting colostomy is Nd:YAG laser ablation of the obstructing tumor and recanalization of the rectum to allow for fluid resuscitation, nutritional assessment, full bowel preparation, full colonoscopic evaluation, and an essentially elective resectional procedure.[78,79] Pre-resectional laser therapy seems to be safe and effective. A large series of patients was first reported in 1986 by Kiefhaber et al.[80] They described 27 patients who underwent resection after laser ablation and recanalization. There was one death (due

Figure 2-7. A 58-year-old man presented with weight loss and change in bowel habits. He was hemoccult positive. Barium enema revealed near-obstructing rectal lesion (*arrow*). CT scan showed liver metastases. He underwent a low anterior resection and primary anastomosis and had an unremarkable recovery.

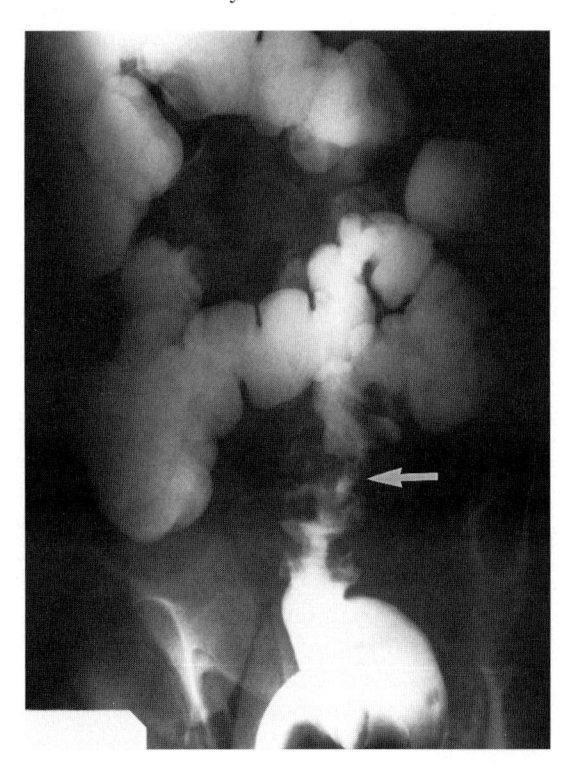

to other medical problems) and two complications related to the laser therapy. Eckhauser et al.[81] have described the use of this technique, initially in 11 patients with obstructing colorectal cancers. Their results were excellent. Their latest cumulative report of 33 patients revealed morbidity rates of 9% and mortality rates of 3% for the combined laser and resectional therapy.[79]

A 58-year-old man presented with weight loss and a change in his bowel habits. The barium enema shown in Figure 2-7 revealed a tight lesion in the upper rectum and abdominal CT scans showed liver metastases. He underwent a low anterior resection with primary anastomosis and had an uneventful recovery.

PALLIATIVE MANAGEMENT OF LOCALLY ADVANCED OR RECURRENT COLORECTAL CANCER

SURGICAL RESECTION OR DIVERSION

Anastomotic and local recurrences occur more commonly with rectal cancer than colon cancer and there does not seem to be a difference between handsewn and stapled anastomoses. The reasons for these higher local recurrence rates may be anatomic and technical, with less room for adequate lateral margins being available for rectal cancers.[82] These lesions should be carefully evaluated colonoscopically and by abdominal and pelvic CT scans prior to an attempt at surgical extirpation. Surgical resection of the involved bowel segment may be possible; diversion alone for unresectable lesions may be necessary, and on occasion, an exenteration procedure may be justified. Anastomotic and local recurrences are often not resectable secondary to invasion into surrounding structures. Resections including partial sacrectomy and cystectomy have been described.[83] This aggressive approach is of unproven long-term benefit, but in the short-term, some groups have shown good results.[83] This aggressive approach should only be for curative intent and should never be undertaken as palliation.

Wanebo et al[83] described 24 patients who underwent composite resection of pelvic recurrences of rectal cancer for curative intent. Twenty-two required formal abdominosacral resection and over half required bladder resection. There were three operative deaths (12%). The actuarial 5-year survival was 25% and recurrence developed in 13 of 21 surviving patients (62%) a mean of 17 months after resection. These authors claimed that this radical approach to a very selected group of patients resulted in improved survival and improved symptoms.

Figure 2-8 shows an abdominal CT scan image from an elderly man who presented with rectal bleeding and pencil-thin stools. He had a near-obstructing lesion on sigmoidoscopy 17 cm from the anal verge. Computed tomographic scan of the abdomen and pelvis revealed a large mass at the rectosigmoid junction adjacent to the right iliac vessels and right ureter. The tumor was unresectable at exploration owing to iliac vessel and ureteral involvement by the tumor. Colostomy was performed and the patient was referred for postoperative chemoradiation therapy.

RADIATION THERAPY AND LOCALLY ADVANCED OR RECURRENT RECTAL CANCER

Radiation therapy plays an important role in the treatment of locally advanced rectal cancer, either primary or recurrent. It is often used in conjunction with initial surgical diversion, in the face of obstruction or impending obstruction, and with concomitant chemotherapy such as 5-FU as a radiation sensitizer. Occasionally, this approach renders an unresectable rectal tumor resectable.

Preoperative radiation therapy has been used in an attempt to decrease tumor size and downstage both T and N tumor classifications of locally advanced rectal cancers. The results regarding conversion of unresectable lesions to resectable ones are promising, but the use of radiation preoperatively does not result in improved survival or local failure rates when compared with postoperative therapy. It is for this reason that its use cannot routinely be recommended and that the recommendation for adjuvant radiation therapy be based on accurate pathologic staging.

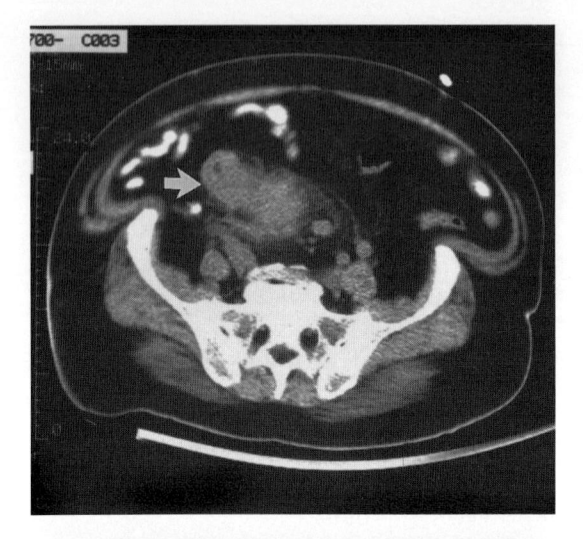

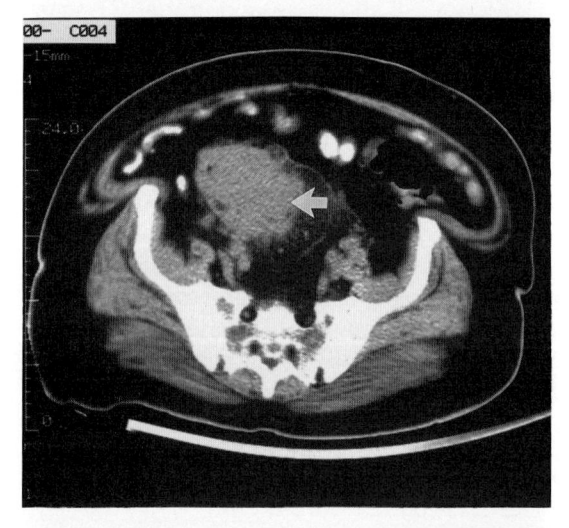

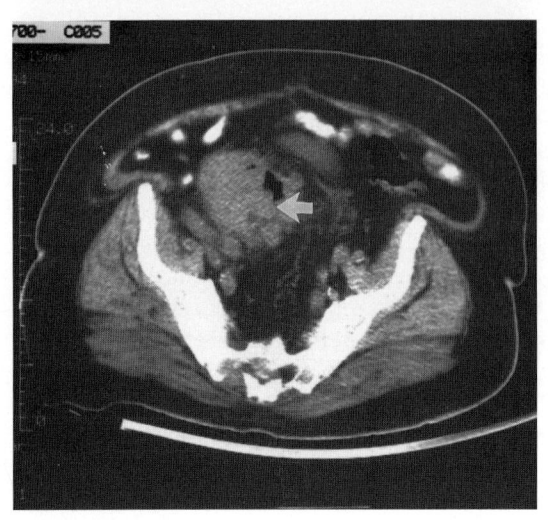

For unresectable, obstructing lesions, exploration with assessment of extent of disease combined with diverting colostomy is the initial approach. Radiation or combined chemoradiation therapy can then be instituted in an attempt to downstage the tumor. The utility of combined chemoradiation in patients with unresectable rectal cancer who are not obstructed has been studied. The Memorial Sloan-Kettering group[73] reported on 20 clinically unresectable patients (7 with recurrent cancer) who underwent preoperative 5-FU and leucovorin chemotherapy (two cycles) with the second cycle given at the completion of 5040 cGy of pelvic irradiation. Resection was performed on 18 patients and chemotherapy continued for a maximum of 10 months. Fifteen of 20 patients received some postoperative chemotherapy. Seventeen patients were converted to resectable status, and one had gross tumor left behind after resection. Three-year failure rates were as follows: local, 29%; abdominal, 42%; and distant, 34%. The three-year disease-free and overall survival rates were 64% and 69%, respectively. Although very promising, this report did not have a parallel comparison group, and none of the patients were deemed unresectable initially based on operative findings. The report does emphasize some very important points: higher doses of preoperative chemotherapy were tolerated when

Figure 2-8. A 69-year-old man presented with rectal bleeding and pencil-thin stools. Sigmoidoscopy revealed a near-obstructing cancer 17 cm from the anal verge. Abdominal and pelvic CT scan revealed a large mass at rectosigmoid junction (*arrows*) adjacent to the right iliac vessels and right ureter. He was unresectable at exploration owing to iliac vessel and ureteral encasement. Colostomy was performed and he was referred for chemoradiation therapy.

compared with postoperative-only chemotherapy groups and enhanced downstaging and resectability rates were possible compared with the use of radiation alone. This work deserves a careful look; however, in the future, unresectability based on clinical findings will need to be more standardized so that different groups, and results from different institutions, can be effectively compared. The use of rectal ultrasound as a staging tool may provide for a more accurate and reproducible determination of resectability than is currently described, and probably should be used in the absence of operative staging and determination of resectability.

Ideally, recurrent rectal cancer should be diagnosed prior to the development of obstruction. Careful evaluation of complaints of new symptoms, such as pain or change in bowel habits, remains important in the diagnosis of recurrent rectal cancer. Evaluation should include pelvic and abdominal CT scan to delineate the extent of recurrent disease and to look for evidence of liver metastases. Sigmoidoscopy should be performed to evaluate the level of the recurrence and to allow for biopsy of the strictured area. Rectal ultrasound may be of use in defining invasion into local structures. If, after this evaluation, the recurrence is felt to be resectable, surgical exploration and resection is the preferred approach.

Most often rectal cancer recurrences in the pelvis are discovered late. If obstruction is impending, then there are few options short of diverting colostomy available to these patients. Laser ablation, described below, may have some palliative benefit, especially in those recurrent obstructions in patients who have already had full dose pelvic irradiation. After diversion, most patients will need pelvic irradiation in an attempt to control symptoms, the most troublesome being pain. The results of palliation of recurrent rectal cancer by radiation are poor. Good pain relief is attained in 60% to 90% of these patients, but the results are usually temporary. The overall survival of these patients is rarely, if ever, affected.

Attempts have been made to improve these results by combining chemotherapy with pelvic irradiation. One group investigated combination 5-FU and mitomycin-C with pelvic irradiation in 15 patients with locally advanced, recurrent rectal cancer.[84] Seven of eight symptomatic patients experienced excellent pain relief. The treatment protocol, however, resulted in significant toxicity, and only six patients completed the protocol without chemotherapy or radiation dose reductions. The results overall were no better than historical controls who received pelvic irradiation alone, and the authors questioned whether the increased toxicity was justified.

LASER ABLATION

The success of laser palliation of esophageal cancers has led some investigators to use the technique for the palliation of obstructing recurrent and primary rectal cancers in those patients who are unresectable, are at high risk, have had pelvic radiation therapy, or who have metastatic disease. By 1986, more than 1,000 patients who had undergone laser ablation of colorectal cancers were reported on in the literature. Success in controlling bleeding or preventing obstruction occurred 97% of the time.

An early report by Russin et al[85] described 24 patients with unresectable colorectal cancers with bleeding or partial obstruction who underwent laser ablation. Nineteen tumors were in the rectum or rectosigmoid colon. An average of 2.5 sessions were required to treat these tumors, with a range of one to nine being reported. Long-term palliation with a single treatment was not described. They were quite successful in treating bleeding and preventing obstruction and only two procedural complications developed—a perforation and a rectovaginal fistula.

Another report of 12 patients with recurrent or metastatic cancer (7), benign stricture (3), and large villous adenomas (2) illustrated the utility of this technique in a variety of difficult clinical situations.[86] There were no mortalities and one microperforation was treated successfully with antibiotics alone. In the seven patients with cancer, four had local recurrences and three had metastases. Only one cancer patient required more than one laser treatment and all remained free of obstruction in follow-up or until death.

Daneker et al[78] reviewed their experience with laser recanalization and specifically addressed three questions:

1. Was the procedure effective in relieving obstruction?
2. Was luminal patency maintained?
3. Did laser ablation allow for the use of preoperative chemoradiation therapy?

Their report summarized the evaluation of 37 patients who underwent Nd:YAG laser therapy for obstructing or near obstructing cancers of the rectosigmoid colon and rectum. Obstructive symptoms were present in 75% of the patients. Ten patients had recurrent disease. Twenty-seven patients were treated palliatively for unresectable or metastatic cancer, six patients were treated specifically in an attempt to allow for preoperative chemoradiation therapy, and four patients were at high risk. Patency was established after an average of one laser session in all patients (range 1 to 3). Luminal patency was maintained in 31 (84%) patients, with additional treatments often being required (range 0 to 18). Six patients ultimately required fecal diversion. Of the 123 laser sessions performed on this group, there were only three complications. Of the six patients treated prior to chemoradiation therapy, four ultimately required low anterior resection. Three were alive without disease 34 to 102 weeks after their initial laser treatment. These authors concluded that laser therapy was an effective, durable, and safe procedure for patients with difficult sigmoid colon and rectal cancers and that laser ablation represented the preferred alternative to diverting colostomy in these patients.

ELECTROCAUTERY FULGURATION OF RECTAL CANCERS

The role of fulguration in the treatment of obstructing rectal cancers is not clear. Fulguration has been used as a palliative measure for the treatment of unresectable rectal cancer and rectal cancer in high-risk patients. The reported results generally have been good.[87] Procedure mortality rates vary between 0% and 5%, with control of symptoms possible in 40% to 80%. Fulguration of rectal cancer has even been described as a potentially curative modality.[88] The method does not allow for accurate staging, thus comparing results of fulguration to surgical resection is not possible.

A large personal series of rectal cancer patients treated by fulguration was reported by Madden and Kandalaft in 1983.[88] The report presented electrocoagulation of primary rectal malignancies as a primary curative method. This view never gained widespread acceptance. The results, however, deserve our attention. Over a 21-year period, they treated 204 patients, average age 66.5 years. Follow-up was long, averaging 9 years in survivors. Patients required an average of four sessions (range: 1 to 13). There were no deaths and 48 complications (23.5%). The main complication was bleeding (38 patients), with half the patients requiring transfusions and half requiring control with cauterization or suture ligation. There were 156 patients who were felt to be suitable for treatment by low anterior or abdominoperineal resection. The 5-year disease-free survival of this group was 62%. The remaining 48 patients were either clinically high risk or unresectable and the 5-year disease-free survival was 35% for these patients. The 5-year disease-free survival for the entire group was 56%.

In this report, larger tumors required more frequent treatment sessions. This fact would seem to preclude the use of fulguration in the initial management of obstructing rectal cancers: the obstruction would likely not be relieved by the initial treatment. Thus, given the lack of acceptance of this modality in the treatment of rectal cancers in most patients, its use in the management of obstructing lesions should not be considered.

SUMMARY: MALIGNANT OBSTRUCTION AND CARCINOMA OF THE LARGE BOWEL

1. Studies consistently show worse overall and disease-free survival and higher local and distant failure rates for patients with obstructing colorectal cancers. These findings hold when patients are controlled for lymph node status and stage.
2. The surgical management of obstructing right-sided colon cancers should be right hemicolectomy with primary ileo-transverse colostomy.
3. The surgical options for managing obstructing left-sided colon cancer (excluding rectal lesions) include extended right hemicolectomy and primary anastomosis, resection and end colostomy, and resection with primary anastomosis. Each of these procedures has its own distinct benefits and risks, and therefore selection of a particular procedure must be individualized for each patient. Extended colectomy is a very attractive option, with the only significant problem being the potential for diarrhea. Resection and colostomy are very safe, but ultimately a second procedure is needed to reverse to colostomy. Resection with anastomosis of unprepared bowel is clearly the least attractive option, despite the promising reports in the literature. Finally, initial diverting colostomy alone is rarely indicated as many of these patients will die with the malignancy in place. This approach should be reserved for patients with limited expected survival and multiple medical problems.
4. Obstructing rectal or rectosigmoid cancers should be treated with initial colostomy and delayed resection. Patients with unresectable or advanced lesions may be treated with chemoradiation therapy in an attempt to shrink and down-stage the cancer. Another approach to obstructing lesions in this area is Nd:YAG laser ablation recanalization followed by elective bowel preparation, resuscitation, and resection.
5. Palliation of unresectable obstructing primary or recurrent rectal carcinoma consists of either radiation therapy, usually combined with fecal diversion; radical exenterative procedures; or laser recanalization. Of these, experience with radiotherapy combined with colostomy is greatest. Results are reasonable, with high rates of symptomatic control, at least in the short term. Treatment with laser ablation and recanalization has the benefit of avoiding the need for colostomy in patients with relatively short life expectancies. Although the procedure is safe and few complications have been reported, multiple applications are typical. Control of bleeding and pain is good. This would be an excellent approach for locally advanced rectal cancer with distant metastases.

CANCER OF THE ANAL REGION

Cancer of the anal region presents most commonly with chronic symptoms: itching, bleeding, and pain, usually mild and usually associated with other anorectal pathology. These cancers do not typically present with obstruction. The treatment of squamous cell cancer of the anal canal has evolved dramatically in the past three decades; routine abdominoperineal resection has now been supplanted by radiation therapy, usually in combination with 5-FU–based chemotherapy.[89,90] Prior to the initiation of therapy, careful examination of the anorectal area is imperative, with mapping of the tumor and careful biopsy needed to confirm the diagnosis and extent of disease. With resection alone, 5-year survival was roughly 50%; with combination chemoradiation therapy, 5-year survival was more than 80% and the need for permanent colostomy is usually obviated. Involved inguinal nodes, usually evaluated by fine-needle aspiration cytology, are included in the radiation port. Six to 8 weeks after the completion of therapy, biopsy of the area should be performed to evaluate for residual malignancy.

Obstructing lesions should be treated by an initial temporary diverting colostomy followed by chemoradiation therapy. Residual disease present after definitive chemoradiation therapy should be treated by either salvage chemotherapy (usually platinum-based) or abdominoperineal resection.

Patients with other histologies (other than squamous cell carcinoma) may require abdominoperineal resection initially. These may include sarcomas, melanoma, adenocarcinomas, and other very rare lesions. It should be emphasized that the primary use of chemoradiation therapy is limited to squamous cell carcinoma.

SUMMARY: CANCER AND MALIGNANT OBSTRUCTION OF THE ANAL REGION

1. Primary squamous cell carcinoma of the anus presenting with obstruction should be treated by an initial diverting colostomy followed by standard chemoradiation therapy. Because response and cure rates are so high, colostomy reversal may be performed at a later date.
2. Recurrent anal cancer presenting with obstruction should be treated by abdominoperineal resection.
3. The treatment of other histologic types of anal cancer is usually primary surgery.

OBSTRUCTION OF THE GASTROINTESTINAL TRACT AND CANCER THERAPY

The use of combined modality therapy in the treatment of many types of malignancies results in a wide variety of complications. Intestinal obstruction may be caused by previous surgical therapy, radiation therapy, or intraperitoneal chemotherapy. The effects of radiation therapy on the intestine and specifically the complication of bowel obstruction are discussed in Chapter 7.

Small Bowel Obstruction after Intraperitoneal Chemotherapy

The use of intraperitoneal chemotherapy remains an important modality in the treatment of certain tumors such as ovarian cancer, peritoneal mesothelioma, as well as several low-grade malignancies such as pseudomyxoma peritonei, which results in serious consequences despite its histologically benign appearance. This modality is being investigated in combination with cytoreductive surgery to maximize tumor destruction. In particular, the use of intraperitoneal chemotherapy is advocated to treat tumor cells that become disseminated on peritoneal surfaces and then entrapped by fibrin resulting in tumor implants.

There are a number of theoretical advantages to this approach, referred to as EPIC (Early Postoperative Intraperitoneal Chemotherapy) by Sugarbaker.[91] Included among these are good distribution of drug, which should approach 100% of affected surfaces; optimal timing of therapy from a tumor-cell kinetic standpoint; minimal tumor burden at the time of treatment; and cost economy gained from treating patients while they are already recovering from the surgical procedure. A number of drugs have been used in this approach, including 5-FU, mitomycin C, doxorubicin, cisplatin, and others.

It is important for the consulting surgeon to be aware of the complications associated with this novel form of therapy. In their series, Sugarbaker et al[91] reported five cases of bowel perforation after receiving intraperitoneal chemotherapy; all five of these patients also had received radiation therapy to the area.

Bowel obstruction has also been reported following intraperitoneal chemotherapy. Markman and colleagues from the University of California at San Diego Cancer Center reported on 1103 patient-months of follow-up in 115 patients who received intraperitoneal chemotherapy for a number of advanced intra-abdominal malignancies.[92] Of interest in this study, all episodes of bowel obstruction occurred within 6 months of the completion of chemotherapy, with a median of 2.5 months. These authors concluded that two of seven were definitely related to intraperitoneal chemotherapy, and five were possibly related. In other patients in this series who developed intestinal obstruction, the cause was the presence of recurrent or residual tumor.

Patients who present with bowel obstruction and a history of having received intraperitoneal chemotherapy must be carefully evaluated. The indications for surgery are similar to those with obstruction from other causes. Patients who have received intraperitoneal chemotherapy and radiation therapy may be at increased risk for bowel perforation (see Chapter 3 for a complete discussion of perforation).

Small Bowel Obstruction after Cancer Surgery

Postoperative bowel obstruction is most often due to adhesions. Small bowel obstruction that develops in patients after cancer surgery or other cancer treatment may have either a benign or malignant cause. It is often difficult preoperatively to differentiate between these two in cancer patients. The most common primary site of malignancy in patients who subsequently develop small bowel obstruction is the colon. In a variety of retrospective studies, a benign cause of obstruction is found approximately one third of the time, with recurrent cancer accounting for most of the remaining obstructions. Rarely, a second unsuspected primary tumor is identified.

The therapeutic dilemma posed by such a patient can be disconcerting. The data, however, support aggressive surgical intervention in the majority of these patients. In one series of 66 cancer patients who subsequently developed bowel obstruction,[93] of the small number treated successfully with tube decompression initially, 41% required readmission and operation for relief of the obstruction. In another group of 73 patients with bowel obstruction secondary to recurrent cancer,[94] tube decompression failed in 50 of 51 patients in whom it was tried, and all went on to laparotomy. Lastly, in a series of 53 cancer patients with bowel obstruction,[95] all underwent surgery for relief of obstruction. Surgery is justified in these patients because the obstruction often can be relieved, either by adhesiolysis, resection of recurrent or new disease, or bypass. Understandably, the operative mortality is high in patients whose obstruction is due to recurrent cancer, and survival is short; however, relief from obstruction is typical.

In one study, operative mortality in patients with recurrent cancer was 19%, but 42% survived longer than 1 year, with a median survival of 11 months.[95] In another, operative mortality was 34% and mean survival was 6 months; operative mortality was less when patients were supported with perioperative total parenteral nutrition.[94] Interestingly, the risk of bowel strangulation in these patients is small. In the Osteen et al series,[93] only 7 of 66 patients required urgent laparotomy, and of those only 1 had gangrenous bowel. These surgeons, however, did not advocate prolonged intestinal decompression and intravenous hydration: spontaneous resolution of the obstruction occurred rapidly (within 3 days), but was associated with a high recurrence rate (42%) necessitating operation.

A recent study that examined the causes of small bowel obstruction after colon resections for benign and malignant conditions provided some very interesting information.[96]

Of the 118 patients evaluated, benign adhesions were the cause of obstruction in 100% of patients operated on for benign colonic disorders (4% operative mortality), in 82.6% of patients with colon cancer without known recurrence (9% operative mortality), and in 30.1% of patients with known recurrent colon cancer (8% operative mortality). These authors concluded that patients with a history of colon cancer who present with small bowel obstruction should be operated on after an appropriate period of resuscitation. A review of 30 patients with malignant bowel obstruction after surgery for colorectal cancer indicated that an aggressive approach should be maintained for all but the terminally ill patient.[97] Sixty-three percent (19 patients) had restoration of normal bowel function. There were five operative deaths and eight complications. Survival for patients who had relief of obstruction averaged 192 days compared with 26 days for those who remained obstructed. These two studies confirm that an aggressive operative approach to selected patients with bowel obstruction after surgery for colorectal cancer can be very rewarding.

In contrast, a review of 54 patients with a history of intra-abdominal and pelvic malignancies who subsequently developed small bowel obstruction was less optimistic.[98] In this paper, the time interval to development of bowel obstruction was much shorter in the group with malignant obstruction (21 months) compared with obstruction from benign causes (61 months; $p<0.01$). Forty patients were treated initially with nasogastric decompression. In this group, only 11 responded, and 5 of these subsequently developed recurrent obstruction. Twenty-six were known to have recurrent cancer and 26 were felt to be cancer-free. Ultimately, 37 patients were operated on: 25 had recurrent cancer, 3 had radiation enteritis, and 9 had other benign causes for bowel obstruction. The 30-day mortality rate was 16% and in-hospital mortality rate was 22%. All deaths except one occurred in the malignant obstruction group. Overall survival was much worse in the malignant obstruction group (mean 7.4 months) compared with the benign obstruction group (53.6 months). These authors concluded that the results of tube decompression and operative intervention were both unsatisfactory because nearly 50% of the patients developed major complications and 17% of discharged patients developed evidence of recurrent obstruction. They recommended early exploration in those patients without known recurrence and with a long interval between the diagnosis of malignancy and the development of small bowel obstruction. In patients with known recurrent cancer, high complication and mortality rates and high rates of recurrent obstruction precluded recommendation for aggressive surgical intervention: a trial of nonoperative decompression was felt to be warranted. If tube decompression fails, laparotomy should be undertaken in all but the most moribund patient.

Finally, when patients with small bowel obstruction from a variety of causes were analyzed for risk of recurrent obstruction, patients with malignant small bowel obstruction and radiation enteritis had the highest recurrence rates.[29] In a study of 309 consecutive patients who presented with small bowel obstruction, 150 underwent operation and 16 were found to have malignancy (42 had a history of cancer).[29] Recurrent obstruction developed in 56%. In the 113 patients with a history of cancer, 59% developed recurrent obstruction (67% after nonoperative therapy and 42% after surgery). Recurrent obstruction developed in 66% of patients with radiation enteritis. Recurrent obstruction developed less commonly after surgery compared with nonoperative therapy, irrespective of the benign or malignant cause of the small bowel obstruction.

In an excellent review of the topic of bowel obstruction in cancer patients, Ripamonti et al[99] conclude that surgery remains the primary treatment for the majority of patients, but that a group of patients with advanced disease or poor medical and nutritional status require alternatives to operation. Their review highlights the importance of patient selection for the therapies available, as well as thoughtful individualization of the management of these challenging problems.

Malignant Gastrointestinal Obstruction

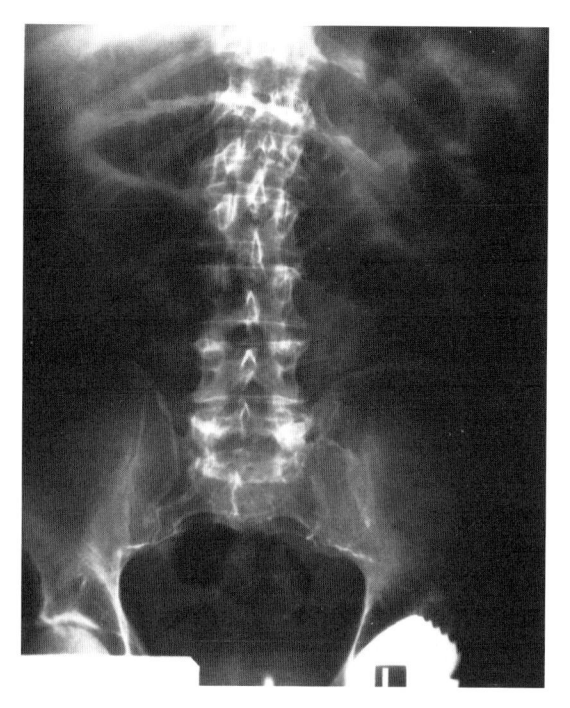

Figure 2-9. An elderly man with a past history of colon cancer presented with obstipation, crampy abdominal pain, and vomiting. Abdominal radiograph revealed dilated loops of small intestine. Carcinomatosis was found at exploration, and the patient was successfully treated with two bypass procedures of the involved segments.

Figure 2-9 is an abdominal radiograph of an elderly man with a history of colon cancer who presented with obstipation and crampy abdominal pain. The film shows dilated small bowel loops. Carcinomatosis was unfortunately found at exploration; however, the patient's obstruction was successfully relieved permanently with two bypass procedures of the involved segments of intestine.

SUMMARY: SMALL BOWEL OBSTRUCTION CAUSED BY CANCER THERAPY

1. Cancer patients who develop small bowel obstruction in the absence of known recurrent disease should undergo exploration after an appropriate period of resuscitation and decompression. A benign cause of obstruction will be found in approximately one third of these individuals.
2. Cancer patients with known recurrence who develop small bowel obstruction should undergo a period of nasogastric decompression. If the obstruction does not resolve, exploration is warranted.
3. Recurrent small bowel obstruction may develop in as many as 60% of patients after successful operative relief of malignant small bowel obstruction. Recurrence rates are much higher after nonoperative therapy.
4. Patients with known peritoneal carcinomatosis and bowel obstruction fare poorly regardless of the approach. Surgery should be avoided because of high morbidity and mortality rates and prohibitive rates of recurrent obstruction (see below).
5. Small bowel obstruction may result from previous intraperitoneal chemotherapy.

PERITONEAL CARCINOMATOSIS: OVARIAN AND OTHER MALIGNANCIES

The development of bowel obstruction in the presence of peritoneal carcinomatosis is a very poor prognostic sign. Under these circumstances, patients have survival times measured in weeks to at most months. In most situations aggressive surgical intervention is not indicated. The difficult decision, then, is to select patients who might benefit from surgical intervention.

There is much reference to concomitant ovarian cancer and bowel obstruction.[100–102] Bowel obstruction occurs in between 15% and 35% of cases of ovarian cancer. Uncured ovarian cancer often presents with late peritoneal carcinomatosis. Surgical treatment rarely improves survival in patients with bowel obstruction secondary to peritoneal ovarian carcinomatosis. The question of adequate palliation of symptoms is central to dealing with these patients; if nonoperative management is successful, operations characterized by high operative morbidity and mortality rates with little chance of long-term obstruction relief can be avoided.

The results of surgical treatment of bowel obstruction caused by carcinomatosis are poor. A report of 34 patients with obstruction secondary to carcinomatosis from a variety of primary tumors revealed a mortality rate of 18%, a morbidity rate of 44%, and a mean survival of 4 months. Six patients required reoperation for recurrent obstruction.[103] This report concluded that surgery may be performed electively and that surgical decompression is often possible in this difficult group of patients. A bypass procedure was the most common operation (in 22 of 39 patients) performed. In contrast, van Ooijen et al[101] concluded that exploration for patients with obstruction from carcinomatosis was rarely successful, with a mean survival time of 36 days. They cautioned that exploration for relief of obstruction should be offered only to those patients without palpable masses and ascites, and to those ovarian cancer patients in whom effective chemotherapy might be available.

Figure 2-10 shows the radiologic evaluation of a 63-year-old man with a locally aggressive and recurrent transitional cell carcinoma of the bladder. He was previously treated with radical cystectomy and ileal conduit urinary reconstruction followed by chemotherapy. A recurrence in the pelvis causing rectal obstruction was treated with diverting colostomy. He subsequently developed bilateral ureteral obstruction requiring bilateral nephrostomy tube placement. Figure 2-10A reveals an unremarkable Kidney/Ureter/Bladder (KUB) film taken after a nephrostomy tube change performed 2 weeks prior to the development of a bowel obstruction. He presented with cessation of colostomy output and distension. Figure 2-10B and Figure 2-10C reveal new small bowel obstruction. A 4-day trial of nasogastric decompression in conjunction with total parenteral nutrition was unsuccessful and the patient underwent exploratory surgery. Carcinomatosis was found. He had a contiguous segment of obstructed transverse colon and ileum resected with the creation of a Brooke ileostomy. He was able to eat and had no further bowel obstruction through the time of his death 3 months later.

Medical management of this group of patients can be successful in carefully selected patients. Colicky pain, nausea, and vomiting need to be controlled. In a review of 40 patients with advanced abdominal and pelvic cancers (colorectal was the most common, followed by ovarian) and bowel obstruction, 38 were treated without surgery.[104] Pain was controlled with smooth muscle relaxing agents (such as loperamide), with celiac block, and with high dose narcotics. Nausea and vomiting were partially relieved with the phenothiazine and butyrophenone antiemetics, but not by metoclopramide. Rarely were nasogastric tubes needed, and most patients continued to take a liquid diet. From the clinical courses described for this group of patients, many clearly had recurrent partial bowel obstruction as the cause of their symptoms. The mean survival time for this group of patients was 3.7 months.

Percutaneous gastrostomy tube placement has been described for palliation of obstruction in patients with advanced ovarian cancers. In one series of 10 patients so treated from the MD Anderson Hospital (Houston, TX) and Tumor Institute,[105] all tolerated the procedure well, and all were discharged. Seven died an average of 35 days after tube placement. In another report, PEG tubes were placed in 12 patients with obstruction from advanced intraperitoneal malignancy.[106] All patients obtained relief of nausea, vomiting, and colicky abdominal pain, and they were encouraged to drink liquids. These patients were also treated with home hyperalimentation. Tubes functioned in most patients; in general, they remained in place until death from the primary malignancy, between 5 and 246 days (median 62 days).

The use of home hyperalimentation is controversial in this group of patients with limited life expectancy. A report from Yale University describes 17 patients with inoperable

Malignant Gastrointestinal Obstruction

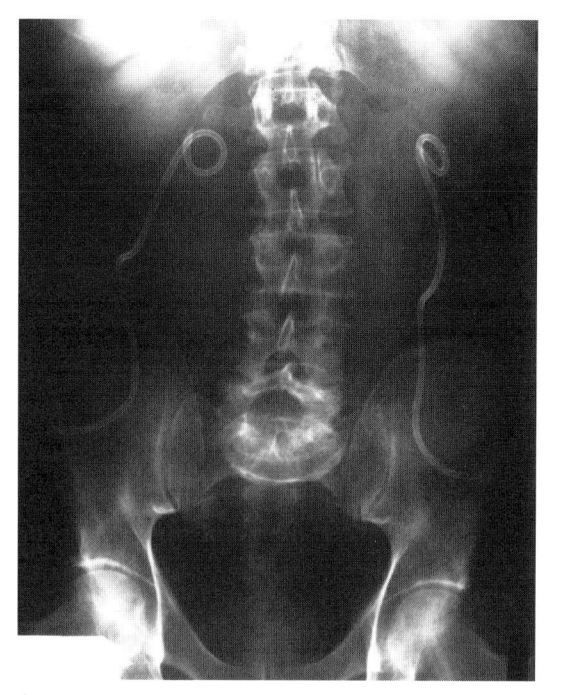

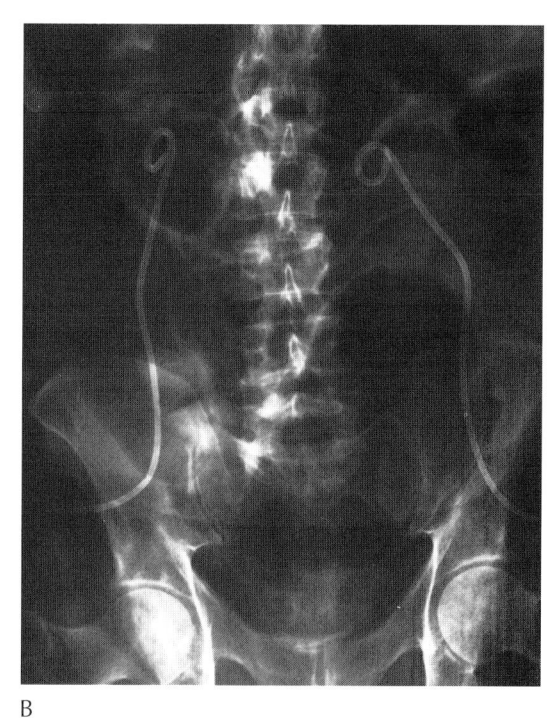

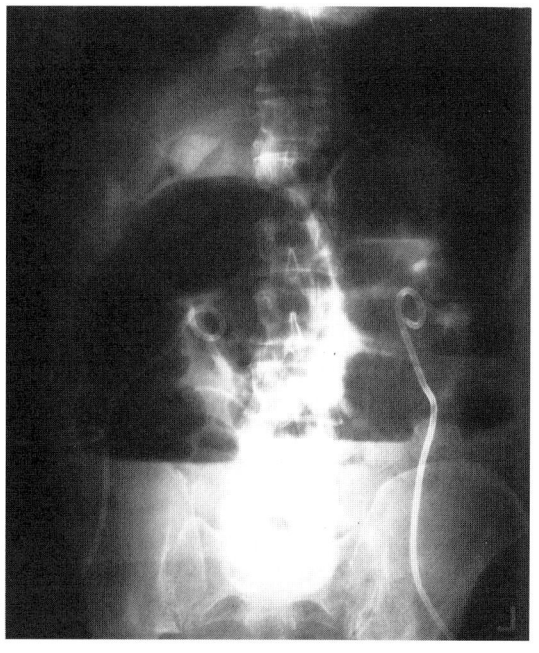

Figure 2-10. A 63-year-old man with known metastatic transition cell carcinoma of the bladder who had previously undergone radical cystectomy and left colectomy with colostomy, presented with cessation of colostomy output and abdominal distension. He did not respond to nasogastric decompression and underwent exploratory surgery. **A**. KUB 2 weeks earlier was normal after nephrostomy tube change. **B**. Flat and (**C**) upright abdominal films were consistent with small bowel obstruction. He underwent resection of obstructed transverse colon and terminal ileum with formation of Brooke ileostomy.

malignant bowel obstruction so treated.[107] They attempted to determine if the therapy provided any benefit to the patients by polling patients and families as well as members of the nutrition support team caring for the individual patients. Median survival for the group was 53 days and there was only one treatment-related complication. This therapy was most beneficial for patients with gastrointestinal primary tumors and least beneficial in patients with ovarian cancer. Fourteen patients and families felt the treatment was beneficial or highly beneficial; the nutrition support team agreed with this assessment in 11 cases. These authors concluded that home hyperalimentation was of palliative benefit and that it provided for and facilitated compassionate home care of these terminally ill patients. Others have agreed with this approach.[108,109]

■
SUMMARY: PERITONEAL CARCINOMATOSIS

1. Bowel obstruction from carcinomatosis is rarely amenable to surgical intervention. Rarely will a bypass procedure be effective in relieving the obstruction long term. In general, surgery should be avoided in these patients.
2. Nonoperative and noninvasive medical therapy for obstruction due to carcinomatosis may be tried, including antiemetic agents and nasogastric decompression; pain may be controlled with narcotics.
3. Patients may obtain significant symptomatic relief with gastric decompression. For relatively long-term decompression, a PEG tube may be placed. Likewise, home hyperalimentation may be beneficial in a selected group of patients (those with known carcinomatosis, recurrent obstruction after recent surgery, persistent symptoms despite pharmacologic intervention, and expected survival greater than 1 month); it allows patients to remain home with their families for the longest possible time period.

■
EXTRINSIC COMPRESSION AND OBSTRUCTION OF THE GASTROINTESTINAL TRACT BY MALIGNANCY

Table 2-1 lists some of the rarer causes of gastrointestinal tract obstruction by cancer secondary to extrinsic compression. Although the list is not exhaustive, it attempts to highlight the fact that cancer may cause obstruction in unusual and therefore diagnostically and therapeutically challenging ways.

An example of extrinsic compression of the rectum causing obstruction is illustrated in Figure 2-11. This elderly man was treated for known metastatic prostate cancer with bilateral orchiectomies. A CT scan to evaluate the extent of the tumor was performed in preparation for pelvic irradiation. Figures 2-11A through 2-11E reveal a massive tumor mass compressing the rectum (arrows). Five days after the CT scan was performed, the patient presented with distension, obstipation, and constipation. Flat (Fig. 2-11F) and upright (Fig. 2-11G) abdominal radiographs revealed dilated bowel loops to the descending colon and no rectal air. He underwent exploratory surgery and a diverting transverse

Table 2-1. Causes of Malignant Gastrointestinal Tract Obstruction by Extrinsic Compression

ESOPHAGUS: Metastatic lymph node involvement (lung cancer, esophageal cancer)

STOMACH: Pancreatic neoplasms

SMALL BOWEL: Colon cancer, metastatic lymph node involvement (lymphoma, colon cancer, carcinoid) Retroperitoneal sarcoma

COLON AND RECTUM: Pancreatic cancer, chordoma, prostatic cancer (adenocarcinoma, sarcoma), retroperitoneal sarcoma

Malignant Gastrointestinal Obstruction 55

A

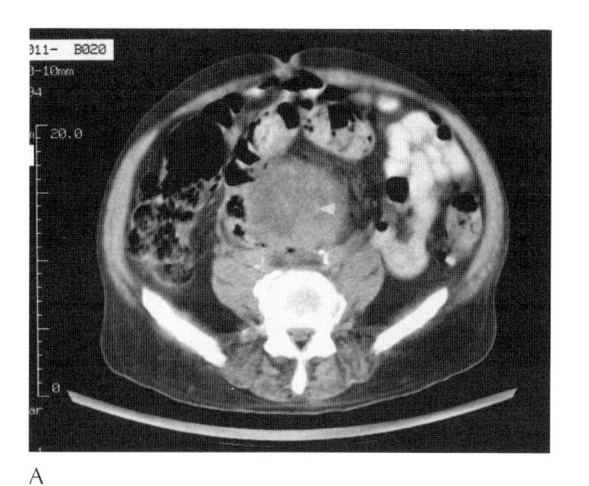

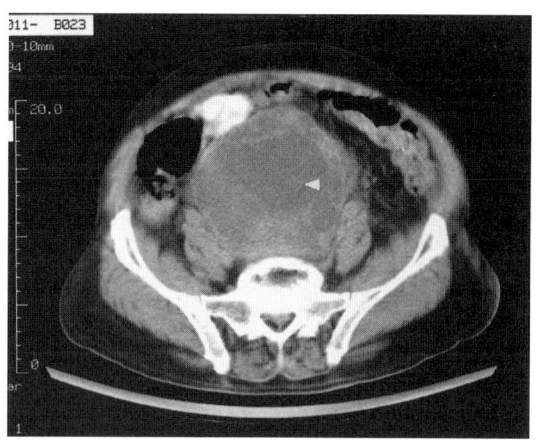

B

C

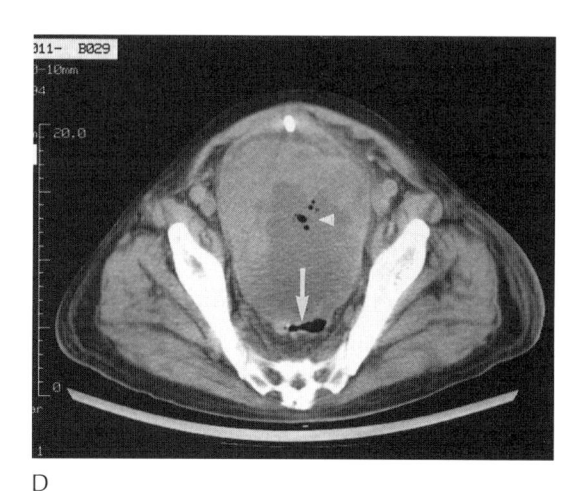

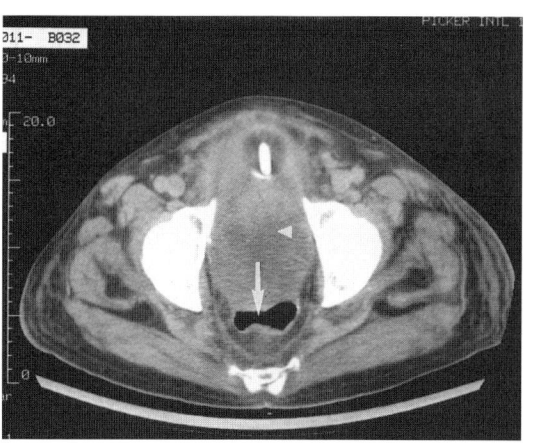

D

E

Figure 2-11. A 74-year-old man with known metastatic prostate cancer presented with obstipation, distension, and vomiting. **A–E.** A CT scan performed the previous week revealed impending obstruction of the rectum by extrinsic compression from a large prostatic mass (*arrows*). **F.** Flat and (**G**) upright abdominal radiographs revealed dilated bowel loops to the descending colon consistent with rectal obstruction. The patient underwent palliative transverse colostomy and mucous fistula with relief of the obstruction and made an unremarkable recovery.

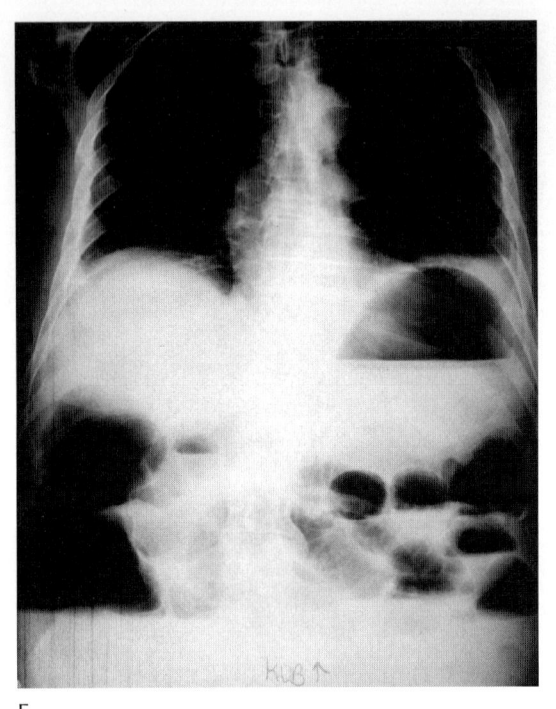

F

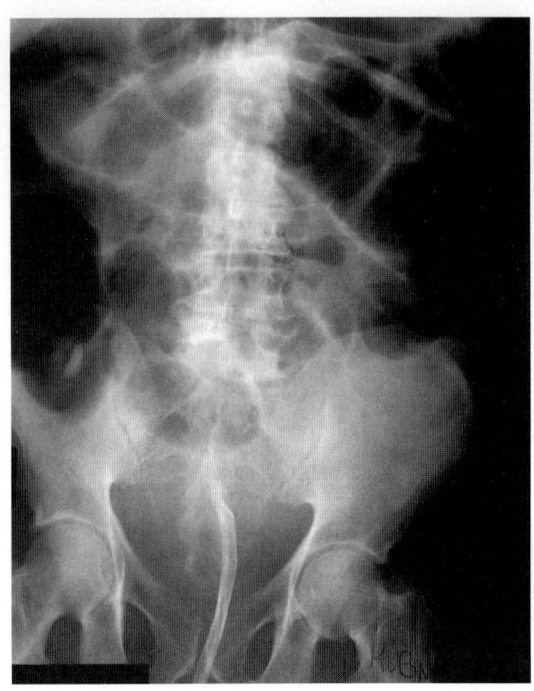

G

Figure 2-11 (continued)

colostomy and mucous fistula were created. His recovery was unremarkable.

SUMMARY

Gastrointestinal tract obstruction can be the initial problem presenting in a patient with cancer or it can be a significant clinical problem in the care of the patient with recurrent or persistent disease. The choice of therapeutic modality used depends on many factors including site of obstruction, cause of obstruction, and overall status of the patient.

Gastrointestinal tract obstruction can result from primary or recurrent tumors in any location from esophagus to anus. Esophageal obstruction is probably best treated by surgical resection, even if only for palliation. Other approaches include stenting of the esophagus, radiation therapy, and laser ablation. Bypass of the esophagus is not recommended. Cancers causing gastric obstruction should be resected whenever possible. Resection for palliation is also indicated. There is no role presently for palliative radiation or chemotherapy in cancer of the stomach. Patients with obstructing carcinomas of the periampullary region should undergo resection for cure whenever possible. Patients with unresectable lesions should have palliative combined biliary and gastric bypass. Resection is the treatment of choice for carcinomas of the small bowel, with chemotherapy in addition for lymphomas.

Obstructing lesions of the colon and rectum show consistently lower survival rates than those in patients without obstruction. Treatment is resection with primary anastomosis if possible, but patients with unprepared bowel should probably undergo colostomy with reversal at a later date if indicated. Colostomy alone is an unattractive option. Obstructing rectal lesions are approached with diverting colostomy and delayed resection. Obstructing anal lesions are treated with colostomy followed by chemoradiation therapy.

The second group of patients with gastrointestinal obstruction are those with obstruction following cancer therapy, rather than as a result of the tumor itself. Postoperative bowel obstruction following surgical resection may be due to benign or malignant causes. In general, an aggressive surgical approach is recommended in these cases, usually following a trial of nonoperative therapy with nasogastric decompression. However, those with advanced disease or poor overall status should probably have other therapeutic interventions. Bowel obstruction with peritoneal carcinomatosis indicates a poor prognosis. Survival is usually short, measured in weeks to months. In general, these patients should be treated nonoperatively. Gastric decompression and home hyperalimentation may help these patients enjoy what time remains. Bowel obstruction following radiation therapy is covered in Chapter 7. Bowel obstruction may also follow the use of intraperitoneal chemotherapy.

Obstruction of the gastrointestinal tract remains a significant problem in the care of the cancer patient, and one for which surgeons are often consulted. As is the case in many interventions, the best approach will be discerned from consideration of the individual situation presented by each patient, keeping in mind the important guidelines presented in this chapter.

REFERENCES

1. Schlag PM. Randomized trial of preoperative chemotherapy for squamous cell cancer of the esophagus. Arch Surg 1992;127:1446.
2. Akakura I, Nakamura Y, Kakegawa T, Nakayama R, Watanabe H, Yamashita H. Surgery with carcinoma of the esophagus with preoperative radiation. Chest 1970;57:47.
3. Stewart JR, Hoff SJ, Johnson DH, Murray MJ, Butler DR, Elkins CC, et al. Improved survival with neoadjuvant therapy and resection for adenocarcinoma of the esophagus. Ann Surg 1993;218:571.
4. Yadava OP, Hodge AJ, Matz LR, Donlon JB. Esophageal malignancies: is preoperative radiotherapy the way to go? Ann Thorac Surg 1991; 51:189.
5. Skinner DB, Ferguson MK, Soriano A, Little AG, Staszak VM. Selection of operation for esophageal cancer based on staging. Ann Surg 1986; 204:391.
6. Lerut T, DeLeyn P, Coosemans W, Van Raemdonck D, Scheys I, LeSaffre E. Surgical strategies in esophageal carcinoma with emphasis on radical lymphadenectomy. Ann Surg 1992; 216:583.
7. Orringer MB. Transhiatal esophagectomy for carcinoma of the thoracic esophagus. Ann Surg 1984;200:282.
8. Gadacz TR. Esophageal carcinoma: an assessment of treatment. Persp Gen Surg 1990; 1:30.
9. Watson DI, Devitt PG, Game PA, Grantley-Gill P, Jamieson G. Surgical bypass for palliation of malignant esophageal obstruction. Aust N Z J Surg 1993;63:333.
10. Orringer MB, Forastiere AA, Perez-Tamayo C. Chemotherapy and radiation therapy prior to transhiatal esophagectomy for esophageal carcinoma. Ann Thorac Surg 1990;49:348.
11. Hartley L, Strong R, Fielding G, Evans E. Morbidity and mortality of operative intubation for malignant esophageal obstruction. Aust N Z J Surg 1985;55:555.
12. Anderson JR, Sorenson SM, Kruse A, et al. Randomized trial of endoscopic endoprosthesis versus operative bypass in malignant obstructive jaundice. Gut 1989;30:1132.
13. Shepard HA, Royle G, Ross APR, et al. Endoscopic biliary endoprosthesis in the palliation of malignant obstruction of the distal common bile duct: a randomized trial. Br J Surg 1988;75:1166.
14. Shaer J, Katon RM, Ivancev K, et al. Treatment of malignant esophageal obstruction with silicone-coated metallic self-expanding stents. Gastrointest Endosc 1992;38:7.
15. Pietrafitta JJ, Dwyer RM. Endoscopic laser therapy of malignant esophageal obstuction. Arch Surg 1986;121:395.
16. Isaac JR, Sim EK, Ngoi SS, Goh PM. Safe and rapid palliation of dysphagia for carcinoma of the esophagus. Am Surg 1991;57:245.
17. Schulze S, Fischerman K. Palliation of oesophagogastric neoplasms with Nd:YAG laser treatment. Scand J Gastroenterol 1990;25: 1024.
18. Alderson D, Wright PD. Laser recanalization versus endoscopic intubation in the palliation of malignant dysphagia. Br J Surg 1990; 77:1151.
19. Ferraro P, Beauchamp G, Aumais G. Endoscopic Nd:YAG laser therapy of malignant esophageal obstruction. Can J Surg 1990;33: 479.
20. Sankar MY, Joffe SN. Endoscopic contact

Nd:YAG laser resectional vaporization (ECLRV) and esophageal dilatation (ED) in advanced malignant obstruction of the esophagus. Am Surg 1991;57:259.
21. Caspers R, Welvaart K, Verkes R, Hermans J, Leer J. The effect of radiotherapy on dysphagia and survival in patients with esophageal cancer. J Rad Ther Oncol 1988;12:15.
22. Welvaart K, Caspers R, Verkes R, Hermans J. The choice between surgical resection and radiation therapy for patients with cancer of the esophagus and cardia: A retrospective comparison between two treatments. J Surg Oncol 1991;47:225.
23. Petrovich Z, Langholz B, Formenti S, Luxton G, Astrahan M. Management of carcinoma of the esophagus: the role of radiotherapy. Am J Clin Oncol 1991;14:80.
24. Ellis H. The diagnosis of benign and malignant pyloric obstruction. Clin Oncol 1976;2:11.
25. Johnson CD, Ellis H. Gastric outlet obstruction now predicts malignancy. Br J Surg 1990;77:1023.
26. Aranha GV, Georgen R. Gastric linitis plastica is not a surgical disease. Surgery 1989;106:758.
27. Bozzetti F, Bonfanti G, Audisio RA, Doci R, Dossena G, Gennari L, et al. Prognosis of patients after palliative surgical procedures for carcinoma of the stomach. Surg Gynecol Obstet 1987;164:151.
28. Boddie AW, Jr, McMurtrey MJ, Giacco GG, McBride CM. Palliative total gastrectomy and esophagogastrectomy. A reevaluation. Cancer 1983;51:1195.
29. Meijer S, DeBakker OJGB, Hoitsma HFW. Palliative resection in gastric cancer. J Surg Oncol 1983;23:77.
30. Ekbom GA, Gleysteen JJ. Gastric malignancy: resection for palliation. Surgery 1980;88:476.
31. Cocconi G, DeLisi V, DiBlasio B. Randomized comparison of 5-FU alone or combined with mitomycin and cytarabine (MFC) in the treatment of advanced gastric cancer. Cancer Treatment Reports 1982;66:1263.
32. MacDonald JS, Schein PS, Wooley PV, et al. 5-Fluorouracil, mitomycin-C, and adriamycin (FAM): a new combination chemotherapy program for advanced gastric carcinoma. Ann Intern Med 1980;93:533.
33. Preusser P, Achterrath W, Wilke H, et al. Chemotherapy of gastric cancer. Cancer Treatment Reports 1988;15:257.
34. Preusser P, Wilke H, Achterrath W, et al. Phase II Study with the combination etoposide, doxorubicin, and cisplatin in advanced measurable gastric cancer. J Clin Oncol 1989;7:1310.
35. Truong S, Bohndorf V, Geller H, Schumpelick V, Gunther RW. Self-expanding metal stents for palliation of malignant gastric outlet obstruction. Endoscopy 1992;24:433.
36. Meinke WB, Twomey PL, Guernsey JM, Frey CF, Higgins G, Keehn R. Gastric outlet obstruction after palliative surgery for cancer of head of pancreas. Arch Surg 1983;118:550.
37. Lillemoe KD, Sauter PK, Pitt HA, Yeo CJ, Cameron JL. Current status of surgical palliation of periampullary carcinoma. Surg Obstet Gynecol 1993;176:1.
38. Weaver DW, Wiencek RG, Bouwman DL, Walt AJ. Gastrojejunostomy: is it helpful for patients with pancreatic cancer? Surgery 1987;102:608.
39. Doberneck RC, Berndt GA. Delayed gastric emptying after palliative gastrojejunostomy for cancer of the pancreas. Arch Surg 1987;122:827.
40. Singh SM, Longmire WP, Jr, Reber HA. Surgical palliation for pancreatic cancer. The UCLA experience. Ann Surg 1990;212:132.
41. Lucas CE, Ledgerwood AM, Bender JS. Antrectomy with gastrojejunostomy for unresectable pancreatic cancer causing duodenal obstruction. Surgery 1991;110:583.
42. Geoghegan J, Delaney PV, Egan TJ. Duodenal obstruction in advanced pancreatic carcinoma: how effective is gastroenterostomy in palliation? Irish J Med Sci 1990;159:13.
43. Keymling M, Wagner HJ, Vakil N, Knyrim K. Relief of malignant duodenal obstruction by percutaneous insertion of a metal stent. Gastrointest Endosc 1993;39:439.
44. Coit DG. Cancer of the small intestine. In: DeVita VT, Jr, Hellman S, Rosenberg SA, eds. Cancer. Principles and practice of oncolgy. 4th ed. Philadelphia: JB Lippincott, 1993:915.
45. Martin RG. Malignant tumors of the small intestine. Surg Clin North Am 1986;66:779.
46. Frost DB, Mercado PD, Tyrell JS. Small bowel cancer: a 30-year review. Ann Surg Oncol 1994;1:290.
47. Shepherd FA, Evans WK, Kutas G, et al. Chemotherapy following surgery for stages IE and IIE non-Hodgkin's lymphoma of the gastrointestinal tract. J Clin Oncol 1988;6:253.
48. Caputy GC, Donohue JH, Goellner JR, Weaver AL. Metastatic melanoma of the gastrointestinal tract. Results of surgical management. Arch Surg 1991;126:1353.
49. Boring CC, Squires TS, Tong T, Montgomery S. Cancer statistics, 1995. CA-Cancer J Clin 1995;45:7.
50. Kaufman Z, Eiltch E, Dinbar A. Completely

obstructive colorectal cancer. J Surg Oncol 1989;41:230.
51. Wolmark N, Wicand HS, Rockette HE, Fisher B, Glass A, Lawrence W, et al. The prognostic significance of tumor location and bowel obstruction in Dukes B and C colorectal cancer. Ann Surg 1983;198:743.
52. Steinberg SM, Barkin JS, Kaplan RS, Stablein DM. Prognostic indicators of colon tumors: the Gastrointestinal Tumor Group experience. Cancer 1986;57:1866.
53. Willett C, Tepper JE, Cohen A, Orlow E, Welch C. Obstructive and perforative colonic carcinoma: patterns of failure. J Clin Oncol 1985;3:379.
54. Chapuis PH, Dent OF, Fisher R, et al. A multivariate analysis of clinical and pathological variables in prognosis after resection of large bowel cancer. Br J Surg 1985;72:698.
55. Gandrup P, Lund L, Balslev I. Surgical treatment of acute malignant large bowel obstruction. Eur J Surg 1992;158:427.
56. Welch JP, Donaldson GA. Management of severe obstruction of the large bowel due to malignant disease. Am J Surg 1974;127:492.
57. Fielding LP, Wells BW. Survival after primary and after staged resection of large bowel obstruction caused by cancer. Br J Surg 1974;61:16.
58. Phillips RKS, Hittinger R, Fry JS, Fielding LP. Malignant large bowel obstruction. Br J Surg 1985;72:296.
59. Irvin TT, Greaney MG. The treatment of colonic cancer presenting with intestinal obstruction. Br J Surg 1977;64:741.
60. Sjodahl R, Franzen T, Nystrom PO. Primary versus staged resection for acute obstructing colorectal carcinoma. Br J Surg 1992;79:685.
61. Morgan WP, Jenkins N, Lewis P, Aubrey DA. Management of obstructing carcinoma of the left colon by extended right hemicolectomy. Am J Surg 1985;149:327.
62. Halevy A, Levi J, Orda R. Emergency subtotal colectomy. A new trend for treatment of obstructing carcinoma of the left colon. Ann Surg 1989; 210:220.
63. Brief DK, Brener BJ, Goldenkranz R, et al. Defining the role of subtotal colectomy in the treatment of carcinoma of the colon. Ann Surg 1991;213:248.
64. Stone JM, Bloom RJ. Transendoscopic balloon dilatation of complete colonic obstruction. An adjunct in the treatment of colorectal cancer: report of three cases. Dis Colon Rectum 1989;32:429.
65. Smith SRG, Connolly JC, Gilmore OJA. The effect of faecal loading on colonic anastomotic healing. Br J Surg 1983;70:49.
66. Bloomquist P, Jiborn H, Zederfeldt B. Effect of diverting colostomy on collagen metabolism in the colonic wall. Studies in the rat. Am J Surg 1985;149:330.
67. MacKenzie S, Thomson SR, Baker LW. Management options in malignant obstruction of the left colon. Surg Obstet Gynecol 1992;174:337.
68. White CM, Macfie J. Immediate colectomy and primary anastomosis for acute obstruction due to carcinoma of the left colon and rectum. Dis Colon Rectum 1985;28:155.
69. Irving AD, Scrimgeour D. Mechanical bowel preparation for colonic resection and anastomosis. Br J Surg 1987;74:580.
70. Mealy K, Salman A, Arthur G. Definitive one-stage emergency large bowel surgery. Br J Surg 1988;75:1216.
71. Dorudi S, Wilson NM, Heddle RM. Primary restorative colectomy in malignant left-sided large bowel obstruction. Ann Royal Coll Surg Eng 1990;72:393.
72. Cohen AM, Minsky BD, Friedman MA. Rectal cancer. In: DeVita VT, Jr, Hellman S, Rosenberg SA, eds. Cancer. Principles and practice of oncology. 4th ed. Philadelphia: JB Lippincott, 1993:978.
73. Minsky BD, Cohen AM, Kemeny N, et al. The efficacy of preoperative 5-fluorouracil, high-dose leucvorin, and sequential radiation therapy for unresectable rectal cancer. Cancer 1993;71:3486.
74. Marks J, Mohiuddin M, Kakinic J. New hope and promise for sphincter preservation in the management of cancer of the rectum. Semin Oncol 1991;18:388.
75. Mendenhall WM, Million RR, Bland KI, et al. Preoperative radiation therapy for clinically resectable adenocarcinoma of the rectum. Ann Surg 1985;202:215.
76. Reed WP, Garb JL, Park WC, et al. Long-term results and complications of preoperative radiation in the treatment of rectal cancer. Surgery 1988;103:161.
77. Frykolm G, Glimelius B, Pahlman L. Preoperative irradiation with and without chemotherapy (MFL) in the treatment of primarily non-resectable adenocarcinoma of the rectum: results from two consecutive studies. Eur J Cancer 1989;25:1535.
78. Daneker GW, Jr, Carlson GW, Hohn DC, et al. Endoscopic laser recanalization is effective for prevention and treatment of obstruction in sigmoid and rectal cancer. Arch Surg 1991;126:1348.
79. Eckhauser ML. Laser therapy of colorectal carcinoma. Surg Clin North Am 1992;72:597.
80. Kiefhaber P, Kiefhaber K, Huber F. Pre-operative neodymium:YAG laser treatment of obstructive colon cancer. Endoscopy 1986;18:44.

81. Eckhauser ML, Imbembo AL, Mansour EG. The role of pre-resectional laser recanalization for obstructing carcinomas of the colon and rectum. Surgery 1989;106:710.
82. Beart RW. Prevention and management of recurrent rectal cancer. World J Surg 1991;15:589.
83. Wanebo HJ, Gaker DL, Whitehill R, et al. Pelvic recurrence of rectal cancer. Options for curative resection. Ann Surg 1987;205:482.
84. Dobrowsky W. Mitomycin C, 5-fluorouracil and radiation in advanced, locally recurrent rectal cancer. Br J Radiology 1992;65:143.
85. Russin DJ, Kaplan SR, Goldberg RI, Barkin JS. Neodymium-YAG laser. A new tool in the treatment of colorectal cancer. Arch Surg 1986; 121:1399.
86. Walfisch S, Stern H, Ball S. Use of Nd-Yag laser ablation in colorectal obstruction and palliation in high-risk patients. Dis Colon Rectum 1989;32:1060.
87. Fritsch A, Seidl W, Walzel C, et al. Palliative and adjunctive measures in rectal cancer. World J Surg 1982;6:569.
88. Madden JL, Kandalaft SI. Electrocoagulation as a primary curative method in the treatment of carcinoma of the rectum. Surg Gynecol Obstet 1983;157:164.
89. Wiebke EA, Niederhuber JE. Anal canal cancer. In: Niederhuber JE, ed. Current therapy in oncology. St Louis: BC Decker, 1993;437.
90. Nigro ND. The force of change in the management of squamous-cell cancer of the anal canal. Dis Colon Rectum 1991;34:482.
91. Sugarbaker PH, Cunliffe WJ, Belliveau J, et al. Rationale for integrating early postoperative intraperitoneal chemotherapy into the surgical treatment of gastrointestinal cancer. Semin Oncol 1089;16(Suppl 6):83.
92. Markman M, Cleary S, Howell SB, Lucas WE. Complications of extensive adhesion formation after intraperitoneal chemotherapy. Surg Gynecol Obstet 1986;162:445.
93. Osteen RT, Guyton S, Steele G, Jr, Wilson RE. Malignant intestinal obstruction. Surgery 1980;87:611.
94. Aranha GV, Folk FA, Greenlee HB. Surgical palliation of small bowel obstruction due to metastatic carcinoma. Am Surg 1981;47:99.
95. Walsh HPJ, Schofield PF. Is laparotomy for small bowel obstruction justified in patients with previously treated malignancy? Br J Surg 1984; 71:933.
96. Ellis CN, Boggs HW, Jr, Slagle GW, Cole PA. Small bowel obstruction after colon resection for benign and malignant diseases. Dis Colon Rectum 1991;34:367.
97. Lau PWK, Lorentz TG. Results of surgery for malignant bowel obstruction in advanced, unresectable, recurrent colorectal cancer. Dis Colon Rectum 1993;36:61.
98. Butler JA, Cameron BL, Morrow M, Kahng K. Small bowel obstruction in patients with a prior history of cancer. Am J Surg 1991;162:624.
99. Ripamonti C, De Conno F, Ventafridda V, et al. Management of bowel obstruction in advanced and terminal cancer patients. Ann Oncol 1993;4:15.
100. Fernandes JR, Seymour RJ, Suissa S. Bowel obstruction in patients with ovarian cancer: a search for prognostic factors. Am J Obstet Gynecol 1988;158:244.
101. van Ooijen B, van der Berg MEL, Planting AST, et al. Surgical treatment or gastric drainage only for intestinal obstruction in patients with carcinoma of the ovary or peritoneal carcinomatosis of other origin. Surg Gynecol Obstet 1993;176:469.
102. Clarke-Pearson DL, Chin NO, DeLong ER, et al. Surgical management of intestinal obstruction in ovarian cancer I. Clinical features, postoperative complications, and survival. Gynecol Oncol 1987;26:11.
103. Annest LS, Jolly PC. The results of surgical treatment of bowel obstruction caused by peritoneal carcinomatosis. Am Surg 1979; 718.
104. Baines M, Oliver DJ, Carter RL. Medical management of intestinal obstruction in patients with advanced malignant disease. A clinical and pathological study. Lancet 1985; 2:990.
105. Malone JM, Jr, Koonce T, Larson DM, et al. Palliation of small bowel obstruction by percutaneous gastrostomy in patients with progressive ovarian carcinoma. Obstet Gynecol 1986;68:431.
106. Adelson MD, Kasowitz MH. Percutaneous endoscopic gastrostomy in the treatment of gastrointestinal obstruction from malignancy. Obstet Gynecol 1993;81:467.
107. August DA, Thorn D, Fisher RL, Welcher CM. Home parenteral nutrition for patients with inoperable malignant bowel obstruction. JPEN 1991;15:323.
108. Moley JF, August DA, Norton JA, et al. Home parenteral nutrition for patients with advanced intraperitoneal cancers and gastrointestinal dysfunction. J Surg Oncol 1986;33:342.
109. Gouttebel MC, Saint-Aubert B, Jonquet O, et al. Ambulatory home parenteral nutrition. JPEN 1987;11:475.

3

Gastrointestinal Bleeding and Perforation in the Cancer Patient

WILLIAM E. BURAK, JR
WILLIAM B. FARRAR

Gastrointestinal bleeding is a complication frequently encountered in the care of patients with cancer. The degree of hemorrhage can range from mild to massive, with life-threatening bleeding requiring immediate surgical attention. There are many different causes of gastrointestinal bleeding, especially in the patient population that is undergoing aggressive treatment for an underlying malignant process. Bleeding may arise from primary gastrointestinal malignancies or metastatic lesions to the gastrointestinal tract; it may occur as a complication related to treatment, or it may be due to progression of the malignancy. In view of the many variables that come into play when managing the bleeding patient (site, cause, degree of hemorrhage), it is important to undertake a rational, systematic approach during the initial work-up and evaluation. However, it must also be kept in mind that treatment strategies vary depending on the general condition and overall prognosis of the patient, making it essential to individualize the approach.

Gastrointestinal bleeding is classified as upper or lower, depending on the site where the hemorrhage originates. Upper gastrointestinal bleeding originates at a site proximal to Treitz's ligament, whereas lower gastrointestinal bleeding occurs distal to this useful landmark. Because the presentation, workup, and subsequent management vary according to the source of bleeding, upper and lower gastrointestinal bleeding will be discussed individually (Fig. 3-1).

UPPER GASTROINTESTINAL BLEEDING

Patients who present with hematemesis or have bleeding that is evident in a nasogastric tube will almost certainly be found to have a bleeding source proximal to Treitz's ligament. However, not all patients with upper gastrointestinal bleeding will present in this fashion; a large number will have melena or hematochezia as the initial symptom. It is crucial to localize the exact bleeding site early in the evaluation of these patients, as treatment options vary accordingly. With this in mind, initial management should include three important phases: resuscitation, identification of the bleeding site, and treatment. It should be emphasized that these three phases often temporally overlap. For example, identification of the bleeding site frequently occurs during the resuscitation phase of management to expedite treatment.

Initial Management

RESUSCITATION

Patients with what is judged to be moderate to severe hemorrhage should undergo placement

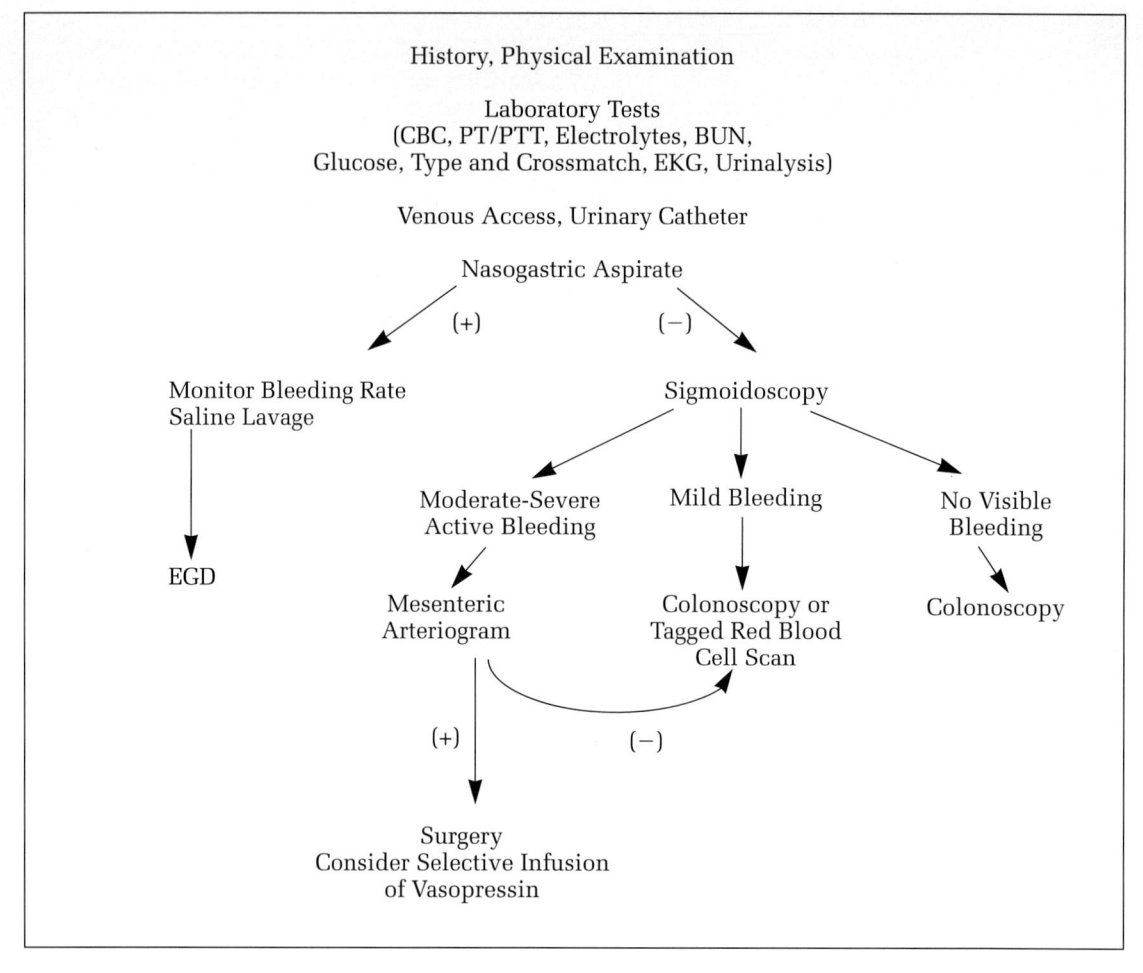

```
                    History, Physical Examination

                           Laboratory Tests
                   (CBC, PT/PTT, Electrolytes, BUN,
              Glucose, Type and Crossmatch, EKG, Urinalysis)

                       Venous Access, Urinary Catheter

                           Nasogastric Aspirate
                         ↙(+)           (−)↘
        Monitor Bleeding Rate                  Sigmoidoscopy
        Saline Lavage                    ↙          ↓          ↘
                 ↓              Moderate-Severe  Mild Bleeding  No Visible
                EGD             Active Bleeding                  Bleeding
                                       ↓              ↓              ↓
                                   Mesenteric    Colonoscopy or   Colonoscopy
                                   Arteriogram   Tagged Red Blood
                                                    Cell Scan
                                    (+)↓    (−)↗
                                       Surgery
                                Consider Selective Infusion
                                      of Vasopressin
```

Figure 3-1. Diagnosis of gastrointestinal bleeding.

of two large-bore intravenous catheters and have blood samples sent for complete blood count, electrolytes, liver function studies, coagulation profile, and most importantly type and cross-match for 4 to 6 units of packed red blood cells. A urinary catheter should be placed and fluids rapidly administered to maintain a urine output of at least 0.5 ml/kg/h. Hypotension that does not respond to 2 L of crystalloid signifies a massive hemorrhage and immediate blood transfusion is necessary. Simultaneously, a nasogastric tube is inserted to relieve vomiting, assess the ongoing bleeding, and to lavage the stomach in preparation for upper endoscopy. Evacuating the clot also plays a role in reducing fibrinolysis at the site of bleeding. In fact, it is evacuation of the clot that does much to help control further bleeding; it also helps relieve distention caused by a large amount of intragastric blood. Whereas iced saline has been used traditionally for lavage, the temperature of the fluid is unimportant and room temperature saline is probably equally effective.

IDENTIFICATION OF THE BLEEDING SITE

During the initial resuscitation, a brief history should be taken and physical examination performed to assist in identifying the bleeding site. A history of similar episodes, heavy alcohol use, or specific medications may also give clues as to the source of bleeding. It is also essential to learn of the patient's treatment (chemotherapy, radiation therapy) schedule as this may provide additional useful information, particularly in relation to the hematologic effects of chemotherapy (see Chapter 17). Physical examination allows the examiner to obtain a general idea of the degree of blood loss that has occurred by measuring vital signs and assessing for orthostatic changes, while facilitating identification of peripheral stigmata of parenchymal liver disease or coagulation defects. The next step in management involves the liberal use of upper endoscopy to localize the bleeding site properly. Again, removal of the intragastric blood is essential to enable this procedure to yield useful information. Fiberoptic esophagogastroduodenoscopy enables visualization of the exact location of hemorrhage in greater than 95% of patients and may provide an avenue by which appropriate therapy can be provided.[1,2] An example of this is endoscopy-guided electrocoagulation of a bleeding duodenal ulcer. There is *no* role for contrast radiographs (barium studies) in the bleeding patient, as the yield is extremely low and the barium may obscure the bleeding point should the patient need additional diagnostic studies.[2]

TREATMENT

Once the cause and the site of the upper gastrointestinal hemorrhage are known, specific therapy may be instituted. Exact treatment is extremely variable and must be individualized according to the patient and to the cause of bleeding. Depending on the underlying disease, rate of bleeding, anatomic region of hemorrhage, the patient's coagulation status, and overall prognosis, therapy may range from simple observation and replacement of blood products to acute surgical intervention. The use of fresh frozen plasma may be indicated if clotting studies are abnormal, whether or not surgery is planned.

SUMMARY: INITIAL MANAGEMENT OF UPPER GASTROINTESTINAL BLEEDING

1. Gastrointestinal bleeding is a frequent occurrence in the cancer patient and may occur for a variety of reasons. Management includes resuscitation, identification of the bleeding site, and treatment.
2. Initial resuscitation involves replacement of fluid volume, nasogastric suction, and other routine measures to maintain hemodynamic stability. Evacuation of the clot is important to slow bleeding and to enable endoscopic examination of the stomach.
3. Abnormal clotting studies usually warrant administration of fresh-frozen plasma, which is especially useful if surgery is planned.

Specific Sites of Upper Gastrointestinal Bleeding

ESOPHAGUS

Esophageal Varices. Varices of the esophagus and stomach commonly result from portal hypertension which is secondary to alcoholic cirrhosis, hepatitis, primary biliary cirrhosis, hepatic vein thrombosis (Budd-Chiari syndrome, see Chapter 5), or portal vein thrombosis. In the cancer patient, primary hepatic malignancies, metastases to the liver, pancreatic cancer, and tumors that invade the portal vein can lead to obstruction resulting in portal venous hypertension and variceal hemorrhage. Splenic vein thrombosis can occur as a result of local invasion of pancreatic cancer leading to splenomegaly and bleeding gastric varices. Budd-Chiari syndrome occurs as a result of thrombosis of the major hepatic veins within the liver or at their junction with the inferior vena cava. This disease entity is further discussed in Chapter 5. Hepatocellular, renal cell, and adrenal carcinoma can be responsible for this syndrome, as can myeloproliferative disorders, leukemia, and lymphoma. The most frequent clinical sign is massive ascites, although the variceal bleeding may occur secondary to portal hypertension from intrahepatic fibrosis.[3-5]

Management of bleeding esophageal varices is very different from the treatment of other causes of upper gastrointestinal bleeding, making it essential to establish a prompt diagnosis. After initial resuscitation and correction of any coagulopathy with fresh frozen plasma, platelets, and parenteral vitamin K, esophagogastroduodenscopy is performed to verify the bleeding varices and to rule out other sources of bleeding (duodenal ulcer), which can mimic variceal bleeding even in the patient with known portal hypertension and varices.

After the variceal bleeding is documented, it is essential to control the hemorrhage through the least invasive method as quickly as possible. Active bleeding should be treated with systemic intravenous vasopressin (pitressin) at a rate of 0.2 to 0.4 U/min for 24 to 48 hours as this drug lowers splanchnic pressures and may aid in slowing or stopping variceal bleeding.[6,7] It may be beneficial to also infuse systemic nitroglycerine to patients with known or suspected coronary artery disease to offset the vasoconstrictive effects of vasopressin on the coronary vasculature.[8] At the time of endoscopy, varices should be visualized, and if bleeding, sclerotherapy should be performed by injecting the responsible varix with a sclerosing agent in an attempt to provide hemostasis.[9-11] If successful, a second session should be performed in 7 to 10 days and then at 4- to 6-week intervals until obliteration of all varices is complete. Failure of sclerotherapy, or rebleeding after sclerotherapy, necessitates more invasive treatment; meanwhile balloon tamponade (*e.g.*, Sengstaken-Blakemore tube) may serve as a temporizing measure until definitive treatment can be provided.[12,13] It should be emphasized that if balloon tamponade is successful in controlling hemorrhage, one should prepare either for another sclerotherapy session (if the first session was initially successful) or surgery. There are a variety of procedures available to the surgeon from which to choose. Decompression of the varices can be provided by reducing portal hypertension through total portal systemic shunts (portacaval, mesocaval), partial portal systemic shunts (portacaval H-graft), or selective shunts (distal splenorenal).[14-18] Because results are similar, the shunt with which the surgeon is most familiar should be used. The distal splenorenal shunt, although more technically demanding, affords a reduction in portal hypertension and maintains hepatic blood flow while avoiding the area of the porta hepatis and is useful when liver transplantation is a future consideration.[16]

Direct ligation of varices, esophageal and gastric transection, and gastroesophageal devascularization have also been used in selected patients but can have a high failure rate because the underlying portal hypertension remains untreated.[19-21] Patients who present with bleeding gastric varices secondary to splenic vein thrombosis should not be treated with sclerotherapy but instead should undergo splenectomy.

Recently, there has been increasing interest in a technique known as *transjugular intrahepatic portosystemic shunt* (TIPS), a nonsurgical technique used to decompress the portal system in the patient with bleeding esophageal varices.[22,23] It is performed by the invasive radiologist and involves transvenously (internal jugular vein) placing an intrahepatic stent between a major hepatic vein and a major branch of the portal vein. This procedure has the advantage of being less invasive than surgery and if it proves to be as effective in relieving hemorrhage, is an attractive option, especially in the cancer patient who may be less able to tolerate a major operation or has a poor overall prognosis. It is particularly useful in the patient for whom liver transplantation is anticipated.

Mallory-Weiss Tear. Cancer patients with protracted vomiting (see Chapter 8) may develop upper gastrointestinal hemorrhage from a mucosal tear near the gastroesophageal (GE) junction, otherwise known as a *Mal-*

lory-Weiss tear.[24] A history of retching and prolonged vomiting suggests the diagnosis. Definitive diagnosis is made at the time of endoscopy when 83% of the nontransmural tears are seen in the stomach just below the GE junction, whereas 10% to 15% either extend across or are above the junction.[25] Only 25% of patients are likely to be actively bleeding at the time of esophagogastroduodenscopy, and 90% will stop bleeding spontaneously without therapeutic intervention. Prior to endoscopy, it is important to distinguish Mallory-Weiss syndrome from Boerhaave's syndrome where there is a transmural injury to the esophagus associated with less bleeding and more pain. If a Mallory-Weiss tear is seen during endoscopy and is not bleeding, treatment should consist of antacids or H_2 blockers, correction of any coagulopathy, and removal of the nasogastric tube to prevent irritation leading to rebleeding.[26] The patient is then observed closely for signs of hemorrhage. If the tear is actively bleeding at the time of endoscopy, an attempt at endoscopic sclerosis can be made along with infusion of systemic intravenous vasopressin, which plays an important role in those patients with associated portal hypertension.[27] Failure of endoscopic therapy necessitates more definitive intervention; either operative or angiographic measures can be successful.

Angiographic identification of the bleeding vessel (usually a branch of the left gastric artery) followed by either embolization or selective infusion of vasopressin has been reported to be successful in selected patients.[26] Otherwise, surgery is the mainstay in the treatment of continued bleeding. The operation is performed through a midline laparotomy (if the tear is confined to below the GE junction), where an anterior gastrotomy is made followed by direct suture ligation of the bleeding vessel. If the tear extends into the distal esophagus and downward traction is ineffective in exposing the injury, a left thoracotomy may be required.

Miscellaneous. Less common causes of esophageal bleeding in the cancer patient include esophageal ulceration secondary to viral infections (cytomegalovirus, herpes), reflux esophagitis, and primary esophageal malignancies. Virus-related ulcerations are relatively common in the immunocompromised patient and should be treated with appropriate antiviral agents after obtaining the necessary cultures. Massive upper gastrointestinal hemorrhage is extremely rare in patients with these lesions.

STOMACH

Erosive Gastritis. Gastritis may arise in the cancer patient as a result of stress, central nervous system insult, or may stem from direct chemical injury to the gastric epithelium from chemotherapeutic agents or analgesics. Gastric erosions that occur in stress gastritis are acute, multiple, shallow, well-demarcated, and involve only the superficial epithelium.[28] They are predominantly found in the body and fundus of the stomach, sparing the antrum. Patients prone to erosive stress gastritis often have some form of major stress (shock, sepsis) preceding the onset of the gastric lesions. Cushing's ulcers are ulcers seen after a major central nervous system insult (*e.g.,* craniotomy) and seem to occur as a result of a marked increase in centrally mediated acid secretion.[29] These ulcerations can be seen anywhere from the distal esophagus to the third and fourth portions of the duodenum and can progress to perforation, in direct contrast to erosive stress gastritis. Probably the most frequently encountered cause of gastritis in the patient with a malignancy is due to chemical insult to the gastric epithelium from nonsteroidal anti-inflammatory drugs (NSAIDs), exogenous corticosteroids, and certain anticancer drugs.[30] These agents cause direct injury to the gastric epithelium, hydrogen ion back-diffusion, and mucosal cell death. The most effective means of controlling bleeding from gastritis is through prevention. Prophylaxis can be achieved in the high risk patient by raising the gastric pH to greater than 4 to 5 with H_2 blockers or antacids.[31,32] In the critically ill cancer patient, this often requires hourly pH measurements with antacid adjustment to achieve adequate pH values.

The diagnosis of erosive gastritis is often made when blood is seen in the nasogastric tube drainage or when the "at-risk" patient presents with painless upper gastrointestinal bleeding. The hemorrhage may be trivial or massive and the cornerstone of diagnosis is upper endoscopy where numerous, small, well-delineated punctate lesions are seen in the acid-secreting portion of the stomach. Initial management includes replacement of blood loss, correction of underlying coagulopathy, evacuation of clots with saline lavage, and gastric pH adjustment (>5.0) with antacids or antisecretory agents. Unfortunately some of these patients will continue to bleed and require more definitive treatment despite maximal medical management.

A number of other therapeutic approaches have been used. There have been reports of successful application of an endoscopic heater probe to the responsible erosions; however, the ulcerations are usually diffuse, making complete hemostasis extremely difficult.[33] Arteriography, followed by selective infusion of vasopressin or embolization has also been reported with mixed results.[34] Again, the diffuse nature of the erosions make these techniques less attractive. In the patient who continues to bleed despite maximal medical therapy, surgery becomes necessary. Some authors recommend that surgery be reserved for those patients who require more than six units of packed red blood cells in a 24-hour period to maintain a stable hematocrit.[35] However, this is not an absolute dictum and the treatment for each patient should be individualized.

Prior to surgery, an effort should be made to correct any coagulopathy that may contribute to unnecessary intraoperative bleeding. There is debate concerning the surgical procedure that should be performed in this situation.[28] Although total gastrectomy has the lowest rate of rebleeding, it is associated with an operative mortality ranging from 20% to 100%.[35,36] Subtotal gastric resection, vagotomy and hemigastrectomy or antrectomy, truncal vagotomy with a drainage procedure, and parietal cell vagotomy all have been used with less operative mortality, but rebleeding rates have been between 25% and 50%. These lesser procedures require that the remaining gastric mucosa be visualized and all bleeding sites be suture ligated. Therefore, a rational treatment strategy should be formulated for each clinical scenario. A patient with diffuse, active bleeding should probably undergo a subtotal gastrectomy, or if all bleeding sites can be incorporated into the resection, a hemigastrectomy with vagotomy. If only several discrete erosions are present and can be suture-ligated without creating a large anterior gastrotomy, a truncal vagotomy and pyloroplasty should be considered. The patient who rebleeds following one of these operations can then be salvaged with a total gastrectomy, although the overall prognosis is poor at this point.

Gastric Ulcers. Unlike erosive gastritis, gastric ulcers that penetrate the superficial layers of the epithelium into the muscularis mucosa are larger and frequently solitary. Although the cause of gastric erosions is thought to be due to diminished mucosal blood flow, gastric ulcers are believed to arise from injury to the mucosal barrier (NSAIDs, viral, bile acid reflux, alcohol, uremia) followed by back diffusion of acid and further injury.[37] Benign gastric ulcers are classified according to their location, with type I located along the lesser curvature at or below the incisura, type II ulcers consist of combined gastric and duodenal ulcers, and type III are prepyloric.[38] Type III gastric ulcers behave as duodenal ulcers in both cause and treatment, thus necessitating acid reduction in their treatment. Occasionally a benign gastric ulcer will erode into a blood vessel and cause brisk upper gastrointestinal hemorrhage that requires surgical treatment, but for the most part bleeding is slow and insidious. Upper endoscopy is the preferred method of diagnosis, allowing accurate diagnosis in greater than 90% of cases.[1,2] The medical management is similar to the management of erosive gastritis in that removing blood from the stomach through lavage and maintenance of the gastric pH greater than 5.0 is the goal. Again, endoscopy-guided coagulation of the bleeding ulcer may be attempted,[39] but patients who have a visible vessel identifiable, are in shock, or require more than 4 to 6 units of blood for resuscitation should be managed surgically.[40] The goal of surgery is to control the bleeding and remove the ulcer with as little morbidity as possible. Because gastric ulcers are most commonly found in the transition zone between acid-secreting and antral mucosa, complete antrectomy will accomplish these goal and also provide the pathologist with the ulcer-containing portion of the stomach so that malignancy can be ruled out and viral cultures can be obtained. Reconstruction can usually be accomplished with a Billroth I gastroduodenostomy. Because these ulcers are probably due to a loss of the gastric mucosal barrier, a vagotomy is usually not indicated in type I gastric ulcers. In the patient that presents in extremis or becomes unstable during surgery, a prolonged operation is not ideal. In this situation, if the patient has not been treated for ulcer disease in the past, simple excision of the bleeding ulcer and postoperative maintenance H_2 blockade is acceptable treatment.

Miscellaneous. Cancer of the stomach can also cause significant upper gastrointestinal bleeding requiring emergency surgery, but usually is responsible for slow, chronic bleeding. Upper endoscopy usually reveals a fungating, ulcerative mass and occasionally it is difficult to distinguish early carcinoma from a benign gastric ulcer. Radical subtotal gastrectomy is the procedure of choice unless extensive disease precludes clear proximal margins, at which time total gastrectomy is required. Leiomyosarcomas, leiomyoma, carcinoid, and lymphoma (gastric and metastatic) also can present with upper gastrointestinal bleeding and can be treated with a less radical gastric resection aimed at obtaining clear margins.[41]

HEMOBILIA

Bleeding arising from anywhere in the biliary system can result in hemobilia. This includes the liver parenchyma, intrahepatic and extrahepatic bile ducts, gallbladder, periampullary region, and pancreas.[42] Primary tumors of the liver rarely cause significant hemobilia and tumors of the bile duct generally cause obstruction before clinically evident bleeding can occur. Gallbladder carcinoma, angiosarcoma, hepatic adenomas, and metastatic lesions to the liver parenchyma, gallbladder, and bile ducts have all been reported to cause hemobilia.[43] The most common cause of hemobilia in the cancer patient is currently iatrogenic, owing to the drastic increase in the number of invasive radiologic procedures being performed on these patients. Specifically, percutaneous transhepatic cholangiography and percutaneous transhepatic placement of stents in patients with bile duct tumors and periampullary carcinoma is now commonly performed for both diagnostic and palliative purposes. Hemobilia follows in 4% to 9% of these patients, whereas therapeutic endoscopic maneuvers can result in some degree of hemobilia in 5% to 10% of patients.[44–46] Percutaneous liver biopsies may give rise to hemobilia directly, or through the creation of a pseudoaneurysm with subsequent rupture into the biliary system.[47–49]

Symptoms of gastrointestinal bleeding, right upper quadrant pain, and jaundice suggest the possibility of hemobilia and warrant further investigation. In the evaluation of the patient with gastrointestinal bleeding of unknown origin, endoscopy will reveal blood arising from the ampulla of Vater, confirming the diagnosis of hemobilia. Gastrointestinal bleeding immediately following percutaneous transhepatic cholangiography is virtually always owing to hemobilia and does not require endoscopic confirmation. Most often this bleeding is slow and can be managed expectantly; however, brisk hemorrhage requires immediate measures be taken.

The patient with suspected hemobilia should be promptly and aggressively resuscitated while plans for arteriography are made as this is the single most important diagnostic test in evaluation of patients in whom bleeding into the biliary tract is suspected.[42] This technique also allows access to the responsible vessel so selective embolization can be undertaken, a maneuver that is usually highly successful[50] (Figure 3-2). If embolization fails to arrest the bleeding, surgery is required as a last resort. At the time of surgery, an effort should be made to identify the underlying pathology as this will influence treatment decisions. Intrahepatic lesions (tumors) should be resected if the patient's condition permits, otherwise ligation of the offending hepatic artery is acceptable. This is generally well tolerated, despite a transient rise in the liver enzymes. If bleeding continues despite arterial ligation in patients with hemobilia due to a percutaneous hepatic procedure, partial hepatectomy (to include the offending vessel) may be required. Bleeding arising from the gallbladder should be treated by cholecystectomy. Lesions of the bile ducts should be resected and reconstructed in a standard fashion (hepaticojejunostomy), whereas hemorrhage following endoscopic sphincterotomy is best managed by a surgical transduodenal sphincteroplasty.

DUODENUM

Although duodenal ulcers are not specifically seen in the oncology patient, they can lead to significant bleeding requiring surgical consultation. A pancytopenic patient with a known or unknown preexisting duodenal ulcer may exhibit signs of gastrointestinal hemorrhage as the initial symptom. Hematemesis, hematochezia, or melena can all be seen depending on the rate and site of bleeding, necessitating further work-up. Esophagogastroduodenoscopy is the diagnostic test of choice and should be performed as soon as

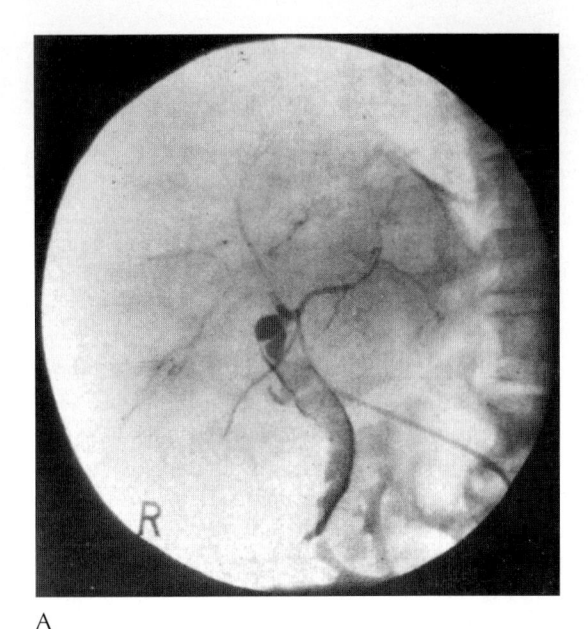

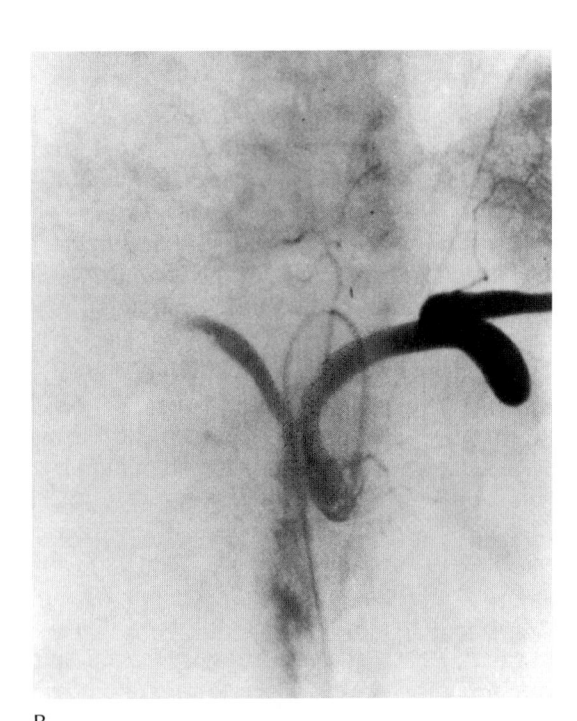

Figure 3-2. Embolization of intrahepatic aneurysm. **A**. Selective celiac injection reveals aneurysm in right hepatic artery bleeding into biliary tree. **B**. Postembolization study. From Allison DJ. Interventional radiology. In: Grainger RG, Allison DJ, eds. Diagnostic radiology: an anglo-American textbook of imaging. New York, Churchill Livingstone, 1986;2121.

possible, even during resuscitation and replacement of blood products. This should result in proper identification of the bleeding site while allowing other potential lesions to be ruled out; it frequently gives the endoscopist a vehicle by which hemostatic techniques can be applied. A heater probe applied to the ulcer is sometimes successful in cessation of the bleeding, but continued bleeding requires surgical therapy.[39] Medical management of bleeding duodenal ulcers includes administration of H_2-receptor antagonists, gastric decompression, and correction of coagulation defects.

Indications for surgery include failure of endoscopic therapy, rebleeding after successful endoscopic treatment, massive bleeding accompanied by shock, and continued bleeding requiring more than 4 to 6 units of packed red cells over a 24-hour period. The patient who undergoes surgery should have two goals accomplished at the end of the operation: the bleeding should be arrested and an acid-reducing ulcer operation should be completed. The pyloroduodenal region is opened in a longitudinal fashion, the ulcer identified and oversewn with transfixion sutures of nonabsorbable material. Because the duodenum is opened to directly oversew the ulcer, a reasonable acid-lowering procedure is truncal vagotomy with pyloroplasty, but oversewing or resection of the ulcer accompanied by an antrectomy and vagotomy is an alternative approach in the stable patient with long-standing ulcer disease or duodenal scarring.[51] Highly selective vagotomy has been advocated as another operation in the treatment of bleeding duodenal ulcers. The very unstable patient should be managed by merely oversewing the ulcer followed by postoperative H_2-blockade.

Duodenitis (as a result of chemotherapy or radiation), duodenal tumors, and periampullar carcinomas can present with slow, chronic bleeding that rarely causes symptoms and is usually discovered when the patient is being evaluated for another complaint.

SUMMARY: SPECIFIC SITES OF UPPER GASTROINTESTINAL BLEEDING

1. Esophageal bleeding can be due to a number of causes including varices, Mallory-Weiss tears, and a number of other causes. Identification of the cause by endoscopic examination is an important step. Variceal bleeding can be controlled by sclerotherapy or surgical decompression with a shunt. Radiographically placed shunts (TIPS) are also available. Mallory-Weiss tears rarely require surgical intervention but must be differentiated from transmural tears of the esophagus (Boerhaave's syndrome).
2. Gastric sources are common in upper gastrointestinal bleeding. Erosive gastritis may be caused by stress, central nervous system insult, or direct chemical injury to the gastric wall. Prevention is an important part of therapy in this condition. The often diffuse nature of the bleeding makes localized therapy less effective. Surgery may eventually be indicated. Type I gastric ulcers may require simple excision of the ulcer or an antrectomy, whereas type II and III ulcers require an acid-reducing procedure.
3. The most common cause of hemobilia is iatrogenic injury. Arteriography is the most important diagnostic test in the evaluation of this condition. Although embolization may be effective, surgery may also be needed.
4. Bleeding duodenal ulcers are not common in the cancer patient but can be a cause of significant upper gastrointestinal bleeding. They usually require an acid-reducing procedure such as vagotomy and pyloroplasty.

Lower Gastrointestinal Bleeding

Patients with active hematochezia or melena and no source of hemorrhage evident on esophogastroduodenscopy almost always have bleeding originating from a site distal to the ligament of Treitz. The rate and duration of bleeding should dictate the aggressiveness of the diagnostic work-up and the need for any resuscitation. For example, when lower gastrointestinal bleeding presents with only a positive fecal occult blood test and there is no immediate threat to the patient, the work-up can be done routinely. In contrast, the patient may present more dramatically with hypotension or circulatory collapse, necessitating prompt resuscitation accompanied by an aggressive diagnostic search to localize the source of hemorrhage. Similar to the clinical management of upper gastrointestinal bleeding, treatment of lower gastrointestinal bleeding involves three phases: resuscitation, identification of the bleeding site, and treatment. Again, these phases should overlap temporally.

RESUSCITATION

Intravenous access is obtained through two large bore catheters and lactated Ringer's solution or normal saline is infused in the rapidly bleeding patient. Response to resuscitation should be judged by the normalization of vital signs and a urinary output of 0.5 mL/kg/h. Hemodynamic monitoring may be required if there is a history of cardiac dysfunction, but this in no way should interfere with or delay the resuscitation. In addition to these measures, any underlying coagulopathy should be corrected and red blood cells infused depending on the degree of bleeding. Frequently the initial hemoglobin measurement does not reflect the true red blood cell volume as it takes time for the fluid compartments of the body to equilibrate, giving the physician a false sense of security.

IDENTIFYING THE BLEEDING SITE

The initial diagnostic maneuver to be performed in all patients with lower tract bleeding should be rigid sigmoidoscopy, which can identify distal rectal sources or evaluate for the presence of bleeding internal hemorrhoids. After this, the three most commonly employed modalities are colonoscopy, arteriography, and the tagged red blood cell scan. The specific test to be used depends on the clinical situation. Rapid *active* bleeding (>0.5 mL/min) is best localized with arteriography, which will demonstrate extravasation of radiopaque dye at the site of hemorrhage.[52] It is extremely specific, but the sensitivity is poor due to the fact that fairly rapid bleeding is required for visualization. Slow bleeding, or rapid hemorrhage that spontaneously ceases, should be evaluated with colonoscopy, which can be performed in the presence or absence of a bowel preparation because of the cathartic effect of blood.[53] Tagged red blood cell scans are more sensitive than arteriography but lack the specificity when the scan is positive, as the exact site of bleeding is often poorly identified.[54] This test may have a role in the patient who is bleeding too slowly to be visualized by arteriography, but too rapidly for colonoscopy. The tagged red cell scan may also be used to screen those patients who would benefit by arteriography. However, the clinician should be familiar with the limitations of a positive scan.

TREATMENT

Treatment strategies vary depending on the individual patient, the long-term prognosis of the underlying malignancy, and the site and severity of bleeding. For example, in a patient with widespread cancer and slow bleeding, the treatment goals should be aimed at comfort and support; this may require occasional blood transfusions but certainly not aggressive surgical therapy. On the other hand, surgery plays a major role in selected patients with advanced disease as a form of palliation and should be considered an option if bleeding is significant.

SUMMARY: INITIAL MANAGEMENT OF LOWER GASTROINTESTINAL BLEEDING

1. The aggressiveness of the work-up is dictated by the rate and duration of blood loss. As with upper gastrointestinal bleed-

ing, patients are treated with three overlapping phases: resuscitation, identification of the site of bleeding, and definitive treatment.
2. The initial diagnostic test is usually rigid sigmoidoscopy. Following this, arteriography, colonoscopy, and tagged red cell scan may be used depending on the rate of blood loss.

Specific Sites of Lower Gastrointestinal Bleeding

JEJUNUM AND ILEUM

The most common causes of hemorrhage from the small bowel include primary and metastatic neoplasms[55] (Table 3-1). Primary small bowel malignancies which may be responsible include adenocarcinoma, lymphoma, and leiomyosarcoma; whereas primary tumors of the cervix, ovaries, kidneys, stomach, and colon are most likely to manifest metastases to the small intestines. Cutaneous melanoma has a propensity to metastasize to the small bowel causing mucosal erosions and subsequent bleeding.[56] (Fig. 3-3). In some cases, the first sign of recurrent disease is a positive stool guaiac test. Adenomas and leiomyomas are the two benign neoplasms most commonly responsible, but bleeding is generally slow and chronic. Alternatively, intra-abdominal tumors may

Table 3-1. Neoplasms Potentially Responsible for Small Intestinal Hemorrhage

BENIGN NEOPLASMS
Adenoma
Angioma
Hemangioma
Telangiectasia
Fibroma, neurofibroma
Leiomyoma
Lipoma
Lymphangioma
Osteoma, osteofibroma, osteochondroma
Teratoma

MALIGNANT NEOPLASMS
Adenocarcinoma
Angiosarcoma
Malignant hemangiopericytoma
Kaposi's sarcoma
Carcinoid
Lymphoma
Leiomyosarcoma
Malignant melanoma
Neurofibrosarcoma
Plasmacytoma
Rhabdomyosarcoma

METASTATIC OR LOCALLY INVASIVE TUMORS

Duarte B, Bohrer S. Small intestinal hemorrhage and angiodysplasia. **In**: Zuidema G, Orringer MB (eds.) Shackelford's surgery of the alimentary tract. 3rd ed. Philadelphia: W.B. Saunders Co., 1991;287, with permission.

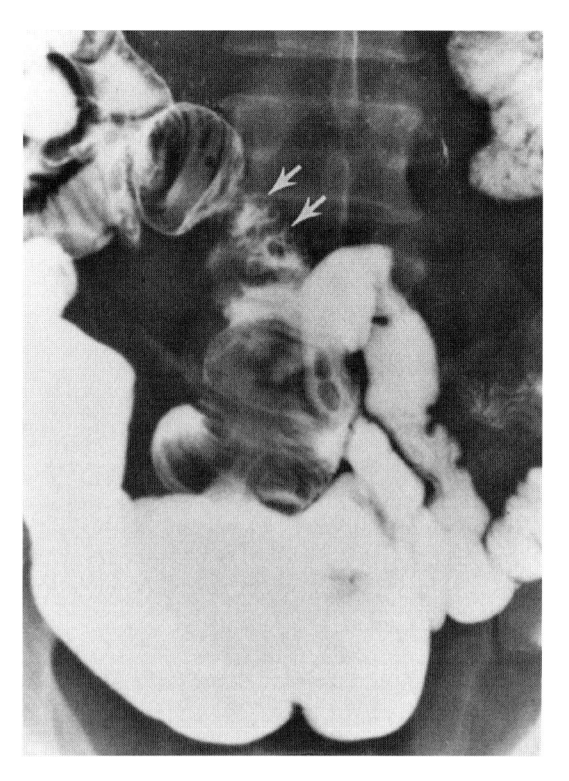

Figure 3-3. Melanoma metastatic to the small bowel in a patient who presented with abdominal distension and melena. An upper gastrointestinal series with small bowel follow-through shows an obstructing metastasis in the ileum with intussusception. From Balch CM, Houghton AN. Diagnosis of metastatic melanoma at distant sites. In: Balch CM, Houghton AN, Milton GW, et al, eds: Cutaneous melanoma. Philadelphia, JB Lippincott, 1992.

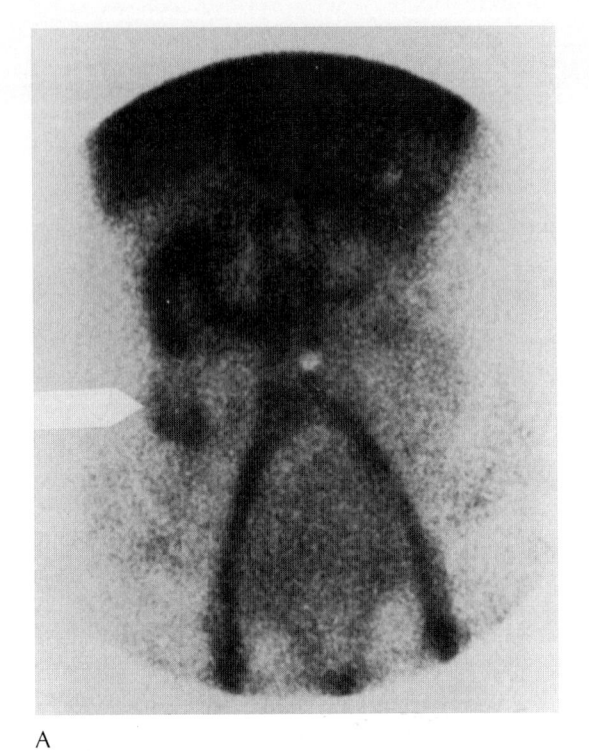

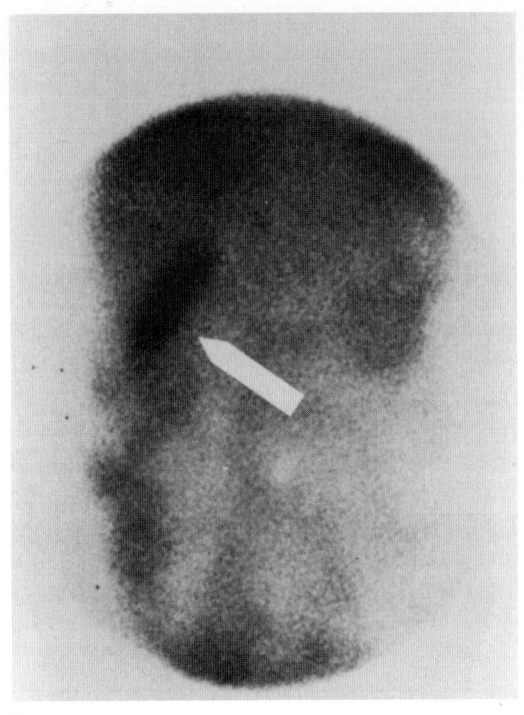

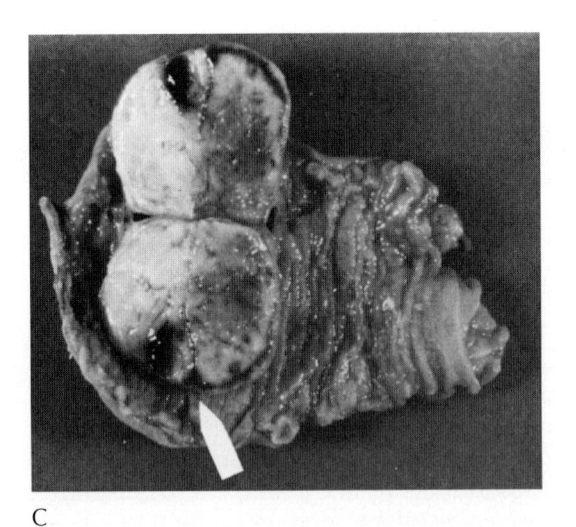

Figure 3-4. A. Delayed imaging 15 hours after injection of Tc-99m labeled red blood cells demonstrates tracer in the right colon. **B.** Repeat red blood cell scan with shortened imaging intervals demonstrated the bleeding source to be in the small bowel. **C.** Tumor hemisected to demonstrate hemorrhage from necrotic area and mucosal ulceration. From Oliver GC, Rubin RJ, Park YH, et al. Localization of small intestinal tumors. Dis Colon Rectum 1987;30:715.

erode through the wall of the small bowel causing necrosis and hemorrhage.

Gastrointestinal hemorrhage arising from the small bowel is one of the most difficult diagnostic problems encountered by the clinician as localization of the bleeding site is hampered by the inaccessibility of the small intestine to routine endoscopic examination. Furthermore, contrast radiography is difficult to perform and interpret owing to the length and redundancy of the small intestines. Endoscopy (EGD and colonoscopy) have a definite role in this patient population as it is essential in ruling out other potential sites of bleeding. Mesenteric arteriography can be helpful in localizing a bleeding site if the rate is greater than 0.5 ml/min, but this is rarely the case with small bowel lesions. Occasionally a small bowel contrast study (enteroclysis) will demonstrate a mucosal lesion; however, this study should not be performed if an arteriogram is anticipated, as the residual barium makes interpretation of the arteriogram difficult. Radionucleotide studies have also been used for localization of slower small bowel bleeding, but positive findings are difficult to interpret as the actual anatomic site of hemorrhage is not known[54,57,58] (Fig. 3-4). Small bowel endoscopy has been evaluated as a technique to address this problem but this technique is difficult to perform owing to the length and mobility of the bowel and the diameter of the fiberoptic scope.[59]

Patients who are bleeding significantly and have a negative diagnostic work-up should undergo surgical exploration. At the time of laparotomy, a thorough exploration should be carried out in an attempt to locate the bleeding small bowel segment. In the cancer patient the lesions should be readily identifiable; however, intraoperative endoscopy is occasionally necessary to help locate small mucosal lesions that are not palpable.[60–62] Segmental small bowel resection with primary anastomosis is the preferred method of treatment for small bowel neoplasms. If the lesion is believed to be a primary malignancy, then the small bowel mesentery should be incorporated into the resection to encompass the draining lymphatics. Metastatic lesions are best treated by a simple sleeve resection.

COLON AND RECTUM

Bleeding arising from the colon or rectum in the general population is most commonly due to diverticular disease and angiodysplasia. In the cancer patient, it can originate from primary colonic neoplasms, metastases to the colon from extracolonic malignancies, local invasion from another intra-abdominal neoplastic process, or from mucosal injury to the large bowel secondary to treatment of an underlying malignant process (i.e., radiation therapy, chemotherapy).

Primary colonic neoplasms (benign and malignant) can present with rectal bleeding; however, it is generally not as massive as that usually seen with diverticular bleeding and angiodysplasia. Hemorrhage from right-sided lesions is usually slow and chronic, often only detected when the patient is found to be anemic or by a fecal occult blood test. Left-sided or rectal colonic polyps and carcinomas more frequently present with visible rectal bleeding, but again, are rarely life-threatening. Occasionally the clinician will be faced with the patient with a bleeding, fungating rectal carcinoma that is unresectable due to local infiltration. Radiation therapy or operative fulguration to control bleeding are viable options for this difficult problem. Unfortunately neither of these palliative treatment modalities are extremely successful in this patient population.

Extracolonic malignancies also can cause lower gastrointestinal bleeding through metastatic spread to the bowel or by direct extension and invasion through the wall of the colon. Intra-abdominal sources include gastric, pancreatic, gallbladder, ovarian, cervical, bladder, renal cell, and prostate carcinomas. This pattern of disease also can be seen with extra-abdominal malignancies such as lymphoma, lung, and breast cancer. The hemorrhage seen in these patients can range from mild to severe and warrants prompt evaluation.

Radiation injuries of the large bowel can cause rectal bleeding in addition to the more common symptoms of nausea, vomiting, cramps, tenesmus, diarrhea, and mucous discharge. (Radiation injury to the bowel is discussed further in Chapter 7.) This injury is most common in the rectum due to its fixed position and its proximity to the primary cancer being radiated (cervix, prostate).

The diagnosis can be confirmed with flexible sigmoidoscopy where the mucosa appears erythematous and ulcerated due to fragile mucosal vascular lesions (telangiectasias) that may accompany other complications of radiation therapy or occur alone. Usually the symptoms of acute radiation proctitis subside shortly after completion of radiation therapy and require no therapy for the small amount of bleeding that may be present. Not infrequently, marked continuous bleeding may require medical treatment of the proctitis (stool bulking agents, softeners, antidiarrheal agents, antispasmodics, and steroid enemas) with periodic blood transfusion. Continued bleeding despite these measures requires more aggressive treatment.

Endoscopic laser photocoagulation has been used in these patients in several centers with reported success.[63,64] If bleeding continues and is severe, then surgical resection of the affected rectum is the last option, as a simple diverting colostomy is often unsuccessful in controlling significant hemorrhage. A primary anastomosis should be avoided in this setting and reconstitution of the gastrointestinal tract can be undertaken after radiation therapy is completed. Less severe bleeding can be managed with a simple diverting colostomy should medical management fail.

Less common causes of rectal bleeding in the patient with cancer include chemotherapy-induced colitis and pseudomembranous colitis secondary to antibiotics. Both syndromes are accompanied by diarrhea and in some cases, bloody diarrhea occurs. Colitis secondary to chemotherapy is most evident at the time of the white blood cell nadir when the mucosal damage to the bowel is associated with local inflammation. Bleeding is usually minor and ceases following mucosal cell recovery. Pseudomembranous colitis, secondary to intestinal overgrowth of *Clostridium difficile*, an anaerobic bacterium that produces a toxin causing colitis and secondary diarrhea, is often accompanied by systemic symptoms. Submucosal hemorrhage can also complicate this disease, leading to bloody diarrhea. Administration of nearly any antibiotic can be responsible for *C. difficile* colitis, and the diagnosis is made with sigmoidoscopy, which will reveal a pseudomembrane on affected areas of the colon. Stool can also be collected and tested for the *C. difficile* toxin, which can confirm the diagnosis. These patients should receive adequate intravenous hydration to compensate for gastrointestinal losses and any antibiotics should be discontinued. Metronidazole or vancomycin is given by mouth to eradicate the offending bacterium.

SUMMARY: SPECIFIC SITES OF LOWER GASTROINTESTINAL BLEEDING

1. Most jejunal or ileal bleeding is due to primary or secondary neoplasms. Localization of the bleeding site can be quite a challenge. Endoscopy helps to rule out other sites of bleeding. Surgical exploration is needed in patients with significant bleeding and a negative diagnostic evaluation. Intraoperative enteroscopy may be helpful.
2. Colonic and rectal bleeding are usually due to diverticular disease or angiodysplasia, but in the cancer patient it obviously can originate from effects of a primary or metastatic neoplasm. Direct extension of extracolonic neoplasms may also cause significant bleeding.
3. Radiation injury may also lead to significant bleeding from the lower intestine. Other causes include chemotherapy-induced colitis and pseudomembranous colitis, usually secondary to antibiotic use with subsequent *C. difficile* overgrowth.

GASTROINTESTINAL PERFORATION

Perforation of the gastrointestinal tract is one of the most devastating events encountered by the clinician involved in the care of cancer patients. This catastrophic event carries a high morbidity and mortality rate in the general population; in the oncology patient this multiplies owing to poor health from underlying disease processes and the immunosuppressive effects of both the malignancy and its treatment. Moreover, delays in presentation and diagnosis worsen the prognosis owing to continued contamination and the septic sequela of this insult.

Esophagus

Esophageal perforation carries the highest morbidity and mortality of all gastrointestinal perforations while also being the most difficult both to diagnose and to manage.[65] Early diagnosis and the prompt initiation of treatment are essential ingredients for a favorable outcome; however, timely intervention does not guarantee successful treatment of this morbid complication. Immediate surgical management is the mainstay of treatment, with the specific goal of preventing further contamination of the mediastinum with bacteria, corrosive fluids, and food. Left untreated, this contamination almost invariably leads to overwhelming sepsis with cardiopulmonary collapse and death.

ETIOLOGY

Perforations can be classified by etiology as iatrogenic, traumatic, spontaneous; and those due to foreign bodies, caustic injuries, and neoplasm (Table 3-2). The incidence of esophageal perforation has increased over the last several decades; a rise that has been thought to be due to the increased use of upper endoscopy and its many applications. Although spontaneous rupture of esophageal tumors accounts for only a small percentage of all perforations, it is important to note that these tumors can perforate as a complication of various endoscopic procedures. Therefore, it is not uncommon to be faced with a patient who has an esophageal perforation and a coexisting carcinoma.

DIAGNOSIS

Pain, fever, and dyspnea are the most common symptoms of esophageal perforation.

Table 3-2. Etiology of Esophageal Perforation in 115 Patients

Cause	Patients (N)
IATROGENIC	65
Endoscopy	29
Dilatation	14
Surgery	13
Sengstaken-Blakemore tube	3
Souttar tube	1
Sclerotherapy	1
Intubation	1
Temperature probe	1
Cantor tube	1
Feeding tube	1
TRAUMATIC	28
SPONTANEOUS	22

Adapted and modified from Nesbitt JC, Sawyers JL. Surgical management of esophageal perforation. Am Surg 1987;53:183.

Cervical or high retrosternal pain is more typical of cervicothoracic perforations, whereas mid- or distal tears produce anterior thoracic, posterior, intrascapular, or epigastric pain.[65] Additionally, cervical perforations can present with subcutaneous emphysema; however, this is rare with intrathoracic and intraabdominal rupture. Pain or fever after esophageal instrumentation are hallmark signs of perforation and when present indicate the need for an emergency contrast esophagogram. Often the diagnosis is not straightforward and requires a high clinical index of suspicion and liberal use of contrast radiographs. This is particularly true with spontaneous perforations, or Boerhaave's syndrome, which is characteristically preceded by episodic vomiting, resulting in a transmural tear in the distal esophagus. If the tear is in the intra-abdominal esophagus, patients usually present with symptoms of acute peritoneal irritation, suggesting the diagnosis. Spontaneous intrathoracic perforations typically present with more subtle signs of pain and fever and can be more difficult to diagnose accurately in a timely fashion.

A chest roentgenogram can be useful in patients suspected of having a perforation;

air in the soft tissues of the neck or mediastinum or a hydropneumothorax adds further support to the diagnosis. Right-sided pleural effusions are more common with tears of the upper or midthoracic esophagus, whereas left pleural effusions are seen with perforations of the distal third.[66] A negative chest roentgenogram does not rule out a perforation and if a high index of suspicion is present, a contrast study using a water-soluble agent should be performed. If this is negative, a study using dilute barium should follow, as this will provide better mucosal detail, enabling a higher degree of sensitivity.

MANAGEMENT

Management of the patient with a perforated esophagus consists of immediate intravenous fluid resuscitation, the institution of broad-spectrum antibiotics, and prompt surgical intervention. The negative intrathoracic pressure allows saliva, food, and gastric contents to pass into the mediastinum resulting in a marked inflammatory response and secondary third-spacing of intravascular volume.[67] Intravenous hydration is essential in restoring this volume deficit and central access may be required to monitor central venous pressure or pulmonary artery pressures, depending on the clinical scenario. Intravenous antibiotics are given that cover oral and gastric flora (*i.e.*, a first generation cephalosporin and an aminoglycoside). At this point a decision should be made regarding optimum definitive treatment. This is a very controversial area in surgery and recommendations range from nonoperative therapy[68–70] to early aggressive surgery.[65,71–73] Esophageal perforations vary in cause and behavior, similar to the patient population, who may respond to the insult in a variety of fashions.

Selective nonoperative management of esophageal perforations has been advocated by some provided strict criteria are met.[68–70] If the leak is contained within the mediastinum, there is free drainage back into the esophagus, there are minimal symptoms, and there are minimal or no signs of systemic sepsis, the patient may be considered for conservative treatment. The patient is given nothing by mouth, broad spectrum intravenous antibiotics are given, and the patient is observed. Preexisting mediastinal fibrosis from the initial disease process may help in containing the leak. A deteriorating clinical course in a patient being treated conservatively requires a more aggressive treatment strategy. Few patients meet these strict criteria, subsequently very few with esophageal perforations are managed nonoperatively.

Once a decision has been made to operate, there should be no delay since morbidity and mortality rise as the interval between perforation and treatment increases.[26,70,74–78] The operative management of perforations depends on the location of the lesion (cervical, thoracic, or abdominal) and the time that has elapsed since the perforation occurred.

Operative Management of Cervical Esophageal Perforations. Perforations of the cervical esophagus are predominantly treated by primary suture repair.[65] This portion of the esophagus is best approached through a left lateral cervical incision, followed by lateral retraction of the sternocleidomastoid muscle and carotid sheath. Following identification of the leak and debridement of nonviable tissue, the esophagus can be closed in either one or two layers, followed by drainage of the retropharyngeal space and upper mediastinum. If the perforation cannot be identified after a thorough exploration, the neck should be drained in a similar fashion and antibiotics continued postoperatively. All patients should have a water-soluble contrast study (followed by barium) prior to the initiation of oral feedings (5 to 7 days).

Figure 3-5. The Grillo flap can be used as a technique of repair for extensive or late perforations. **A,** The pleural mediastinum is opened to expose the esophagus and perforation. **B** and **C,** A generous flap of pleura is raised. **D** and **E,** This flap is then wrapped around the perforation and sutured in place. From Grillo HG, Wilkins EW. Esophageal repair following late diagnosis of intrathoracic perforation. Ann Thorac Surg 1975;20:387.

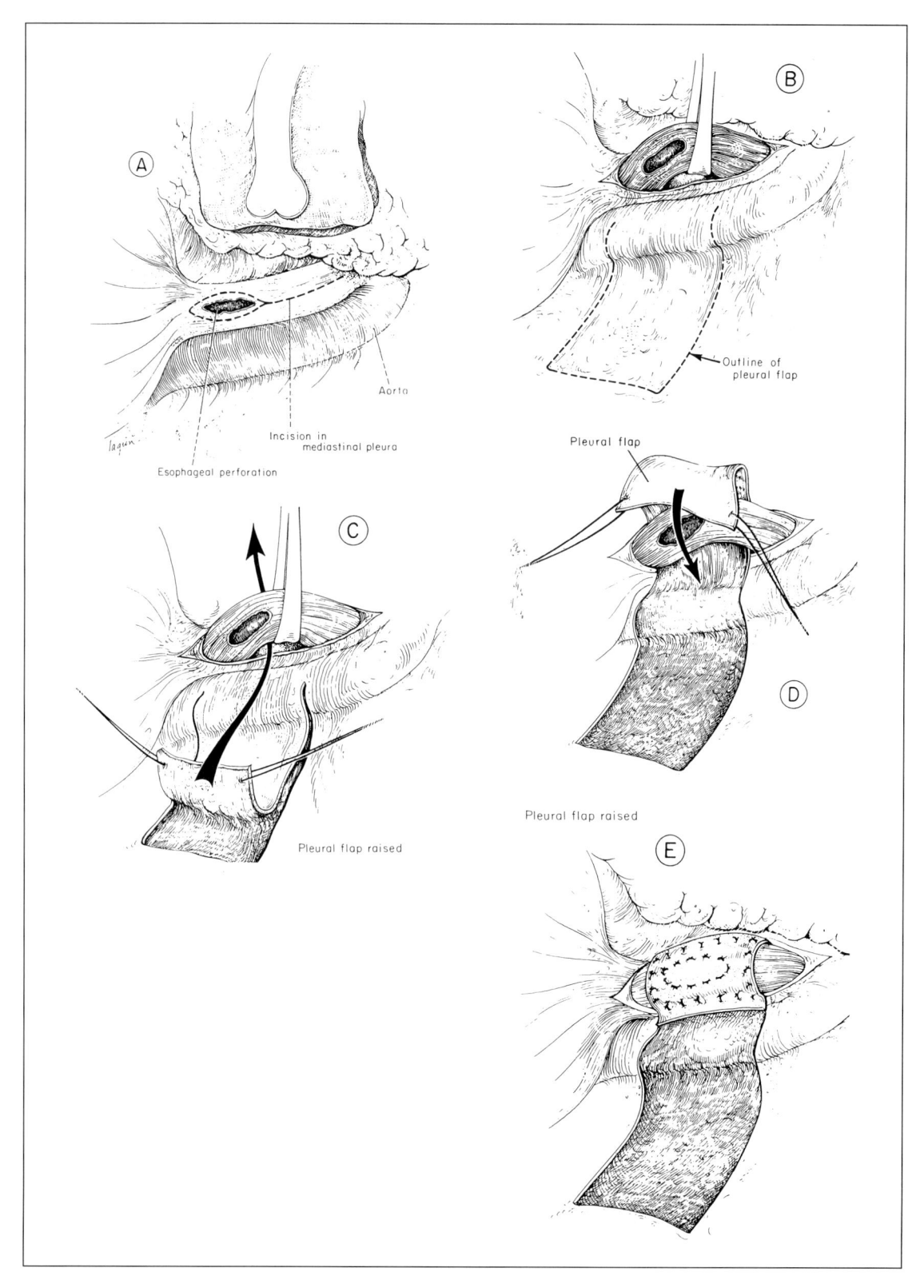

Gastrointestinal Bleeding and Perforation in the Cancer Patient　　　　77

Figure 3-5

Operative Management of Thoracic Esophageal Perforations. Perforations of the lower cervical and upper thoracic esophagus (above the level of the carina) are approached through the neck, whereas optimal exposure of the mid and lower esophagus requires a thoracotomy. Distal esophageal perforations are best managed through a left posterior-lateral thoracotomy, whereas a right posterior-lateral thoracotomy is required to gain exposure to the midesophagus. The decision concerning the type of operation to be performed depends on several factors; these include the amount of time from the actual time of the injury, the underlying disease process, and the patient's general condition.

With early recognition and treatment (less than 24 hours) of the perforation, direct suture closure and mediastinal drainage generally provides satisfactory results.[65] When recognition of a perforation has been delayed, the presence of a massive inflammatory response in the esophagus and surrounding tissues makes simple suture closure extremely difficult and fraught with complications. It is in this patient population that sound judgement and decision-making are essential. Grillo et al[79] have popularized the concept of using a vascularized pedicle of pleura (pleural flap) to cover the perforation even if it can be closed primarily, in essence allowing the pleura to "seal" the injury (Fig. 3-5). Other pedicles that can be used include an intercostal muscle flap,[80,81] omentum, pericardium,[82,83] or diaphragm.[84–86] This technique requires that the entire mediastinal pleura be opened to ensure adequate drainage and that large chest tubes be left to control an esophageal leak should disruption of the repair occur. Oral feedings are not initiated until a water-soluble contrast study (followed by thin barium) confirms integrity of the repair. The insertion of a gastrostomy tube and feeding jejunostomy tube should also be performed at the time of surgery.

If repair of an injury is delayed to the point where the inflammatory changes do not allow a secure closure, the repair can be protected by esophageal exclusion.[87–89] Total

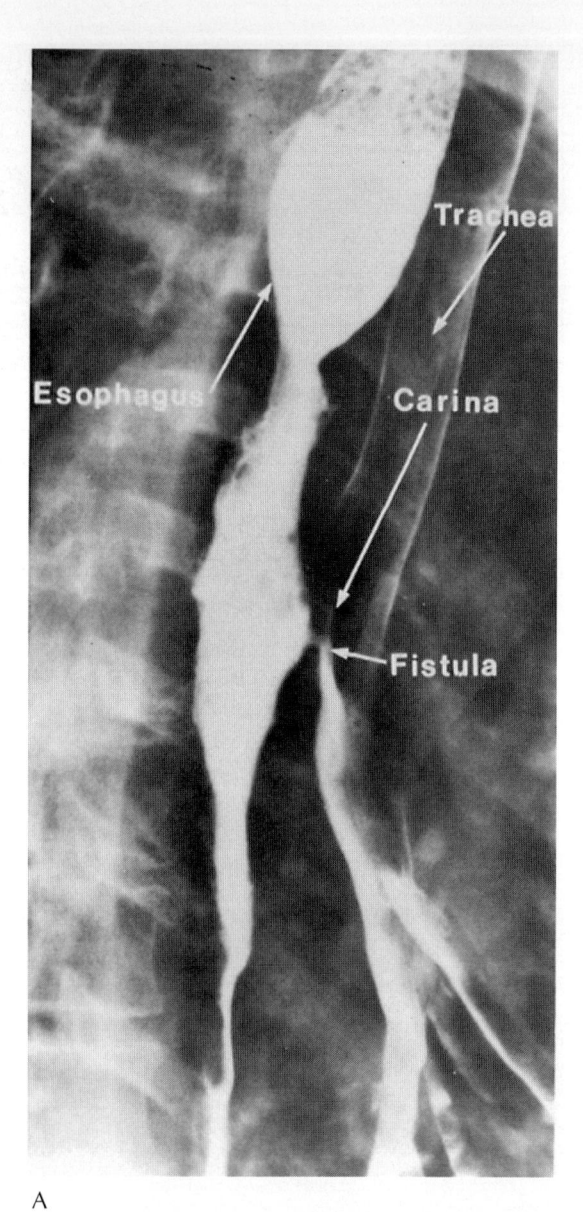

A

Figure 3-6. Representative barium contrast study of a patient with a respiratory tract fistula secondary to a squamous cell carcinoma of the esophagus treated with radiation therapy. **A.** Fistula is present between the esophagus and right main-stem bronchus. **B.** Representation of a substernal bypass. From Little AG, Ferguson MK, DeMeester TR. Esophageal carcinoma with respiratory tract fistula. Cancer 1984;53:1322.

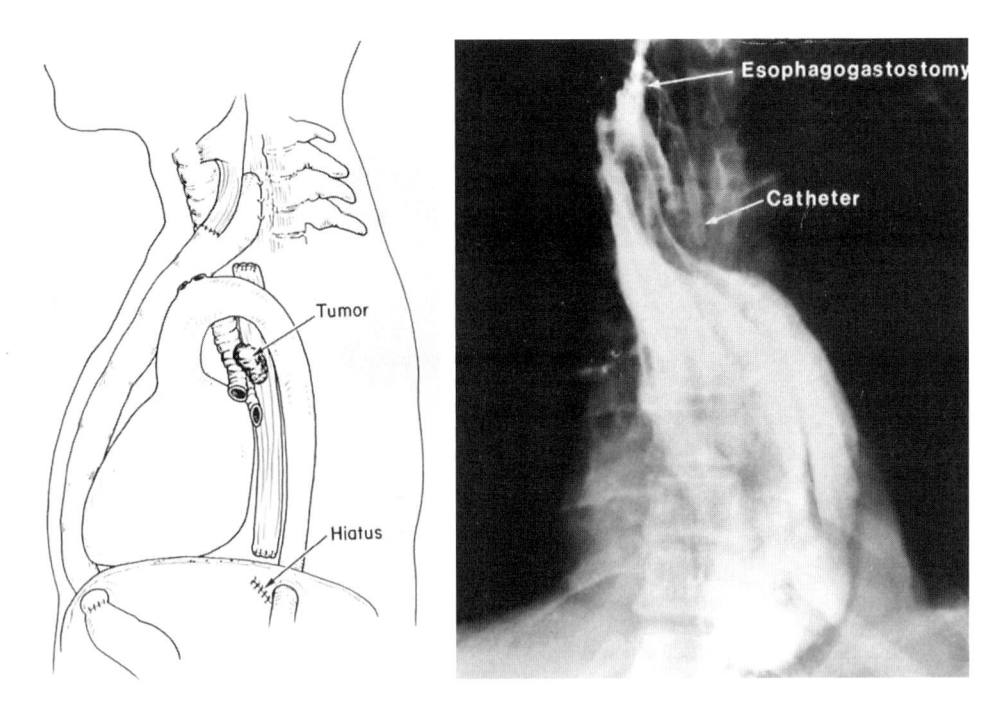

Figure 3-6. (*continued*)

exclusion entails a cervical esophagostomy and oversewing of the gastroesophageal junction, which will divert any saliva or gastric contents from the repair, allowing better healing. This diversion can be reversed once the esophagus is healed. If surgery is undertaken more than 48 hours after the perforation, the likelihood of successful primary closure is minimal and total esophageal exclusion with mediastinal drainage should be considered.

Esophageal perforations that occur proximal to a malignancy or stricture require a different treatment strategy, as simple repair almost invariably will break down owing to the distal obstruction. Aggressive diagnostic and therapeutic endoscopy, as well as dilatation, can be complicated by perforation in this patient population. Because this complication is generally recognized early and contamination minimal, resection of the malignancy can be undertaken, either with immediate or delayed reconstruction, depending on the patient's condition and the amount of inflammation present. Options for a conduit include stomach, colon, and less desirably, a jejunal free flap. Immediate reconstruction should be reserved for the stable patient with an early, contained perforation, as this adds significantly to the time and morbidity of the procedure. A benign stricture (*i.e.*, secondary to gastroesophageal reflux) also may need to be resected, but in the case where it can be successfully dilated intraoperatively, primary esophageal repair is a reasonable option.

Operative Management of Abdominal Esophageal Perforations. Perforation of the intra-abdominal segment of the esophagus is less common, occurring most frequently secondary to iatrogenic injuries caused during surgery, but also occurring spontaneously. Direct closure at the time of recognition is effective for these iatrogenic injuries. Spontaneous rupture can be treated by primary closure of the defect; if the closure appears tenuous, the fundus can be used as a serosal patch (fundic wrap), as in a Nissen procedure.[90,91]

Management of Tracheoesophageal Fistula. A fistula between the esophagus and the respiratory tract, referred to as a *tracheoesophageal fistula*, can occur in the patient with advanced esophageal carcinoma. The malignant process can erode through the wall of the esophagus and into the trachea or bronchus resulting in significant respiratory complications such as aspiration pneumonia. The site of the fistula in the airway is usually in one of the divisions of the left bronchus, but may be in the trachea in 50% of patients.[92,93] Commonly these patients present with episodic coughing and choking while eating or drinking. This complication can develop spontaneously in the course of the disease, or more commonly as a complication of radiotherapy when it is used to treat the primary tumor. The diagnosis is best made with a barium swallow; bronchoscopy often fails to visualize the fistulous tract (Fig. 3-6). The presence of locally advanced or metastatic disease precludes a curative procedure in this patient population, so providing palliation is the main intent of the clinician.[92] Because failure to provide palliative treatment results in a mean survival of only 4 to 6 weeks, efforts should be made to approach this complication aggressively in selected patients.[94] Those patients with poor pulmonary reserve or in poor health will not tolerate general anesthesia, hence effective nonoperative means of palliation should be employed in this circumstance. Esophageal intubation with an indwelling prosthetic tube is a reasonable alternative to surgery in this group and can provide effective palliation in most patients, allowing them to eat semisolid food and avoid the respiratory problems associated with this fistula.[95] The main problem with these tubes is erosion and bleeding, often requiring tube replacement and manipulation. Continued respiratory difficulties can also occur owing to reflux around the tube and aspiration.

Those patients who are able to tolerate general anesthesia can be more effectively palliated through one of two surgical techniques, namely esophageal bypass[96,97] and esophageal exclusion.[92] Esophageal bypass procedures involve using a conduit, usually placed extra-anatomically, to bypass the diseased esophagus. Stomach, colon, or a prosthetic tube can be placed retrosternally and anastomosed end to end to the cervical esophagus, in essence excluding the esophagus and allowing palliation of dysphasia, leading to a median survival of more than 20 weeks.[96-99] Another option is esophageal exclusion, which can be useful when no organ is available for use as a conduit. This technique uses an end cervical esophagostomy, esophageal decompressing tube (for the isolated thoracic esophagus), and division of the gastroesophageal junction. A feeding tube is also placed to provide nutrition. This less desirable form of operative palliation carries a moderate risk of morbidity and mortality and provides the same median survival time as bypass.

SUMMARY: ESOPHAGEAL PERFORATION

1. Diagnosis and management of this potentially life-threatening complication remain difficult at best. Overall, survival depends partly on the rapidity with which the diagnosis is established.
2. Patients present with chest pain, fever, and dyspnea. Contrast radiography is often useful in establishing the diagnosis.
3. Management includes resuscitation, antibiotics, and prompt surgical intervention. Surgical repair is sometimes accompanied by use of a pleural flap. In cases where repair is not deemed appropriate, esophageal exclusion is performed with a cervical esophagostomy and oversewing of the gastroesophageal junction with gastrostomy tube placement.
4. Tracheoesophageal fistulae occur with advanced carcinoma of the esophagus, and can be treated surgically with esophageal bypass or exclusion. This condition is associated with significant morbidity and usually limited survival.

Stomach and Duodenum

ETIOLOGY

Gastric perforation in the cancer patient can be caused by many factors including benign gastric ulcers, primary tumors of the stomach, a complication of the treatment of gastric malignancy, and iatrogenic insults.

Cancer patients receiving treatment for their malignancy are often undergoing therapeutic regimens, which increase their susceptibility to ulceration of the stomach. Systemic high-dose steroids and nonsteroidal anti-inflammatory drugs are two such agents that can lead to gastric ulcers which heal poorly in the immunocompromised host.[30] Despite the use of H_2-blockers, transmural perforation is not uncommon and can result in high morbidity and increased mortality in this patient population.

Unrecognized primary gastric adenocarcinomas, lymphomas, and sarcomas occasionally present with acute perforation, often surprising the unsuspecting clinician. Not infrequently the diagnosis is made during surgery at which time it is often difficult to discern tumor from surrounding inflammatory tissue. The long-term prognosis of patients who present in this manner is poor since these tumors are usually locally advanced, and patients often harbor unrecognized metastatic disease. The difficulty in obtaining negative margins and the theoretical peritoneal seeding of tumor cells make this situation particularly bothersome, especially for adenocarcinomas and sarcomas.

Increasingly, gastric lymphomas are being treated with primary chemotherapy and or radiation therapy instead of surgery.[100] One of the more worrisome complications of this modality is that the treatment will result in gastric perforation, especially in locally advanced disease, as the tumor responds to chemotherapy. This situation is much less common in adenocarcinoma of the stomach, as this histologic subtype is primarily treated surgically, responding suboptimally to chemotherapy, even when used in the primary or neoadjuvant setting.

Other causes of gastric perforation in the patient with cancer are iatrogenic. Diagnostic and therapeutic endoscopic mishaps as well as complications of percutaneous endoscopic gastrostomy placement can result in perforation and require surgical consultation.

Duodenal perforation is most commonly associated with peptic ulcer disease, although infrequently a malignant process, such as periampullary carcinoma or lymphoma, may be responsible.

DIAGNOSIS

When entertaining the diagnosis of gastric or duodenal perforation, a succinct history and physical examination are crucial. A history of chronic upper abdominal pain, early satiety, and weight loss point to a diagnosis of gastric cancer; whereas the patient with a benign gastric ulcer typically has a history of prolonged epigastric discomfort, often made worse with the ingestion of food. A patient with duodenal ulcer disease often also has a history of prolonged, episodic epigastric discomfort relieved by food intake. Physical examination will reveal an acute abdomen with guarding and muscular rigidity, localized to the epigastrium. An upright chest radiograph will reveal pneumoperitoneum in a large percentage of these patients. If the diagnosis of perforation remains uncertain at this point, air can be injected into the nasogastric tube and the chest radiograph repeated. If this maneuver fails to demonstrate free air, an upper gastrointestinal contrast study (with a water-soluble agent) can be helpful in the patient with an equivocal physical examination. A posterior perforation may not present with free air under the diaphragm, but air in the lesser sac can often be seen on an upright abdominal radiograph.

MANAGEMENT

The management of the patient with a perforated upper gastrointestinal tract viscus is usually surgical. Vigorous fluid resuscitation should be undertaken to correct underlying hypovolemia (and often shock), which is frequently present due to both third-space losses in the peritoneal cavity and as a response to sepsis. Placement of central lines may be necessary to obtain hemodynamic parameters and measure central pressures; however, these maneuvers should not delay surgical intervention. Broad-spectrum antibiotics should be instituted immediately and should provide coverage for gastric and upper intestinal flora. There may be a place for the nonoperative management of perforated duodenal ulcers if strict criteria are met. In particular, the continued leak of gastric contents must be shown to have stopped by a contrast radiograph demonstrating sealing at the site of perforation.

Benign Gastric Ulcer. The surgical treatment of a perforated benign gastric ulcer depends on several factors including the age and general health of the patient, the amount of preoperative shock, the length of time from perforation, and the degree of inflammation and contamination present. Optimal treatment includes resection of the perforated ulcer with antrectomy or hemigastrectomy. This not only removes the source of the perforation, but allows the pathologist to examine the resected ulcer for carcinoma, which may be present in a significant number of cases.[38] Reconstruction can be performed with a Billroth I or II reconstruction depending on the amount of stomach that is resected and if duodenal scarring is present. An extended antrectomy or hemigastrectomy requires a gastrojejunostomy, whereas an antrectomy can be satisfactorily reconstructed using a gastroduodenostomy. A vagotomy should be included if there is an associated duodenal ulcer (type II) or the patient requires ulcerogenic drugs.

Both simple excision of the perforated ulcer with primary closure and omental patching of the perforation (without resection) have been advocated as primary treatment in patients with the forementioned risk factors that might increase the morbidity and mortality of a longer operation, such as gastrectomy. These procedures may abbreviate the length of the operation, but are less definitive and often do not allow the diagnosis of a malignant ulcer to be ruled out. Moreover, up to 20% of patients treated in this manner require eventual reoperation.[101]

Gastric Neoplasm. Most commonly, the perforated gastric neoplasm is not recognized as a neoplasm until the time of surgery when inflammation due to contamination make operating conditions particularly undesirable. The goal of surgery is resection of the tumor with gastrectomy. Frozen section may be helpful in determining the cell type, but more often than not a firm diagnosis cannot be made until permanent sections are available. Furthermore, because these operations are done in an emergency setting, a pathologist is not always available for assistance. If adenocarcinoma is suspected, then subtotal or total gastrectomy should be undertaken along with omental resection, splenectomy, and regional lymphadenectomy. Posterior perforations may require partial pancreatectomy if the tumor is contiguous with this structure, whereas partial hepatectomy is sometimes needed for those malignancies that invade the liver.

A less common neoplasm that occasionally presents with perforation is a soft tissue tumor of the stomach. Gastric sarcomas will require a hemigastrectomy with the aim of obtaining a margin of several centimeters, and because they infrequently metastasize to regional lymph nodes, an extended lymph node dissection is not indicated. Benign sarcomas are generally smaller and infrequently perforate, but are difficult to discern intraoperatively, thus they should be treated similarly.

The presenting symptoms of gastric lymphoma are mainly epigastric pain and gastrointestinal bleeding. Perforation is extremely uncommon as an initial clinical presentation, seen in only 1 of 33 patients in a recent review.[100] More commonly perforation is seen in the patient receiving chemotherapy and radiation as primary treatment for this disease, and is reported to be 3% to 13%.[100] When surgery is undertaken for perforation, the tumor should be resected to obtain histologically negative margins, although the prognostic significance of positive surgical margins is controversial.[100] Usually subtotal or total gastrectomy is required and the gastrointestinal continuity is restored with a Roux-en-Y limb of jejunum or a gastrojejunostomy.

Iatrogenic Injuries. Perforations caused by endoscopy should be immediately operated on at which time the perforation should be debrided and closed primarily. Occasionally, following the placement of a percutaneous endoscopic gastrostomy (PEG) tube, the stomach will fall away from the abdominal wall resulting in a free perforation into the peritoneal cavity. This complication can be addressed through a small laparotomy in which the abdomen is irrigated and the PEG converted to a conventional Stamm gastrostomy. A laparoscopic approach could also be used in this situation, accomplishing the same goals.

Duodenal Ulcer. Perforation of a duodenal ulcer is an indication for surgery for nearly all patients presenting in this fashion. The two surgical options recommended are simple closure versus definitive ulcer treatment. The decision regarding which procedure should be performed depends on the presence or absence of three factors: serious underlying medical illnesses, ongoing shock, and perforations present for more than 24 hours based on a careful history. Simple closure should be performed when two or more factors are present. If one factor only is present, then a definitive procedure may be performed. The duration of ulcer symptoms is also to be considered. In patients with a short history (<3 months), simple closure with intensive postoperative medical therapy is adequate therapy. Those patients with a history of ulcer symptoms less than 3 months have a lower incidence of recurrence than those with a longer history.

A simple closure consists of primary closure of the perforated ulcer with an omental patch (Graham patch).[102] Intensive postoperative acid-reducing measures (H_2-blockers) are given to promote ulcer healing. In the patient who arrives to the operating room in stable condition, with a fresh (<24 hours) perforation and no serious underlying medical conditions, consideration should be given to performing a definitive ulcer operation. This is especially true if the patient has a long ulcer history or is currently taking H_2-blockers, suggesting that this ulcer is less likely to heal if treated medically; in addition, this group of patients is at a high risk of ulcer recurrence, even if the current ulcer heals. The most common operation performed in this situation is truncal vagotomy and pyloroplasty. The perforation can be incorporated into the pyloroplasty and closed in a Heineke-Mikulicz fashion. Another option that can be considered is parietal cell vagotomy with omental patching of the perforation, which has the advantage of lowering acid secretion with little effect on gastric motility. This operation is best performed on the very stable patient, as it adds time to the operation, but in the proper hands appears to be as effective as vagotomy and pyloroplasty.

There have been scattered reports in the literature of "selective" nonoperative treatment of perforated duodenal ulcers, a technique that can actually be performed in very rare clinical circumstances.[103] Patients who are poor operative risks (due to concurrent illnesses) and have radiographically documented sealed perforations, occasionally will be considered for this type of treatment. Broad-spectrum antibiotics, intravenous hydration, nasogastric decompression, and H_2-blockers are instituted promptly and the patient observed, preferably in an intensive care setting. If there are any signs of clinical deterioration during this period of close observation, surgery should be undertaken.

SUMMARY: GASTRIC AND DUODENAL PERFORATION

1. Gastric perforation can be due to benign ulcers, primary gastric tumors, therapy of gastric tumors, or iatrogenic causes. Un-

recognized tumors can be identified only at the time of surgery in some cases.
2. Diagnosis is often established by the appearance of free air on an upright chest radiograph. Patients are often able to precisely state the time of onset of symptoms as it is often sudden. Contrast studies are sometimes needed.
3. Benign gastric ulcers are usually excised, which may necessitate an antrectomy. Gastric neoplasms require resection of the lesion and regional lymph nodes. Perforation of gastric lymphomas may be associated with therapy. Iatrogenic injuries usually are noted at the time of injury and are treated with immediate surgical intervention.
4. The treatment of perforated duodenal ulcers is either simple repair or a definitive ulcer operation. The choice of procedure depends on the presence of concurrent medical illnesses, preoperative shock, and perforations present for more than 24 hours. The presence of two or more of these usually dictates performance of a simple closure only, whereas the presence of one factor alone may permit the safe conduct of a definitive procedure. A short history of ulcer symptoms suggests that simple closure is adequate therapy. Nonoperative therapy is reserved for few patients.

Perforation of the Small Intestine

ETIOLOGY

Perforation of the small intestine can stem from a multitude of causes but will result in free communication with the peritoneal cavity, skin (enterocutaneous fistulae), or with other intra-abdominal or pelvic organs. If a fistula does not form, and the patient receives no treatment, the free perforation usually will be walled off by another intraperitoneal structure resulting in an abscess cavity, should the patient survive the initial septic insult.

Intestinal wall perforation may be due to a variety of causes, including operative trauma, tumor, obstruction, inflammation, and radiation. During any abdominal or pelvic surgical procedure the small bowel is at risk for iatrogenic injury; this risk is further increased during reoperative surgery. Small bowel perforation also can be seen after an intestinal operation, when the anastomosis is at risk for postoperative breakdown.

Approximately 10% of patients with malignant small bowel tumors present with an acute abdomen resulting from bowel perforation and peritonitis.[104] Carcinoma of the lung, cervix, esophagus, and ovary, and melanoma all can be responsible for small bowel metastases and patients with these neoplasms occasionally present with small bowel perforation, although gastrointestinal bleeding and obstruction are more common symptoms.

Small bowel obstruction, if untreated, can lead to serious consequences including intestinal strangulation, with full thickness necrosis and perforation. The cause of small intestinal obstruction in the patient with cancer includes adhesions, hernia, intussusception, and tumor (primary or metastatic). Of particular danger are closed-loop obstructions, which by definition do not allow the small bowel to be decompressed proximally, resulting in increased intraluminal pressure, decreased venous return of the bowel wall, ischemia, and necrosis with perforation. This form of obstruction is seen in 10% to 49% of patients with small bowel obstruction and demands immediate surgical intervention.[105]

Inflammatory lesions of the gastrointestinal tract can lead to small bowel perforation, particularly if they involve the full thickness of the bowel wall. Free perforation with peritonitis occurs in 1% to 2% of patients with Crohn's disease, with 90% of the perforations found in the distal ileum and the remaining 10% in the proximal ileum.[106,107] Other inflammatory lesions in the peritoneal cavity also may be responsible for small bowel perforation, although free perforation is generally seen only in primary inflammatory lesions of the small bowel, whereas fistula development is more common when other intra-abdominal viscera are responsible for the inflammation.

Fistula formation can be seen as a complication of radiation therapy in the period referred to as the *late acute phase* when superficial mucosal ulcerations fail to heal owing to compromised blood supply, leading to perforation. Free perforation is also uncommon in this setting as surrounding structures tend to wall off the injury, resulting in the formation of a fistula. Intestinal complications of radiation therapy are further discussed in Chapter 7.

DIAGNOSIS

Patients with free perforations of the small intestine tend to present with a more clear clinical picture than those with contained perforations. A history of an **acute** onset of abdominal pain coupled with a physical examination suggestive of peritonitis (rigid abdominal wall muscles, rebound tenderness) will be present in the majority of these patients. A plain flat abdominal radiograph and upright chest radiograph will often be helpful by demonstrating pneumoperitoneum, leading the clinician to the diagnosis of a perforated viscus. Not until the time of surgery will the location of the perforation be confirmed.

More commonly, a small bowel perforation will present as a fistula or abscess. When the fistula is enterocutaneous, as in patients who have recently undergone abdominal surgery (60% to 90% of patients with enterocutaneous fistulae), the diagnosis is straightforward.[108] Succus entericus draining from the anterior abdominal wall is characteristic and the anatomic location of the fistula can be ascertained by obtaining a fistulogram, which may provide useful information concerning the cause of the fistula.[109] Enterovesical fistulae are characterized by pyuria, dysuria, and hematuria and best confirmed through cystoscopy, although even with a careful cystoscopy the lesion may not be visible. Sometimes all that is seen is an area of inflammation. Enteroenteric fistulae are perhaps the most difficult to diagnose and can result in electrolyte imbalances and nutritional deficiencies due to resulting short bowel syndrome. Small bowel follow-through contrast radiographs are most helpful in confirming the diagnosis and can give information regarding the anatomic location and cause of the fistula. Enterovaginal fistula can be investigated during a careful pelvic examination.

It is important to point out that prior to any type of treatment it is important to determine the status of the remaining distal gastrointestinal tract either through preoperative radiographs or at the time of surgery to rule out a more distal obstruction.

Intestinal perforation followed by the formation of an intra-abdominal abscess can have an impressive clinical presentation, or it can be a more subtle, elusive diagnosis to make. A history of abdominal pain followed by some relief of this discomfort generally precedes the onset of fever by several days. Localized abdominal tenderness, fever, and leukocytosis are characteristic. A computed tomographic scan of the abdomen and pelvis with both intravenous and oral contrast media may reveal an intra-abdominal or pelvic fluid collection suggestive of an abscess in the majority of cases.

MANAGEMENT

When determining the management of the patient with intestinal perforation, many factors are important. The cause of the perforation, the general health and nutritional status of the patient, any underlying disease processes, and the anatomic location of the perforation all play important roles when formulating a decision concerning the future management of this complication.

Free Perforation. Patients with a clinical history suggestive of a perforated viscus (intestinal or otherwise) present with peritonitis and demand immediate surgical intervention. The exact location of the perforation is not definitely known until the time of laparotomy; therefore, preoperative measures are limited to intravenous hydration, institution of broad-spectrum antibiotics aimed at covering gastrointestinal flora, and insertion of a nasogastric tube to decompress the proximal small bowel and theoretically minimalize spillage. Surgery should be conducted through a midline incision as this provides optimal exposure to the entire abdominal cavity. A thorough exploration should be carried out to determine the exact location and cause of the perforation. Once the perforation is identified, the portion of small bowel containing this injury should be resected and primary anastomosis performed.

Enterocutaneous Fistula. The management of a patient with an enterocutaneous fistula is not nearly as straightforward. Postoperative enterocutaneous fistulae generally occur 7 to 10 days after abdominal surgery, often preceded by leukocytosis, low grade fevers, and abdominal pain. They are associated with significant morbidity and mortality. Major causes of death in patients with fistulae include sepsis, electrolyte imbalance, and malnutrition. Although there is considerable disagreement in the literature about the exact definition, fistulae are characterized as high-output or low-output. A high-output fistula is defined as 500 mL or more drainage over a 24-hour period. These fistulae are characterized by greater incidence of associated electrolyte imbalance and malnutrition than low-output fistulae with less than 500 mL drainage per day.

Characteristic bile-stained fluid may appear in the wound or be evident in an abdominal drain left at the time of surgery. Immediate measures should be aimed at restoring fluid and electrolyte imbalances, control of sepsis, initiating bowel rest, skin protection, and nutritional support. If the patient is stable, a computed tomographic scan of the abdomen and pelvis should be obtained to rule out the possibility of any undrained intra-abdominal fluid collections. If present, these should be drained either percutaneously or operatively, depending on the accessibility and number of collections present. If percutaneous drainage can be performed safely and effectively, an effort should be made to accomplish this. However, if there are multiple abscess cavities or the collection is in an area that cannot be safely aspirated, the patient should be taken to the operating room for open drainage. If the patient appears septic with diffuse peritonitis, a single, contained abscess is unlikely and surgical intervention should be undertaken. Otherwise, broad-spectrum antibiotics should be instituted until all abscesses are completely drained and there are no signs of continued sepsis.

Once these initial priorities are addressed, measures should be taken to provide good wound management as continued soilage with intestinal contents ultimately leads to poor wound healing and continued skin breakdown. Collection bags not only provide skin protection, but also enable the clinician to measure the fistula output, an important parameter by which to gauge fluid and electrolyte replacement. The use of an ileostomy bag with a karaya ring placed around the fistula is usually effective in controlling drainage, whereas more advanced drainage control systems can be devised aimed at protecting uninvolved skin. A fistulogram should then be performed to delineate the anatomy and provide clues to the cause of the fistula, which should aid in formulating a treatment plan.

Several factors have been found to be associated with failure of a fistula to close including radiated bowel, inflammatory bowel disease, abscess, epithelization of the tract, carcinoma, foreign body, or distal obstruction. If these are not present, most fistulae will close within 1 month if treated nonoperatively.[110] During the course of nonoperative treatment, total parenteral nutrition should be provided; enteral feedings with an elemental diet can be instituted if the fistula is in the distal small intestine and there is no evidence of distal obstruction. Careful management of fluid and electrolyte balance is extremely important during this trial of nonoperative therapy and cannot be ignored if a successful outcome is to occur.

If operative management is chosen, the operation should be individualized to each patient. An emergency operation is required when the postoperative patient presents with peritonitis and an associated fistula, suggesting diffuse contamination. The operation should be carried out with the goal of providing adequate external drainage of the leak and efforts at primary repair of the fistula are not advisable when diffuse contamination is present as anastomotic breakdown occurs with a high frequency. Exteriorization of the proximal and distal bowel segments after resection of the involved segment is advisable in this situation.[111] These enterostomies can be taken down once the patient is more stable and in better nutritional condition.

When the patient is being operated on in a more elective setting, such as is the case for failure of the fistula to close, then resection with primary anastomosis can be safely performed after resection of the involved bowel. Primary closure of the fistula without resection is associated with a high percentage of postoperative recurrences.[110] A careful exploration should be carried out to ensure that there is no distal obstruction or other factor that may be responsible for this failure to heal. When there is an associated abscess present, the surgeon must use judgement in determining whether an anastomosis should be undertaken. Generally, if the patient is stable and the abscess contained and effectively drained, primary small bowel anastomosis is safe and desirable.

Enteroenteric Fistula. Enteroenteric fistulae are most commonly due to Crohn's disease and are unusual in the cancer patient. When they do occur, they are usually the consequence of a perforated colon cancer as a result of radiation therapy. In patients with fistulae arising unassociated with Crohn's disease, management should be operative, consisting of resection of the involved bowel with primary intestinal anastomosis. In the case of perforated adenocarcinoma of the colon, this is ideally done through an *en bloc* resection of the primary large bowel lesion with the attached small bowel segment. Enteroenteric fistulae secondary to radiation therapy require no intervention if no symptoms are present.

Enterovesical Fistula. Surgery plays the major role in managing the patient with an enterovesical fistula. Although these fistulae are also seen most commonly in patients with Crohn's disease, they can also be seen as a complication of radiation therapy or as a result of a perforating colon cancer or diverticulum. Resection of the involved bowel with primary anastomosis and resection of the involved bladder with primary closure is the procedure of choice. If the large bowel is responsible for the fistula and it is not prepared preoperatively, then resection with colostomy and mucous fistula is advised.

Enterovaginal Fistula. Enterovaginal fistulae in cancer patients are usually a result of radiation therapy or pelvic surgery (with associated small bowel injury). The management is similar to the management of patients with enterocutaneous fistulae. If there is no sepsis present and the drainage can be well-controlled, nonoperative treatment can be instituted. If this is not the case, or if nonoperative measures fail to close the fistula, then surgery is indicated. Resection of the involved bowel and diseased vaginal cuff is performed, usually accompanied by primary small bowel anastomosis. The vaginal cuff can either be closed or left open to function as a drain.

SUMMARY: SMALL INTESTINAL PERFORATION AND FISTULAE

1. Perforation is a presenting problem in 10% of patients with a small bowel malignancy. The diagnosis is usually straightforward as patients present with frank peritonitis.
2. Free perforations are generally treated

with immediate surgery including resection of the affected area, and usually re-anastomosis of the bowel with copious irrigation of the abdominal cavity.

3. The management of enterocutaneous fistulae is directed at control of sepsis, control of fistula drainage, restoration of fluid and electrolyte imbalances, bowel rest, and nutritional support. High-output (>500 mL/d) fistulae are associated with greater morbidity and mortality than low-output fistulae.

Perforation of the Large Intestine

ETIOLOGY

Colonic perforation can occur as a result of a variety of disease processes. Perforating carcinomas, obstructing lesions, diverticulitis, iatrogenic injuries, appendicitis, colitis, radiation therapy, and trauma all have been associated with perforation of the large intestines. Whatever the cause, the result is usually the same: fecal spillage with peritonitis resulting in intra-abdominal sepsis.

Colon cancers can cause perforation either by direct extension through the bowel wall or by causing luminal obstruction resulting in a functional closed-loop obstruction, cecal distension, and ultimately perforation. Additionally, adenocarcinoma of the large bowel can perforate directly into other abdominal viscera, including small bowel, vagina, and bladder[112,113] (Table 3-3).

Although more common in the general population than in the cancer population, diverticulitis is a common cause of perforation, occurring in 4% to 15% of patients undergoing operation for complicated diverticular disease.[114–116] In patients receiving steroid therapy, diverticular perforation may be the most common presenting symptom of diverticulitis because the inflammatory response that normally allows diverticulitis to "seal off" is lost. Immunocompromised patients made up 11% of the overall population with perforated diverticulitis in a recent review.[116]

Iatrogenic injuries can complicate diagnostic colonoscopy, polypectomy, or therapeutic colonoscopic treatment (i.e., laser therapy for obstructing malignancies). Perforation occurs in 0.2% to 0.4% of cases of diagnostic colonoscopy and can be due to direct tip injury, shaft injury during scope flexion, and distension of the colon with resultant perforation.[117]

Appendicitis, if unrecognized and untreated, will eventually result in perforation of the appendix, leading to increased morbidity and mortality, especially in the debilitated patient. It often goes unrecognized in this patient population owing to either their underlying disease processes or therapy (i.e., leukopenia, steroids), both of which can mask an inflammatory response and delay the diagnosis.

Other inflammatory lesions of the colon, in addition to diverticulitis, can result in colonic perforation. Typhlitis and *C. difficile* colitis, both of which are seen more frequently in cancer patients, can involve the full-thickness of the colon wall resulting in

Table 3-3. Perforative Carcinoma of the Colon Fixation and Organ Involvement

Adherent Organ	Patients (N)	5-year Survival (%)
Prostate	17	17.6
Sacrum, anterior or posterior abdominal wall	74	23.0
Bladder	19	21.1
Small intestine	18	27.8
Colon	7	42.9
Stomach	2	100.0
Ovary	4	25.0
Uterus	8	12.5
Liver	1	0
Gallbladder	2	50.0
Spleen	2	50.0
Diaphragm	1	0
Vagina	4	50.0
Multiple structures	54	27.8

Adapted from Miller LD, Buruchow IB, Fitts WT. An analysis of 284 patients with perforative carcinoma of the colon. Surg Gynecol Obstet 1966;123:1212, with permission.

free perforation. The existence of right lower quadrant pain in the neutropenic patient suggests the possibility of typhlitis, and is further discussed in Chapter 1. Although the colon and rectum are the most common segments of the gastrointestinal tract to be injured by radiation, perforation of the large intestines is not a common complication. Both free perforation and fistula formation can be seen with severe radiation injuries of the colon (discussed in Chapter 7); however, because of the retroperitoneal location of the rectum, free perforation is not seen; fistulization and abscess formation are more frequent occurrences. The rectum also receives a higher dose of radiation owing to its proximity to other pelvic organs that are purposely being irradiated.

DIAGNOSIS

A thorough history and physical examination give the clinician clues to the diagnosis and cause of a colonic or rectal perforation in most patients. In cancer patients, however, the correct diagnosis may be more difficult to obtain due to confounding factors, including the underlying disease and treatment side effects.

A history of several days of left lower quadrant abdominal pain that suddenly worsened is a typical history of a patient with perforated diverticulitis, whereas the patient with a malignant perforation would perhaps complain of vague abdominal pain, weight loss, and constipation followed by acute diffuse abdominal pain. A cecal perforation due to a malignant obstruction is preceded by constipation, obstipation, and crampy abdominal pain. The physical examination will reveal diffuse peritoneal signs if the perforation is in communication with the peritoneal cavity, as is the case with acute perforations, whereas the pain will be more localized if the perforation has been sealed off by surrounding structures. Laboratory studies usually show a leukocytosis, and upright chest or abdominal radiograph will demonstrate free intraperitoneal air in most cases of free perforation, but this will not be present with a "sealed" perforation. If the diagnosis is still in doubt, as is often the case with a walled-off or subacute perforation, a water-soluble enema may be helpful, whereas an abdominal and pelvic computed tomography (CT) scan with water-soluble contrast media introduced per rectum is a better alternative in most cases.

Acute abdominal pain during or immediately following colonoscopy is a perforation until proved otherwise. Often the endoscopist will be able to see the perforation, but if not, physical examination and abdominal and chest radiographs will confirm the diagnosis revealing either peritonitis or pneumoperitoneum. A water-soluble contrast enema can be performed if the diagnosis is still in question.

Often the patient with a colon or rectal perforation will present with a fistula. Colovesical, colovaginal, and coloenteric fistulae are seen in cases of diverticulitis, perforated carcinoma, or less frequently associated with radiation therapy. The diagnosis of a colovesical fistula is made after the patient complains of dysuria, pyuria, or pneumaturia. It can be confirmed by cystoscopy, which will reveal an area of bullous edema, usually located on the posterior lateral wall or the fundus of the bladder. Charcoal or indigo carmine given orally will give the urine a characteristic color if a fistula is present. Colovaginal fistulae are confirmed by visualization on vaginal speculum examination. Coloenteric fistulae are difficult to diagnose but can often be demonstrated on a small bowel contrast study or barium enema (Figure 3-7).

MANAGEMENT

Perforated Diverticulitis. As previously mentioned, free perforation is relatively uncommon in the immunocompetent host owing to the response of the surrounding tissue during the slow progression of the disease with subsequent "walling-off" of the transmural process. Free perforation is seen when the perforation is in direct continuity with the

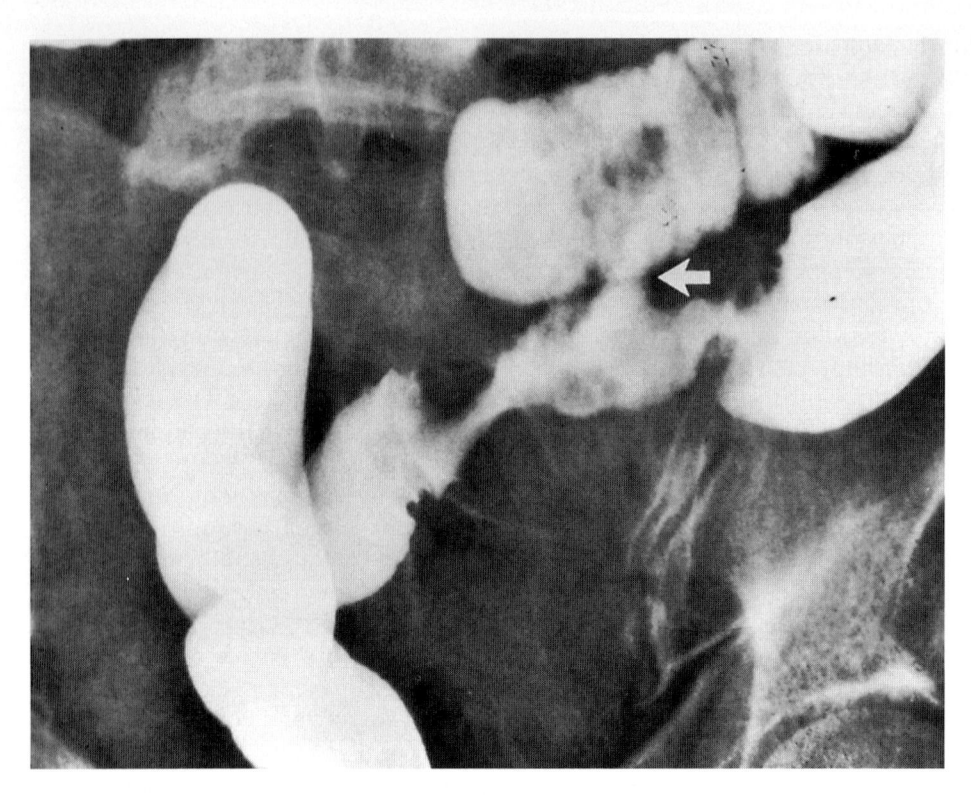

Figure 3-7. Ileocolic fistula (*arrow*) secondary to carcinoma of the sigmoid colon as demonstrated by barium contrast study. From Eisenberg RL, ed. Gastrointestinal radiology: a pattern approach. Philadelphia, JB Lippincott, 1983.

peritoneal cavity, as is the case with the immunocompromised patient. Patients with free perforation demand immediate attention and surgical intervention. Intravenous fluids should be given along with broad-spectrum antibiotics prior to surgery. Laparotomy should be performed emergently with the goal of removing the septic process and this is best done with a sigmoid resection accompanied by end colostomy. The distal segment of bowel can be brought to the skin as a mucous fistula, but more commonly is left as a Hartmann closure owing to insufficient length. Colostomy take-down can safely be performed 6 to 12 weeks later, after evaluation of the remaining colon and rectum by endoscopy or contrast radiography. Resection with primary anastomosis and proximal diverting colostomy[114] or resection, on table colonic irrigation, and primary anastomosis[118] have been advocated in selected clinical situations. These procedures should not be performed when gross fecal contamination is present, or when the host is immunocompromised or unstable.

Occasionally a patient will present with fevers and abdominal pain with a CT scan revealing a well-defined abscess cavity and sealed off diverticular perforation. This can be safely managed with percutaneous drainage, intravenous antibiotics, and sigmoid colon resection once the inflammation has subsided (generally several weeks).

Perforated Carcinoma. A diagnosis of perforated carcinoma may not be made prior to surgery because these patients often end up in the operating room with a presumed diagnosis of perforated peptic ulcer or diverticulum. The goal of surgery is to resect the large bowel containing the carcinoma in a curative fashion, to include the mesentery and draining lymph nodes, as the 5-year survival rate can approach 44% in this group of patients.[119] The abdominal cavity should be evaluated for additional disease as occult liver and peritoneal metastases are not uncommon findings. Intestinal continuity can be restored in patients with right-sided carcinomas in the absence of a large degree of fecal contamination and with a physiologically stable patient; otherwise an end colostomy and mucous fistula should be created. Carcinomas in the remaining colon usually are best managed with end colostomy and mucous fistula following resection.

Obstructing Lesions. Obstructing carcinomas, colonic volvulus, diverticulitis, carcinomatosis, and postradiation strictures all can cause obstruction of the large bowel. Most commonly, the symptoms of colonic obstruction will bring the patient to seek medical attention prior to cecal perforation. The condition of colonic obstruction is discussed extensively in Chapter 2. Occasionally a patient will present with a perforated cecum secondary to obstruction or one may perforate while being observed with a colonic obstruction if a competent ileocecal valve is present. Again, treatment is surgical, aimed at removing the perforated cecum while addressing the underlying obstructing lesion. This is best accomplished by right colon resection and ileostomy, reserving resection of the obstructing lesion for a time when the patient is more stable. A transverse mucous fistula must be created to avoid the creation of a closed loop of colon.

Perforated Appendicitis. Treatment of perforated appendicitis consists of appendectomy with drainage only if there is a localized, contained abscess cavity. Perioperative antibiotics should be used and continued until the abscess is completely drained and there are no signs of continued sepsis.

Colonic Fistulae. Colovesical fistulae are most commonly due to diverticulitis and are treated with sigmoid resection and closure of the bladder defect. Carcinomas that perforate into the bladder should be managed with a formal colon resection accompanied by *en bloc* resection of the bladder wall. This often requires complete cystectomy to ensure adequate margins, as the fistula is frequently near the trigone. Five-year survival rates are reported to be 56% in this group of patients.[120] Coloenteric fistulae require formal colon resection with *en bloc* resection of the attached small bowel, whereas colovaginal fistulae can be treated with colon resection to include the vaginal wall or cuff. Closure of the cuff is performed or it may be left open to act as a drain.

Iatrogenic Injuries. Because patients who undergo colonoscopy usually have had a complete mechanical bowel preparation, resection and primary anastomosis or direct repair of the perforation can often be safely performed. The underlying disease process that necessitated the colonoscopy should be addressed at the time of surgery.

SUMMARY: LARGE INTESTINAL PERFORATION

1. Colonic perforation can be a result of carcinomas, diverticular disease, iatrogenic injury, radiation therapy, and a variety of other conditions. Diagnosis is usually established by history and physical examination. A CT scan may be helpful.

2. Therapy is usually surgical. A two-step procedure (drainage and resection followed by reanastamosis in the future) is most commonly performed. The distal end may be exteriorized as a mucous fistula, or oversewn and left in the pelvis (Hartmann procedure).

3. Patients with perforation due to an iatrogenic injury may be treated with a single operation including resection and anastomosis because they often have undergone bowel preparation prior to the procedure.

SUMMARY

Gastrointestinal bleeding is frequently encountered in the cancer patient. Bleeding can arise from primary tumors, metastatic lesions, or causes unrelated to their underlying tumor. It is important to consider the hematologic effects of the therapy these patients are receiving (refer to Chapter 17). Bleeding is defined as upper (proximal to the Treitz's ligament) or lower (distal to the ligament). In all cases of gastrointestinal bleeding, it is important to correct any coexistent coagulopathy as an adjunct to definitive surgical therapy that is anticipated.

Many patients with upper gastrointestinal bleeding will have blood in a nasogastric tube or hematemesis. Patients with gastrointestinal bleeding must first be resuscitated with intravenous fluids, and initial blood work should be obtained including type and cross match. A urinary catheter should be placed. Evacuation of gastric blood is important to decrease gastric distention and to allow further diagnostic evaluation. Definitive therapy may be undertaken once the site is identified.

Esophageal varices may be caused by a number of conditions, including cirrhosis, hepatitis, Budd-Chiari syndrome (see Chapter 5), or portal vein thrombosis. Management includes fluid resuscitation and control of hemorrhage with sclerotherapy or portalsystemic shunting. Other esophageal sources of bleeding include Mallory-Weiss tears, ulcerations, and malignancies. Gastric bleeding sources include erosive gastritis, gastric ulcers, and primary gastric tumors. Gastritis is best treated preventively. Gastric ulcers may require resection. Hemobilia is commonly iatrogenic in nature and is diagnosed by the observation of blood arising from the ampulla of Vater. Arteriography is the most important diagnostic test in the work-up of hemobilia. Duodenal bleeding is often caused by peptic ulcer disease which, when surgical therapy is indicated, usually necessitates control of the bleeding with sutures and an antiulcer operation to limit recurrence.

The treatment of lower gastrointestinal bleeding also involves the three phases of resuscitation, identification of the bleeding site, and definitive therapy. Rigid sigmoidoscopy is performed first and will aid in the identification of distal rectal bleeding sources such as hemorrhoids. Following this, colonoscopy, arteriography, and tagged red blood cell scan are used depending on the rate and site of bleeding. Small bowel sources of lower gastrointestinal bleeding are a diagnostic challenge. Colonic bleeding may be caused by a variety of factors including diverticular disease, angiodysplasia, tumors, infection, prior radiation therapy, or inflammatory bowel disease.

The presentation of gastrointestinal perforation is usually not subtle. Prompt diagnosis and therapy is essential to reduce the morbidity and mortality associated with this devastating problem. Patients with esophageal perforation usually present with chest pain, fever, and dyspnea. Contrast radiography may be useful in establishing the diagnosis. Surgical repair is the treatment of choice, often with a pleural flap. In cases where the perforation is longer than 24 hours, esophageal exclusion may be indicated. Gastric and duodenal perforation may be due to benign causes such as peptic ulcer disease or malignancy. The treatment in almost all cases is prompt surgical repair. Small bowel perforation may be due to malignancies. Enterocutaneous fistulae require control of sepsis, control of enteric drainage, restoration of fluid and electrolyte imbalances, nutritional support, and bowel rest. Although some enterocutaneous fistulae may close spontaneously, surgical intervention with resection and anastomosis is often required. Perforations of the colon may be due to diverticular disease, malignancy, or iatrogenic injury. Although a two-stage procedure is often required, some patients may be treated with simple repair or a single-stage resection.

Abdominal problems are a major reason for surgical consultation in the cancer patient, and gastrointestinal bleeding and perforation are fairly common in the cancer patient. Although these problems also occur in the noncancer population, they are perhaps more urgent in the cancer patient. Patients receiving chemotherapy often have coagulation and hematologic side effects of their therapy that will exacerbate any gastrointestinal bleeding. These changes in the hematologic system must be considered (see Chapter 17). Cancer patients, simply because they have a tumor, may be immunocompromised compared with the healthy population. This may adversely affect their ability to deal with the devastating physiologic sequelae of gastrointestinal perforation. Thus, the surgeon consulted to deal with gastrointestinal perforation and bleeding in the cancer patient must be prepared to deal with a host of factors.

REFERENCES

1. Katon RM, Smith FW. Panendoscopy in the early diagnosis of acute upper gastrointestinal bleeding. Gastroenterology 1973;65:728.
2. McGinn FP, Guyer PB, Wilken BJ, et al. A prospective comparative trial between early endoscopy and radiology in acute upper gastrointestinal hemorrhage. Gut 1975;16:707.
3. Cameron JL, Herlong HF, Sanfey H, et al. The Budd-Chiari syndrome: Treatment by mesenteric-systemic venous shunts. Ann Surg 1983;198:335.
4. Wang Z, Zhu Y, Wang S, et al. Recognition and management of Budd-Chiari syndrome: Report of one hundred cases. J Vasc Surg 1989;10:149.
5. Henderson JM, Warren WD, Millikan WJ, et al. Surgical options, hematologic evaluation, and pathologic changes in Budd-Chiari syndrome. Am J Surg 1990;159:41.
6. Johnson W, Widrich W, Ansell J, et al. Control of bleeding varices by vasopressin: A prospective randomized study. Ann Surg 1977;180:369.
7. Chojkier M, Groszmann R, Atterbury C, et al. A controlled comparison of continuous intraaterial and intravenous infusion of vasopressin in hemorrhages from esophogeal varices. Gastroenterology 1979;77:540.
8. Groszmann RJ, Kravetz D, Bosch J, et al. Nitroglycerin improves the hemodynamic response to vasopressin in portal hypertension. Hepatology 1982;2:562.
9. Rikkers LF, Burnett DA, Volentine GD. Shunt surgery versus endoscopic sclerotherapy for long-term treatment of variceal bleeding. Ann Surg 1987;206:261.
10. Warren WD, Henderson JM, Millikan WJ, et al. Distal splenorenal shunt versus endoscopic sclerotherapy for long-term management of variceal bleeding: Preliminary report of a prospective, randomized trial. Ann Surg 1986;203:454.
11. Teres J, Bordas JM, Bravo D, et al. Sclerotherapy versus distal splenorenal shunt in the elective treatment of variceal hemorrhage: A randomized controlled trial. Hepatology 1987;7:430.
12. Chojkier M, Conn HO. Esophageal tamponade in the treatment of bleeding varices. Dig Dis Sci 1980;25:267.
13. Sarin SK, Mundy S. Balloon tamponade in the management of bleeding esophageal varices. Ann R Coll Surg Engl 1984;66:30.
14. Orloff MJ, Bell RH, Hyde PV, et al. Long-term results of emergency portacaval shunt for bleeding esophageal varices in unselected patients with alcoholic cirrohosis. Ann Surg 1980;192:325.
15. Sarfeh IJ, Rypins EB, Mason GR. A systematic appraisal of portacaval H-graft diameters: clinical and hemodynamic perspectives. Ann Surg 1986;204:356.
16. Warren WD, Zeppa R, Fomon JJ. Selective transplenic decompression of gastroesophageal varices by distal splenorenal shunt. Ann Surg 1967;166:437.
17. Drapanas T. Interposition mesocaval shunt for treatment of portal hypertension. Ann Surg 1972;176:435.
18. Sarr MG, Herlong HF, Cameron JL. Long term patency of the mesocaval C shunt. Am J Surg 1986;151:98.
19. Matory WE, Sedgwick CE, Rossi RL. Nonshunting procedures in management of bleeding esophogeal varices. Surg Clin North Am 1980;60:281.
20. Bothe A, Stone MD, McDermott WV, Jr. Portoazygous disconnection for bleeding esophageal varices. Am J Surg 1989;149:546.
21. Burroughs AK, Hamilton G, Phillips A, et al. A comparison of sclerotherapy with staple transection of the esophagus for the emergency control of bleeding from esophageal varices. N Engl J Med 1989;321:857.
22. Richter GM, Noeldge G, Roessle M, et al. Transjugular intra-hepatic porto-syndrome stent shunt (TIPSS). Radiology 1990;174:1027.
23. Rogers CG, Paolini RM, O'Leary JP. Intrahepatic vascular shunting for portal hypertension: Early experience with the transjugular intrahepatic porto-systemic shunt. Am Surg 1994;60:114.
24. Mallory GK, Weiss S. Hemorrhages from

lacerations of cardiac orfice of the stomach due to vomiting. Am J Med Sci 1929;178:506.
25. Sugawa C, Benishek D, Walt AJ. Mallory-weiss syndrome: A study of 224 patients. Am J Surg 1983;145:30.
26. Michel L, Serrano A, Malt RA. Mallory-Weiss syndrome: Evolution of diagnostic and therapeutic patterns over two decades. Ann Surg 1980;192:716.
27. Paquet KJ, Mercado-Diaz M, Kalk JF. Frequency, significance, and therapy of Mallory-Weiss syndrome in patients with portal hypertension. Hepatology 1990;11:879.
28. Cheung LY. Pathogenesis, prophylaxis, and treatment of stress gastritis. Am J Surg 1988;156:437.
29. Cushing H. Peptic ulcers and the interbrain. Surg Gynecol Obstet 1932;55:1.
30. Fromm D. Drug-induced gastric mucosal injury. World J Surg 1981;5:199.
31. Peura DA, Johnson LF. Cimetidine for prevention and treatment of gastroduodenal mucosal lesions in patients in an intensive care unit. Ann Intern Med 1985;103:173.
32. Zinner MJ, Zuidema GS, Smith PL, et al. The prevention of upper gastrointestinal tract bleeding in patients in an intensive care unit. Surg Gynecol Obstet 1981;153:214.
33. Gaisford WD. Endoscopic electro hemostasis of active upper gastrointestinal bleeding. Am J Surg 1979;137:47.
34. Conn HO, Ramsby GR, Storer EH, et al. Intra-arterial vasopressin in the treatment of uppergastrointestinal hemorrhage: a prospective, controlled clinical trial. Gastroenterology 1975;68:211.
35. Hubert JP, Kiernan PD, Welch JS, et al. The surgical management of bleeding stress ulcers. Ann Surg 1980;191:672.
36. Cheung LY. Treatment of established stress ulcer disease. World J Surg 1981;5:235.
37. Baron JH. Current views on pathogenesis of peptic ulcer. Scand J Gastroenterol 1982;80:1.
38. Adkins RB Jr., DeLozier JB, Scott HW, et al. The management of gastric ulcers: a current review. Ann Surg 1985;201:741.
39. Lin HJ, Lee FY, Chan CY, et al. Heat probe thermocoagulation as a substitute for surgical intervention to arrest massive peptic ulcer hemorrhage: an experience in 153 cases. Surgery 1990;108:18.
40. Hunt PS. Bleeding gastroduodenal ulcers: selection of patients for surgery. World J Surg 1987;11:289.
41. Hanks JB, Jones RS. Tumors at the Stomach and Duodenum. In: Zuidema GD, Ritchie WP, eds. Shackleford's surgery of the alimentary tract. 3rd ed. Philadelphia, WB Saunders, 1991.
42. Goodnight JE, Jr, Blaisdell FW. Hemobilia. Surg Clin North Am 1981;61:973.
43. Sandblom P. Hemobilia (Biliary Tract Hemorrhage): history, pathology, diagnosis, treatment. Springfield Il: Charles C Thomas, 1972.
44. Cahow CE, Burell M, Greco R. Hemobilia following percutaneous cholangiography. Ann Surg 1977;185:235.
45. Sarr MG, Kaufman SL, Zuidema GD, et al. Management of hemobilia associated with transhepatic internal biliary drainage catheters. Surgery 1984;95:603.
46. Monden M, Okamura J, Kabayashi N, et al. Hemobilia after percutaneous transhepatic biliary drainage. Arch Surg 1980;115:161.
47. Hoevels J, Nilsson U. Intrahepatic vascular lesions following non-surgical percutaneous transhepatic bile duct intubation. Gastrointest Radiol 1980;5:127.
48. Hellenkaut C. Vascular complications following needle puncture of the liver: Clinical angiography. Acta Radiol 1976;17:209.
49. Okuda K, Musha H, Nakajima Y. Frequency of intrahepatic arteriovenous fistula as a sequela to percutaneous needle puncture of the liver. Gastroenterology 1978;71:1201.
50. Curet P, Baumer R, Roche A, et al. Hepatic hemobilia of traumatic or iatrogenic origin: Recent advances in diagnosis and therapy, review of the literature from 1976-1981. World J Surg 1984;8:2.
51. Herrington JL Jr., Davidson J. Bleeding gastroduodenal ulcers: Choice of operations. World J Surg 1987;11:304.
52. Wright HK, Pelliccia O, Higgins EF Jr., et al. Controlled semielective, segmental resection for massive colonic hemorrhage. Am J Surg 1980;139:535.
53. Todd GJ, Forde KA. Lower gastrointestinal bleeding with negative or inconclusive radiographic studies; the role of colonoscopy. Am J Surg 1979;138:627.
54. Friedman HI, Hilts SV, Whitney PJ. Use of technetium-labeled autologous red blood cells in detection of gastrointestinal bleeding. Surg Gynecol Obstet 1983;156:449.
55. Wilson JM, Melvin DB, Gray GF, et al. Primary malignancies of the small bowel: A report of 96 cases and review of the literature. Ann Surg 1974;180:175.
56. Jorge E, Harvey HA, Simmonds MA, et al. Sympromatic malignant melanoma of the gastrointestinal tract: Operative treatment and survival. Ann Surg 1984;199:328.
57. Yamamoto Y, Sano K, Shigemoto H. Detec-

tion of the bleeding source from small intestine: intraopertive endoscopy and preoperative abdominal scintigraphy by technetium 99m pertechnetate. Am Surg 1985;51:658.
58. Oliver GC, Rubin RJ, Park YH, et al. Preoperative localization of intermittently bleeding small intestinal tumors using Tc-99m labeled red blood cell scanning: Report of two cases. Dis Col Rectum 1987;30:715.
59. Lewis BS, Waye JD. Chronic gastrointestinal bleeding of obscure origin: Role of small bowel enteroscopy. Gastroenterology 1988;94:1117.
60. Lau WY, Fan ST, Chu KW, et al. Intra-operative fibreoptic enteroscopy for bleeding lesions in the small intestine. Br J Surg 1986;73:217.
61. Myers RT. Diagnosis and management of occult gastrointestinal bleeding: Visualization of the small bowel lumen by fiberoptic colonscope. Am Surg 1976;42:92.
62. Apelgren KN, Vargish T, Al-Kawas F. Principles for use of intraoperative enteroscopy for hemorrhage from the small bowel. Am Surg 1988;54:85.
63. Ahlquist DA, Gostout CJ, Viggiano TR, et al. Laser therapy for severe radiation-induced rectal bleeding. Mayo Clin Proc 1986;61:927.
64. Berken CA. Nd:YAG laser therapy for gastrointestinal bleeding due to radiation colitis. Am J Gastroenterol 1985;80:730.
65. Nesbitt JC, Sawyers JL. Surgical management of esophageal perforation. Am Surg 1987;53:183.
66. Orringer MB. Complications of esophogeal surgery. In: Zuidema GD, Orringer MB, eds. Shackelford's surgery of the alimentary tract. 3rd ed. Philadelphia: W.B. Saunders Co, 1991.
67. Loop FD, Groves LK. Esophageal perforations. Ann Thorac Surg 1970;10:571.
68. Cameron JL, Kieffer RF, Hendrix TR, et al. Selective nonoperative management of contained intrathoracic esophageal disruptions. Ann Thorac Surg 1979;27:404.
69. Brown RH, Cohen PS. Nonsurgical management of spontaneous esophageal perforation. JAMA 1978;240:140.
70. Lyons WS, Seremetis MG, deGuzman VC. Ruptures and perforations of the esophagus: The case for conservative supportive management. Ann Thorac Surg 1978;25:346.
71. Mayer JE, Murray CA, Varco RL. The treatment of esophageal perforation with delayed recognition and continuing sepsis. Ann Thorac Surg 1977;23:568.
72. Hendren WH, Henderson BM. Immediate esophagectomy for instrumental perforation of the thoracic esophagus. Ann Surg 1968;168:997.
73. Symbas PA, Hatcher CR, Harlaftis N. Spontaneous rupture of the esophagus. Ann Surg 1978;187:634.
74. Sawyers JL, Lane CE, Foster JH, et al. Esophageal perforation. Arch Surg 1975;110:233.
75. Sandrasagra FA, English TAH, Milstein BB. Prognosis and management of oepophageal perforations. Thorax 1978;33:131.
76. Schulze S, Pederson VM, Hoier-Madsen K. Iatrogenic perforation of the esophagus. Acta Chir Scand 1982;148:679.
77. Skinner DB, Little AG, DeMeester TR. Management of esophageal perforation. Am J Surg 1980;139:760.
78. Triggiani E, Belsey R. Oesophageal trauma: incidence, diagnosis and management. Thorax 1977;32:241.
79. Grillo HC, Wilkins EW, Jr. Esophageal repair following late diagnosis of intrathoracic perforation. Ann Thorac Surg 1975;20:387.
80. Bryant LR. Experimental evaluation of intercostal pedicle graft in esophageal repair. J Thorac Cardiovasc Surg 1965;50:626.
81. Dooling JD, Zick HR. Closure of an esophageal fistula using only intercostal pedicle graft. Ann Thorac Surg 1967;3:553.
82. Hooper CL, Berk PD, Howes EL. Strength of esophageal anastomoses repaired with autogenous pericardial grafts. Surg Gynecol Obstet 1963;117:83.
83. Millard AH. "Spontaneous" perforation of the oesophageal treated by utilization of a pericardial graft. Br J Surg 1971;58:70.
84. Rao KV, Mir M, Cogbill CL. Management of perforation of the thoracic esophagus. Am J Surg 1974;127:609.
85. Westaby S. An improved method for primary repair after spontaneous oesophageal perforation. Br J Surg 1980;67:801.
86. Jara FM. Diaphragmatic pedicle flap for treatment of Boerhaave's syndrome. J Thorac Cardiovasc Surg 1979;78:931.
87. Johnson J, Schwegman CW, Kirby CK. Esophageal exclusion for persistent fistula following spontaneous rupture of the esophagus. J Thorac Surg 1956;32:827.
88. Urschel HC, Razzuk MA, Wood RE, et al. Improved management of esophageal perforation: exclusion and diversion in continuity. Ann Surg 1979;179:587.
89. Appleton DS, Sandrasagra FA, Flower CDR. Perforated esophagus: A review of twenty-eight conservative cases. Clin Radiol 1979;30:493.

90. Thal AP, Hatafuku T. Impoved operation for esophageal rupture. JAMA 1964;188:826.
91. Bush RG. Treatment of perforation of the esophagus associated with stricture. Surg Gynecol Obstet 1984;158:498.
92. Martini N, Goodner JT, D'Angio GJ, et al. Tracheoesophageal fistula due to cancer. J Thorac Cardiovasc Surg 1970;59:319.
93. Angorn IB. Intubation in the treatment of carcinoma of the esophagus. World J Surg 1981;5:535.
94. Duranceau A, Jamieson GG. Malignant tracheoesophageal fistula. Ann Thorac Surg 1984;37:346.
95. Hegarty MM, Angorn IB, Bryer JV, et al. Palliation of malignant esophago-respiratory fistulae by permanent indwelling prosthetic tube. Ann Surg 1977;185:88.
96. Kirschner MB. Ein neues Verfahren der Oeophagoplastie. Arch Klin Chir 1920;114:606.
97. Wong J, Lam KH, Wei WI, et al. Results of the Kirschner operation. World J Surg 1981;5:547.
98. Skinner DB, DeMeester TR. Permanent extracorporeal esophagogastric tube for esophageal replacement. Ann Thorac Surg 1976;22:107.
99. Orringer M. Substernal gastric bypass of the excluded thoracic esophagus for palliation of esophageal carcinoma. J Thorac Cardiovac Surg 1975;70:826.
100. Rackner VL, Thirlby RC, Ryan JA, et al. Role of surgery in multimodality therapy for gastrointestinal lymphoma. Am J Surg 1991;161:570.
101. Cameron JL, Barquist E, Zinner M. Peptic ulcer disease. In: Cameron JL, ed. Current surgical therapy. 4th ed. St Louis: Mosby, 1992.
102. Graham RR. The treatment of perforated duodenal ulcers. Surg Gynecol Obstet 1937;64:235.
103. Donovan AJ, Vinson TL, Maulsby GO, et al. Selective treatment of duodenal ulcer with perforation. Ann Surg 1979;189:627.
104. Darling RC, Welch CE. Tumors of the small intestine. New Eng J Med 1959;260:397.
105. Shatila AH, Chamerlain BE, Webb WR. Current status of diagnosis and management of strangulation obstruction of the small bowel. Am J Surg 1976;132:299.
106. Steinberg DM, Cooke WT, Alexander-Williams J. Free perforation in Crohn's disease. Gut 1973;14:187.
107. Abascal J, Rojas FD, Jorge J, et al. Free perforation of the small bowel in Crohn's disease. World J Surg 1982;6:216.
108. Coutsoftides R, Fazio VW. Small intestine cutaneous fistulas. Surg Gynecol Obstet 1979;149:33.
109. Goldfarb WB, Monafo W, McAlister WH. Clinical value of fistulography. Am J Surg 1964;108:902.
110. Reber HA, Roberts C, Way LW, et al. Management of external gastrointestinal fistulas. Ann Surg 1978;188:460.
111. Goligher JC. Resection with exterioriation in the management of faecal fistula originating in the small intestine. Br J Surg 1971;58:163.
112. DeLeon ML, Schoetz DJ Jr., Coller JA, et al. Colorectal cancer: Lahey clinic experience, 1972 to 1976. Dis Colon Rectum 1987;30:237.
113. Miller LD, Boruchow B, Fitts WT. An analysis of 284 patients with perforative carcinoma of the colon. Surg Gynecol Obstet 1966;123:1212.
114. Hackford AW, Schoetz DJ Jr., Coller JA, et al. Surgical management of complicated diverticulitis: The Lahey clinic experience, 1967 to 1982. Dis Colon Rectum 1985;28:317.
115. Parks TG. Natural history of diverticular disease of the colon. A review of 521 cases. Br Med J 1969;4:639.
116. Rodkey GV, Welch CE. Changing patterns in the surgical treatment of diverticular disease. Ann Surg 1984;200:466.
117. Schrock TR. Complications of gastrintestinal endoscopy. In: Sleisenger MH, Fordtran JS, eds. Gastrointestinal disease: pathophysiology, diagnosis, management. 4th ed. Philadelphia: WB Saunders, 1989:216.
118. Koruth NM, Krukowski ZH, Youngson GG, et al. Intra-operative colonic irrigation in the management of left-sided large bowel emergencies. Br J Surg 1985;72:708.
119. Willett C, Tepper JE, Cohen A, et al. Obstructive and perforative colonic carcinoma: Patterns of failure. J Clin Oncol 1985;3:379.
120. Aldrete JS, ReMine WH. Vesicocolic fistula: a complication of colonic cancer. Arch Surg 1967;94:627.

4

Inflammatory Lesions of the Gastrointestinal Tract

WILLIAM E. FISHER
WILLIAM E. BURAK, JR
WILLIAM B. FARRAR

Inflammatory lesions of the gastrointestinal tract are frequent complications of cancer therapy. These lesions have a great impact on the patient's quality of life during treatment and frequently interfere with the delivery of optimal therapy. Ionizing radiation causes the formation of free radicals within the cell which damage DNA. Chemotherapeutic agents damage dividing cells through a variety of mechanisms. Alkylating agents such as cyclophosphamide cause cross-linking of DNA. Antimetabolites interfere with nucleic acid synthesis. For example, 6-mercaptopurine blocks purine ring biosynthesis and 5-fluorouracil blocks the synthesis of thymidylic acid from deoxyuridylic acid. The vinca alkaloids bind tubuli and destroy the spindle thus producing mitotic arrest. The frequently dividing tumor cells therefore are more sensitive to radiation and chemotherapy than less frequently dividing cells such as neurons. Unfortunately, the cells of the gastrointestinal tract and the hematopoietic stem cells are also rapidly dividing and are often injured along with the tumor cells. Thus, chemotherapy and radiation cause inflammation of the gastrointestinal tract by two mechanisms. One mechanism is by direct damage to the mucosal cells. The second is by damage to the hematopoietic cells causing immunosuppression and subsequent infection of the gastrointestinal tract. The effects of chemotherapy on hematopoietic cells are further discussed in Chapter 17.

Inflammatory lesions of the gastrointestinal tract occur anywhere from mouth to anus in the cancer patient. Stomatitis is a frequent complication of head and neck radiation and systemic chemotherapy that can become a life-threatening source of sepsis. Esophagitis usually results from an opportunistic infection with *Candida* species due to myelosuppression. In addition to direct damage by radiation or infection, the stomach in the cancer patient is vulnerable to inflammatory lesions caused by nonsteroidal anti-inflammatory drugs, the stress of major surgery and sepsis, or even displaced hepatic arterial chemotherapy infusion catheters. Nausea with chemotherapy may be caused by inflammatory lesions of the small intestine. This common problem is fully discussed in Chapter 8.

Less common are the late sequelae of fistulous tracts, abscesses and strictures that can be caused by radiation. The colon, being a partially fixed retroperitoneal organ, is particularly susceptible to radiation injury. Also, acute colitis in the cancer patient can result from opportunistic infection. Prompt recognition and treatment of inflammatory lesions of the gastrointestinal tract in the cancer patient are essential to ensure optimal results from antineoplastic regimens and to avoid major morbidity and even mortality.

STOMATITIS

Stomatitis is an inflammatory response of the oral mucosa and is frequently a significant complication of cancer therapy. In addition to interfering with the ability to eat, stomatitis can become a source of sepsis in the immunocompromised cancer patient. Unless recognized early and managed correctly, stomatitis will preclude further anticancer treatment or even imperil the life of the patient. Radiation induces stomatitis by decreasing mucosal cell renewal resulting in atrophic changes in the epithelium. The patient complains of pain and drying of the oral mucosa. Erythema is usually present and even minor trauma can cause ulceration. Lesions are discrete initially but can progress to confluent ulceration. Stomatitis usually resolves spontaneously several weeks after cessation of radiation treatment. However, severe episodes may require temporary cessation of radiation. Treatment also includes the use of topical anesthetic agents and avoidance of mucosal trauma. Benadryl and Kaopectate can be beneficial. Patients often find ice chips soothing. The use of ice chips just before and 30 minutes after injection of 5-fluorouracil may reduce subsequent stomatitis.[1] As a last resort, systemic analgesics are sometimes necessary.

Almost all patients develop oral complications after receiving head and neck radiation but stomatitis can affect patients with more distant disease who receive chemotherapy. Chemotherapy induces stomatitis either by direct effect on the rapidly dividing mucosal cells or indirectly by myelosuppression and opportunistic infection (Table 4-1). Direct stomatoxicity is usually seen about 7 days after starting chemotherapy because oral mucosal cells undergo renewal by division of basal epithelial cells approximately every week. Stomatitis secondary to myelo-

Table 4-1. Chemotherapy Agents Associated With Inflammatory Lesions of the GI Tract

AGENTS COMMONLY ASSOCIATED WITH IMMUNOSUPPRESSION
Alkylating agents
  Cyclophosphamide
  Mechlorethamine
  Chlorambucil
  Busulfan
  Melphalan
  Thiotepa
Antimetabolites
  5-flourouracil
  Floxuridine
  Cytosine arabinoside
  6-mercaptopurine
  6-thioguanine
  Methotrexate
Antibiotics
  Adriamycin
  Daunomycin
  Actinomycin D
  Mithramycin
  Mitomycin C
Plant alkaloids
  Vincristine
  Vinblastine
Nitrosoureas
  BCNU
  CCNU
  Methyl CCNU
Miscellaneous
  Dicarbazine
  Procarbazine
  Hydroxyurea

AGENTS COMMONLY ASSOCIATED WITH DIRECT STOMATOXICITY
  5-Fluorouracil
  Fluxuridine
  Methotrexate
  Adriamycin
  Daunomycin
  Actinomycin D
  Mitomycin C
  Mithramycin
  Hydroxyurea

AGENTS THAT INCREASE SENSITIVITY TO RADIOTHERAPY
  Cytosine arabinoside
  Adriamycin
  Vincristine
  Bleomycin
  Actinomycin D

Inflammatory Lesions of the Gastrointestinal Tract

Table 4-1. *(Continued)*

AGENTS ASSOCIATED WITH COLITIS
  Cytosine arabinoside
  Cyclophosphamide
  Methotrexate
  Fluorouracil

Table adapted from Sonis ST. Oral complications of cancer therapy In Devita VT, Hellman S, Rosenberg SA, eds. Cancer: principles and practice of oncology. 4th ed. Philadelphia: JB Lippincott 1993;2389.

suppression usually occurs at the time of the blood count nadir, which is usually later, about 2 weeks after chemotherapy was initiated. This topic is further discussed in Chapter 17.

Oral bleeding and infection is caused by bacterial, fungal, or viral pathogens. These patients present with oral lesions, lymphadenopathy, fever, and pain. Empiric treatment with intravenous antibiotics covering gram-positive and gram-negative bacteria should be started promptly and adjusted based on culture results from the lesion and blood. The most common organisms are gram-negative including *Pseudomonas*, *Klebsiella*, *Serratia*, *Enterobacteriaceae*, *Proteus*, and *Escherichia*.

The diagnosis of an oral fungal infection is based on the lesion's appearance. The lesions begin as small pearly white patches that are firmly adherent to the underlying epithelium and which subsequently enlarge and coalesce. Removal of the lesion leaves abraded superficial ulcerated surfaces with bleeding points. Fungus can be demonstrated in potassium hydroxide smears of scrapings from the necrotic surface of the lesion. Treatment can be with topical mycostatin for early cases,[2] or with agents such as fluconazole[3] or amphotericin B. Herpes simplex infections can be primary but are usually reactivation of latent virus and are characterized by a viral syndrome of fever, anorexia, and malaise and vesicles on the mucosa. Herpes may play a role in as much as 48% of oral infections in patients undergoing chemotherapy.[4] The lesions begin as painful, itching vesicles that rupture and become encrusted with dried exudate. They usually cover the labial mucosa and extend to the circumoral skin. Treatment is with acyclovir.[5] Prophylactic acyclovir should be considered for bone marrow transplant patients and leukemia patients who are herpes simplex virus seropositive.[6,7] Regardless of the causative organism, every oral infection in such patients is extremely dangerous and potentially lethal. The mucosa serves as a portal of entry to the blood stream that can lead to widespread hematogenous dissemination.[2]

SUMMARY: STOMATITIS

1. Stomatitis usually resolves several weeks after cessation of radiation therapy.
2. Treatment includes prevention of oral trauma and the use of topical anesthetic agents.
3. Chemotherapy induces stomatitis by its direct effects on the rapidly dividing mucosal cells or by myelosuppression with accompanying opportunistic infection. Infection can be caused by bacterial, fungal, or viral pathogens and can lead to systemic sepsis.

ESOPHAGITIS

As in stomatitis, esophagitis from radiation and chemotherapy may result from a direct attack on the dividing basal cells or as a result of myelosuppression and subsequent infection. Esophagitis occurs in as many as 80% of patients undergoing combined chemotherapy and chest radiation.[8] In addition to viscous lidocaine and a bland diet, the standard treatment of radiation esophagitis is to decrease the daily dose by 10%, modify fields, or perhaps interrupt treatment. The incidence of radiation-induced esophagitis has been decreased with hyperfractionation or multiple doses per day.[9] In one study, anti-inflammatory agents protected the esophagus

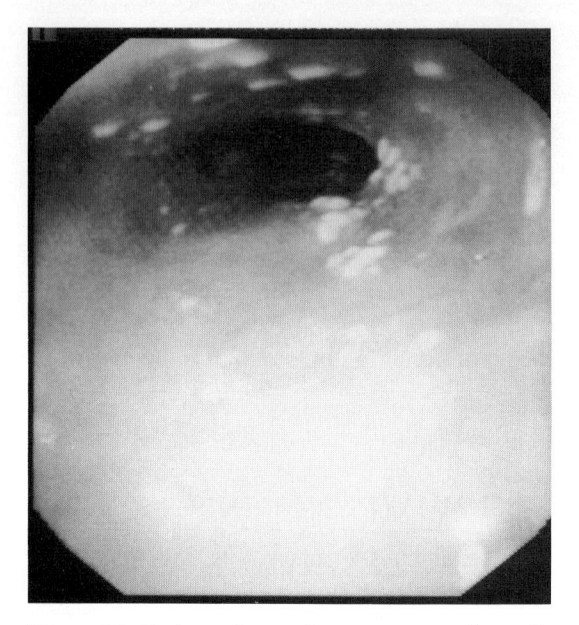

Figure 4-1. Early endoscopic appearance of *candida* esophagitis.

during radiotherapy.[10] The pain of radiation esophagitis may be due to spasm and has been reported to respond to nifedipine.[11]

In patients undergoing radiation and chemotherapy, opportunistic esophageal infection is sometimes indistinguishable from radiation-induced esophagitis. *Candida* species are the most frequent cause of infection of the esophagus in the immunocompromised patient. The patient presents with dysphagia or odynophagia. Esophagoscopy and biopsy with brushings for culture and histologic examination should be performed. The endoscopic appearance ranges from a few white plaques to a dense white-gray pseudomembrane overlying friable and ulcerated mucosa (Figs. 4-1 and 4-2).

Endoscopic examination is the most sensitive and specific way of diagnosing esophageal candidiasis. Brushings alone are often not sufficient to establish a definitive diagnosis. Biopsy is often necessary for culture and to assess intranuclear inclusion of viruses and invasion by *Candida* (Figs. 4-3 and 4-4).

However, it is not always safe to do a biopsy in thrombocytopenic patients making empiric treatment the only alternative. This can be done with oral nystatin and fluconazole or low dose amphotericin B. Intravenous miconazole has been used successfully in patients who cannot tolerate amphotericin B. There have been reports of success with oral ketoconazole prophylactically and as a treatment for diagnosed infection.[12,13] Also, oral clotrimazole has been reported to be successful in treating chronic resistant esophageal candidiasis.[14] If this is ineffective, a fungal infection is unlikely to be the cause and prophylactic acyclovir is recommended because the second most likely pathogen is herpes simplex virus. Endoscopically, herpes esophagitis appears as discrete punched out ulcers. However, bullous formation or coalescence of ulcers may give the mucosa an erosive, hemorrhagic appearance with exudates that may mimic esophageal candidiasis. Esophageal candidiasis and herpes esophagitis can occur concomitantly.[15,16] Also, in immunocompromised cancer patients, a bacterial cause of infectious esophagitis should be considered.[17] In addition to appropriate antibiotics, a semi-solid diet and analgesia with

Figure 4-2. Late endoscopic appearance of *candida* esophagitis.

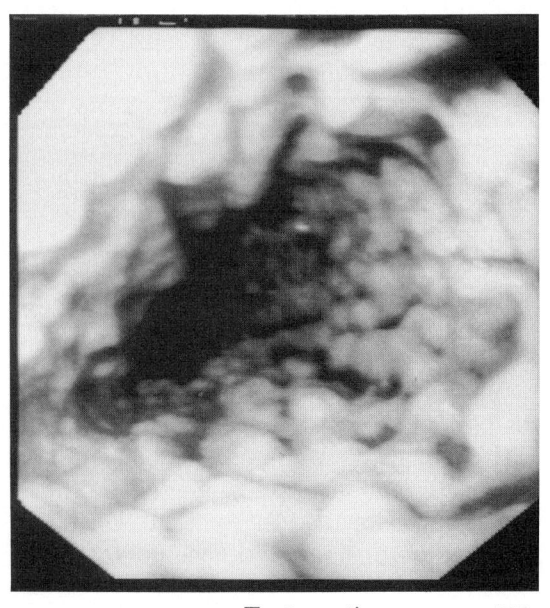

Text continues on p. 102.

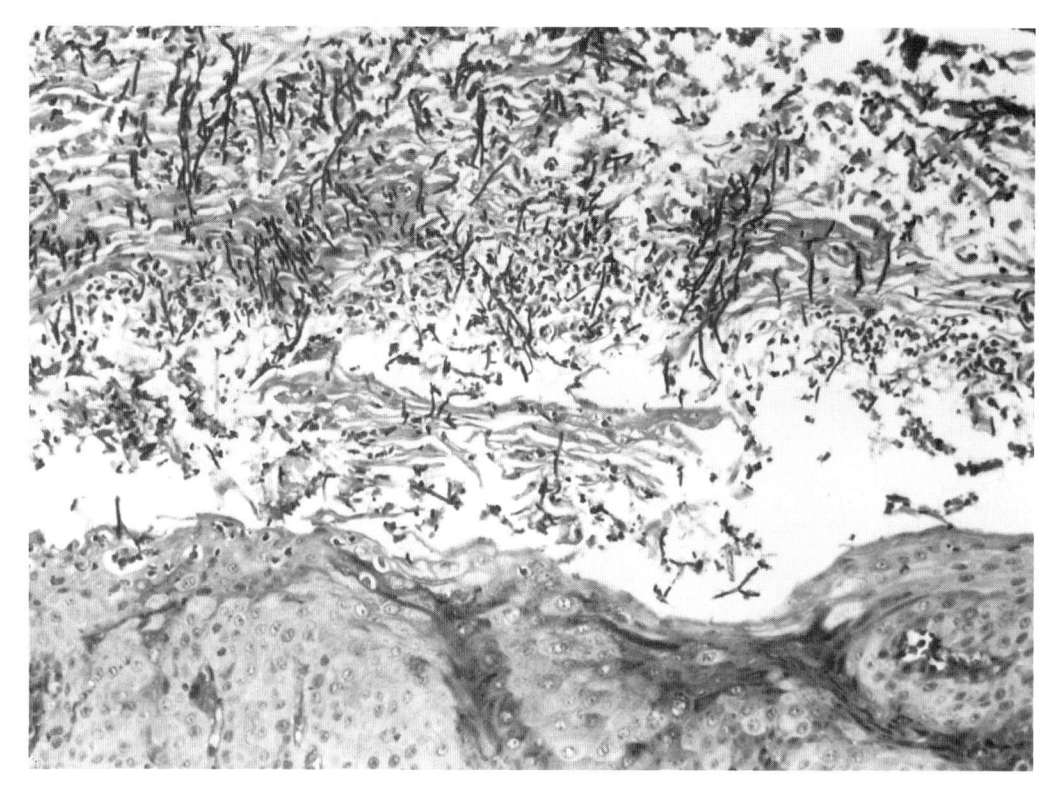

Figure 4-3. Invasive *Candida albicans* in an esophageal biopsy specimen (×100, PAS).

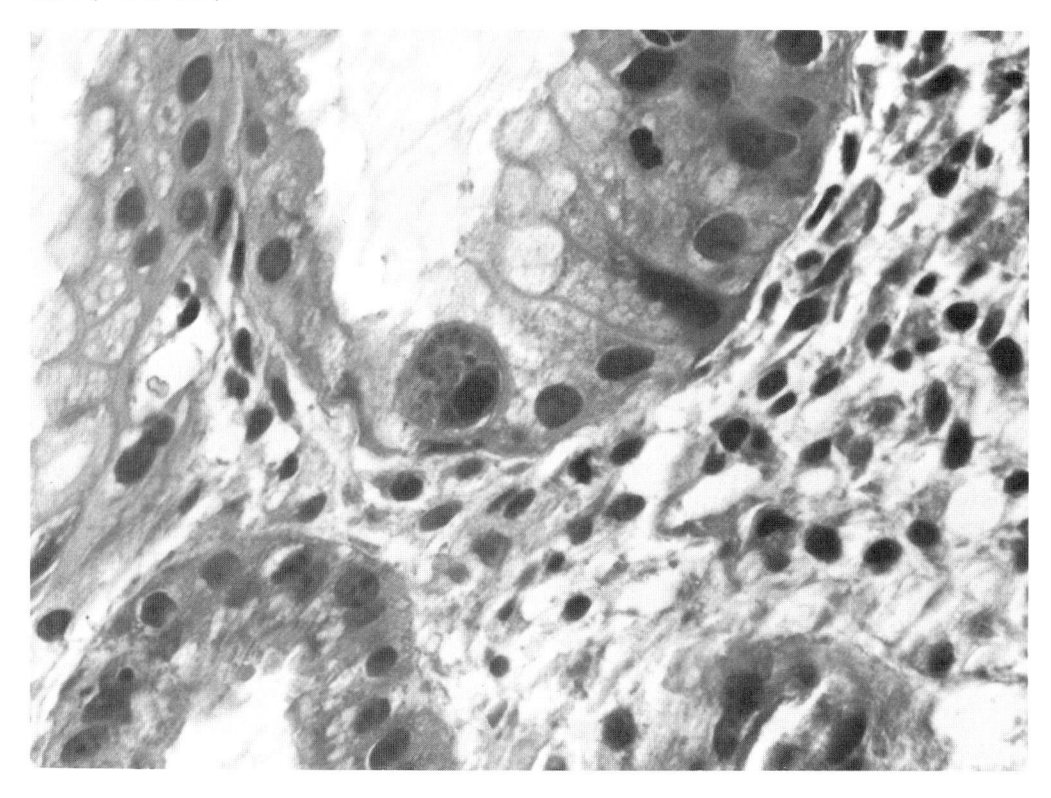

Figure 4-4. Gastric biopsy demonstrating the hallmark viral intranuclear inclusion of CMV (×400, H&E).

2% viscous lidocaine suspension are often helpful.

Late effects of radiation esophagitis are stenosis and strictures, fistulas, sinus tracts, and ulcers. There has been some success with hydrocortisone injection of strictures.[18] However, standard treatment of a stricture is dilation, although the risk of rupture is high. The poor prognosis of most patients with thoracic malignancies usually precludes surgical resection of an esophageal stricture when dilation is unsuccessful. Nasogastric feeding tubes or gastrostomy tubes may then be used to provide nutritional support.

SUMMARY: ESOPHAGITIS

1. Esophagitis is a result of direct effects on the mucosal cells or myelosuppression with opportunistic infection, as in stomatitis. It occurs in as many as 80% of patients receiving chemotherapy and thoracic irradiation.
2. *Candida* species are the most common cause of opportunistic infection of the esophagus. Biopsy may be necessary to make a definitive diagnosis.
3. Treatment is with oral nystatin and fluconazole or low dose amphotericin B.
4. Late effects of esophagitis include stenoses, strictures, fistulae, and ulcers.

GASTRITIS

Gastritis induced by nonsteroidal anti-inflammatory drugs (NSAIDs) may be the most common cause of gastritis in the cancer patient. Many cancer patients are treated with NSAIDs for pain, which may induce gastric mucosal injury. The pathogenesis is believed to be through inhibition of prostaglandin synthesis; these are important components of the gastric mucosal defense against acid. Chemotherapy and radiation also affect the mucosal barrier and increase the risk of NSAID-induced gastritis and ulceration. In patients with endoscopically documented ulceration, it is recommended that NSAIDs be discontinued and conventional antiulcer therapy with histamine-receptor antagonists be initiated.

Stress gastritis is a common occurrence in the cancer patient undergoing extensive surgery, especially in the presence of shock, sepsis, or organ failure. The erosions develop rapidly, usually within the first postoperative day and tend to begin in the proximal stomach and progress distally. Endoscopically, acute superficial bleeding gastric erosions are seen that range from petechiae to superficial ulceration. Treatment is aimed at raising the intraluminal gastric pH above 5.0. Histamine-receptor antagonists have been demonstrated to prevent stress gastritis as well as prevent established gastroduodenal stress lesions from progressing in severity and diminish bleeding.[19,20] However, success is often determined by the rapidity and effectiveness with which the underlying stressful conditions can be ameliorated. The most effective therapy for stress gastritis is prophylaxis. Surgery may be required for severe hemorrhage. If the bleeding sites cannot be sutured or excised by partial gastrectomy, total gastrectomy is warranted because there is a high incidence of rebleeding with lesser operations.

Cancer patients who have undergone partial gastrectomy, especially with a Billroth II anastomosis, frequently develop erosive gastritis. This usually develops near the anastomosis, and chronic atrophic gastritis commonly develops in the gastric remnant. In addition to radiation and chemotherapy, the pathogenesis of the gastritis is likely related to the antrectomy with the loss of antral G cells and the trophic hormone gastrin. Also, reflux of damaging intestinal juices that contain bile and pancreatic secretions may play a role. Operations designed to prevent reflux, such as conversion to Billroth I or Roux-en-Y diversion, are helpful in selected patients.

Cancer patients with myelosuppression from chemotherapy are susceptible to infectious gastritis due to viral pathogens. Cytomegalovirus (CMV) may cause gastritis; however, the virus is so prevalent in the immunocompromised host, its recovery from the stomach does not prove that it is the cause of observed inflammation and erosions. Identification in gastric biopsy specimens of classic cytomegalic cells with intranuclear inclusions along with positive cultures provides the diagnosis (see Fig. 4-4). Treatment is with gancyclovir.

With hepatic chemoembolization or totally implanted systems for hepatic arterial chemotherapy infusion, symptomatic gastric injury can occur. This is caused by direct flow of these toxic agents to the stomach through vessels distal to the catheter tip. Improper catheter placement with the tip migrating distal into the left gastric artery or proximal to the right gastric or gastroduodenal arteries increases the likelihood of this complication.[21] Gastritis secondary to hepatic arterial chemotherapy can be minimized by meticulous dissection of vessels between the hepatic artery and the stomach and proper placement of the catheter tip distal to gastric collateral vessels.[22] The catheter is usually placed through the gastroduodenal artery and it is critically important to ligate all branches of the common hepatic artery distal to this to avoid inadvertent infusions of chemotherapy. Intraoperative fluorescein injection through the catheter using a Woods lamp to examine the abdominal viscera can help detect and eliminate all direct flow of infused chemotherapy to the stomach.

■ **SUMMARY: GASTRITIS**

1. Most commonly caused by NSAIDs.
2. Stress may cause gastritis in patients undergoing major operative procedures. Treatment is directed at elevating the gastric pH.
3. Marginal ulcerations near the site of anastomosis, particularly in patients who have undergone Billroth II anastomoses, also are a common cause of gastritis.
4. Gastritis may result from the use of hepatic artery chemotherapy through vessels (*e.g.*, the right gastric artery) that were inadvertently not ligated at the time of catheter placement or through a catheter that has migrated.

■

ENTERITIS

Acutely after radiation, abnormal epithelial cell replication results in villous atrophy and a decrease in mucosal thickness that is accompanied by hyperemia, edema, and inflammation of the intestinal mucosa. The dose of radiation that causes radiation enteritis is close to that producing tumor eradication. The margin of safety between the therapeutic and toxic doses is small. The patient presents with diarrhea, nausea, and vomiting usually during the second week of therapy. The watery diarrhea usually resolves about 6 weeks after treatment is completed. Early symptoms of nausea and vomiting usually respond to phenothiazines or dopamine antagonists. The pathophysiology and treatment of chemotherapy-induced emesis are fully discussed in Chapter 7.

Diarrhea and abdominal cramps associated with acute enteritis usually respond to conventional antidiarrheal drugs such as loperamide and diphenoxylate. These drugs act by slowing intestinal transit, thereby allowing more effective absorption. Some patients respond to bile salt-sequestering agents such as cholestyramine.[23] Hydrophilic mucilloids may give more bulk to the stool if mild diarrhea exists. A 10% reduction in the daily radiation dose may produce significant relief in some patients without risking the chances for cure. Malnourished patients may benefit from an elemental diet or parenteral nutrition before and during radiation treatment. When the intestinal mucosal barrier has been impaired by radiation, normal flora can cause infection. If bacterial overgrowth is the cause of the diarrhea, broad-spectrum antibiotics alter the course and decrease abdominal pain.

The interval from time of completion of radiation therapy to development of chronic radiation bowel damage is 3 months to 30 years (see Chapter 7 for further discussion of intestinal complications of radiation therapy). Months after radiation therapy, epithelial cells of small arterioles in the submucosa may undergo degeneration and thrombosis resulting in progressive ischemia. The serosa can develop hyalinization with collagen, and adhesions can develop between loops of intestine. Ischemic necrosis in such areas can lead to formation of fistulous tracts, abscesses, and strictures.[24]

The treatment of enteritis includes parenteral nutrition, bowel rest, and occasionally steroids.[25] Fortunately, these complications rarely require surgical intervention because surgery in the face of severe radiation injury has very high morbidity and mortality rates. In one study, 30% suffered mortality and all patients experienced morbidity.[26] When operation is required, resection of the affected intestines and primary anastomosis using uninvolved bowel is preferred (further discussion is found in Chapter 7). Resection with anastomosis between the ascending, transverse, or descending colon and uninvolved bowel is preferred by some to colostomy or bypass. The decision to resect or perform a bypass must be individualized as there are some situations where bypass is preferred. In fact, the complication rates of resection and bypass are similar.

Without resection, the progression of radiation injury that leads to late complications is not prevented.[27,28] A sigmoid colostomy, although providing solid stool, may be followed by more complications than a transverse colostomy placed in a nonirradiated colon. With extensive distal disease, where even the anal canal is damaged, abdominalperineal resection or colonal pull-through may be useful options in select patients.[29] Avoiding extensive lysis of adhesions and tacking the omentum around anastomoses performed on irradiated bowel have been shown to decrease fistula formation.[28] Factors that increase the incidence of radiation-induced enteritis include thin physique, mesenteric vascular occlusive disease, and previous abdominal surgery. Elderly women with thin physiques have been reported to have an increased amount of small bowel in the pelvis making the amount of small bowel exposure greater in pelvic irradiation.[30] Mesenteric vascular disease increases the vulnerability to small vessel injury caused by radiation. Previous abdominal surgery increases the susceptibility to radiation-induced enteritis because adhesions cause loops of bowel to be fixed in one position, allowing excessive radiation to be delivered to a localized area of intestine.[31] These factors often have a greater effect on the development of small bowel damage than radiation dose and interval. In patients with these risk factors, consideration may be given to alternative modes of treatment when feasible.[32] A polyglycolic acid mesh sling placed at the original cancer operation has been used to prevent bowel descent into the true pelvis and decrease the rate of radiation enteritis[24] (See Chapter 7 for further discussion of intestinal complications of radiation therapy, including Figures 7-4A and 7-4B). This can also be accomplished by suturing the bladder to the rectum, uterus, or sacrum.[28] Some chemotherapeutic agents cause intestinal epithelial injury and increase sensitivity to radiotherapy (see Table 4-1).

SUMMARY: ENTERITIS

1. Radiation therapy is a common cause of enteritis in the cancer patient because of direct effects on rapidly dividing mucosal cells in acute toxicity and because of effects on vessels in chronic toxicity.

2. Prevention is the best approach. Elevating the small bowel out of the pelvis by using a mesh sling may be an effective preventive measure. Initial nonoperative treatment includes parenteral nutrition and bowel rest.
3. Surgical treatment may include resection or bypass depending on individual circumstances. Obstruction is the most common indication for surgery.

COLITIS

In patients receiving systemic chemotherapeutic agents for treatment of malignancy, it is often difficult to discern the cause of acute colitis from a variety of potential causes including infectious, antibiotic-associated, radiation-induced, primary disease induced, or chemotherapy-related. Several chemotherapeutic agents have a primary toxic effect on the colon (see Table 4-1).

Clostridium difficile can colonize the colon of cancer patients whose flora has been altered with antineoplastic agents or antibiotics. *C. difficile* produces colonic mucosal damage by release of a potent exotoxin. The infection can be hospital-acquired; the organism has been cultured 5 months after an infected patient has moved from a hospital room.[33,34] The symptoms of diarrhea and crampy abdominal pain usually begin during the first week of chemotherapy, although there is a wide range of time during which they may occur. Some patients complain of diffuse lower abdominal pain. Fever, chills, and dehydration may accompany severe episodes. Abdominal distention and diffuse tenderness are the usual physical findings. Small excrescences on the rectal mucosa due to pseudomembranes sometimes can be palpated. The diagnosis can be made by endoscopic examination, which reveals the characteristic yellow-white, raised plaques, approximately 2 to 5 mm in diameter, scattered over the mucosal surface. However, the diagnosis is not excluded by the absence of pseudomembranes on sigmoidoscopy because the findings may be limited to the more proximal colon.[35] Pseudomembranes will be noted on rigid sigmoidoscopy in 77% and by flexible sigmoidoscopy to 60 cm in 91%. Colonoscopy beyond 60 cm is necessary to make the diagnosis in the remaining 9%.[36] The presence of *C. difficile* and its toxin in stool samples is a more rapid and cost-effective diagnostic method. The new latex *C. difficile* toxin test provides immediate and specific results.[37] Oral vancomycin and metronidazole have equivalent efficacy and are tolerated to a similar extent, but metronidazole is considerably more economical.[38–40] The stool should be cultured to prove the absence of *C. difficile* and to identify patients prone to relapse.[41] These patients should be treated with tapering doses of vancomycin.[42] Chemotherapy may need to be stopped temporarily. (Infectious colitis is discussed in Chapter 16.)

Serologic prevalence rates for CMV are high in the general population. In most people, the infection is not a significant clinical illness and enters a latent phase that is lifelong. Those who are immunocompromised may suffer episodes of viral reactivation. The colonic picture of CMV is variable and includes erythema, petechial hemorrhage, and occasionally vesicles or ulcerations are seen. The hallmark of CMV infection is histologic demonstration of the viral intranuclear inclusion (see Fig. 4-4). Ganciclovir, which is structurally related to acyclovir, inhibits CMV replication and has been demonstrated to prolong survival.[43] (Viral infections are discussed in Chapter 16.)

Another inflammatory condition of the colon seen in the cancer patient is diversion colitis, a recently described inflammatory disease that occurs in a segment of colon from which the fecal stream has been diverted.[44] The prevalence of this disorder in patients with such anatomy is unknown. The mucosal inflammatory changes in the diverted segment of colon may be common with about 30% of those with colitis becoming symptomatic. Symptoms are purulent discharge, abdominal cramps, tenesmus, and bleeding.[44] The symptoms can occur months to years postoperatively. Endoscopically and histologically, the inflammatory changes resemble ulcerative colitis. The cause of this inflammation is unknown. Overgrowth of normal flora or development of invasive pathogenic organisms in the excluded segment have not been demonstrated. Diversion of short-chain fatty acids present in stool, the preferred energy source for colonic epithelial cells, may be the cause of this condition.[44] Instillation of a solution containing short-chain fatty acids twice daily resulted in the disappearance of symptoms and the inflammatory changes observed at endoscopy over a period of 4 to 6 weeks. Remission has been maintained up to 4 months by continued enemas but relapse is rapid if treatment is stopped.[45] The inflammatory process and symptoms resolve promptly after reanastomosis, which is the treatment of choice whenever possible. There also have been recent case reports of successful treatment with corticosteroid and 5-amino-salicylate enemas.

The colon, being relatively immobile due to its partial retroperitoneal position, can receive significant doses of radiation. Acute radiation effects on the colon and rectum are nearly universal, and are thoroughly reviewed in Chapter 7. As with the small bowel, the radiation tolerance limits of the colon and tumoricidal doses are similar making the achievement of a therapeutic dose without toxicity difficult. Symptoms of diarrhea, tenesmus, cramping, and abdominal and rectal pain occur in three fourths of the patients receiving 4000 cGy or more of external radiotherapy.[46] Symptoms usually respond to antispasmodics or antidiarrheals and resolve promptly with completion of radiation therapy. Although the symptoms occur within 1 year in 65% of cases, the late manifestations of radiation colitis can present years after treatment.[46] The most common chronic radiation-induced injury to the colon and rectum is radiation proctitis. Patients usually present with hematochezia, change in bowel habits, and pain. Chronic slow blood loss may necessitate transfusion. Colonoscopy is indicated for diagnosis and exclusion of other entities such as recurrent colon cancer and infectious colitis. In most cases, symptoms are reversible and respond to a low residue, lactose-free diet, and antispasmodics. Other medical treatments include systemic steroids, steroid suppositories and enemas, sucralfate enemas, and oral sulfasalazine.[47] In some cases, chronic slow bleeding can be treated with laser coagulation of bleeding telangiectasias.[48,49] Cholestyramine has also been shown to control radiation-induced diarrhea.[50] Resection is reserved for resistant cases because the morbidity and mortality rates are increased in the face of prior irradiation. Indications for surgery include perforation, bleeding, obstruction, fistula, and intractable colitis or proctitis. Regardless of the indication, resection of all radiation-damaged colon with anastomosis of nonirradiated bowel is the operation of choice and diversion should be avoided. If an aggressive operation is planned, the preoperative placement of ureteral catheters may be useful to aid in the intraoperative identification of the ureters, especially in patients who have had previous extensive surgical procedures.

SUMMARY: COLITIS

1. Several chemotherapeutic agents have direct colonic toxicity, but colitis may also result from a variety of other causes: infectious, radiation-induced, and antibiotic-associated.
2. *Clostridium difficile* is a common nosocomial infection causing colonic symptoms and toxicity. It can be detected in stool samples and is treated with oral vancomycin or metronidazole.
3. Colonic CMV infections are also common in the immunocompromised patient.

4. Radiation induced colonic injury is also common. Most patients respond to nonoperative therapy. Resection may be necessary in some cases.

SUMMARY

Inflammatory lesions in the gastrointestinal tract of the cancer patient are quite common and can occur anywhere from mouth to anus. There are two mechanisms usually implicated: direct mucosal injury and myelosuppression with accompanying opportunistic infection. Radiation-induced injury is usually a direct effect of radiation on the involved mucosa. Stomatitis commonly accompanies head and neck irradiation and when due to infection may be of bacterial, fungal, or viral origin. Esophagitis is commonly caused by *Candida* infection and is treated with oral nystatin and fluconazole or low dose amphotericin B. Gastritis is commonly caused by NSAID use, stress gastritis associated with major resections, Billroth II anastomoses with marginal ulceration, and viral infections. Poorly placed or migrated hepatic artery infusion catheters can lead to inadvertent gastric infusion with high concentrations of chemotherapeutic agents and resultant gastritis. Enteritis is commonly caused by radiation therapy. Prevention is the best approach, and elevating the bowel out of the pelvis may reduce the incidence of this complication. Treatment usually is nonoperative with bowel rest and parenteral antibiotics. Surgical therapy is undertaken only when necessary and, although resection is performed when possible, bypass of the diseased segment may be appropriate in some situations. The complication rate in patients undergoing bypass and resection are similar. Colitis may be due to radiation effects, *C. difficile* infection, CMV infection, or other causes. Most patients respond to nonoperative therapy.

REFERENCES

1. Mahood DJ, Dose AM, Loprinzi CL, et al. Inhibition of fluorouracil-induced stomatitis by oral cryotherapy. J Clin Oncol 1991;9(3):449.
2. Epstein JB, Pearsall NN, Truelove EL: Oral candidiasis: effects of antifungal therapy upon clinical signs and symptoms, salivary antibody, and mucosal adherence of Candida albicans. Oral Surg 1981;51(1):32.
3. Drcmery V, Koza I, Hornikova M, et al. Fluconazole in the treatment of mycotic oropharyngeal stomatitis and esophagitis in neutropenic cancer patients. Chemotherapy 1991;37:343.
4. Montgomery MT, Redding SW, LeMaistre CF. The incidence of oral herpes simplex virus infection in patients undergoing cancer chemotherapy. Oral Surg Oral Med Oral Pathol 1986;61:238.
5. Wade JC, Vewton B, McLaren C, et al. Intravenous acyclovir to treat mucocutaneous herpes simplex virus infection after marrow transplantation. Ann Intern Med 1982;96(3):265.
6. Saral R, Burns WH, Laskin OL, et al. Acyclovir prophylaxis of herpes-simplex-virus infections. A randomized double-blind, controlled trial in bone-marrow-transplant recipients. N Engl J Med 1981;305:63.
7. Woo SB, Sonis ST, Sonis AL. The role of herpes simplex virus in the development of oral mucositis in bone marrow transplant recipients. Cancer 1990;66:2375.
8. Umsawasdi T, Valdivieso M, Barkley HT, et al. Esophageal complications from combined chemoradiotherapy (cyclophosphamide + adriamycin + cysplatin + XRT) in the treatment of non-small cell lung cancer. Int J Radiat Oncol Biol Phys 1985;11(3): 511.
9. Seydel HG, Eiener-West M, Urtasun R, et al. Hyperfractionation in the radiation therapy of unresectable non-oat cell carcinoma of the lung: Preliminary report of a RTOG pilot study. Int J Radiat Oncol Biol Phys 1985;11(10):1841.
10. Northway MG, Eastwood GL, Libshitz HI, et al. Anti-inflammatory agents protect opossum esophagus during radiotherapy. Dig Dis Sci 1982;27(10):923.
11. Finkelstein E. Nifedipine for radiation oesophagitis. Lancet 1986:1205.
12. Fazio RA, Wickremesinghe PC, Arsura EL. Ketoconazole treatment of candida esophagitis-A prospective study of 12 cases. Am J Gastroenterol 1983;78(5):261.
13. Hann IM, Corringham R, Keaney M, et al. Ketoconazole versus nystatin plus amphotericin B for fungal prophylaxis in severely immunocompromised patients. Lancet 1982;1(8276): 826.

14. Ginsburg CH, Braden GL, Tasuber AI, et al. Oral clotrimazole in the treatment of esophageal candidiasis. Am J Med 1981;71:891.
15. Brayko CM, Kozarek RA, Sanowski RA, et al. Type I herpes simplex esophagitis with concomitant esophageal moniliasis. J Clin Gastroenterol 1982;4:351.
16. Mirra SS, Bryan JA, Butz WC, et al. Concomitant herpes-monilial esophagitis: Case report with ultrastructural study. Hum Pathol 1982;13(8):760.
17. Walsh TJ, Belitsos NJ, Hamilton SR. Bacterial esophagitis in immunocompromised patients. Arch Intern Med 1986;146:1345.
18. Nelson RS, Hernandez AJ, Goldstein HM, et al. Treatment of irradiation esophagitis. Value of hydrocortisone injection. Am J Gastroenterol 1979;71:17.
19. Peura DA, Johnson LF. Cimetidine for prevention and treatment of gastroduodenal mucosal lesions in patients in an intensive care unit. Ann Intern Med 1985;103(2):173.
20. Basso N, Bagarani M, Materia A, et al. Cimetidine and antacid prophylaxis of acute upper gastrointestinal bleeding in high-risk patients. Controlled, randomized trial. Am J Surg 1981;141:339.
21. Narsete T, Ansfield F, Wirtanen G, et al. Gastric ulceration in patients receiving intrahepatic infusion of 5-fluorouracil. Ann Surg 1977;186(6):734.
22. Hohn DC, Stagg RJ, Price DC, et al. Avoidance of gastroduodenal toxicity in patients receiving hepatic arterial 5-fluoro-2-deoxyuridine. J Clin Oncol 1985;3(9):1257.
23. Kinsella TJ, Bloomer WD. Tolerance of the intestine to radiation therapy. Surg Gynecol Obstet 1980;151:237.
24. Devereux DF, Davanah MT, Feldman MI, et al. Small bowel exclusion from the pelvis by a polyglycolic acid mesh sling. J Surg Oncol 1984;26:107.
25. Loiudice TA, Lang JA. Treatment of radiation enteritis: A comparison study. Am J Gastroenterol 1983;78(8):481.
26. O'Brien PH, Jenrette JM, Garvin AJ. Radiation enteritis. Am Surg 1987;53:501.
27. Makela J, Nevasaari K, Kairaluoma MI. Surgical treatment of intestinal radiation injury. J Surg Oncol 1987;36:93.
28. Deitel M, To TB. Major intestinal complications of radiotherapy. Management and nutrition. Arch Surg 1987;122:1421.
29. Galland RB, Spencer J. Natural history and surgical management of radiation enteritis. Br J Surg 1987;74:742.
30. Green N, Iba G, Smith WR. Measures to minimize small intestine injury in the irradiated pelvis. Cancer 1975;35:1633.
31. LoIudice T, Baxter D, Balint J. Effects of abdominal surgery on the development of radiation enteropathy. Gastroenterology 1977;73:1093.
32. Potish RA. Importance of predisposing factors in the development of enteric damage. Am J Clin Oncol (CCT) 1982;5:198.
33. Kim KH, Fedety R, Batts DH, et al. Isolation of clostridium difficile from the environment of contacts of patients with antibiotic-associated colitis. J Infect Dis 1981;143(1):42.
34. Fekety R, Kim KH, Brown D, et al. Epidemiology of antibiotic-associated colitis. Isolation of clostridium difficile from the hospital environment. Am J Med 1981;70:906.
35. Tedesco FJ. Antibiotic associated pseudomembranous colitis with negative proctosigmoidoscopy examination. Gastroenterology 1979;77:295.
36. Tedesco FJ, Corless JK, Brownstein RE. Rectal sparing in antibiotic-associated pseudomembranous colitis: A prospective study. Gastroenterology 1982;83:1259
37. Peterson LR, Holter JJ, Shanholtzer CJ, et al. Detection of clostridium difficile toxins A (enterotoxin) and B (cytotoxin) in clinical specimens. Evaluation of a latex agglutination test. Am J Clin Pathology 1986;86(2):208.
38. Teasley DG, Olson MM, Gebhard RL, et al. Prospective randomized trial of metronidazole versus vancomycin for clostridium-difficile-associated diarrhea and colitis. Lancet 1983;1:1043.
39. Cherry RD, Portnoy D, Jabbari M, et al. Metronidazole: an alternate therapy for antibiotic-associated colitis. Gastroenterology 1982;82:849.
40. Tedesco F, Markham R, Gurwith M, et al. Oral vancomycin for antibiotic-associated pseudomembranous colitis. Lancet 1978;2(8083):226.
41. Walters BAJ, Roberts R, Stafford R, et al. Relapse of antibiotic associated colitis: endogenous persistence of clostridium difficile during vancomycin therapy. Gut 1983;24:206.
42. Tedesco FJ, Gordon D, Fortson WC. Approach to patients with multiple relapses of antibiotic-associated pseudomembranous colitis. Am J Gastroenterol 1985;8(11):867.
43. Erice A, Chou S, Biron KK, et al. Progressive disease due to ganciclovir-resistant cytomegalovirus in immunocompromised patients. N Engl J Med 1989;320(5):289.
44. Glotzer DJ, Glick ME, Goldman H. Proctitis and colitis following diversion of the fecal stream. Gastroenterology 1981;80:438.

45. Ona FV, Boger JN. Rectal bleeding due to diversion colitis. Am J Gastroenterol 1985;80(1):40.
46. Jao SW, Beart RW, Gunderson LL. Surgical treatment of radiation injuries of the colon and rectum. Am J Surg 1986;151:272.
47. Goldstein F, Khoury J, Thornton JJ. Treatment of chronic radiation enteritis and colitis with salicylazosulfapyridine and systemic corticosteriods. Am J Gastroenterol 1976;64(3):201.
48. Ahlquist DA, Gostout CJ, Viggiano TR, et al. Laser therapy for severe radiation-induced rectal bleeding. Mayo Clin Proc 1986;61:927.
49. Berken CA. Nd:YAG Laser therapy for gastrointestinal bleeding due to radiation colitis. Am J Gastroenterol 1985;80(9):730.
50. Heusinkveld RS, Manning MR, Aristizabal SA. Control of radiation-induced diarrhea with cholestyramine. Int J Radiat Oncol Biol Phys 1978;4:687.

Hepatobiliary Disease in the Cancer Patient

JAMES V. SITZMANN

The management of hepatobiliary disease in the cancer patient can be broadly divided into two main categories. The first is the treatment of primary hepatocellular processes associated with either primary or secondary damage to the liver from either a tumor's direct effects or the toxicity of antitumor therapy. Secondly, the treatment of biliary tract disease, which may be calculous disease or biliary tract disease due to primary or secondary effects of tumors or tumor therapy.

MALIGNANT BILIARY TRACT OBSTRUCTION: CHOLANGIOCARCINOMA

Malignant biliary tract obstruction can occur as a result of either primary hepatic tumors or metastatic disease. The most straightforward biliary obstruction is the primary biliary tract tumor. Almost all primary biliary tumors are adenocarcinomas arising from the bile duct epithelium. All are classified broadly as cholangiocarcinomas.[1] The site of occurrence determines in large part the treatment and ultimate prognosis. Distal common bile duct cholangiocarcinomas, in fact, have a rather good prognosis.[2] They tend to obstruct the bile duct early and are localized tumors that are amenable to resection via the Whipple procedure. Several groups have documented significant long-term (5-year) survival using the Whipple procedure in the treatment of distal common bile duct cholangiocarcinomas[3–5] (Fig. 5-1), as distal common bile duct adenocarcinomas may also be confused with duodenal or pancreatic adenocarcinomas. Histologically they may be quite difficult to distinguish. These tumors are also discussed in Chapter 2.

The clinical work-up of such tumors is fairly straightforward, as they tend to present with asymptomatic jaundice. Upper abdominal 3-dimensional (3-D) imaging with either computed tomography (CT) scan, magnetic resonance imaging (MRI), or ultrasonography shows a dilated common bile duct in the absence of a pancreatic-head mass. Typically in the absence of a pancreatic-head mass, endoscopic retrograde cholangiopancreatography (ERCP) demonstrates the absence of a duodenal mass or lesion, a patent pancreatic duct, and a tightly obstructed common bile duct with a typical "crow's beak" deformity. There is some debate in the literature as to whether there is a role for preoperative biliary drainage in this setting. Certainly in most patients the obstruction is acute, the patient is afebrile, and there is little need to invade the duct with either an endoscopically placed transhepatic biliary stent or a transhepatic percutaneously placed biliary stent. If the bilirubin is markedly elevated (>12 mg/dL),

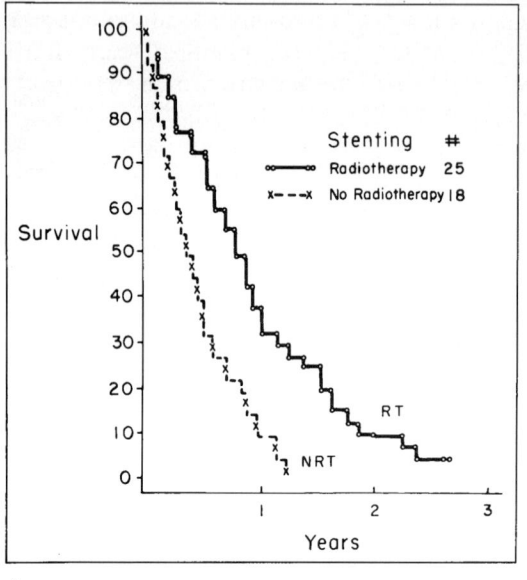

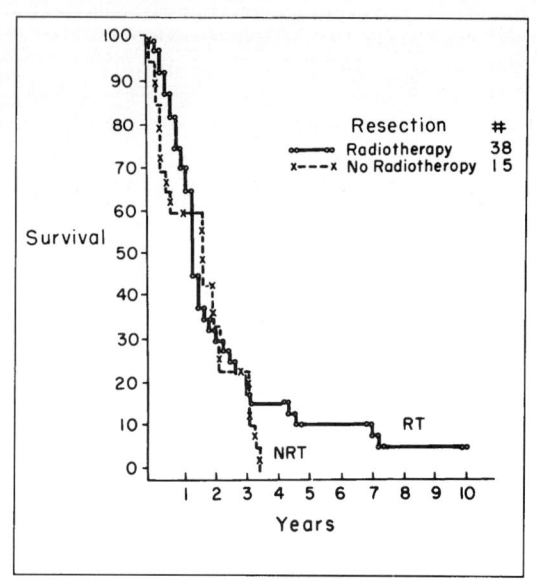

Figure 5-1. A. Actuarial survival of 43 surgically palliated patients managed with postoperative radiation (RT, n=25) or no radiation therapy (NRT, n=18) at The Johns Hopkins Hospital. This retrospective analysis, as with many others in the literature, suggests improved survival for patients receiving radiotherapy. However, no prospective randomized data have proved that radiotherapy is beneficial. **B.** Actuarial survival of 53 surgically resected patients managed with postoperative radiation (RT, n=38) or no radiotherapy (NRT, n=15) at The Johns Hopkins Hospital. Although no statistically significant difference was present between the two groups, only long-term survivors received radiation therapy after resection. From Cameron JL, Pitt HA, Zinner MJ, et al. Management of proximal cholangiocarcinomas by surgical resection and radiotherapy. Am J Surg 1990;159:91.

some surgeons feel more comfortable with a preoperative biliary drain, with the knowledge that there are risks to the drainage procedure. A CT scan of the chest should be obtained to rule out pulmonary metastasis and visceral renal angiography to rule out splanchnic renal involvement.

Proximal biliary duct cholangiocarcinomas involving the biliary bifurcation are classically known as *Klatskin tumors*. Although rare, they also present with asymptomatic jaundice. Because of the close proximity to the portal vein, which is immediately subjacent to the bile duct and the common hepatic artery, the tumors frequently involve these structures. For this reason, visceral angiography and percutaneous transhepatic cholangiography are useful in staging these tumors. In a study at The Johns Hopkins Hospital, of 85 patients with proximal cholangiocarcinomas, 32% had arteriographic evidence of venous or arterial encasement. Obtaining a CT or MRI scan is also important in these patients to determine if there is a mass lesion involving either right or left lobes. Lesions that involve a lobe or occlude or impinge on a lobar branch of the portal vein, require a lobectomy. The decision should be made preoperatively whether these lesions are resectable and whether or not to treat the patient palliatively with bilateral transhepatic stents and chemo- or radiotherapy, as opposed to operative exploration.

Operative exploration involves resection of the tumor mass in the porta hepatis or proximal bile duct, with or without a synchronous hepatic lobectomy. All attempts are made to obtain negative margins, although this can be very difficult to achieve, as cholangiocarcinoma tends to grow proximally in the duct and involve the duct wall outside of the tumor mass itself. Therefore, although the surgical procedure's intent is to achieve "negative margins," frequently it is only palliative for the patient with resection of the tumor mass and restoration of biliary continuity. It is possible at the time of laparotomy to determine that the patient is not a candidate for resection, even with a palliative intent. Postoperatively, patients can receive intrahepatic radiotherapy, with or without chemotherapy. Although several studies suggest that there is improved survival for patients receiving radiotherapy, either postoperatively or in the palliative setting, there has been no prospective randomized trial to document this.

Nonoperative management of cholangiocarcinomas generally involves placement of percutaneous transhepatic stents.[6] Endoscopic stents can be used for distal bile duct lesions; however, in general, endoscopically placed stents are difficult to maintain and establish adequate bilateral lobar drainage because of the more proximal position of these tumors.[7] Thus, the percutaneous approach tends to be the most commonly used modality.[8]

The prognosis of patients with cholangiocarcinoma is quite poor because of the usually advanced stage of the tumor at the time of diagnosis (see Fig. 5-1). In general, patients who have unresectable tumors with or without operative procedures have a mean survival less than 2 years, and the survival of patients managed with operative therapy in most series is not significantly better. The most common nonsurgical therapy in either the adjuvant or in the treatment setting in cholangiocarcinomas is 5-fluorouracil (5-FU) plus radiation therapy.[9]

Gallbladder cancer and peripheral bile duct cholangiocarcinoma are also two rare forms of biliary tract cancer. Gallbladder cancer occurs generally in the elderly, and there is a slight association with calcification of the gallbladder wall.[10] In general, gallbladder cancer is found incidentally following a routine cholecystectomy for stone disease, or following biliary duct obstruction due to tumor growth into the porta hepatis. This latter situation is almost invariably a late-stage disease, which is unresectable for cure. The most aggressive approach has been delineated by Japanese surgical groups who have advocated a wide *en bloc* resection (combined gallbladder plus liver resection) and perihepatic nodal dissection.[11–13] This is effective palliative therapy for early stage disease (*i.e.*, that found incidentally in cholecystectomy for other reasons) (see Table 5-1).[14]

Peripheral cholangiocarcinomas generally present as a liver mass in conjunction with biliary obstruction above the porta hepatis. These tumors tend to be very aggressive, with diffuse involvement of the biliary tree. Although technically resectable, these lesions carry a 2-year survival not significantly different from that of cholangiocarcinoma of the major extrahepatic biliary tree.

SUMMARY: MALIGNANT BILIARY TRACT OBSTRUCTION: CHOLANGIOCARCINOMA

1. Obstruction of the biliary tree can result from primary tumors or metastatic disease. Primary biliary tract tumors are classified as cholangiocarcinomas. Tumors of the distal common duct have a rather good prognosis.
2. Evaluation of these patients usually includes a CT scan or MRI scan and imaging of the tumor with ERCP if possible. Visceral angiography is useful in Klatskin tumors to evaluate vascular involvement.
3. Resection is carried out if possible, although it may be only palliative. Percutaneous or endoscopically placed stents may be good palliation in the patient for whom resection for cure is not possible.

Table 5-1. Carcinoma of the Gallbladder

STAGING AND PROGNOSIS BY THE NEVIN CLASSIFICATION

Nevin Stage	Depth	5-Year Survival (%)
Stage I	Mucosa only	50–97
Stage II	Muscularis	57–72
Stage III	All layers	0–25
Stage IV	Lymph node involvement	0–20
Stage V	Liver invasion Adjacent organs Distant metastasis	0–15

TNM STAGING SYSTEM FOR GALLBLADDER CARCINOMA

Stage I	T1 N0 M0	Tumor limited to mucosa and muscularis No lymph nodes No metastasis
Stage II	T2 N0 M0	Tumor invading subserosa
Stage III	T3 or N1 M0	Tumor into liver (less than 2 cm) or one adjacent organ Lymph node involvement
Stage IV	T4 N0 or N1 or M1	Tumor more than 2 cm into liver or invading two or more adjacent organs Distant metastasis

INFECTIONS OF THE BILIARY TREE

The major infectious processes involving the biliary tree in cancer patients are either acalculous cholecystitis or cholangitis. Calculous disease is a common source of infection of the biliary tree in the general population.[15] It is well described in any general surgery textbook, and its management will not be discussed in this chapter. Rather, this section will concentrate on acalculous cholecystitis and cholangitis in the cancer population.

Acalculous cholecystitis

Acalculous cholecystitis in patients with cancer occurs following intensive high-dose chemotherapy following bone marrow transplantation, and following intrahepatic arterial or regional chemotherapy of the liver, or chemoembolization. Acalculous cholecystitis can be a life-threatening complication. It is particularly dangerous because it can be easily misdiagnosed and because of its potential to rapidly progress to frank gallbladder necrosis, gangrene, and bile peritonitis. In general, with an intact hemopoietic and immune system, patients present with an exquisitely tender mass in the right upper quadrant, accompanied by high fever and leukocytosis. In the aplastic or the compromised patient, which occurs frequently in oncologic patients, the leukocytosis is frequently relative or completely absent. Therefore, the surgeon must be acutely aware of shifts in the white blood cell count leading to more immature forms or, in a patient following bone marrow transplant, any upper right quadrant pain associated with fever, which would mandate a sonographic evaluation.

Most surgeons obtain a sonogram in all patients. The typical sonographic appearance of acalculous cholecystitis includes a thickened gallbladder wall, with or without sludge. A particularly worrisome variant is the emphysematous gallbladder, which is the appearance of gas in the wall of the gallbladder or in the gallbladder fossa. This denotes the presence of gas-forming organisms such as *Escherichia coli* or *Clostridium* species. The diagnosis of acute cholecystitis (calculous or acalculous) may also be made by nonvisualization of the gallbladder on a Tc-HIDA scan.

In general, if the diagnosis of acalculous cholecystitis is entertained, the patient should be treated with broad-spectrum antibiotics to cover both aerobic and anaerobic organisms. Most surgeons use a combination of ampicillin and an aminoglycocide and metronidazole or clindamycin, which should be combined with a biliary drainage procedure. The drainage procedure can either be a transhepatic cystostomy, which is a transhepatic drainage of the gallbladder, or open cholecystectomy.[16] Although, laproscopic cholecystectomy is usually the surgeon's choice, in patients with acute gangrenous cholecystitis, the gallbladder is frequently so frankly necrotic, enlarged, and friable that it cannot be safely removed laproscopically and requires an open cholecystectomy.[17-19]

Chronic cholecystitis also occurs in the cancer patient. This was initially described following intra-arterial chemotherapy with 5 floxuridine (FUDR) through Infusaid™ pumps caused by high concentrations of chemotherapy in the cystic artery with the typical infusion in the gastroduodenal artery. For this reason, most patients who now undergo placement of hepatic artery infusion catheters (with or without pumps) undergo cholecystectomy at the time of catheter placement to avoid this complication. Typically, the patient presents with chronic right upper quadrant pain occasionally aggravated by a meal; a very small, shrunken, thickened gallbladder is seen on sonogram. On exploration, these patients have a woody, indurated, shrunken, and scarred gallbladder. Chronic or acute acalculous cholecystitis can occur following chemoembolization procedures. This is especially frequent if the blood supply to the right hepatic lobe is compromised during embolization with subsequent synchronous compromise of gallbladder blood flow. The diagnosis and management are the same as outlined above.

Cholangitis

Cholangitis is one of the more feared, rapidly progressive, and potentially lethal bacterial infections in the cancer patient. Originally described by Charcot in 1887 (for whom the triad of fever, abdominal pain, and jaundice is named), it is proportionally less common owing to the natural history of calculous disease, and it increasingly becomes an iatrogenic complication following instrumentation of the biliary tree.[20] Cholangitis is most commonly caused by calculous disease or it occurs following malignant duct strictures or benign duct strictures (such as sclerosing cholangitis following intra-arterial chemotherapy), or after prolonged internal endoscopic or transhepatic stent placement (Table 5-2).[21] A recent series at The Johns Hopkins Hospital indicated that over the last 40 years the incidence of calculous cholangitis had diminished markedly, whereas the incidence of malignant duct strictures causing cholangitis had doubled. The clinical presentation, however, remains remarkably similar to that described by Charcot, and expanded by Reynolds who coined a pentad that included

Table 5-2. Changing Etiology (%) of Cholangitis at The Johns Hopkins Hospital

Etiology	1952–1974 n=76	1976–1978 n=40	1983–1985 n=48	1986–1989 n=48
Choledocholithiasis	70	70	32	28
Benign duct strictures	13	18	14	12
Malignant duct strictures	17	10	30	57
Sclerosing cholangitis	0	3	24	3

Modified from Lipsett PA, Pitt HA. Acute cholangitis. Surg Clin N Am 1991;70:1297.

Charcot's triad of jaundice, fever, and abdominal pain, as well as mental confusion and hypotension.[22]

In addition to the physical findings noted above, the laboratory examination reveals leukocytosis, positive blood cultures, and elevation of the bilirubin and other liver function tests including alkaline phosphatase and serum transaminases. Imaging tests should include sonography or 3-D imaging, such as a CT scan of the abdomen to document dilated intrahepatic bile ducts. If the patient has previously been instrumented and has an indwelling biliary stent, this may be a redundant step and the dilatation may be problematic (Fig. 5-2). Therefore, patients with biliary stents should be studied immediately by their respective specialists; endoscopists should replace the endoscopic stent and the invasive radiologist should use a guidewire to exchange the transhepatic stents. If the patient does have a transhepatic stent, it can be opened and flushed and then left to open exterior drainage as a short-term immediate technique to decompress the biliary tree. In patients who have not been previously instrumented, cholangiography is indicated. If there appears to be an ampullary lesion with combined common bile duct and gallbladder dilatation, endoscopic evaluation is the choice of most surgeons. Whereas if the lesion appears higher in the biliary tree on sonography or CT scan, intrahepatic ducts are probably better stented percutaneously.[23,24]

Therapy after decompression of the biliary tree following replacement of the transhepatic or endoscopically placed stent should also include appropriate antibiotic coverage.[25] The most common organisms causing cholangitis are *Escherichia coli* or *Klebsiella*. Other organisms include *Enterobacter*, *Bacteroides* and *Pseudomonas*. Bile cultures are almost always positive in all patients, and in the majority of patients multiple organisms will be cultured. This bacteriology dictates empiric antibiotic coverage, which most physicians employ prior to obtaining the culture results. Most surgeons start triple drug therapy including an aminoglycocide, penicillin, and metronidazole or clindamycin. There has been a recent suggestion that the broad-spectrum third generation cephalosporins, or new synthetic penicillins[26,27] could be used *in lieu* of the nephrotoxic aminoglycosides. This also has some theoretic advantage in that cephalosporins and synthetic penicillins are excreted in high quantities in the bile.

Most patients resolve their cholangitis following adequate biliary drainage and antibiotic therapy. Following the resolution of biliary sepsis, the recovery of adequate liver function, and the resolution of jaundice, the surgeon can address the underlying cause of the cholangitis. If it is a malignant stricture, plans for operative management or chemoradiation therapy should be made. If it is due to long-term instrumentation of the biliary tree, the surgeon should review the possible treatment variations available, such as a larger stent, more stents, or more frequent stent changing in an effort to reduce the risk of future cholangitis.

SUMMARY: INFECTIONS OF THE BILIARY TREE

1. Acalculous cholecystitis is commonly found in patients following the chemotherapy administered with bone marrow transplantation. Leukocytosis may be absent in these immunocompromised patients. Patients with right upper quadrant pain and fever should be evaluated sonographically. A Tc-HIDA scan may also be useful in establishing the diagnosis. Patients are generally treated with antibiotics and drainage of the gallbladder with cholecystostomy or cholecystectomy.
2. Patients with cholangitis present with fever, jaundice, and right upper quadrant pain (Charcot's triad), which can be caused by stones or strictures. Patients with stents in place should have them studied radiographically. Principles of

Hepatobiliary Disease in the Cancer Patient

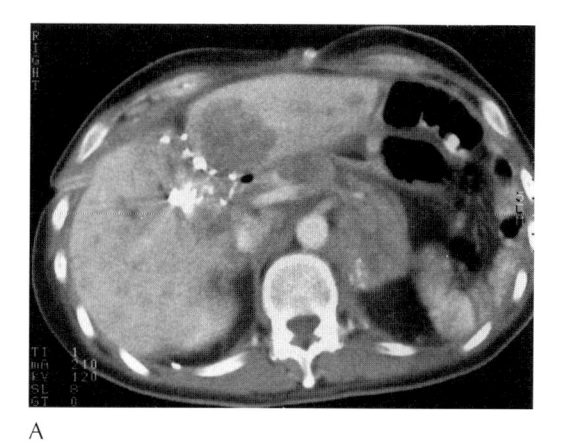

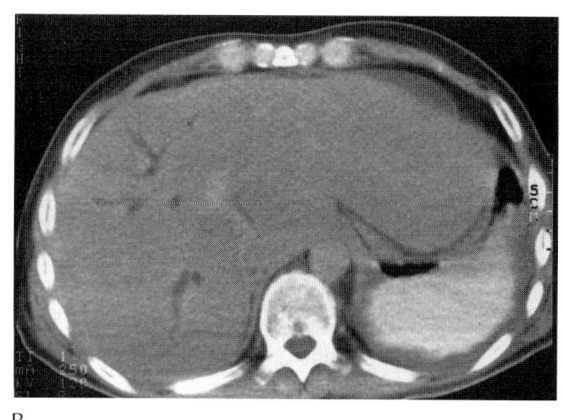

Figure 5-2. A. A patient with a large, centrally located hepatic metastasis causing bilateral biliary obstruction. **B.** Despite bilateral transcutaneous hepatic stents, the patient has undrained biliary ducts, which are a source of continued biliary sepsis.

therapy include decompression of the biliary tree and antibiotics.

PANCREATITIS

Inflammation of the pancreas gland can occur in the oncologic patient, and can be either acute or chronic. It can frequently be confused with an ileus or simple chemotherapeutic-related gastrointestinal toxicity. In particular, pancreatitis has been associated with certain chemotherapeutic agents including L-asparaginase and Ara-C. It is a fairly common cause of abdominal pain in the cancer patient and is further discussed in Chapter 1. An extensive list of causes of pancreatitis is found in Table 1-2.

A typical presentation is one of abdominal distention, vague diffuse abdominal pain with some localization to the upper abdomen associated with profuse nausea, vomiting, fever, with or without diarrhea. If it becomes severe necrotizing pancreatitis, the classic signs of volume deficit, oliguria, hypotension, and association with rising amylase, falling calcium, serum calcium, and rising blood urea nitrogen (BUN) and creatinine are present. The diagnosis is made by radiographic examination, including a CT scan of the abdomen showing an edematous or swollen pancreas with or without parapancreatic fluid collections in association with an elevation in the serum amylase or lipase, or elevation in the urine amylase to creatinine ratio measurement (Fig. 5-3). In almost all cases pancreatitis should be treated nonoperatively with nasogastric suction, intravenous fluids, progressive intravenous nutritional support, and a search for a correctable

Figure 5-3. A patient with postoperative pancreatitis following a colectomy for cancer in a familial adenomatus polyposis patient. CT scan shows a swollen, edematous pancreas gland.

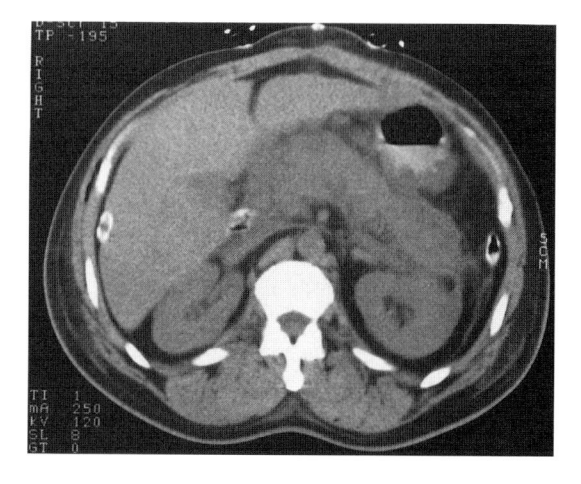

cause of the pancreatitis, such as calculous disease, recent instrumentation, or tumor.

SUMMARY: PANCREATITIS

1. Pancreatitis can affect the cancer patient, and is associated with L-asparaginase and Ara-C therapy. It may easily be confused with ileus or other causes of abdominal pain.
2. Patients present with abdominal pain and a variable range of other symptoms. Evaluation usually includes abdominal computed tomography scan and serum amylase and lipase, which usually are elevated. Treatment is usually nonoperative with supportive care, but in cases of necrotizing pancreatitis, surgical debridement may be needed.

BUDD-CHIARI SYNDROME AND PORTAL VEIN OCCLUSION

Occlusions of the splanchnic outflow tract occur in the cancer patient at any site including intrahepatic occlusions, the portal vein, the confluence of the splenic and superior mesenteric veins to form the portal vein, or an extrahepatic venous obstruction.[21] This latter group of occlusions of the major hepatic vein (*i.e.*, extrahepatic venous obstruction) are known as the Budd-Chiari syndrome. The obstruction of the hepatic outflow (as opposed to the splanchnic outflow) can be in either the major hepatic vein or the suprahepatic vena cava. In the cancer patient, this is almost always due to tumor or due to membranous occlusion of the vessel secondary to busulfan toxicity. The occlusive disease is also associated with the use of oral contraceptives, herbal teas containing pyrolizidine alkaloids, or with chemotherapy such as busulfan used in the treatment of hemopoietic tumors. It can also occur after chemo- or radiation therapy and bone marrow transplantation. One series reported that up to 11% of bone marrow transplantation patients developed Budd-Chiari syndrome.[28,29]

Budd-Chiari syndrome secondary to malignant tumors can occur with metastatic disease, but more commonly occurs with hepatoma. Malignant hepatoma has a frequent predilection for venous thrombus formation; hence, it has actually been reported in one patient to have presented with a right-sided heart thrombus composed of hepatoma tumor.[30,31]

Intrahepatic tumor can also cause obstruction to the splanchnic outflow. This typically follows complete or near complete replacement of the liver with tumor, or the combination of aggressive tumor in a cirrhotic fibrotic liver. The functional results of this are the same as a hepatic venous outflow obstruction or a portal venous obstruction. The cause of splanchnic outflow obstruction tends to be slower and more insidious than the pre- or posthepatic causes.

The prehepatic cause of splanchnic outflow obstruction is portal vein obstruction. In cancer patients this can occur from either direct tumor invasion, as seen in cholangiocarcinomas and ampillary or pancreatic tumors; or secondary to wide-spread perihepatic nodal disease, which occurs most commonly in pancreatic and biliary tumors, but also occurs with pancreatic lymphoma or in metastatic disease from colorectal cancer.

The clinical presentation of the patient with an acute splanchnic outflow obstruction can be dramatic with patients developing rapidly progressive ascites in the absence of abdominal pain. In portal venous obstruction this can also be associated with lower extremity edema or anasarca and oliguria. In the patient with Budd-Chiari syndrome, there can be progessive abdominal pain with associated oliguria to the point of overt renal failure. It is associated with deteriorating liver function and the development of hepatic encephalopathy within days or months. On average, patients rarely have symptoms more than 1 month before they seek medical attention.[32] Although the acute onset of encephalopathy is relatively rare, patients will present with abdominal pain, jaundice, and variceal bleeding. Radiologic evaluation should be directed toward documenting the patency of the splanchnic venous outflow tract.[33] In all patients, new onset of ascites should be the clinical development that triggers the clinician to obtain a magnetic resonance imaging scan or duplex sonogram of the portal vein to determine if it is patent.[34,35] If the portal vein is patent and the liver does not have extensive tumor involvement, splanchnic angiography should be performed with synchronous inferior vena cavography and direct visualization of the hepatic veins. The classic appearance of a spiderlike web showing the occluded hepatic vein should be seen in patients with Budd-Chiari syndrome. In patients with prehepatic portal obstruction, splenomegaly and gastric varices will be visible. Most patients with portal venous obstruction, however, will not require angiography, as the diagnosis should be made with the duplex sonogram or MRI showing the presence of a bulky, portahepatic mass, and occlusion of the portal vein (Fig. 5-4).

In general, treatment is directed at symptomatic palliation of the increased portal pressure and ascites.[32] Most oncologic patients who develop either portal venous obstruction or Budd-Chiari syndrome are in the end-stages of disease and need palliative and supportive care before their ultimate demise, typically in weeks to months after the diagnosis is made. In patients in whom this is the presenting sign or symptom of a malignancy, it is generally an indication of a poor prognosis, and severely limits the surgeon's options.

Prehepatic portal venous obstruction is generally treated symptomatically. The ascites is first treated with the standard medical therapies of diuresis, fluid and salt restriction, and possibly a beta blocker to reduce splanchnic inflow in the hemodynamically stable patient. If the patient has encephalopathy, protein restriction is indicated. If the

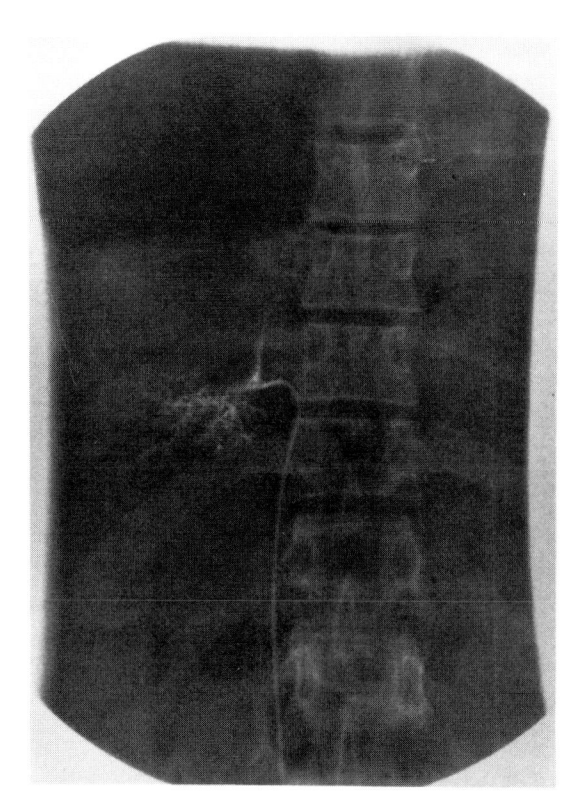

Figure 5-4. "Spiderweb" view of classic Budd-Chiari syndrome due to hepatic venous thrombosis. From Sitzmann JV, Klein AS, Cameron JL. Budd-Chiari syndrome. In: E Rypins, LM Nyhus, eds. Problems in general surgery. Philadelphia: JB Lippincott, 1992.

patient has chronic portal venous obstruction, is expected to survive a long time, and is resistant to medical management, peritoneal venous shunting (which is further discussed in Chapter 6) is an option. Patients with the Budd-Chiari syndrome due to hepatic venous outflow obstruction can sometimes be treated with a TIPS procedure (transjugular intrahepatic portosystemic shunt). In these patients, it is frequently possible to pass a catheter through the obstructed hepatic vein and through a secondary catheter identified as the portal venous inflow. Under flouroscopy, the three hepatic venous catheters can be advanced into the portal venous system and a TIPS performed. The drawbacks of using a TIPS in patients with

Budd-Chiari syndrome secondary to tumor is that it is possible to place the stent through a tumor-bearing region, thus potentially leading to tumor dissemination. Organ transplantation is of use in the management of Budd-Chiari syndrome due to benign conditions, but not in patients with the disease from malignant causes.[36]

SUMMARY: BUDD-CHIARI SYNDROME AND PORTAL VEIN OCCULSIONS

1. The Budd-Chiari syndrome is associated with bone marrow transplantation, but may also be due to primary or metastatic hepatic tumors. Prehepatic obstruction (of the portal vein) can result from direct vascular invasion by tumor or adenopathy. Intrahepatic obstruction is usually a result of massive involvement of the liver by tumor.
2. These patients usually present with massive ascites in the absence of abdominal pain. Evaluation includes determination of portal vein patency; if it is patent, then angiography is indicated.
3. Therapy is usually directed at symptomatic palliation. Ascites is treated with diuretics and salt restriction. Peritoneovenous shunting may be indicated (see Chapter 6). The TIPS procedure may be beneficial.

RUPTURE OF HEPATIC TUMORS

Primary hepatic tumors occur in approximately 10,000 patients per year in the United States.[37] The incidence of benign hepatic tumors such as hemangiomas, adenomas, and multifocal nodular hyperplastic lesions adds to this total. Any and all of these tumors can present with spontaneous rupture. Spontaneous rupture of liver tumors was rarely reported until the late 1930s, and more recently has been reported owing to the advent of the 3-D imaging techniques, such as CT scan, MRI scan, and ultrasonography. Hepatic adenomas can rupture and have been described most commonly in women.[38] Although metastatic malignancies can rupture, this is extraordinarily rare and it is more common for hepatocellular carcinomas or hepatic adenomas to rupture.[39,40] Rupture of hepatic tumors can occur spontaneously or can be caused by therapy, such as embolization. Lai et al,[41] reported the largest series of ruptured hepatocellular carcinomas occurring in 56 patients; hepatoma remains the single most common cause of hepatic tumor rupture. Other tumors that have been reported to cause spontaneous bleeding include lung cancer metastases, or melanoma metastases.[42,43]

The presentation of spontaneous rupture is rarely subtle; it is characterized by severe abdominal pain following by frank shock and hypotension. Radiographic evaluation includes a plain abdominal film, which in general shows a nonspecific ground glass appearance, and 3-D imaging of the abdomen with either sonography or CT scan. CT scan is the preferred diagnostic modality, and it typically shows a large tumor with frank perihepatic blood. In addition to profound anemia and hypovolemia, laboratory examinations typically show liver compromise with varying degrees of jaundice and elevations of alkaline phosphatase and serum transaminases. The treatment is initially symptomatic, rather than curative. The patients in frank shock with ruptured hepatic tumors are poor candidates for major hepectomy. It is best to stabilize and volume resuscitate these patients, and then correct any abnormalities in serum coagulation factors with fresh frozen plasma. If the patient continues to show evidence of bleeding following this, most surgeons would use angiography to determine the site of bleeding, followed by embolization. An alternative route could be selective vasospastic therapy *in lieu* of embolization therapy, with pitressin infused intra-arterially. If this is not successful, open exploration is required with suture and packing, or resection, or arterial ligation. In most series, the mortality of patients who undergo operative exploration ranges from 28% to 60%.[39,44] In general, the long-term survival of any patient who presents with a bleeding hepatic tumor is extraordinarily poor, and few survive more than a year even with subsequent elective resection.

■ SUMMARY: RUPTURE OF HEPATIC TUMORS

1. Hepatocellular carcinomas and hepatic adenomas are the tumors most associated with spontaneous rupture. The clinical presentation of tumor rupture is that of abdominal pain and shock. A CT scan is the preferred diagnostic modality.
2. Treatment is symptomatic and involves aggressive volume resuscitation and correction of coagulopathy. Patients who are still bleeding should undergo angiography and embolization. Mortality rates for exploration are high.

SUMMARY

Hepatobiliary disease resulting from the direct effect of a tumor or as a result of anticancer therapy can be a major source of morbidity in the cancer patient. Although hepatobiliary disease is common in all patients, there are a number of conditions and causes that are particularly common in the cancer patient which may deserve special consideration.

Malignant biliary tract obstruction can occur from tumors of the biliary duct or from metastatic lesions. Surgical resection offers the only chance for cure of these lesions, with patients with tumors of the distal common bile duct having a fairly good prognosis. Percutaneously placed stents offer palliation in those patients for whom resection is not technically possible.

Infections of the biliary tree are also an important source of morbidity in the cancer patient. Acalculous cholecystitis occurs following intensive high-dose chemotherapy after bone marrow transplant and following intra-arterial chemotherapy of the liver. Cholangitis is also a problem; it is usually due to stones or strictures but has also been associated with the prolonged stenting of the common bile duct. Patients with cholangitis usually present with the classic findings of fever, jaundice, and right upper quadrant abdominal pain. This condition requires decompression of the biliary tree and antibiotics.

Pancreatitis is associated with the use of several chemotherapeutic agents (e.g., L-asparaginase and Ara-C), and may also be due to calculi or other causes. It is usually treated with supportive care and withdrawal or treatment of the cause if one exists and can be identified.

Budd-Chiari syndrome can be a significant problem and is associated with hepatoma or as a result of bone marrow transplantation. Obstruction can be prehepatic (portal vein obstruction), intrahepatic (primary or metastatic tumors), or posthepatic (suprahepatic vena cava obstruction). Treatment is usually symptomatic palliation. Peritoneovenous shunting may be used to palliate the ascites in some of these patients.

Spontaneous rupture of hepatic tumors is reported with a wide variety of lesions including benign and malignant tumors of the liver. Patients usually present with shock. Treatment is first directed at stabilization with volume resuscitation. Angiography followed by embolization is probably the preferred course as these patients are usually poor candidates for major liver resection.

REFERENCES

1. Longmire WP. Tumors of the extrahepatic biliary radicals. Curr Probl Surg 1976;2:1.
2. Kopelson G, Galdabini J, Warshaw AL, et al.

Patterns of failure after curative surgery for extrahepatic biliary tract carcinoma: implications for adjuvant therapy. Int J Rad Oncol Biol Phys 1980;7:413.
3. Crist DW, Sitzmann JV, Cameron JL. Improved hospital morbidity, mortality and survival following the Whipple procedure. Ann Surg 1987;206:358.
4. Cameron JL, Pitt HA, Zinner MJ, et al. Management of proximal cholangiocarcinomas by surgical resection and radiotherapy. Am J Surg 1990;159:91.
5. Reding R, Buard JL, Lebeau G, et al. Surgical management of 552 carcinomas of the extrahepatic bile ducts (gallbladder and periampullary tumors excluded). Ann Surg 1991;213:235.
6. McLean GK, Burke DR. Role of endoprostheses in the management of malignant biliary obstruction. Radiology 1989;170:961.
7. Ring EJ, McLean GK, eds. Interventional radiology: principles and techniques. Boston: Little Brown, 1981.
8. Speer AG, Russell RC, Hatfield ARW, et al. Randomized trial of endoscopic versus percutaneous stent insertion in malignant obstructive jaundice. Lancet 1987;2:57.
9. Gunderson LL, Martin JK, Earle JD, et al. Intraoperative and external beam irradiation +/− resection. 1983 ASTR Proceedings. Int J Rad Oncol Biol Phys 1983;9:111.
10. Koga A, Watanabe K, Fukuyama T, et al. Diagnosis and operative indications for polypoid lesions of the gallbladder. Arch Surg 1988;123:26.
11. Ogura Y, Mizumoto R, Isaji S, et al. Radical operations for carcinoma of the gallbladder: present status in Japan. World J Surg 1991;15:337.
12. Todoroki T, Iwasaki Y, Orii K, et al. Resection combined with intraoperative radiation therapy(IORT) for stage IV(TNM) gallbladder carcinoma. World J Surg 1991;15:357.
13. Nakamura S, Sakaguchi S, Suzuki S, et al. Aggressive surgery for carcinoma of the gallbladder. Surgery 1989;106:467.
14. Nevin JE, Morgan TJ, Kay S, et al. Carcinoma of the gallbladder: staging, treatment, and prognosis. Cancer 1976;37:141.
15. Barbara L, Sama C, Lebate AMM, et al. A population study on the prevalence of gallstone disease: the Sermione study. Hepatology 1987;7:913.
16. Vogelzang RL, Nemcek AA Jr. Percutaneous cholecystostomy: diagnostic and therapeutic efficacy. Radiology 1988;168:29.
17. Gadacz TR, Talamini M, Lillemoe K, et al. Laparoscopic cholecystectomy. Surg Clin N Am 1990;70:1249.
18. Peters JH, Ellison EC, Innes JT, et al. Safety and efficacy of laparoscopic cholecystectomy: a prospective analysis of 100 initial patients. Ann Surg 1991;213:3.
19. Zucker KA, Bailey RW, Gadacz TR, et al. Laparoscopic guided cholecystectomy. Am J Surg 1991;161:36.
20. Lipsett PA, Pitt HA. Acute cholangitis. Surg Clin N Am 1990;70:1297.
21. Sitzmann JV, Klein AS, Cameron JL. Budd-Chiari syndrome. In: Rypins E, Nyhus LM, eds. Problems in general surgery. Philadelphia:JB Lippincott, 1992.
22. Gigot JF, Leese T, Dereme T, et al. Acute cholangitis: multivariate analysis of risk factors. Ann Surg 1989;209:435.
23. Pessa ME, Hawkins IF, Vogel SB. The treatment of acute cholangitis: percutaneous transhepatic biliary drainage before definitive therapy. Ann Surg 1987;205:389.
24. Lai EC, Lo CM, Choi TK, et al. Urgent biliary decompression after endoscopic retrograde cholangiopancreatography. Am J Surg 1989;157:121.
25. Thompson JE Jr, Pitt HA, Doty JE, et al. Is a broad spectrum penicillin adequate therapy for cholangitis? Surg Gynecol Obstet 1990;171:275.
26. Gerecht WB, Henry NK, Hoffman WW, et al. Prospective randomized comparison of mezlocillin therapy alone with combined ampicillin and gentamicin therapy for patients with cholangitis. Arch Intern Med 1989;149:1279.
27. Calhoun P, Brown KP, Strunk R, et al. Experimental studies of biliary excretion of piperacillin. Ann Surg 1987;205:420.
28. Woods WG, Dehner LP, Nesbit ME, et al. Fatal veno-occlusive disease of the liver following high dose chemotherapy, irradiation and bone marrow transplantation. Am J Med 1980;68:285.
29. Shulman HM, McDonald GB, Mathews D, et al. An analysis of hepatic veno-occlusive disease and centrilobular hepatic degeneration following bone marrow transplantation. Gastroenterology 1980;79:1178.
30. Cardell BS, Merill DAF, Williams R. Leiomyosarcoma of inferior vena cava producing Budd-Chiari syndrome. J Pathol 1971;104:283.
31. Justiniani FR, Cohen GH, Roen SA, et al. Budd-Chiari syndrome due to leiomyosarcoma of the inferior vena cava. Dig Dis 1973;18:337.
32. Klein A, Sitzmann J, Coleman J, et al. Current management of the Budd-Chiari syndrome. Ann Surg 1990;212:144.
33. Maguire R, Doppman J. Angiographic abnormalities in partial Budd-Chiari syndrome. Radiology 1977;122:629.
34. Stark DD, Hohn PF, Trey C, et al. MRI of the Budd-Chiari syndrome. AJR 1986;146:1141.
35. Hosoki T, Kuroda C, Tokunaga K, et al. Hepatic venous outflow obstruction: evaluation with

pulsed duplex sonography. Radiology 1989; 170:733.
36. Half G, Todo S, Tsakio AG, et al. Liver transplantation for the Budd-Chiari syndrome. Ann Surg 1990;211:430.
37. Murphy GP, ed. CA-A cancer journal for clinicians: cancer statistics. American Cancer Society, 1995, p. 7.
38. Antoniades K, Brooks CE. Hemoperitoneum from liver cell adenoma in a patient on oral contraceptives. Surgery 1976;77;137.
39. Spector J, Chodoff RJ. Massive intraperitoneal hemorrhage from carcinoma of the liver. Surgery 1950;27:457.
40. Ahmed A, Metcalfe-Gibson C. Haemoperitoneum complicating secondary carcinoma in the liver. Br J Surg 1972;59:576.
41. Lai EC, Wu KM, Choi TK, et al. Spontaneous ruptured hepatocellular carcinoma. Ann Surgery 1989;210:24.
42. Dousei T, Miyata M, Yamaguchi T, et al. Rupture of liver metastasis of malignant melanoma: a case of hepatic resection. Surg Today 1991;21:480.
43. Mittleman RE. Hepatic rupture due to metastatic lung carcinoma. Am J Clin Pathol 1987; 88:506.
44. Chen MF, Hwang TL, Jeng L, et al. Surgical treatment for spontaneous rupture of hepatocellular carcinoma. Surg Gyn & Obst 1988;167:99.

Management of Malignant Ascites

ERIC A. WIEBKE

Malignant ascites complicates the clinical course of many patients with cancer and represents a grave prognostic sign. The most common tumors causing malignant ascites are breast and ovarian cancers in women, and colorectal, pancreatic, and rarely other gastrointestinal (GI) malignancies in men. Malignant ascites may rarely be the initial presenting sign in these patients, and it may present without a known primary tumor site. Survival in these situations is particularly dismal, with one report of 14 patients with malignant ascites and an unknown primary tumor having a mean survival of only 43 days.[1] Malignant ascites has been a notoriously difficult problem to treat, with regimens from diuretics, to paracentesis, to shunting, to instillation of chemotherapeutic agents all being described with varying results and complications.

Defining malignant ascites is difficult. Ascites secondary to malignancy may be from two causes: massive liver involvement by tumor, where the ascitic fluid does not contain malignant cells; and peritoneal carcinomatosis, where malignant cells would be commonly found in the peritoneal fluid. For this discussion, we will define malignant ascites as that due to peritoneal involvement by metastatic cancer. Ascites secondary to hepatic venous outflow obstruction (Budd-Chiari syndrome) in the patient with cancer is discussed in Chapter 5. This chapter focuses on the causes of malignant ascites, including the pathophysiology and complications when left untreated, the indications and rationale for treatment, as well as the multiple treatment modalities described in the literature. The complications of interventions will be assessed and the results and patient survival examined. Intervention is based on the severity of symptoms and an estimate of short-term survival.

ETIOLOGY

The accumulation of protein-rich fluid in the abdominal cavity often follows tumor implantation and growth on peritoneal surfaces. Not all cases of peritoneal carcinomatosis are complicated by malignant ascites, however, and our understanding of the mechanism of fluid accumulation remains incomplete. Fluid accumulation may result from two general problems with the peritoneal surface: first, exudate formation (fluid influx) may be enhanced, and second, lymphatic drainage (fluid efflux) may be impeded. It is likely that abnormalities in both fluid influx and efflux are present in patients with peritoneal carcinomatosis, resulting in ascites formation.[2]

Animal and laboratory models of malignant ascites have provided us with some explanations regarding these abnormalities. Recent studies reveal that many tumor cells produce factors that allow for local matrix digestion and neovascularization, thus permitting local tumor progression and possibly metastasis formation. The neovasculature induced by tumor cells is not normal. Frequently identified is the lack of normal basement membrane and endothelial support. These defects result in a more leaky vasculature that may in part account for the increased fluid efflux into the peritoneum with widespread peritoneal tumor implantation. In fact, many solid and ascitic tumors produce a protein, vascular permeability factor, that enhances normal blood vessel permeability to circulating macromolecules.[3,4]

Increased fluid influx cannot account for ascites formation alone, however, given the tremendous resorptive capacity and lymphatic drainage of the peritoneum. Animal studies have confirmed impedance to normal peritoneal lymphatic drainage in models of malignant ascites. In addition, increased intracavitary oncotic and hydrostatic pressures inevitably affect the influx and efflux rates. Initial thoughts on malignant ascites formation centered around lymphatic obstruction by cancer cells and impaired fluid absorption via diaphragmatic lymphatics as the principal defect. One of the first reports to question this explanation appeared in 1987.[5] These workers looked at a rat model of malignant ascites. Cell-free fluid obtained from rats with malignant ascites was placed into the peritoneal cavities of rats without cancer and the results compared to the infusion of serum or saline. The permeability of the omentum to protein was evaluated. The study demonstrated that rats treated with the cell-free ascitic fluid developed a significant increase in omental permeability compared with those treated with serum or saline. These investigators correctly postulated that the tumor cells produced a substance that resulted in increased capillary permeability, which could explain the development of ascites in the absence of lymphatic obstruction. A recent study examined the relative contributions of altered influx and efflux in the formation of malignant ascites using murine models of ovarian and breast cancer.[2] In this elegant series of experiments, influx into and efflux from the peritoneal cavity was studied by following ^{125}I-radiolabeled human serum albumin. Efflux through lymphatics was followed by using ^{51}Cr-labeled red blood cells, which act more like particulates. These authors found that efflux of both markers was markedly reduced within 1 day of intraperitoneal tumor injection. This decrease preceded a detectable increase in tumor cell number and was not caused by lymphatic obstruction by tumor cells. The albumin tracer influx, on the other hand, did not increase detectably until 5 to 7 days after tumor injection. At that time, there was a 10 to 100 times increase in the number of tumor cells. Only at this stage did ascites begin to accumulate, indicating that impaired efflux alone could not account for ascites formation.

In humans, malignant ascites is the end result of a variety of abnormalities including lymphatic obstruction by tumor cells, enhanced peritoneal fluid production due to tumor-derived substances, and liver disease. The relative contributions of each of these processes in the pathogenesis of malignant ascites results in the wide range of ascites seen clinically: high or low protein, cellular or cell-free, and bloody or blood-free. Thus, malignant ascites from one patient to another may vary dramatically in composition. It is this heterogeneity in the composition of malignant ascites that makes generalizations about its treatment difficult, and probably what explains the variability in the results of treatment from one institution to another. Successful treatment, therefore, depends on careful diagnosis and ascitic fluid analysis, and individualization of the type of therapeutic intervention.

DIAGNOSIS

The differentiation between malignant and benign ascites is often difficult even in patients with known cancer. When cytologic examination of ascitic fluid reveals malignant cells, the diagnosis is virtually assured. However, positive cytology results are obtained in only 50% to 75% of cases of true malignant ascites.[6,7]

When cytologic examination of ascitic fluid is negative or inconclusive in a cancer patient with suspected malignant ascites, other laboratory and radiologic tests may help confirm the diagnosis. All patients should undergo routine liver function testing, as benign ascites associated with severe liver disease often is associated with other evidence of hepatic dysfunction.

In addition to these basic tests (fluid cytology and serum chemistries), other tests are available to help establish the diagnosis of malignant ascites, although many have not gained widespread acceptance and use. These include ascites protein and albumin determinations; serum-ascites albumin difference; ascites pH, lactate dehydrogenase (LDH), glucose, carcinoembryonic antigen (CEA), cholesterol, and fibronectin determinations; and ascites flow cytometric analysis. Radiologic studies include ultrasonographic appearance of the gallbladder and technetium-99m accumulation.

Ascitic fluid chemistry determinations are relatively easy to perform, with the rationale for their use being similar to the use of such measurements to distinguish between transudative and exudative pleural effusions. High protein content is a consistent finding in malignant ascites, yet upwards of 25% of those patients with ascites secondary to liver disease have such elevations. Similarly, high LDH, low pH, and low glucose do not reliably distinguish between benign and malignant ascites.

Jungst et al[8] looked at cholesterol, phospholipid, and triglyceride concentrations in ascitic fluid from 40 patients with chronic liver disease and 51 patients with various neoplasms. Application of a cholesterol cutoff value of greater than 48 mg/dL for malignant ascites provided a diagnostic efficiency of 92% for elevated cholesterol (sensitivity 90% and specificity 95%). These authors concluded that cholesterol determination of ascitic fluid was a cost-effective and excellent way to discriminate between malignant and benign ascites.

Prieto et al[6] evaluated ascitic fluid fibronectin and cholesterol levels and the serum-ascites albumin difference in an effort to differentiate benign from malignant ascites. They compared these results with those of LDH and total protein determinations; LDH was the least reliable test for distinguishing benign from malignant ascites. Diagnostic accuracy was excellent for elevated ascitic fluid cholesterol (above 46 mg/dL)(97%) and fibronectin (above 50 mg/mL)(97%), as was a low serum-ascites albumin difference (under 1.1 g/dL)(94%) and a high total protein (above 2.5 g/dL)(93%). These authors concluded that ascitic fluid cholesterol determination was the preferred test to differentiate between benign and malignant ascites because of its low cost and easy availability. Other studies have looked at fibronectin determinations and have found them to be specific but not sensitive when high levels are found.[9] Given the lack of availability and high cost of fibronectin determinations, they should not be a routine part of the evaluation of ascitic fluid. The low serum-ascites albumin difference, on the other hand, as with the cholesterol determination, represents a reliable and readily available measurement with both high sensitivity and specificity.

There has been one report describing the efficacy of gallbladder ultrasonography in distinguishing malignant from benign ascites.[10] Patients with ascites due to benign disease such as portal hypertension or hypoproteinemia were found to have gallbladders characterized by a "double wall" appearance, or an echo-free zone within the wall. In contrast, patients with malignant ascites had normal, thin-walled gallbladders. We have no clinical experience with this technique and other studies have not confirmed this finding.[11] Similarly, technetium-99m has been found to accumulate in malignant ascites as it does in malignant pleural effusions, but the clinical utility of this study in differentiating benign from malignant ascites has not been carefully evaluated.[12] Neither ultrasonography nor nuclear medicine evaluations play a significant role in the evaluation of ascites.

Lastly, the role of ascitic fluid analysis with flow cytometry has been evaluated in an attempt to enhance the diagnostic yield of 60% to 90% described using cytologic analysis of large fluid volumes.[13] This technique may be used if confirmation of the diagnosis is critical to decisions regarding therapy. Weissman et al[13] analyzed 33 ascitic fluid samples, 13 in patients with known malignancies. Of the patients with malignancies, aneuploidy was demonstrated in 10. Six patients with proved peritoneal carcinomatosis and normal cytologic examination had abnormal DNA histograms on flow cytometry. The overall accuracy was high, with flow cytometry having a sensitivity of 77% and a specificity of 100%. The technique is labor intensive, expensive, and useful for nondiploid tumors. Its general use, therefore, cannot be recommended.

SUMMARY: DIAGNOSIS OF MALIGNANT ASCITES

1. Cancer patients with new ascites should undergo paracentesis for diagnosis.
2. Fluid samples should be sent for the following:
   a. cytologic examination
   b. chemistries including total protein, albumin, and cholesterol
3. Blood samples should be sent for serum determinations of total protein, albumin, and liver function tests.
4. If the diagnosis of malignant ascites will result in a therapeutic change (systemic or intraperitoneal chemotherapy; immunotherapy protocol), and cytologic examination is negative, flow cytometric DNA analysis may be performed.
5. Other studies, such as fibronectin determinations or radiologic procedures, should not be performed.

NATURAL HISTORY AND COMPLICATIONS OF MALIGNANT ASCITES

Untreated malignant ascites becomes symptomatic because of the pronounced mechanical effects of the ascitic fluid load. Dyspnea and respiratory compromise are common owing to diaphragmatic pressure and decreased chest excursion. Abdominal wall hernias may develop, typically at umbilical and inguinal sites, because of increased intra-abdominal pressure. These are difficult and dangerous to treat prior to obtaining control of the ascites; ascitic leaks have a very high mortality rate and recurrent hernias are common in this situation. Malnutrition develops secondary to anorexia, which is very common due to increased intra-abdominal pressure; there may be associated nausea and vomiting. All of these problems are indications to decrease the volume of the ascites. Spontaneous bacterial peritonitis almost never occurs in malignant ascites, perhaps because good liver function is generally maintained.[14]

TREATMENT OF MALIGNANT ASCITES

The Need for Intervention

Initiating therapy for malignant ascites is not always indicated. The survival of patients with malignant ascites is less than 6 months in most cases. Patients with ovarian cancer and those without liver metastases at the time of diagnosis of malignant ascites fare best. Each intervention carries its own set of complications. The decision to intervene is based on level of patient discomfort and estimates of survival, which are routinely measured in weeks with only rare exceptions. Untreated ascites can cause anorexia, pain from distension, and dyspnea from diaphragmatic pressure; and these represent the general indications for intervention. Except for possible chemotherapy for ovarian cancer and possibly breast cancer, intervention is symptomatic only and will not prolong survival in the majority of patients. In some patients, then, no intervention is the appropriate course of action.

Symptomatic Treatment: Paracentesis

Frequent large volume paracentesis provides short-term symptomatic relief of the pressure-related effects of malignant ascites. Paracentesis is usually followed by rapid reaccumulation of fluid; it depletes the patient of electrolytes and protein and therefore does not represent a good solution to symptomatic ascites in patients with reasonable function and survival. Sonographic guidance of paracentesis in 43 patients with malignant ascites was described,[15] with 109 therapeutic paracenteses performed with three procedure complications, two of which were fatal. Symptomatic relief was obtained in 87% of patients, with duration of relief ranging from 4 to 45 days (mean 10.4 days). Drains were left in place from 1 to 6 days (mean 36 hours) for inpatients; outpatients were drained for 15 to 30 minutes only. Initial paracentesis volume averaged 3.5 L. Only one paracentesis was required by 29 patients; the remaining 14 patients underwent 2 to 31 paracenteses. The effects of paracentesis on serum electrolytes and protein in these patients were not discussed by the authors.

A modification of paracentesis is placement of a permanent peritoneal drain, such as a Tenckhoff catheter.[16] Obviously, the problems with electrolyte abnormalities and hypoproteinemia that occur with multiple paracenteses remain, and there is the added risk of bacterial peritonitis. In one report of 17 patients with malignant ascites treated by peritoneal drainage,[17] two patients developed cellulitis at the catheter site and one developed peritonitis; however, symptomatic relief was excellent and significant electrolyte and protein abnormalities were surprisingly nonexistent. These patients also showed decreasing drainage volume requirements with time. Although promising in one report, this method cannot be recommended for general use until results are confirmed in additional studies.

External drainage of fluid as described above represents a simple way to obtain symptomatic relief of tense malignant ascites. It is reasonable to attempt this as the initial therapy for malignant ascites with repeat drainage if fluid reaccumulation is slow; rapid reaccumulation of fluid in an individual with reasonable function and survival should preclude further attempts at external drainage and consideration should be given to peritoneovenous shunting.

Symptomatic Treatment: Diuretics

In general, malignant ascites is refractory to medical treatment with sodium and fluid restriction and diuretics. One report of 15 patients with malignant ascites, however, claimed an excellent response to spironolactone in 13 of the patients (150 to 600 mg/dL divided).[18] These patients were initially treated as inpatients with bedrest and were discharged on two thirds of the maximal dosage required to control the ascites. In contrast, an evaluation of 16 patients with cancer-related ascites revealed no ascitic fluid mobilization in response to spironolactone with or without furosemide.[19]

A brief trial of escalating-dose spironolactone therapy may be warranted in individuals with normal renal function and symptomatic malignant ascites, especially given the lack of side effects of the drug. Attempts at fluid and salt restriction are neither useful nor necessary.

Symptomatic Treatment: Peritoneovenous Shunting

The peritoneovenous shunt was introduced by LeVeen and colleagues in 1974.[20] The initial description of its use for the continuous drainage of ascites in cirrhotic patients was quickly adopted for use in malignant ascites. Initial concerns regarding dissemination of cancer using the shunt seem unwarranted, in retrospect, given the poor survival of these patients overall.

Selecting patients appropriate to undergo peritoneovenous shunting is difficult. The operative mortality for peritoneovenous shunting is roughly 25%. Patients who may benefit from chemotherapy, such as ovarian and breast cancer patients, should not undergo placement of a peritoneovenous shunt initially. Patients with expected survival times of less than 2 months and those patients with pseudomyxoma peritonei should not receive a shunt. Other general contraindications to shunt placement include evidence of severe liver dysfunction (rising bilirubin, elevated protime), as the risk of postprocedure coagulopathy is high; evidence of infected ascites (positive culture, organisms on gram stain, or greater than 400 leukocytes/mL ascitic fluid) on preoperative sampling; and congestive heart failure. Reviews describing the important features of preoperative assessment, operative techniques to minimize shunt occlusion and dysfunction, and postoperative monitoring and care are available.[21-23]

Operative Approach. Table 6-1 summarizes the preoperative assessment, operative approach, and postoperative care of the patient undergoing placement of a peritoneovenous shunt. Briefly, preoperative evaluation should include an estimate of short-term survival. Expected survival of less than 2 months should preclude shunt placement. The diagnosis may be confirmed as described above, however, the decision to treat malignant ascites is based on severity of symptoms, not the presence of malignant cells. Diagnostic paracentesis must be performed to exclude the presence of infected ascites. Evaluation of clotting function should be performed as should liver function tests as part of the preoperative evaluation. Evidence of severe hepatic dysfunction, such as an elevated serum bilirubin, is associated with increased bleeding complications after peritoneovenous shunting procedures. All patients should receive a broad-spectrum antibiotic prophylactically, and antibiotics should continue for 48 hours after shunt placement.

The procedure may on occasion be performed under local anesthetic, however, a general anesthetic is clearly more desirable. The procedure includes a small abdominal incision with access to the peritoneal cavity gained through a rectus-splitting approach. The venous end of the catheter may be placed

Table 6-1. Perioperative Management of Patients Undergoing Peritoneovenous Shunt Placement

PREOPERATIVE ASSESSMENT
Symptomatic ascites
Estimation of short-term survival: >2 months
Diagnostic paracentesis: infected ascites contraindication to procedure
 • positive gram stain
 • positive culture
 • WBC >400/mL ascitic fluid
Coagulation parameters: prothrombin time, platelet count, fibrinogen
Prophylactic antibiotics: cover staphylococci and gram-negative enteric organisms

OPERATIVE APPROACH
General anesthetic preferred
Rectus muscle-splitting abdominal incision
Drain ascites and replace with 1 to 2 L warm lactated Ringer's solution
Posterior sheath pursestring of nonabsorbable suture material
Counter-incision along chest wall
Venous limb placed centrally via internal jugular or cephalic vein cutdown
Confirm correct venous and peritoneal limb position by intraoperative fluoroscopy
Confirm shunt function intraoperatively

POSTOPERATIVE CARE
Continue prophylactic antibiotics for 48 hours
Abdominal binder; abdominal girth measurements
Incentive spirometry
Supplement oxygen and elevate head of bed
Induce brisk diuresis with intravenous doses of furosemide
Daily laboratory determinations:
 • hematocrit
 • platelet count
 • prothrombin time
 • fibrinogen
 • fibrin split products
 • serum electrolytes

into the superior vena cava via a cephalic or internal jugular cutdown, or via a percutaneous internal jugular or subclavian approach. Most surgeons employ the internal jugular cutdown approach. Drainage of the abdominal cavity of the ascites, with replacement with 1 to 2 L of warmed lactated Ringer's solution, may decrease the incidence of coagulopathy and early shunt occlusion by eliminating a large protein load. Meticulous attention must be paid to detail in maintaining sterile technique and hemostasis. Shunt function should be confirmed in the operating room. This is relatively easy with a Denver™ shunt where fluid flow through the shunt can be monitored as the pumping mechanism is activated. A small amount of methylene blue may be injected into the peritoneal limb of the shunt, and flow of the blue dye observed into the venous limb. Figure 6-1 shows the configuration of a shunt after placement. Note that the pump is placed over the ribs to allow for easy use by the patient.

Postoperatively, these patients must be closely monitored, usually in an intensive care unit setting. Most surgeons apply an abdominal binder to the patient to maintain high intra-abdominal pressure. Incentive spirometry will cause negative intrathoracic pressure and contribute to the flow of ascites through the shunt. The patient should be kept in a head-up position, oxygen should be supplemented by nasal cannula, and a brisk diuresis should be induced with low doses of intravenous furosemide to prevent fluid overload and pulmonary edema. Laboratory determinations should include daily hematocrit, protime, platelet count, and electrolytes. A functioning shunt often causes a dilutional drop in the hematocrit, as well as evidence of mild coagulopathy, such as an elevated protime, decreased fibrinogen, elevated fibrin split products, and a drop in platelet count. These need not be treated in the absence of clinical bleeding and in fact represents evidence of shunt function. Patients are instructed to pump the device several times daily. Function of the pump chamber is ascertained by palpation. Easy refill of the chamber, indicating a functioning peritoneal limb, can be felt as the chamber fills under the palpating finger. Similarly, a functioning venous limb can be ascertained by easy egress of the chamber's contents.

Figure 6-1. This schematic shows a peritoneovenous shunt in place. Note the placement of the pump (or one-way valve in this diagram) directly over the inferior ribs in the midclavicular line (reprinted with permission from DeVita V, Hellman S, Rosenberg S. Principles and practice of oncology. 4th ed. Philadelphia: JB Lippincott, 1994;2259.)

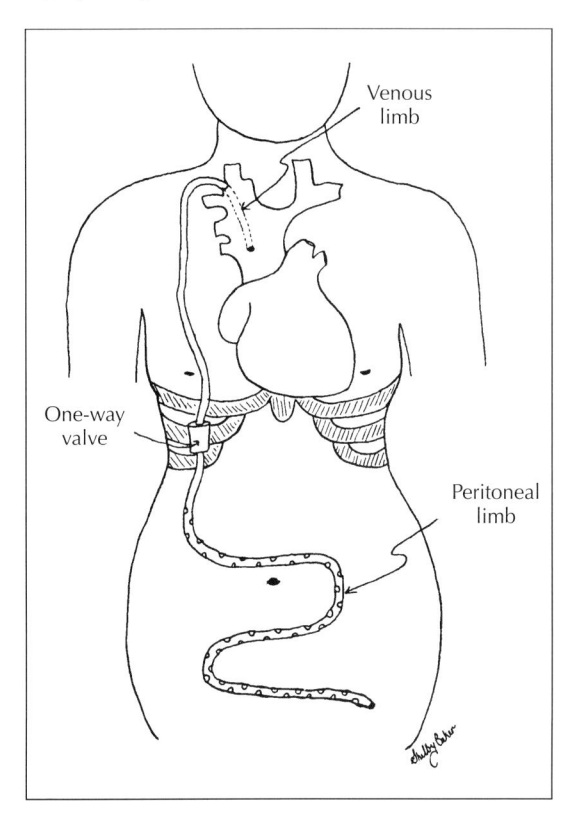

RESULTS IN MALIGNANT ASCITES

LeVeen™ shunting has largely been supplanted by use of the Denver™ shunt. Some of the original work points to higher failure rates with the LeVeen™ shunt, thought to be due to valve occlusion secondary to the high protein and cellular content of malignant ascites. Direct comparisons are rare, but one study compared the two and concluded that short-term function of Denver shunts was better, but that long-term function and patency for both types of shunt were similar for malignant ascites.[24] These authors concluded that the Denver™ shunt was marginally better than the LeVeen shunt. In a prospective, randomized study, the Denver shunt was felt to be superior to the LeVeen shunt for the treatment of ascites secondary to cirrhosis.[25]

A careful review of the results of peritoneovenous shunting with LeVeen and Denver shunts is warranted. Caution is always required in evaluating the reports in the literature; follow-up is often short, selection criteria are never clearly described, and the type of ascites (from metastatic liver involvement or peritoneal carcinomatosis) is rarely identified. Thirty-five patients with documented malignant ascites (35% ovarian, 12% endometrial, 8% each colon, gastric, breast) intractable to medical management were palliated with the LeVeen shunt.[26] Twenty-seven had good palliation until time of death; eight patients had early shunt malfunction and no palliation, many related to grossly bloody ascitic fluid. Survival of the group overall was poor: mean survival was 12 weeks. These authors described few significant complications, although nine patients died within 1 month of shunt placement, three related to shunt complications. They concluded that shunting provided effective palliation, but that bloody ascites represented a contraindication to shunting.

Another report on the effectiveness of LeVeen shunting in five patients is somewhat suspect.[27] Two patients died within 8 days of shunt placement, and two others died within 1 and 2 months of placement, respectively. The remaining patient had late failure requiring revision. Clearly, no selection criteria were used in this small group of patients and the results were poor.

Ten patients were treated with the LeVeen shunt in another small series reported early on from Ohio State University.[28] Four patients were alive from 4 to 16 weeks after shunt placement; all had patent shunts. Of the six patients who died, time to death was 1 to 13 weeks; two had patent shunts at the time of death; two failed in less than 24 hours; two failed at 5 and 7 weeks after placement. Overall follow-up time was short, with a patency rate of 60% reported.

A small group of six patients treated with the Denver shunt was described.[29] There was only one early failure, and this patient died 2 weeks after shunt placement; the remaining five resulted in good clinical response, with a duration of observation between 3 and 10 months. No patient required subsequent paracentesis. There were no significant complications reported in this study.

An attempt was made to distinguish between the results of shunting procedures in patients with cell-free malignant ascites and those with cellular ascitic fluid.[30] Twenty-two patients were evaluated, and 27 shunts were placed; most were LeVeen shunts. Overall survival averaged 32 days. Ten of 18 patients were cytologically positive for malignant cells. There were 16 complications, 12 (75%) in the cytologically positive group. Also, shunt function fared much better in the cytologically negative group. These authors concluded that shunting was indicated in patients with intractable, symptomatic ascites with rapid reaccumulation of fluid after therapeutic paracentesis. They also considered malignant cell-positive ascites to be a relative contraindication to shunting because of high shunt failure rates. Recommendations for shunting based on survival estimates, and alternatives to shunting in patients with cellular malignant ascites, were not presented.

Two other smaller series of patients looked specifically at outcome of shunts (mostly LeVeen) placed in a total of 48 patients with intractable malignant ascites.[31,32] Twenty-seven patients underwent 29 shunting procedures.[31] All patients were dead within 4 months, and three died of potential shunt complications. No selection based on estimated survival was described. In the other study, 21 patients underwent 25 LeVeen shunts or revisions.[32] There were no shunt-related deaths in this group and no coagulopathy developed. Thirty-day mortality was 38%, and all deaths were due to disease progression, with a mean survival of 82 days. Four patients were alive with good palliation 25, 169, 177, and 233 days after the procedure. Shunt occlusion occurred in four patients (19%). Both groups felt that the procedure provided effective palliation in a majority of patients, and that shunt failure and complications were rare.

The larger series of patients treated with peritoneovenous shunting stressed the importance of patient selection contributing to a good outcome. Table 6-2 summarizes the results of seven studies of greater than 35 patients each, for a total of 334 patients, published between 1982 and 1989. Three studies compared the results of shunting malignant and benign ascites,[33–35] whereas the remaining four looked specifically at the results in malignant ascites.[24,36–38]

Comparisons of results for shunts placed for benign versus malignant ascites reveal similar failure and patency rates. Death was rarely shunt-related in patients with malignant ascites, who typically died of cancer progression. In cirrhotic patients, however, death was frequently related to shunt placement (disseminated intravascular coagulation [DIC] related to shunt placement or sepsis). In cirrhotic patients who survived the procedure, long-term palliation was quite good. In two of the reports, patients whose underlying malignancy originated from the gastrointestinal tract had very poor survival rates, low enough to question the use of peritoneovenous shunting in these patients. On the other hand, patients with ovarian cancer survived longer, some for well over a year.

Four studies looked specifically at larger numbers of patients with malignant ascites treated with peritoneovenous shunts. A total of 171 patients were evaluated in these studies. The earliest study[38] looked at LeVeen shunt palliation in 40 patients (28 with ovarian cancer). The shunt functioned effectively in 28 patients, although revision was required in eight. The remaining 12 patients obtained no benefit. There were no significant complications or shunt-related deaths. Roussel et al[37] looked at the Denver shunt in 1986. Thirty-six patients had shunts placed for control of malignant ascites; of these, 12 had ovarian cancer, 11 had breast cancer, and 10 had gastrointestinal malignancies. Outcome was no different in cytology-positive ascites compared with cell-free ascites. Median survival for all patients was 13 weeks. Ultimately, 13 shunts (56.5%) failed. These authors concluded that because of the short life expectancy of these patients and the unpredictable results obtained with shunting, this method should be chosen as a last resort. In another study, 45 patients received shunts for malignant ascites, with a near equal distribution between Denver and LeVeen shunts.[24] No difference in shunt patency was noted. The majority of patients had gastrointestinal cancers underlying their ascites; 75% had effective palliation. Patients with gastrointestinal malignancies had short survival times (10 weeks) compared with those with gynecologic malignancies (71 weeks). The shunt revision rate was 18%, there were no cases of DIC, and there were no shunt-related deaths. Three patients required placement of an additional shunt because of high ascitic fluid production rates. These authors concluded that the patients best suited for peritoneovenous shunting for ascites control were those who still had reasonable treatment options for their malignant disease, notably ovarian and breast cancer patients. Although they found no differences in patency between the two types of devices, they favored the extra-high-flow Denver shunt as the device of choice. Finally, 50 patients were evaluated by Smith et al in 1989.[36] Again, gastrointestinal primary tumors predominated. In this analysis, women did better than men, even excluding gynecologic malignancies. Shunt occlusion occurred in 16 patients (32%). Half of the LeVeen shunts occluded, whereas only 26% of the Denver shunts occluded. DIC occurred in three patients, with bleeding occurring at surgical incisions only.

Table 6-2. Comparison of Results of Peritoneoenous Shunt Procedures in Malignant versus Benign Ascites

Author(s)	Ref.	Number of Patients Benign	Number of Patients Malignant	Shunt Failure Rates Benign	Shunt Failure Rates Malignant	Median (Mean) Survival Benign	Median (Mean) Survival Malignant	Other Complications[a] Benign	Other Complications[a] Malignant	Comments
Soderlund	34	30	24	6/30	9/24	3.5 months	1.7 months	11/30	11/24	Symptomatic improvement in 50%
Kostroff et al.	35	28	32	8/28	7/32	10 months	2 months	23/28	10/32	7 shunt-related deaths in cirrhotics
Holm et al.	33	41[b]	13	8/41	3/13	N/R[c]	N/R	N/R	N/R	Operative mortality: 31% cirrhosis; 15% malignant
Roussel et al.	37	N/A[d]	36	N/A	15/36	N/A	13 weeks	N/A	9/36	Shunt: last resort
Qazi et al.	38	N/A	40	N/A	12/40	N/A	N/R	N/A	5/40	High cellularity contributed to shunt failure
Smith et al.	36	N/A	50	N/A	14/50	N/A	12.2 weeks	N/A	18/50	Shunt failure did not affect survival; no shunt-related deaths
Edney et al.	24	N/A	45	N/A	10/45	N/A	33.3 weeks	N/A	6/45	No shunt-related deaths

[a] Some patients had more than one complication.
[b] Includes patients with nephrogenic ascites.
[c] N/R = not reported
[d] N/A = not applicable

Shunt outcome was as follows: three were removed or ligated for infection or DIC; 16 became occluded, 11 of which were not reopened; and 31 functioned without problems. Thus, 36 (72%) shunts ultimately provided effective palliation. Mean survival after shunt placement was 12 weeks. Interestingly, breast cancer patients had the longest survival time (24 weeks), whereas ovarian cancer patient survival was the same as for patients with gastric malignancies. Patients with primary tumors of the colon and pancreas fared the worst (3 to 5 weeks). At 8 weeks postoperatively, only 34% of the women and 14% of the men were still alive. The most striking finding of this report was related to the duration of ascites prior to the initiation of shunt therapy. Patients with ascites present for greater than 6 months had a mean survival of over 24 weeks, whereas those with presumably rapidly progressive ascites present for under 6 months had a mean survival of just over 9 weeks.

A study from Australia compared 42 patients with malignant ascites treated with a shunt with 43 patients treated medically.[39] Primary tumors were similar between the two groups, however, the shunted patients required larger volume paracenteses indicating more rapidly progressive ascites. Shunted patients had variable survival times; however, after placement of the shunt, survival was not affected by location of primary tumor. Overall survival time from the time of diagnosis of ascites was not different between the two groups (mean survival 209 days for shunted patients and 267 days for medically treated patients). The number of days of hospitalization from diagnosis of ascites until death was not different (25 days for shunted patients and 21 days for medically managed patients). A quality of life score was assigned to each patient after completion of a questionnaire. There was no difference between the two groups. Regarding shunt function, there were no differences in patency noted based on type of shunt (Le-Veen or Denver), quality of ascites, or cellularity of ascites. Half the shunts functioned well and did not require revision. Six had temporary occlusions, nine were blocked, and six were patent but did not control the ascites. This study was not controlled or randomized, but it is the only study available comparing peritoneovenous shunting with medical therapy. These researchers found that a trial of diuretics should be performed in all patients after their first paracentesis, and that beneficial results can be expected in up to one third of the patients. Shunting controlled ascites in two thirds of the patients, but survival was not altered. The authors concluded that shunts should be considered for those individuals with rapidly accumulating, difficult to control ascites, whose survival time would exceed 1 month.

There are no reports that widespread tumor dissemination occurs frequently as a result of peritoneovenous shunting for malignant ascites, or that this contributes to decreased survival. Estimates of tumor embolization reveal a rate of well under 5%. Most people do not consider this problem a legitimate reason to withhold peritoneovenous shunting from the patient with symptomatic, intractable malignant ascites.

COMPLICATIONS OF PERITONEOVENOUS SHUNTING

The complications of peritoneovenous shunting in general are summarized in Table 6-3. Compared with shunting for ascites due to liver disease, complications for malignant ascites are more rare. The most common complication after shunting for malignant ascites is shunt malfunction and occlusion.[40,41] Notably, DIC and systemic infectious complications are rare.[21,41–43] Infectious complications may not manifest themselves because of short patient survival times. It is interesting to note that spontaneous bacterial peritonitis is rare even in unshunted malignant ascites.[14] DIC does seem to be related to the level of hepatic dysfunction, and patients with evidence of poor hepatic synthetic function and those with an elevated or rising bilirubin are at highest risk for bleeding complications.[42]

Table 6-3. Complications of Peritoneovenous Shunt Procedures

Disseminated intravascular coagulation: rare with malignant ascites
Infectious:
  • wound infection
  • device infection
  • bacteremia
Fluid overload: pulmonary edema may be life threatening
Shunt occlusion or malfunction
Tumor embolization: < 5% of patients with malignant ascites
Twenty-five percent mortality rate: usually from disease progression
Central venous thrombosis
Ascitic leak

Coagulation abnormalities in the absence of clinical bleeding are common and represent evidence of shunt function.[44]

True DIC occasionally requires shunt ligation but most cases will resolve with supportive care, sometimes requiring fresh frozen plasma and heparin therapy. Abnormalities in coagulation parameters and platelet counts are common after peritoneovenous shunt placement, but clinical bleeding (DIC) is rare. Laboratory abnormalities need not be treated. One study looked at the development of postoperative coagulopathy in 35 patients who received Denver peritoneovenous shunts.[45] The majority of patients had gastrointestinal primary tumors and all were refractory to a trial of diuretics. Coagulation indices were measured preoperatively and on postoperative days 1 and 3. Levels of platelets, antithrombin III, plasminogen, antiplasmin, fibrinogen, and factors V and VIII were lower on day 1 but did not decrease further by day 3. Fibrin split products also increased by day 1, but decreased somewhat by day 3. A correlation was found between hematocrit reduction and platelet count reduction. The authors concluded that thrombocytopenia after peritoneovenous shunt was dilutional. Coagulopathy, on the other hand, was related to plasminogen activation and could be controlled by ascitic fluid removal at the time the shunt was placed. DIC did not occur in any patient. As this study reveals, coagulopathy after shunting for malignant ascites rarely leads to clinical DIC. Should this happen, temporary shunt occlusion by clamping the shunt at the chest counter-incision provides time to address the laboratory abnormalities and correct the bleeding. If bleeding recurs when the shunt is opened again, the device should be removed.

Fluid overload may occur, with acute pulmonary edema occasionally leading to death. Diuretics are usually needed to induce a brisk diuresis, but this is almost never needed past the immediate postoperative period. Mild fluid overload is common. Although some patients are able to diurese on their own, most require furosemide to increase urine output. Pulmonary edema is best prevented by careful postoperative monitoring and judicious use of diuretics. Careful observation and care postoperatively will limit clinically significant fluid overload, thus pulmonary edema should be a very rare occurrence.

Shunt malfunction is common. The suspect shunt may be studied with a radionuclide scan after intraperitoneal injection of a small amount of tracer. Occlusion may occur at either end or at the valve mechanism. Early shunt malfunction may occasionally be successfully treated with shunt revision. The manufacturer has a repair kit with extra shunt components and connectors allowing replacement of the peritoneal limb, the pump chamber, or the venous limb. Such repair procedures often can be undertaken under local anesthesia.

Early shunt occlusion, however, is indicative of unfavorable ascites and usually not of a technical problem. Occasionally, occlusion of the venous end of the shunt may be treated with thrombolytic agents such as streptokinase. Ascitic fluid leaks at the abdominal site may resolve as the ascites decreases and should initially be treated nonoperatively. Persistent leak justifies revision of the peritoneal purse string suture.

Shunt infections are not common. Prophylactic antibiotics should be used to cover gram-negative enteric organisms and staphylococci. Infections, both bacteremia and local, initially should be treated with culture-directed antibiotics. If the infection does not clear, the shunt must be removed. Soderlund[34] compared the complications of shunt placement for cirrhotic versus malignant ascites. He noted seven episodes of sepsis, all in cirrhotic ascites. Antibiotics were successful in treating the infection in four of the seven patients. No patients receiving a shunt for malignant ascites in this series developed serious infectious complications.

SUMMARY: SYMPTOMATIC TREATMENT OF MALIGNANT ASCITES

1. All patients with suspected malignant ascites should undergo a large volume of diagnostic and therapeutic paracentesis. Time to reaccumulation and recurrent symptoms should be determined.
2. A trial of spironolactone is justified in all patients. Patients with rapid reaccumulation of ascites despite diuretic therapy will require an alternative form of intervention.
3. An estimate of patient survival should be made. If expected survival is under 2 months or the patient has a very poor performance status, consideration should be given for repeating paracenteses only.
4. Patients with ovarian or breast cancer and malignant ascites should be considered for systemic (breast) or intraperitoneal (ovarian) chemotherapy, phase I or phase II trials, or immunotherapeutic trials.
5. Patients with malignant ascites from GI primary tumors, or ovarian and breast cancer patients who have no other therapeutic options, should undergo placement of a peritoneovenous shunt.

CANCER THERAPIES AND CYTOREDUCTION

Systemic Chemotherapy

Systemic chemotherapy is ineffective in treating malignant ascites in patients with gastrointestinal primary tumors. Its role in treating ascites in patients with metastatic breast or ovarian cancer is unclear.

Women with breast cancer develop malignant ascites very rarely. Application of regimens used for treating the more common malignant pleural effusions to malignant ascites is not justified. The palliative treatment of a malignant pleural effusion centers around intracavitary instillation of agents that result in pleurodesis (refer to Chapter 12); similar treatments for ascites may result in significant pain and small bowel obstruction from adhesions and therefore are not recommended. Systemic chemotherapy is the treatment of choice, but the therapy is directed at the usually widely metastatic disease, not at the malignant ascites *per se*. Combination therapies based on cyclophosphamide plus either doxorubicin or methotrexate, with or without other agents, remain a standard regimen in the treatment of advanced breast cancer and may be used in women who have failed hormonal therapy. Patients who have already been subjected to these agents pose a challenging situation, and some type of salvage chemotherapy (*e.g.*, doxorubicin alone after cytoxan–methotrexate–5-FU adjuvant therapy) or a phase I or II trial may be offered. Combinations or trials that include taxol may be justified; given the short expected survival of patients with malignant ascites, autologous bone marrow transplantation after very high-dose chemotherapy does not seem reasonable at this time. Lastly, hormonal therapy with tamoxifen may be tried in patients who have failed chemotherapy, have low performance status and thus may not be candidates for trials, and in patients who have estrogen receptor-positive tumors. For those who originally had a response to tamoxifen, a second line agent such as aminoglutethimide may be tried.

Ovarian cancer patients with advanced stage disease often have been treated with tumor debulking followed by cisplatin-based systemic chemotherapy. Patients who develop malignant ascites subsequent to systemic chemotherapy have few good options. Patients who relapse after standard chemotherapy often are treated with experimental combinations, including carboplatin, taxol, and ifosfamide. Toxicity may be very high in previously treated patients. Single agents with less toxicity, such as oral hexamethylmelamine, may be tried. Total abdominal radiation therapy after chemotherapy adds nothing to survival in patients with advanced ovarian cancer and probably should play no part in the treatment of malignant ascites.

INTRAPERITONEAL CHEMOTHERAPY

The use of intraperitoneal chemotherapy for the treatment of malignant ascites has been very disappointing. As stated above, much of the therapy has been based on results with intracavitary therapy for malignant pleural effusions, but the results have not been comparable.

Intraperitoneal chemotherapy for the treatment of malignant ascites in advanced cancer is experimental. It is described most commonly in patients with ovarian cancer and consideration for its use should probably be limited to these patients. Patients with minimal residual disease after ovarian cancer debulking may have complete responses to intraperitoneal chemotherapy up to 40% of the time.[46] Responses in patients with bulky disease are less common.[47] Cisplatin has been the drug of choice and there is no evidence that combination therapy given intraperitoneally improves results. Three patients with malignant ascites due to advanced ovarian cancer were reported in 1988.[48] All three failed systemic chemotherapy regimens. All three were treated with intraperitoneal cisplatin-based chemotherapy and all three had either resolution of ascites or dramatic reduction in rate of ascites accumulation and symptoms. The regimen described did not significantly reduce tumor burden in these patients. It is not clear that intraperitoneal chemotherapy affected survival in these patients, but it may play a useful role in otherwise controlling symptoms.

Immunotherapy and Biologic Response Modifiers

The first reports of biologic response modifiers in the treatment of malignant ascites centered on the unimpressive results of intraperitoneal administration of *Corynebacterium parvum*.[49] Immunotherapy and the administration of biologic response modifiers, such as interferon and tumor necrosis factor, have been applied to patients with malignant ascites. These therapies most commonly have been given intraperitoneally.

Intraperitoneal immunotherapy has consisted of instillations of the inteferons, tumor necrosis factor, interleukin-2 (IL-2), and lymphokine-activated killer (LAK) cells, specific antibodies, and of immunostimulatory preparations such as the streptococcal preparation OK-432. The rationale for intraperitoneal administration of many of these agents has been twofold: first, very high doses of agents may be applied directly to the tumor site; and second, drug-induced toxicities are decreased despite high doses. Both interferon-gamma (IFN-γ) and alpha (IFN-α) have been used to treat malignant ascites from multiple causes. Patients with ovarian cancer with malignant ascites and no bulky disease seem to respond best.[50] Intraperitoneal instillation of IFN-α-2b resulted in partial or complete responses (negative cytologic findings or ascites control only, respectively) in three of eight patients, and slowing of the rate of accumulation of ascites in two additional patients.[51] These responders had malignant ascites only. There were no responders in the ascites plus bulky tumor group. In another report, the combination of intraperitoneal IFN-α and cisplatin proved to be more effective than cisplatin alone in controlling ascites.[50] The response rate for the combination therapy was five of seven (77%) and for cisplatin alone was two of nine (22%). Again, the responders all had ascites in the absence of bulky disease. Most recently, 10 patients with advanced ovarian cancer and ascites were treated with intraperitoneal IFN-α-2b at a dose of 10 M U/m².[52] Seven of the 10 patients had received previous cisplatin or carboplatin therapy systemically. The benefits of IFN-α were minimal and palliation of ascites did not occur in half the patients.

Intraperitoneal administration of recombinant human tumor necrosis factor-alpha (TNF-α) was used to treat 29 patients with malignant ascites secondary to metastases from a variety of primary sites including the ovary, breast, liver, colon and rectum, stomach, and pancreas.[52] Patients with refractory ascites, reasonable performance status, and expected survival of greater than 2 months were selected. In this phase I trial, escalating dosages of TNF-α were used up to 350 mg/m², with no limiting toxicities.[53] Twenty-two responded with complete (16) or partial (6) resolution of their ascites. Only six patients had minimal or no response; one died of disease progression early during the trial. All 10 patients with ovarian cancer had complete responses. Median survival was 139 days. Nine of 15 with GI primary tumors had complete (5) or partial (4) responses. Median survival for nonovarian cancer patients was 56 days. Given the lack of side effects of this therapy and the promising palliative results, further trials of intraperitoneal TNF-α appear to be justified.

The use of intraperitoneal IL-2 and LAK cells has been described. In a report of two patients with gynecologic malignancies and malignant ascites, instillation of IL-2 and allogeneic LAK cells resulted in complete disappearance of malignant cells from peritoneal fluid and a marked reduction in the volume of ascites.[54] There was no prolongation of survival. The patients died 61 and 63 days after initiation of therapy.

Autologous LAK cells and IL-2 were given intraperitoneally to 24 patients with peritoneal space malignancies.[55] Ten patients had ovarian cancer and 12 had colorectal cancer. Toxic side effects (hypotension, oliguria, thrombocytopenia, fluid retention) were frequent but resolved quickly with discontinuation of therapy. One patient suffered both a treatment-induced grand mal seizure and colonic perforation. Severe adhesions developed in 14 patients, limiting repeat treatment cycles in five. Two of 10 ovarian cancer patients and 5 of 12 colorectal cancer patients had partial responses. Given the logistic difficulties and expense of producing LAK cells for therapy, their use in palliative efforts does not seem justified.

Radiolabeled monoclonal antibodies have been used in patients with refractory malignant ascites secondary to metastatic breast and ovarian cancer. Previously, authors had hinted that ascites might be reduced using such therapy.[56] In the most recent report, a radioiodinated (^{131}I) monoclonal antibody to mucin, 2G3, was used.[57] Eleven patients were enrolled, but only nine received therapeutic doses. Of this nine, three received moderate to significant palliation and the remainder had progression of disease. Side effects, which were minor, were felt to be due to prolonged retention of the radioisotope in the peritoneal cavity. These results were disappointing given the results of the other palliative interventions available.

Lastly, in 1983, Torisu et al[58] reported on the use of a nonspecific immune stimulant in the treatment of malignant ascites. The *Strep pyogenes*-derived preparation OK-432 was injected intraperitoneally weekly, for 1 to 6 weeks, into 134 patients with malignant ascites. The origin of the ascites was stomach cancer in 121 patients and colon cancer in 13 patients. Ascites disappeared in 76 patients and was reduced in an additional 8, representing a 63% response rate. When a blind comparison of 48 untreated patients was made to 99 treated patients, all of whom died, these authors found an increased mean survival, from 3.1 months to 10.2 months. They also found the best responses in those patients with highly cellular ascites. Japanese investigators have used OK-432 for the treatment of other advanced malignancies, including lung cancer. It has direct toxic effects on tumor cells and immunostimulatory effects on the host.

Subsequent studies revealed induction

of a peritoneal influx of neutrophils, activated macrophages, and lymphocytes.[59] The number of infiltrating leukocytes was indirectly proportional to the number of tumor cells in the ascites. *In vitro* evaluation revealed recruitment of natural killer cells to the peritoneum by a neutrophil-derived chemotactic factor.[60] Although these results were very promising, there has been little additional experience with the agent outside of Japan.

SUMMARY: CYTOTOXIC AND IMMUNOTHERAPY FOR MALIGNANT ASCITES

1. Standard systemic cytotoxic chemotherapy should be reserved for patients with malignant ascites secondary to breast or ovarian cancer:
   a. Breast cancer therapy should be adriamycin-based if the patient has not been previously treated with this agent.
   b. Taxol-based therapeutic trials should be considered for patients with malignant ascites from breast or ovarian primary tumors and who have been previously treated with standard agents.
2. Intraperitoneal chemotherapy should be reserved for patients enrolled in clinical studies. Current agents are not effective for GI primary tumors. Intraperitoneal cisplatin-based therapy may be considered for ovarian cancer patients.
3. Intraperitoneal immunotherapy with IL-2 and LAK cells is expensive and toxic and the current results cannot justify their use outside of a controlled trial.
4. Intraperitoneal therapy with IFN-α and TNF-α is promising, with excellent results described for ovarian cancer patients with malignant ascites. In addition, intraperitoneal TNF-α seems to be effective in controlling malignant ascites associated with GI primary malignancies.
5. Other immunologic agents (radiolabeled antibodies, nonspecific immune stimulators) have not been adequately evaluated to justify their use outside of a study setting.

SUMMARY

Patients with a history of malignancy who develop ascites should undergo a diagnostic paracentesis. The differentiation of benign from malignant ascites can be difficult because positive cytology is found in only 50% to 75% of cases. Fluid cholesterol may aid in establishing a diagnosis, with levels greater than 48 mg/dL being highly suggestive of malignant ascites.

The decision to intervene in patients with malignant ascites is not straightforward. A trial of diuretic therapy should be initiated. Patients with poor expected survival should undergo paracentesis only. Patients with ascites secondary to ovarian or breast tumors should be considered for chemotherapy. Other patients will probably benefit from peritoneovenous shunt placement.

Intraperitoneal chemotherapy should be reserved for use in clinical trials. Currently available agents are not effective against gastrointestinal primary tumors.

The management of patients with malignant ascites requires careful clinical judgement, as this problem often develops late in the course of disease. The decision to treat these patients, especially with surgical therapy such as peritoneovenous shunt placement, must be made carefully after considering a wide range of factors both medical and social. Clearly, this must be a highly individualized decision.

REFERENCES

1. Ringenberg QS, Doll DC, Loy TS, Yarbro JW. Malignant ascites of unknown origin. Cancer 1989;64:753.
2. Nagy JA, Herzberg KT, Dvorak JM, Dvorak HF. Pathogenesis of malignant ascites formation: initiating events that lead to fluid accumulation. Cancer Res 1993;53:2631.
3. Senger DR, Connolly DT, Van De Water L, Fed-

er J, Dvorak HF. Purification and NH$_2$-terminal amino acid sequence of guinea pig tumor-secreted vascular permeability factor. Cancer Res 1990;50:1774.
4. Senger DR, Peruzzi CA, Feder J, Dvorak HF. A highly conserved vascular permeability factor secreted by a variety of human and rodent tumor cell lines. Cancer Res 1986;46:5629.
5. Garrison RN, Galloway RH, Heuser LS. Mechanisms of malignant ascites production. J Surg Res 1987;42:126.
6. Prieto M, Gomez-Lechon MJ, Hoyos M, Castell JV, Carrasco D, Berenguer J. Diagnosis of malignant ascites. Comparison of ascitic fibronectin, cholesterol, and serum-ascites albumin difference. Dig Dis Sci 1988;33:833.
7. Lee CM, Changchien CS, Shyu WC, Liaw YF. Serum-ascites albumin concentration gradient and ascites fibronectin in the diagnosis of malignant ascites. Cancer 1992;70:2057.
8. Jungst D, Gerbes AL, Martin R, Paumgartner G. Value of lipids in the differentiation between cirrhotic and malignant ascites. Hepatology 1986;6:239.
9. Adamsen S, Jonsson P, Brodin B, Lindberg B, Jorpes P. Measurement of fibronectin concentration on benign and malignant ascites. Eur J Surg 1991;157:325.
10. Tsujimoto F, Miyamoto Y, Tada S. Differentiation of benign from malignant ascites by sonographic evaluation of gallbladder wall. Radiology 1985;157:503.
11. Callen PW, Marks WM, Filly RA. Computed tomography and ultrasonography in the evaluation of the retroperitoneum in patients with malignant ascites. J Comput Assist Tomogr 1979;3:581.
12. Borzutzky CA, Spinuzza TJ, Turbiner EH. Technetium-99m MDP accumulation in malignant ascites. Clin Nucl Med 1985;10:731.
13. Weissman GS, McKinley MJ, Budman DR, Schulman P, Grueneberg D, et al. Flow cytometry. A new technique in the diagnosis of malignant ascites. J Clin Gastroenterol 1987;9:599.
14. Kurtz RC, Bronzo RL. Does spontaneous bacterial peritonitis occur in malignant ascites? Am J Gastroenterol 1982;77:146.
15. Ross GJ, Kessler HB, Clair MR, Gatenby RA, Hartz WH, Ross LV. Sonographically guided paracentesis for palliation of symptomatic ascites. AJR 1989;153:1309.
16. Lomas DA, Wallis PJW, Stockley RA. Palliation of malignant ascites with a Tenckhoff catheter. Thorax 1989;44:828.
17. Belfort MA, Stevens PJD, Dehaek K, Soeters R, Kringe JEJ. A new approach to the management of malignant ascites; a permanently implanted abdominal drain. Eur J Surg Oncol 1990;16:47.
18. Greenway B, Johnson PJ, Williams R. Control of malignant ascites with spironolactone. Br J Surg 1982;69:441.
19. Pockros PJ, Esrason KT, Nguyen C, Duque J, Woods S. Mobilization of malignant ascites with diuretics is dependent on ascitic fluid characteristics. Gastroenterology 1992;103:1302.
20. LeVeen HH, Christoudias G, Moon IP, Luft R, Falk G, Grosberg S. Peritoneovenous shunting for ascites. Ann Surg 1974;180:580.
21. Lacy JH, Wieman TJ, Shively EH. Management of malignant ascites. Surg Gynecol Obstet 1984;159:397.
22. Lund RH, Newkirk JB. Peritoneovenous shunting systems for surgical management of malignant ascites. Contemp Surg 1979;14:31.
23. Reinhardt GP, Stanley MM. Peritoneovenous shunting for ascites. Surg Gynecol Obstet 1977;145:419.
24. Edney JA, Hill A, Armstrong D. Peritoneovenous shunts palliate malignant ascites. Am J Surg 1989;158:598.
25. Fulenwider JT, Galambos JD, LeVeen HH, et al. LeVeen vs. Denver peritoneovenous shunts for intractable ascites of cirrhosis: a randomized, prospective trial. Arch Surg 1986;121:351.
26. Straus AK, Roseman DL, Shapiro TM. Peritoneovenous shunting in the management of malignant ascites. Arch Surg 1979;114:489.
27. Raaf JH, Stroehlein JR. Palliation of malignant ascites by LeVeen peritoneovenous shunt. Cancer 1980;45:1019.
28. Kudsk K, Fabian TC, Minton JP. LeVeen shunts in patients with intractable malignant ascites. J Surg Oncol 1980;13:61.
29. Holman JM, Albo D. Peritoneovenous shunting in patients with malignant ascites. Am J Surg 1981;142:774.
30. Cheung DK, Raff JH. Selection of patients with malignant ascites for a peritoneovenous shunt. Cancer 1982;50:1204.
31. Sonnenfeld T, Tyden G. Peritoneovenous shunts for malignant ascites. Acta Chir Scand 1986;152:117.
32. Martin GW, Cogbill TH. Peritoneovenous shunting for malignant ascites. Wis Med J 1988;87:31.
33. Holm A, Halpern NB, Aldrete JS. Peritoneovenous shunt for intractable ascites of hepatic, nephrogenic, and malignant causes. Am J Surg 1989;158:162.
34. Soderlund C. Denver peritoneovenous shunting for malignant or cirrhotic ascites. A prospective consecutive series. Scand J Gastroenterol 1986;21:1161.
35. Kostroff KM, Ross DW, Davis JM. Peritoneovenous shunting for cirrhotic versus malignant ascites. Surg Gynecol Obstet 1985;161:204.

36. Smith DAP, Weaver DW, Bouwman DL. Peritoneovenous shunt (PVS) for malignant ascites: an analysis of outcome. Am Surg 1989;55:445.
37. Roussel JGJ, Kroon BBR, Hart GAM. The Denver type for peritoneovenous shunting of malignant ascites. Surg Gynecol Obstet 1986;162:235.
38. Qazi R, Savlov ED. Peritoneovenous shunt for palliation of malignant ascites. Cancer 1982;49:600.
39. Gough IR, Balderson GA. Malignant ascites. A comparison of peritoneovenous shunting and nonoperative management. Cancer 1993;71:2377.
40. Souter RG, Wells C, Tarin D, Kettlewell MGW. Surgical and pathologic complications associated with peritoneovenous shunts in management of malignant ascites. Cancer 1985;55:1973.
41. Vo NM, Tortora MJ, DeMaio JT, Aseltine DT. Complications of peritoneovenous shunting for malignant ascites. Conn Med 1981;45:1.
42. Tempero MA, Davis RB, Reed E, Edney J. Thrombocytopenia and laboratory evidence of disseminated intravascular coagulation after shunts for ascites in malignant disease. Cancer 1985;55:2718.
43. Lokich J, Reinhold R, Silverman M, Tullis J. Complications of peritoneovenous shunt for malignant ascites. Cancer Treat Rep 1980;64:305.
44. Harmon DC, Demirjian Z, Ellman L, Fischer JF. Disseminated intravascular coagulation with the peritoneovenous shunt. Ann Intern Med 1979;90:774.
45. Gleysteen JJ, Hussey CV, Heckman MG. The cause of coagulopathy after peritoneovenous shunt for malignant ascites. Arch Surg 1990;125:474.
46. Cohen CV. Surgical considerations in ovarian cancer. Semin Oncol 1985;12:53.
47. Markman M, Howell S, Cleary S, et al. Survival following cisplatin (DDP)-based intraperitoneal chemotherapy for refractory ovarian carcinoma. Proc Am Soc Clin Oncol 1986;5:113.
48. Lind SE, Cashavelly B, Fuller AF. Resolution of malignant ascites after intraperitoneal chemotherapy in women with carcinoma of the ovary. Surg Gynecol Obstet 1988;166:519.
49. Best RC, Berek JS, Obrist R. Intraperitoneal immunotherapy of human ovarian carcinoma with Corynebacterium parvum. Cancer 1983;43:1395.
50. Bezwoda WR, Golombick T, Dansey R, Keeping J. Treatment of malignant ascites due to recurrent/refractory ovarian cancer: the use of interferon-α or interferon-α plus chemotherapy *in vivo* and *in vitro*. Eur J Cancer 1991;27:1423.
51. Bezwoda WR, Seymour L, Dansey R. Intraperitoneal recombinant interferon-alpha 2b for recurrent malignant ascites due to ovarian cancer. Cancer 1989;64:1029-1033.
52. Stuart GCE, Nation JG, Snider DD, Thunberg P. Intraperitoneal interferon in the management of malignant ascites. Cancer 1993; 71:2027.
53. Rath U, Kaufmann M, Schmid H, Hofmann J, Wiedenmann B, Kist A, et al. Effect of intraperitoneal recombinant human tumor nercosis factor alpha on malignant ascites. Eur J Cancer 1991;27:121-125.
54. Kamada M, Sakamoto Y, Furumoto H, Mori K, Daitoh T, Irahara M, et al. Treatment of malignant ascites with allogeneic and autologous lymphokine-activated killer cells. Gynecol Oncol 1989;34:34.
55. Steis RG, Urba WJ, VanderMolen LA, Bookman MA. Intraperitoneal lymphokine-activated killer-cell and interleukin-2 therapy for malignancies limited to the peritoneal cavity. J Clin Oncol 1990;8:1618.
56. Epenetos AA, Hooker G, Krausz T, Snook D, Bodmer WF, Taylor-Papadimitriou J. Antibody-guided irradiation of malignant ascites in ovarian cancer: a new therapeutic method possessing specificity against cancer cells. Obstet Gynecol 1986;68:71S-74S.
57. Ward B, Mather S, Shepherd J, Crowther M, Hawkins L, Britton K, et al. The treatment of intraperitoneal malignant disease with monoclonal antibody guided ^{131}I radiotherapy. Br J Cancer 1988;58:658-662.
58. Torisu M, Katano M, Kimura Y, Itoh H, Takesue M. New approach to management of malignant ascites with a streptococcal preperation, OK-432. I. Improvement of host immunity and prolongation of survival. Surgery 1983;93:357.
59. Katano M, Torisu M. New approach to management of malignant ascites with a streptococcal preparation OK-432. II. Intraperitoneal inflammatory cell-mediated tumor cell destruction. Surgery 1983;93:365.
60. Hayashi Y, Torisu M. New approach to management of malignant ascites with a streptococcal preparation OK-432. III. OK-432 attracts natural killer cells through a chemotactic factor released from activated neutrophils. Surgery 1990;107:74.

Intestinal Complications of Radiation Therapy

PAULINE W. CHEN
WILLIAM F. SINDELAR

Radiation therapy has evolved into a powerful modality in the treatment of the cancer patient since Roentgen's description of ionizing radiation in 1895. It is estimated that more than half of all patients with cancer receive radiation therapy at some time during the management of their disease, either as primary treatment, as adjuvant or neoadjuvant therapy, or as palliation.[1] Irradiation of cancers can consistently inflict damage on neoplastic tissue. However, normal tissues within the radiation portals also can sustain damage, with the possibility of clinical complications. The gastrointestinal tract can be especially sensitive to radiation damage.[1,2] Just as Walsh's first description of radiation-induced enteropathy in 1897[3] closely followed Roentgen's discovery, intestinal radiation injury and its management has plagued many patients of surgical, radiation, and medical oncologists.

By damaging cellular DNA and thereby the overall process of cell replication, acute effects are manifested only after irradiated cells have undergone unsuccessful attempts at mitosis. Thus, the actively mitotic cells of the gastrointestinal tract, particularly the mucosal layers, manifest acute toxicity, which appears earlier than in tissues with less actively dividing cell populations such as bone or nerve. Chronic radiation effects appear late following irradiation, often after many months, and are postulated to be secondary to radiation-induced vascular injury with progressive ischemia.[4]

The delivery of radiation therapy to malignancies must be tempered by the dose limitations of normal surrounding tissue. The major factors involved in normal tissue tolerance include the daily dose fraction administered, the total dose delivered, and the volume of normal tissue within the radiation field. Although the term *dose* generally refers to a specified point in space, typically the midpoint of the tumor volume, tissues along the entire radiation path receive radiation energy, depending on their differing depths, which can vary from a fraction of to substantially more than the estimated dose to the specified point. Absorbed radiation is measured in units termed the Gray (Gy), defined as 1 joule absorbed energy per kilogram of tissue (equivalent to 100 rad). Acute radiation effects on tissue typically correlate with the daily dose (dose rate) and the total dose delivered, whereas chronic effects are generally determined by the total dose and volume of tissue within the radiation field.[5]

Early efforts at therapeutic radiation using low-voltage sources typically produced acute erythematous and sometimes exfoliative dermatitis as the major toxicity to normal tissues, due to the high level of energy absorption at the skin surface and to the necessity to deliver large surface doses to ensure adequate energy penetration to deeper-seated tissues. In the early 1960s, however, high-energy radiation sources were introduced into clinical use. These megavoltage units offered several advantages over the previously utilized kilovoltage sources. Not only did high-energy radiation provide sparing of the skin and diminished absorption in bone, it also decreased absorption by healthy tissue and allowed for greater tissue penetration which permitted the treatment of deeply seated tumors.[6,7] Because of the increased skin sparing with megavoltage techniques, radiation-induced injury to the small intestine came to replace radiation dermatitis as the dose-limiting factor in the treatment of tumors of the abdomen and pelvis.

Acute effects such as vomiting and diarrhea are commonly observed during abdominal and pelvic radiation and are generally self-limited following the conclusion of therapy. *Acute* toxicity can be defined as that occurring during or within 1 month of radiation therapy. Toxicity that appears between 1 and 3 months following radiation is often termed *subacute*, whereas *chronic* toxicity appears later than 3 months following treatment. There may be considerable overlap in the appearance of acute, subacute, and chronic toxicity, and the categoric definitions are somewhat arbitrary. Often acute and subacute complications are grouped together and are considered distinct from chronic toxicity. A generally convenient operational definition may be that acute and subacute effects are self-limited and uncommonly lead to difficult or unmanageable clinical problems, whereas chronic effects tend to be permanent and often progressive leading to circumstances that are difficult to manage clinically. Chronic effects and their more life-threatening sequelae, such as intestinal obstruction and perforation, are rare but can occur up to 20 years after therapy.[8] Although much experience has accrued over the years with this entity, radiation enteritis remains a clinical enigma because of its unpredictable occurrence and its difficulty to manage clinically.

Radiation tolerance to specific sites can be used to quantitate the toxicity of varying doses. The minimal tolerance dose (TD 5/5) represents the dosage that produces complications in 5% of patients within 5 years. The maximal tolerance dose (TD 50/5) produces complications in 50% of patients within 5 years. The small and large intestine are regarded as having a TD 5/5 of 45 Gy and a TD 50/5 of 65 Gy. The rectum has a TD 5/5 of 55 Gy and a TD 50/5 of 80 Gy.[9,10]

External beam radiation can be delivered in combination with intracavitary and interstitial brachytherapy, or with intraoperative electron-beam radiotherapy. By utilizing these specialized modalities in the treatment of intra-abdominal tumors, the external beam dose can be held to below 50 Gy while providing a potentially tumoricidal total dose, thus decreasing the likelihood of radiation-induced injuries to intestine and other normal intra-abdominal tissues. Brachytherapy and intraoperative radiation therapy can deliver high doses of radiation to limited and well-circumscribed areas, thereby limiting the radiation received by adjacent normal tissues. External beam radiation, by comparison, must necessarily traverse normal tissues to reach deeply seated tumor sites and it can deliver substantial doses to normal tissues in the vicinity of the tumor site. These specialized modalities, however, have their own associated complications and do not totally eliminate the risk of radiation-related bowel injury.[11,12]

The vast majority of patients receiving radiation therapy complain of acute radiation-induced symptoms. Most of these manifestations resolve spontaneously upon cessation or completion of therapy. The incidence of chronic radiation injury to the gastrointestinal tract reported in the medical literature ranges from 0.5% to 36%. "Clinically significant" injury is reported in 5% to 15% of patients,[10,13,14] although the parameters of what denotes clinically significant problems often remain variable and undefined in the literature.[15] Moreover, the incidence of radiation enteropathy may be increasing as more patients, whose malignant disease is controlled and who survive for longer periods, begin to manifest the late-appearing symptoms of chronic radiation injury.[15,16]

ACUTE AND SUBACUTE RADIATION INJURY

Acute and subacute radiation-induced toxicity occurs in up to 75% of all patients receiving radiotherapy,[17] especially those receiving abdominal irradiation. Patients are usually affected during their course of radiation therapy delivery and complain of vomiting, nausea, abdominal cramping, and intermittent diarrhea. Although varying in severity in most individuals, these symptoms may become sufficiently troublesome to require the cessation of therapy in up to 20% of patients.[18] Children, in particular those younger than 2 years of age and those receiving combined modality therapy, are especially susceptible to severe radiation-induced enteropathy.[19]

The symptoms of acute radiation enteritis are usually due to the direct effects of radiation on the rapidly dividing intestinal mucosal cells. Pathologic changes include transient mucosal atrophy, crypt dilatation, and loss of villi. Regeneration of injured mucosal cells can occur to some degree between doses, and an interruption of treatment can result in substantial replenishment of the mucosal cell population. As a result of the radiation-induced mucosal injury, the intestinal absorption of nutrients and fluids decreases and fluid efflux can occur. The symptoms of acute radiation enteritis typically end with the completion of therapy. The symptoms may extend beyond the duration of treatment for varying lengths of time, often being classified as subacute enteritis. Subacute symptoms are usually self-limited in such cases.

As therapy progresses, plasma cells and polymorphonuclear cells densely infiltrate the lamina propria. Normal intestinal motility is disrupted. Luminal contents, such as bile salts or trypsin,[20] and luminal pH[21] may affect the severity of injury. Eventually over the course of therapy, patients may begin to exhibit nutritional wasting with decreased absorption of vitamin B_{12} and bile acids.[22]

Radiologic findings during acute and subacute radiation enteritis include dilated and atonic small bowel.[23] These findings, as with the overall constellation of symptoms, generally resolve after the cessation of therapy.

Treatment of Acute and Subacute Radiation Enteritis

Most symptoms of acute and subacute radiation enteritis are self-limited, usually resolving after the completion of therapy. Most commonly, patients complain of diarrhea, abdominal cramping, and nausea. Anticholinergic medications and opiates often can provide symptomatic relief. Those patients with symptoms unresponsive to these agents may benefit from cholestyramine and bile salt sequestrating agents.[15]

Changes in dose rate and in the volume of intestine irradiated also can ameliorate acute radiation-induced symptoms. Decreasing the daily dose rate by as little as 10% can improve symptoms.[5] The volume of normal bowel in the irradiation portal is highly variable and is dependent on multiple factors: proportion of the abdomen irradiated, inclusion of the pelvis, body habitus, and previous abdominal or pelvic surgery which can result in adhesions that fix bowel loops within the radiation field. Methods used to decrease the amount of bowel within the radiation field include: bladder distension (Fig. 7-1) to displace bowel loops cephalad, multiple fixed or rotational fields, and varying patient position.[24]

Various pharmacologic agents have been used in the treatment of acute and subacute radiation enteritis. Increased activity of gut prostaglandins has been shown to have a role in the evolution of symptoms associated with radiation enteritis. Multiple studies have examined the role of prostaglandin inhibitors, such as indomethacin, in alleviating

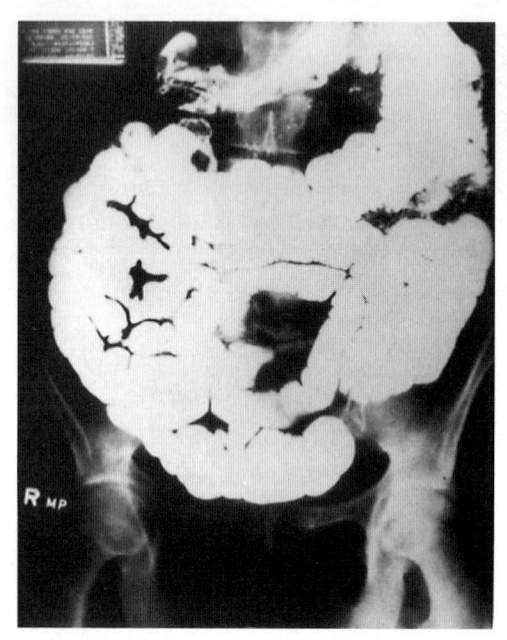

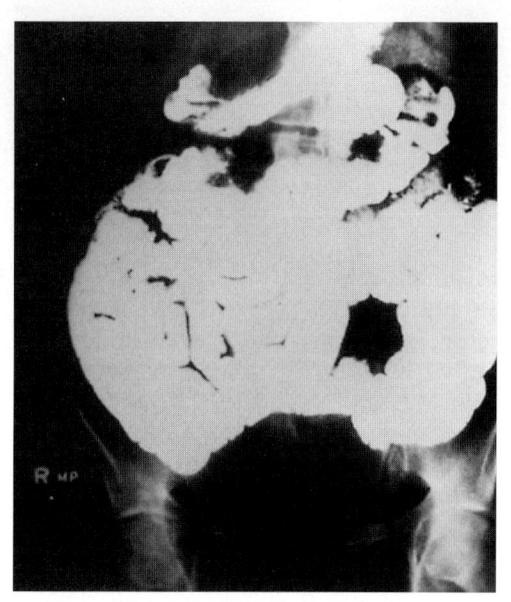

Figure 7-1. Radiographs demonstrating the position of bowel loops before (*left*) and after (*right*) bladder distention. This technique may be useful in preventing radiation-induced bowel injury. (Reprinted with permission from Ahlgren JD and MacDonald JS. Gastrointestinal oncology. Philadelphia, JB Lippincott, 1992;369.)

the symptomatology of acute radiation enteritis.[25-27] However, not all pharmacotherapeutic agents that inhibit eicosanoid synthesis have been demonstrated to be clinically beneficial, and the respective roles of each of the prostaglandins, the thromboxanes, and the leukotrienes remain unclear.[28]

The role of antioxidants has also been explored during irradiation of the gastrointestinal tract. The cytotoxic effects on the small bowel are, for the most part, believed to be secondary to the oxygen free radicals generated during radiation therapy. Ionizing radiation generates free radicals from intracellular water, which can interact with cellular DNA to prevent replication and transcription. Despite intact cellular repair mechanisms, the free radical–induced nuclear injuries may be too numerous or too severe. These lethal injuries tend to affect cells with high turnover rates, such as those of the small intestine.[29] The administration of antioxidants could then, at least in theory, reverse some of the radiation-induced effects. Vitamin E, an antioxidant, administered intraperitoneally to the rat model, has been shown to protect against radiation-induced fluid absorption injury.[30] Delaney et al[31,32] have examined intraluminal administration of antioxidant agents on the presumption that higher concentrations of the agents could be achieved with this method of delivery. However, whether this intraluminal concentration gradient can affect the serosa, typically the most severely injured portion of the bowel, remains unknown.

The use of nutritional therapy with gut rest through the administration of total parenteral nutrition has been advocated both to lessen the severity of radiation damage and to maintain optimal nutritional status through treatment despite radiation intestinal injury.[14] Given the role of glutamine as a primary energy source for the intestinal tract, glutamine-enriched diets have been proposed as methods to accelerate mucosal healing and to prevent injury in the irradiated gut. Such diets rich in glutamine have been investigated in animal models and have shown some benefit.[33,34]

Neurotensin, a trophic gut hormone, has been proposed as a potential radioprotectant. In the rat model, intraperitoneal neurotensin reduced bacterial translocation and aided in preserving mucosal integrity.[18] Whether this and other trophic hormones for the gut have a role in the treatment of acute radiation enteritis in the clinical setting remains to be determined by further investigation.

■ SUMMARY: ACUTE AND SUBACUTE RADIATION INJURY

1. Radiation injury to the intestine is observed in up to 75% of patients receiving radiotherapy, and varies in severity. Acute and subacute radiation enteritis can result in the clinically troubling picture of nausea, vomiting, diarrhea, and food intolerance. In fact, almost all patients undergoing abdominal or pelvic radiotherapy will experience such symptoms to at least some degree during the course of their therapy.
2. Radiologic findings include dilated and atonic loops of small bowel.
3. Symptoms can be ameliorated with a variety of measures including alteration of treatment schedule, temporary interruption of treatment, dietary modifications, and intestinal rest.
4. For most patients, acute and subacute toxicity is a transient phenomenon without significant or lasting sequelae. ■

CHRONIC RADIATION INJURY

By definition, radiation enteritis becomes chronic when gastrointestinal symptoms such as nausea, diarrhea, and abdominal cramping persist for at least 3 months following the cessation of radiotherapy or appear more than 3 months following treatment.[15] These chronic symptoms generally are manifest within 6 to 18 months of the completion of therapy[2] but have been known to present after latent periods of up to 20 years.[8]

The onset of symptoms of chronic radiation enteritis is usually insidious, typically presenting initially with a prodromal phase characterized by colicky abdominal pain, progressing over a variable time course to bloody diarrhea, steatorrhea, tenesmus, and weight loss. On occasion, these symptoms can evolve acutely and patients may present with a perforated viscus or bowel obstruction.[35] Chronic radiation enteritis occurs in 5% to 15% of patients who have undergone abdominal or pelvic irradiation. Operative intervention for the treatment of complications of chronic radiation enteritis is required in 2% to 17% of patients.[36–40] This is fully discussed in the next section of this chapter.

Multiple factors are associated with increased frequency of these chronic radiation-related intestinal complications. Prior abdominal surgery, producing adhesions which fix loops of small bowel within the irradiated field, can increase the incidence of chronic injuries. Patients who have a slender habitus, are elderly, and are female also can be at increased risk because of a small abdominal cavity and consequent close proximity of a large proportion of the intestinal tract to the tumor volume. Comorbid disease, such as diabetes mellitus, hypertension, or idiopathic vasculitis, are also predisposing factors.[5,8,41] Concomitant chemotherapy during radiation therapy can exacerbate the potential for delayed complications.[9] Evidence exists as well for *recall* enteritis, recurrent symptoms following remote radiation that develop during subsequent administration of chemotherapy with actinomycin or doxorubicin.[42]

Grossly, intestine that has chronic radiation-induced injury appears mottled red and gray with numerous fibrous adhesions. These adhesions often fuse loops of bowel, occasionally causing kinks and sites of obstruction. Tapered intestinal strictures can be pre-

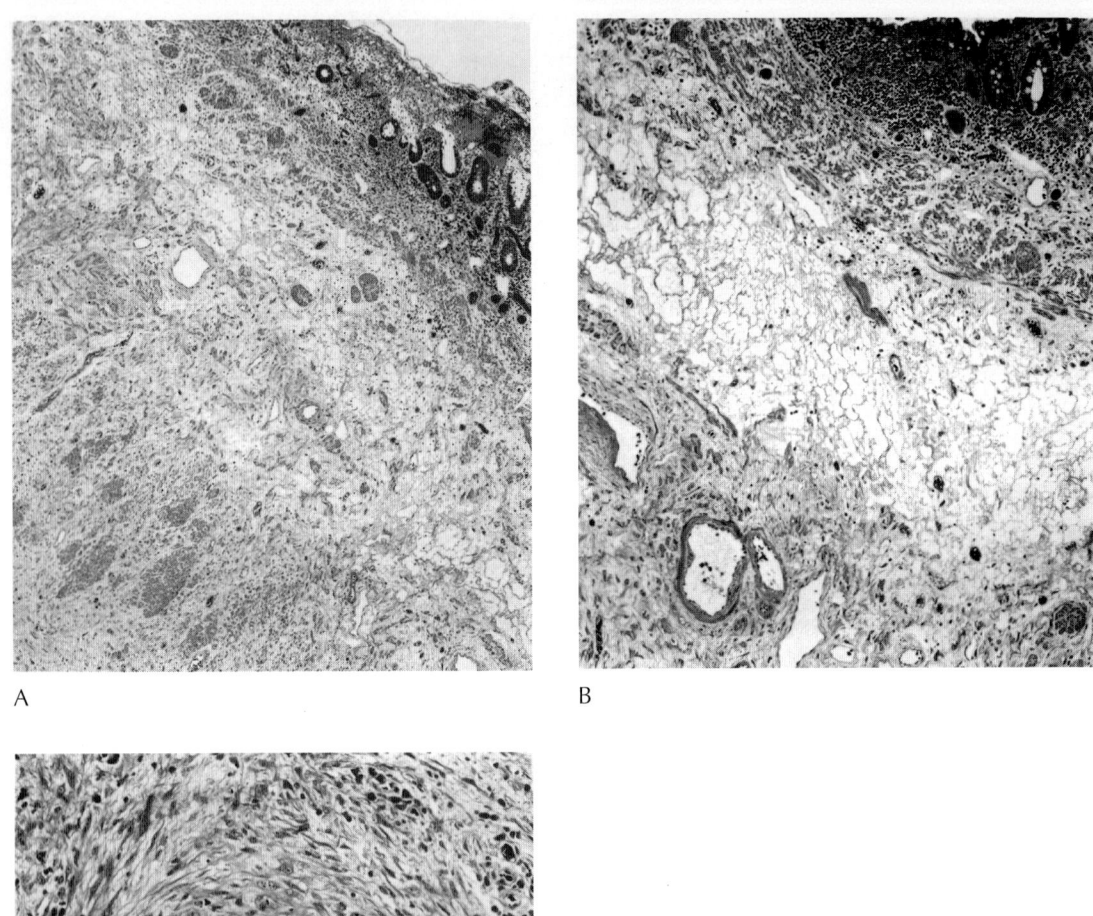

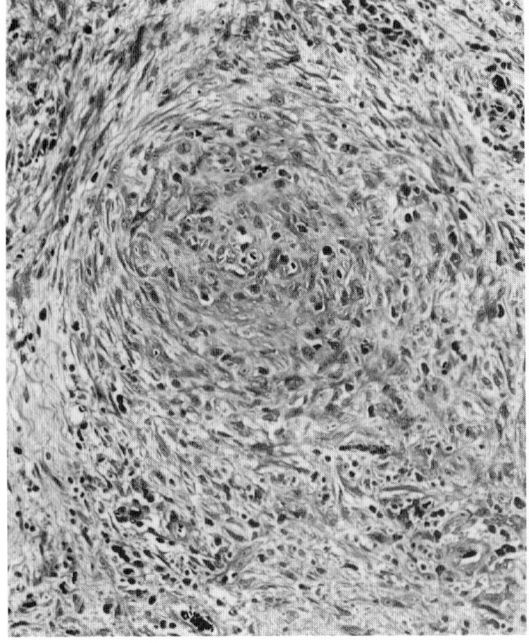

Figure 7-2. Histologic appearance of chronic radiation enteritis involving the small intestine. **A.** Intestinal wall showing atrophy and ulceration of the mucosa, edema of the submucosa, and fibrosis of the muscularis (magnification ×50). **B.** Intestinal wall showing edema and fibrosis (magnification ×100). **C.** Intestinal arteriole obliterated by radiation-induced vasculitis (magnification ×200).

sent. Multiple internal as well as external fistulae can be present within the amalgamation of bowel loops and thickened adhesions. The intestinal serosa and submucosa appear gray and fibrous. Mucosal folds frequently contain ulcerations.[43] Microscopic changes include an atrophic mucosa either with thickened blunted villi or with the absence of villi altogether. Distinct brush borders are lost and the lamina propria exhibits telangiectatic vessels. The submucosa and the serosa, the intestinal layers most severely affected, are thickened and edematous. Serosal and mesenteric arteries show severe myointimal proliferation, which is typical of a late radiation effect on small vessels. Fibrous plaques form on the intima, narrowing the vessel lumen. Some vessels may show full-thickness lesions, with organized thromboses and with occasional occlusion.[44] Figure 7-2 illustrates histologic changes that develop in chronic radiation enteritis.

Vascular injury has been implicated as the principal mechanism for late radiation effects. Irradiated small vessels can show early vascular spasm with a progressive obliterative vasculitis that can result in bowel ischemia. Carr et al[44] examined normal and postradiation colectomy specimens. After intramural perfusion with barium sulfated suspension, microradiography and radiographic fluorescence were used to examine the microvasculature. In sites of radiation-induced stricture, a reduction in vascularity was seen affecting all layers of the bowel. In sites adjacent to perforations, avascular zones were visualized, either transmural or localized to part of the bowel wall. In sites more peripheral to the most severely injured areas, nonocclusive intimal fibrosis, decreased vascularity, and straightening of the submucosal vessels were seen. Some sections of small and large intestinal mucosa were nonperfused, secondary to capillary microthrombi in the mucosal vessels.[44]

The importance of this vascular cause of chronic radiation injury also can be seen in the close relationship between comorbid disease states and the evolution of radiation enteritis. In DeCosse and colleagues'[41] analysis

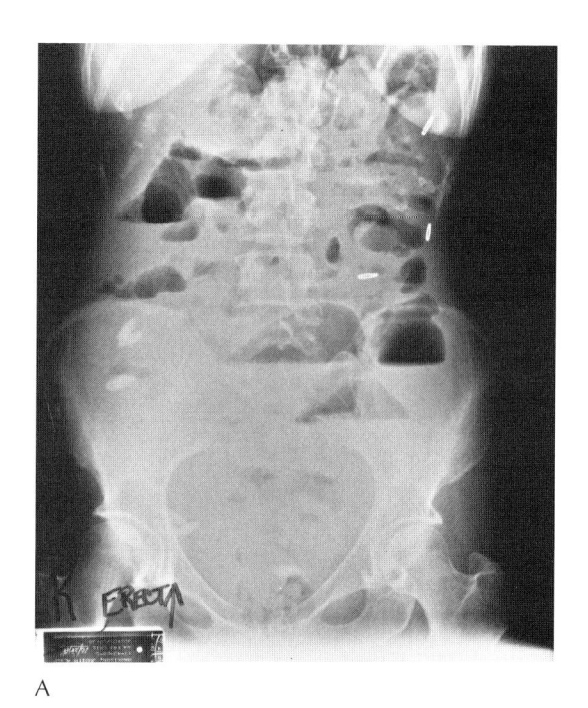

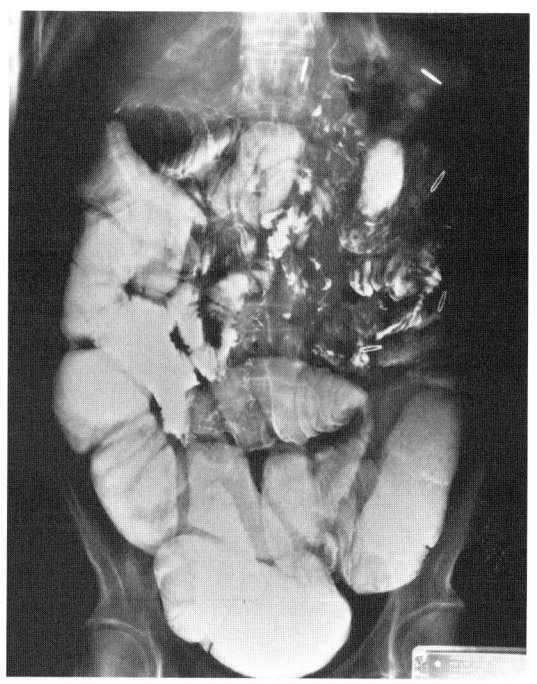

Figure 7-3. Radiographic appearance of chronic radiation enteritis resulting in partial small intestinal obstruction. **A.** Upright radiograph showing multiple air-fluid levels characteristic of intestinal obstruction. **B.** Small bowel follow-through showing intestinal dilatation, intestinal edema with thickening of mucosal folds, and segmental stenosis in the left lower quadrant.

of 100 patients who sustained radiation injury, a significant excess of patients was found who had histories of hypertension, diabetes, or cardiovascular disease. These patients with presumably decreased splanchnic blood flow were found to have a higher incidence of complications from their radiotherapy than patients without medical conditions potentially affecting the intestinal blood flow. This increased propensity of chronic injury underlines the role of inadequate intestinal blood flow in the development of radiation enteritis.[41]

Radiologic features of chronic radiation enteritis on barium studies include bowel wall thickening, chiefly submucosal, often appearing as nodular defects from localized thickening of the submucosa. Frequently, dilatation is present secondary to distal functional or mechanical obstruction. In more advanced stages, the intestine is seen as a rigid pipelike structure with kinks and sharp angulations. Pools of barium, which can often be visualized, are caused by loops of small bowel matted together and encased in a fibrous capsule.[23] Although submucosal thickening is the most frequent change seen on barium studies, it is not totally specific for radiation enteritis. Some of the radiographic changes seen in radiation enteritis also can be present in inflammatory bowel disease, infiltrative neoplasms, carcinoids, lymphoma, and intramural hemorrhages.[45] Figure 7-3 illustrates the radiologic features of chronic radiation enteritis.

Bowel Obstruction After Pelvic Irradiation

Radiation therapy is commonly used as adjunctive or definitive therapy in the treatment of many gynecologic, genitourinary, and rectal cancers. In addition to its anticancer effects, radiation therapy to the pelvis may produce injury to unprotected small bowel and rectum. The mechanism of injury appears to be through the destruction of rapidly dividing mucosal cells in acute injury and through an obliterative arteritis to the bowel wall in chronic injury. The acute changes are typically short-lived and usually are successfully treated symptomatically. Chronic injuries may present months to decades after the radiation dose. Strictures, bleeding, obstruction, perforation, and fistula formation after radiation therapy can be difficult clinical problems to treat successfully. Chronic intestinal injury after pelvic irradiation requiring surgery seems to occur in 2% to 17% of patients treated with radiation,[36-40,46] and may be higher after radiation for cervical cancer.[47] Small intestinal obstruction due to stricture formation after radiotherapy is common. In a study of 70 patients who developed 97 radiation-induced gastrointestinal lesions, there were 63 strictures, 14 fistulas, 12 perforations, and 8 bleeds.[48] The small bowel was the site of injury for 55 radiation-induced lesions, followed by 46 lesions induced in the sigmoid colon and rectum. Sixty-one patients required one or more operations. The high incidence of anastomotic failure in irradiated bowel led these authors to recommend that anastomosis be performed to a segment of healthy, nonirradiated bowel. Another series of 71 patients with radiation injury had predominantly large bowel injuries.[49] Fifteen patients were treated nonoperatively and 54 required surgery, many needing more than one operation. Strictures or adhesions represented the most common radiation-induced lesions in this series, resulting in 42 operative procedures. All clinical anastomotic leaks in this group occurred in patients with ileal anastomoses; there were suspected leaks in only 3 of 28 colonic anastomoses.

Predisposing factors for the development of radiation enteritis or colitis[50] include previous surgery and adhesion formation. Atherosclerosis, hypertension, and diabetes-induced vascular disease may all predispose to increased radiation injury. Radiation dose is critical, and the concomitant use of chemotherapeutic agents thought to be radiation sensitizers, most notably 5-fluorouracil

(5-FU), may increase the risk of developing radiation injury to the bowel.

Attempts at preventing bowel injury from radiotherapy have fallen into two broad categories: pharmacologic and surgical. Pharmacologic interventions have had limited success in the short-term, but the long-term benefits remain to be proved. Agents have included intravenous glutamine,[51] a presumed enterocyte energy source (no benefit in rats); intraluminal glutamine,[52] which is beneficial in rats; systemic and intraluminal misoprostol, a prostaglandin analogue that shows some benefit in minimizing enteric radiation injury in rats;[53] sulfasalazine; 5-aminosalicylic acid,[54] the active moiety in sulfasalazine (no benefit in a randomized trial); vitamin E,[55] which may be protective in rats; steroids; and elemental diets. In contrast, the long-term benefits of surgical prevention of radiation enteritis are well described. The most commonly used procedures include formation of a mesh sling at the pelvic brim and formation of an omental pedicle for placement in the pelvis. Each of these procedures represents an attempt to isolate the small intestine out of the pelvis. In a recent report of 60 patients treated with a polyglycolic acid mesh sling, the rate of radiation enteritis was 7% (4 cases) with an average follow-up of 18 months.[56] Another report of 45 patients treated with an absorbable mesh sling[57] had similarly good results. Forty-four patients received postoperative radiation therapy to a mean dose of 56.8 Gy. With a median follow-up of 34 months, there were no documented cases of radiation injury. Use of pedicalized omentum to pack the pelvis has been used for decades in an attempt to prevent injury to the small bowel by excluding it from the pelvis.[58]

The surgical management of radiation-induced bowel obstruction can be very challenging. The outcome, in general, is good if management is individualized for each patient. For example, gastrointestinal complications requiring surgery developed in 28 patients with radiation injury.[47] All patients were well from 3 to 120 months after surgery.

In contrast, however, other reports describe more dismal outcomes: Almost half the patients surviving surgery required subsequent operations, and upward of 25% of patients with radiation enteritis or colitis died from complications of the injury or the intervention.[46,48,49,59] Obstruction may be treated by resection, with or without anastomosis, or by bypass or diversion. Some authors claim much lower morbidity and mortality rates after bypass when compared with resection and anastomosis.[60] Subsequent reports addressed the high anastomotic failure rates seen in earlier series.[48,61] These authors showed that when nonirradiated bowel was used for one limb of an anastomosis, leaks were uncommon, and they recommended aggressive resection where feasible to prevent the ongoing complications (bleeding, fistula formation, and perforation) of diseased bowel left *in situ* during bypass or diversion. Multiple previous operations or a frozen abdomen or pelvis would preclude such an aggressive approach; under these circumstances bypass or diversion should be used.

■ SUMMARY: BOWEL OBSTRUCTION AFTER PELVIC IRRADIATION

1. Radiation therapy to the pelvis results in bowel injury requiring operation in 2% to 5% of treated patients.
2. Prevention of radiation enteritis is principally surgical: techniques to exclude the small bowel from the pelvis, such as mesh sling construction or creation of an omental pedicle, are successful in preventing small bowel injury from radiotherapy. Pharmacologic methods are as yet unproved in the prevention of chronic radiation injury to the bowel.
3. A high percentage of patients (70% to 80%) who develop symptomatic chronic radiation-induced bowel injury will require surgery, often more than one procedure. Bowel obstruction by adhesion or stricture formation is common. Resection

of affected bowel with anastomosis to healthy, nonirradiated bowel and meticulous adhesiolysis is the surgical procedure of choice. Where this is neither safe nor possible, bypass or diversion is a reasonable alternative.

Therapeutic Considerations in Chronic Radiation Injury

Unlike acute radiation-induced injury, chronic radiation enteritis can be unrelenting and difficult to treat. Medical management is used most frequently for mild to moderate symptoms. However, severe radiation injury is usually refractory to all types of medical management, and these patients, although few, require surgical intervention. Surgery can be effective in dealing with the complications of intestinal obstruction, fistulization, or perforation; but given the typically diffuse intestinal injury in chronic radiation enteritis, the clinical results of surgical intervention are not always uniformly satisfactory. Because of the magnitude and spectrum of complications seen with chronic radiation enteritis, much effort has been expended on the prevention of radiation-induced injury as well as on therapeutic methods to be used once the condition has been manifested.

PREVENTION

Efforts to prevent radiation-induced injury have focused on both medical and surgical methods. Bile salts and trypsin have been postulated to have a role in the development of radiation injury. It has been experimentally demonstrated that neutralization of pancreatic and intestinal proteases as well as bile salts decreases the amount of radiation injury sustained by the intestine.[14,20,62] The significance of these findings and their applicability to the clinical arena remain to be determined.

The role of eicosanoids in inflammatory processes has brought about the possible use of prostaglandin inhibitors as intestinal protective agents.[25-27] Antioxidants have been successful in an animal experimental model in reducing intestinal injury to radiation.[30] Steroids have been proposed as anti-inflammatory and lysosomal-stabilizing agents if given concomitant with radiotherapy.[13] However, caution should be exercised with the clinical use of steroids given the predisposition to intestinal perforation and fistula formation in this patient population. Although some benefits have been seen in patients with proved radiation enteritis who have been given steroids, their prophylactic role is wholly undetermined.[63]

Surgical prophylaxis had generally focused on methods to physically elevate and partially exclude the small intestine from the pelvis, where it may become fixed and particularly prone to radiation injury. Some studies have proposed creating a new extrapelvic peritoneal cavity by using omentum, rectus sheath, bladder, or peritoneal leaflets to suspend the small bowel above the irradiated field.[64-66] Lechner and Cesnik[66] used the greater omentum to form a bag in which to house the small bowel. Among 43 patients followed for an average of 38 months and given between 55 Gy and 60 Gy of radiation, none had complications related to radiation-induced small bowel injury. Three patients, however, did have clinical and endoscopic biopsy-proved radiation colitis, which resolved with low-fiber diets and rectal steroids. Eleven patients had cystitis, some of whom required chronic symptomatic medical treatment. There were no reported postoperative complications.[66]

Prosthetic mesh has been used with some success to suspend the small intestine out of a pelvic radiation portal. Polyglycolic acid mesh has been placed intraoperatively in such a way to elevate the small bowel contents from the pelvis (Fig. 7-4). The use of such a prosthetic mesh theoretically eliminates the need to use local native tissues for bowel elevation such as omentum, which may be attenuated by the necessary resection.

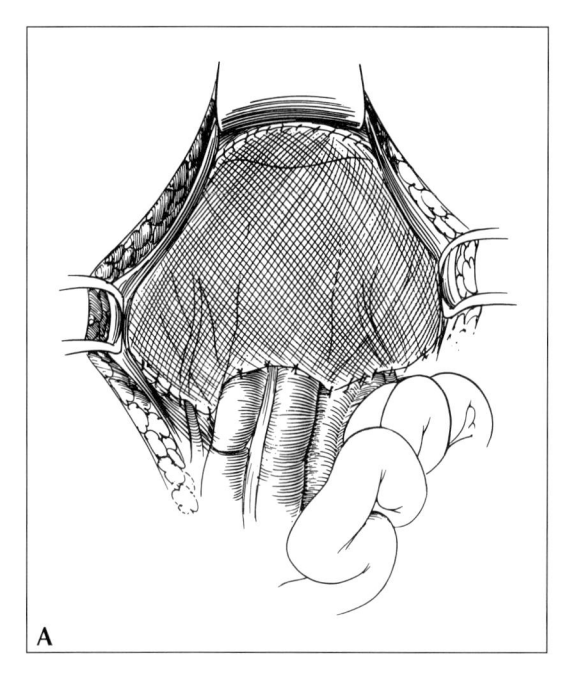

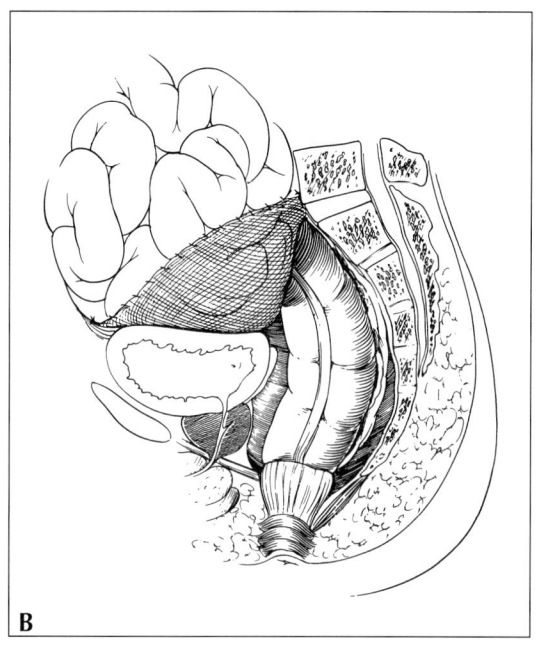

Intestinal Complications of Radiation Therapy 153

Figure 7-4. A. Intraoperative anterior view of mesh placed in the pelvic floor to prevent prolapse of the small bowel into the pelvis and thus limit bowel toxicity. **7-4. B.** Sagittal view of mesh placed in the pelvic floor to prevent caudad displacement of small bowel after a resection for rectal cancer. (Reprinted with permission from Daly JM and Cady B. Atlas of surgical oncology. St Louis, CV Mosby, 1992;519.)

Polyglycolic acid mesh is a foreign body that can precipitate a local inflammatory reaction. However, the mesh is thought to be completely absorbed within 90 days and consequently does not act as a permanent nidus for continuing inflammation. Several studies have examined the use of polyglycolic acid mesh,[67,68] as well as the associated inflammatory response.[69] Rodier et al[68] prospectively studied 60 patients who had received mesh implants. With an average follow-up of 18 months, no patient had debilitating symptoms of acute radiation enteropathy. Four patients (7%) developed chronic radiation enteritis, with surgical intervention ultimately being required in two of those patients. Five patients had mesh-related intestinal obstruction, one of whom required operation and mesh removal. One patient developed a pelvic abscess and three developed asymptomatic pelvic lymphoceles. Whereas these surgical techniques do hold promise, prospective randomized studies with long-term follow-up remain to be performed, with particular attention paid to complications of mesh placement, before the true clinical utility of these techniques is determined.

TREATMENT METHODS

The selection of methods to treat the late effects of radiation enteritis depends on the tumor status, the degree of radiation-induced injury, the presence of comorbid disease, and the severity of symptoms. Given the nonspecific nature of radiation-related symptoms, a clinical work-up of the patient with complaints suspected of being radiation enteritis should be conducted meticulously to evaluate for other disease states with similar presentations, such as recurrent tumor, mechanical intestinal obstruction, or inflammatory bowel disease.

Most of the patients in whom a diagnosis

of chronic radiation enteritis is made will undergo an initial trial of medical treatment. Frequently, medical management will suffice for the reasonable control of symptoms. The patients who fail to respond to medical management, a group comprised of those with the most serious complications, generally require surgical therapy.

Parenteral nutrition and complete bowel rest often have been advocated in the setting of malnutrition secondary to radiation-induced malabsorption. Although its potential value in treating the mucosal ulcerative lesions induced by radiation is unclear and controversial, total parenteral nutrition clearly does play an important role in the management of the malnutrition which frequently follows severe radiation enteritis[70] and in the initial management of patients with enteric fistulae.[29] Indeed, the general management of these patients should concentrate on the re-establishment of optimal nutritional status.[71] Lactose-free diets for demonstrated lactose intolerance, low-fat diets for steatorrhea, and cholestyramine for bile acid malabsorption are all part of the medical armamentarium for patients with radiation enteritis and associated absorption or motility disorders.[71] Loperamide-oxide and anticholinergics have been used with some success to slow the rapid small bowel transit associated with radiation enteritis.[72]

Because of the relentless nature of radiation enteritis, many patients have symptoms that remain refractory to medical management. The decision to proceed to surgery, however, should be cautious and well-considered. Surgery can be technically demanding, dissection can be difficult, and postoperative complications can be frequent. Among patients undergoing operation for radiation enteritis, morbidity rates affecting greater than 60% of patients and mortality rates of up to 37% have been reported.[36] Irradiated bowel heals poorly due to its compromised blood supply and to its fibrous noncompliant wall layers. Complications related to anastomotic breakdown are reasonably frequent. The dense fibrous adhesions and matting of bowel loops within which fistulae, stenoses, or obstructive lesions occur can be technically challenging to lyse surgically without injuring or compromising the intestinal wall. Even the gross identification of intestinal anatomic structures can be difficult during dissection.

Thus, surgical intervention is usually reserved for the most clinically refractory situations and for emergent complications. Generally, the most frequent indication for operation in severe radiation enteritis is intestinal obstruction.[14,36,73] Other surgical indications, in varying orders of frequency, include: bleeding, fistulae, sinus tracts, ulceration, and perforation. Although conservative (i.e., non-operative) management is usually preferred as a first-line treatment given the chronicity of radiation enteritis and the technical difficulty of most surgical interventions,[74] there is also evidence that early surgical intervention in selected patients may prevent progressive deterioration from repeated symptomatic episodes and thereby decrease long-term morbidity.[75] Early surgical intervention may also determine if other treatable causes of intestinal pathology exist, such as tumor recurrence.[13]

Rarely, instead of resulting from radiation enteritis, gastrointestinal symptoms may be due to the appearance of a new primary cancer. There are reports in the literature of a small but significant risk of the development of a second cancer secondary to changes induced by therapeutic radiation.[76-78] Radiation-induced malignancies have a prolonged latency, with most having been reported to occur at least 5 or more years after the course of radiotherapy. The risk of developing colorectal cancer in women who have received pelvic irradiation is estimated to be up to eightfold greater than for the general population.[43] Because of these increased risks, some authors have advocated routine surveillance flexible sigmoidoscopic examinations in women who are greater than 10 years beyond their radiation therapy course.[76]

In those patients who are brought to operation, the pattern of visceral injury can vary considerably and can involve both the small and large intestine, with skip areas forming a geographic pattern. Up to 17% of patients have been reported to have concomitant small and large bowel lesions.[35] Ideally, patients who are operative candidates should be brought to their optimal nutritional status prior to surgery. For those patients presenting with intestinal obstruction, preoperative decompression with nasogastric and intestinal tubes is highly desirable. Moreover, exhaustive preoperative radiographic contrast studies, performed through intestinal tubes if necessary, should be completed to aid the surgeon in attempting to define the site of pathology.

The prospect of exploring an abdomen with dense radiation-induced adhesions, matting of bowel loops, and poorly compliant tissues can be daunting, even for the most experienced of surgeons. When exploration is clinically advised, certain precautionary principles should be observed. Exceptional care in dissection must be exercised when such explorations may jeopardize the genitourinary system because of retroperitoneal encasement by radiation-induced fibrosis, when the bowel is matted and fixed in the pelvis to prevent adequate exposure, and when the intestinal vascular integrity is marginal.[79] Overly aggressive lysis of adhesions can cause focal devascularization of what may already be marginally vascularized bowel. These sites can result in postoperative perforations, fistulae, or sinus tracts. Instilling air or saline through a previously placed intraluminal long tube has been advocated to assure the intestinal integrity following such explorations. Intraoperative endoscopy of the small bowel via enterotomy also recently has been proposed as a method to detect small bowel damage.[80]

When the diseased segment of bowel presumably responsible for symptoms is identified intraoperatively, the management of the affected segment can involve intestinal resection or bypass with exclusion of the segment. Considerable controversy has surrounded the question of resection or bypass in the setting of radiation enteritis. Those who advocate bypass cite the difficulty and potential problems caused by the aggressive dissection and mobilization needed to resect bowel.[14] However, retention of the diseased segment in patients who have undergone bypass can lead to the late development of fistulae, abscesses, sinus tracts, blind loop syndromes, and closed loop obstructions. Other authors, therefore, have advocated wide resection of the radiation-damaged intestinal segments.[25,81,82] Quite reasonably, most authors currently advocate tailoring the surgical management to the severity of disease. Given that intestinal anastomoses are required both in bypasses and in resections, it is hardly surprising that the rates for anastomotic failure are nearly similar for both approaches.[5]

Wide resection is generally recommended when it is surgically feasible to sufficiently mobilize the affected portion of the gut to perform resection and reanastomosis with acceptable morbidity. By resecting the diseased portion, the potential for complications secondary to retained defunctionalized bypassed loops is eliminated. Internal bypass of affected bowel segments is generally reserved for those patients with an adhesion-filled "frozen pelvis," for those with recurrent disease, or for those for whom resection would be felt to yield an unacceptable risk for postoperative complications. The lowest leak rates have been observed in anastomoses where nonirradiated bowel is used for at least one limb.[37]

Intestinal fistulae and sinus tracts occurring in regions of chronic radiation enteritis usually fail to respond to bowel rest and expectant conservative management. Consequently, radiation-induced intestinal fistulae regularly come to operation. Although some authors advocate routine bypass of the fistulized intestinal segment,[36] others promote resection of the fistula and the involved portion of bowel, with reanastomosis of intestinal segments that are less involved with inflammation or radiation-associated fibrosis.[5] Generally, resection is recommended whenever it is technically feasible to safely mobilize, remove, and reconstruct the affected intestinal segments. Bypass of fistulae should be reserved for situations where resection is difficult or impossible because of factors such as extensive fibrosis or inflammation and for situations wherein patients have comorbid medical conditions that significantly increase the risk of complicated surgical interventions. Overall, the rate of surgical complications is similar for patients undergoing resection and bypass, in part possibly because higher-risk patients typically have simpler bypass procedures and thereby raise the overall morbidity of the bypass approach. However, aside from surgical complications, bypass procedures for radiation-induced intestinal fistulae typically have higher rates of failure than resection, with frequent episodes of refistulization, reobstruction, hemorrhage, or perforation. An exception to the general preference of resection over bypass for radiation-related fistulae is in the case of rectovaginal fistula, in which repair without diversion has been shown to lead to higher morbidity and recurrence rates, even when the fistulized intestinal segment is resected.[5,36,83]

Radiation proctitis may become severe enough in some patients to result in significant rectal hemorrhage or to cause incontinence secondary to damage to the internal anal sphincters.[84,85] In such situations, chronic radiation proctitis may require surgical management. Up to 67% of patients who have received radiation therapy for uterine carcinoma have been reported to develop substantial radiation injury to the rectum.[86] Several techniques have addressed the restoration of continence. Resection with pull-through coloanal anastomosis has been used since 1978.[87] However, the pull-through procedure has been plagued with postoperative strictures or with persistent anorectal incontinence, complications that can be easily documented on manometry and electrophysiologic studies.[88] Other techniques have included resection with endoanal or coloanal anastomosis[89] and utilization of bypassed colon as a patch for the diseased area.[90] Although some of these techniques have been promising, patients undergoing such procedures should be chosen carefully because of the associated morbidity and the possibility of a poor functional result.

SUMMARY: CHRONIC RADIATION INJURY

1. Radiation injury becomes chronic when symptoms persist for at least 3 months following the cessation of treatment or appear more than 3 months following treatment. They usually manifest within 6 to 18 months of therapy, but can present as late as 20 years following radiation.
2. Vascular injury has been postulated as the mechanism in this condition. Radiologic features include bowel wall thickening, areas of stricture or dilatation, and pooling of contrast.
3. Prevention is an important mode of therapy. Surgical prophylaxis includes small bowel suspension, sometimes using prosthetic mesh.
4. Medical management of this condition, once present, includes bowel rest with parenteral nutrition, low-fat diets, and cholestyramine.
5. The use of surgical intervention in the treatment of radiation enteritis must be considered very cautiously. Morbidity and mortality rates are high due to the abnormal nature of the tissue and the complex dissection required. The use of resection or bypass is generally tailored to the individual situation.
6. Radiation-induced fistulae regularly come to operation and resection is generally recommended when technically feasible.

SUMMARY

Radiation therapy has evolved into a powerful modality in the treatment of the patient with cancer. However, with its frequent use, there is a high incidence of side effects caused by this therapy. Radiation enteritis is perhaps the most troubling of these complications and presents a difficult clinical management situation for both patient and physician. Fraught with persistent and often progressively evolving complications, radiation enteritis can become a chronic and sometimes life-threatening problem. Clinical attention and investigative work needs to be done both in prevention and in treatment.

Acute and subacute radiation enteritis is a result of DNA damage to the rapidly-dividing mucosal layer, resulting in nausea, vomiting, cramping, and diarrhea. Generally, only symptomatic treatment is required, and the condition becomes self-limited within 3 months of radiotherapy. Steroids, prostaglandin inhibitors, and antioxidants have been suggested as possible agents to protect against the development of radiation damage.

Chronic radiation enteritis evolves late, probably as a result of progressive radiation-induced vasculitis and ischemia of the intestinal wall. This process can lead to mucosal atrophy and intestinal wall fibrosis, with resultant absorption and motility disorders. In severe cases, obstruction, fistulization, and perforation can occur, which typically require surgical intervention to resect or bypass the affected intestinal segments.

By addressing radiation enteritis, its causes and its treatment, abdominal radiation therapy may be viewed both as a valuable curative and palliative tool of the oncologist and as a treatment with potential toxicity that must be balanced against its potential benefit.

REFERENCES

1. DeCosse JJ. Radiation injury to the intestine. In: Sabiston DC, ed. Textbook of Surgery. The Biologic Basis of Modern Surgical Practice. 14th ed. Philadelphia: WB Saunders, 1991:880.
2. Kinsella TJ, Bloomer WD. Tolerance of the intestine to radiation therapy. Surg Gynecol Obstet 1980;151:273.
3. Walsh D. Deep tissue traumatism from roentgen ray exposure. Br Med J 1897;2:272.
4. Withers HR. Biologic basis of radiation therapy. In: Perez CA, Brady LW, eds. Principles and Practices of Radiation Oncology. 2nd ed. Philadelphia: JB Lippincott, 1992:64.
5. Kinsella TJ, Sindelar WF, Bloomer WD. Radiation enteritis: Pathophysiology, clinical manifestations, and management. In: Nelson RL, Nyhus LM, eds.Surgery of the Small Intestine. Norwalk CT: Appleton & Lange, 1987:193.
6. Hellman S. Principles of radiation therapy. In: DeVita VT, Hellman S, Rosenberg SA, eds. Principles & Practice of Oncology. 4th ed. Philadelphia: JB Lippincott, 1993:248.
7. Arbeit J, Hohn DC, Ridge A, et al. Oncology & cancer chemotherapy. In: Current Surgical Diagnosis & Treatment. 10th ed. Way LW, ed. Norwalk CT: Appleton & Lange, 1994:1239.
8. Cox JD, Byhardt RW, Wilson JF, et al. Complications of radiation therapy and factors in their prevention. World J Surg 1986;10:171.
9. Rubin P. The Franz Buschke lecture: Late effects of chemotherapy and radiation therapy: A new hypothesis. Int J Radiat Oncol Biol Phys 1984;10:5.
10. Nelson H, Wolff BG. Radiation enteritis and coloproctitis. In: Cameron JL, ed. Current Surgical Therapy. 4th ed. St. Louis: BC Decker, 1992:181.
11. Cromack DT, Maher MM, Hoekstra H, Kinsella TJ, Sindelar WF. Are complications in intraoperative radiation therapy more frequent than in conventional treatment? Arch Surg 1989;124:229.
12. Sindelar WF, Kinsella TJ, Chen PW, et al. Intraoperative radiotherapy in retroperitoneal sarcomas: Final results of a prospective, randomized clinical trial. Arch Surg 1993;128:402.
13. Shamblin JR, Symmonds RE, Sauer WG, Childs DS. Bowel obstruction after pelvic and abdominal radiation therapy: Factitial enteritis or recurrent malignancy? Ann Surg 1964;160:81.
14. Morgenstern L, Thompson R, Friedman NB. The modern enigma of radiation enteropathy: Sequelae and solutions. Am J Surg 1977;134:166.
15. Yeoh EK, Horowitz M. Radiation enteritis. Surg Gynecol Obstet 1987;165:373.
16. Allen-Mersh TG, Wilson EJ, Hope-Stone HF, Mann CV. Has the incidence of radiation-induced bowel damage following treatment of uterine carcinoma changed in the last 20 years? J R Soc Med 1986;79:387.
17. Tsioulias GJ, De Cosse JJ. Radiation enteritis: Diagnosis and treatment. In: McKenna RJ,

Murphy GP, eds. Cancer Surgery. Philadelphia: JB Lippincott, 1994:201.
18. Vagianos C, Karatzas T, Scopa CD, et al. Neurotensin reduces microbial translocation and improves intestinal mucosa integrity after abdominal radiation. Eur Surg Res 1992;24:77.
19. Donaldson SS, Jundt S, Ricour C, et al. Radiation enteritis in children. A retrospective review, clinicopathologic correlation, and dietary management. Cancer 1975;35:1167.
20. Delaney JP, Bonsack M. Acute radiation enteritis in rats: Bile salts and trypsin. Surgery 1992;112:587.
21. Delaney JP, Kimm GE, Bonsack ME. The influence of lumenal pH on the severity of acute radiation enteritis. Int J Radiat Biol Phys 1992;61:381.
22. Yeoh EK, Lui D, Lee NY. The mechanism of diarrhea resulting from pelvic and abdominal radiotherapy; a prospective study using selenium-75 labelled conjugated bile acid and cobalt-58 labelled cyanocobalamin. Br J Radiol 1984;57:1131.
23. Mason GR, Dietrich P, Friedland GW, Hanks GE. The radiological findings in radiation-induced enteritis and colitis. A review of 30 cases. Clin Radiol 1970;21:232.
24. Bertelrud K, Mehta M, Shanahan T, Utrie P, Gehring M. Bellyboard device reduces small bowel displacement. Radiol Technol 1991;62:284.
25. Sher ME, Bauer J. Radiation-induced enteropathy. Am J Gastroenterol 1990;85:121.
26. Summers RW, Glenn CE, Flatt AJ, Elahmady A. Radiation and indomethacin effects on morphology, prostaglandins, and motility in dog jejunum. Am J Physiol 1991;261:G145.
27. Rose PG, Halter SA, Cheng MS. The effect of indomethacin on acute radiation induced gastrointestinal injury: A morphologic study. J Surg Oncol 1992;49:213.
28. Baughan CA, Canney PA, Buchanan RB, Pickering RM. A randomized trial to assess the efficacy of 5-aminosalicylic acid for the prevention of radiation enteritis. Clin Oncol (R Coll Radiol) 1993;5:19.
29. Smith DH, DeCosse JJ. Radiation damage to the small intestine. World J Surg 1986;10:189.
30. Empey LR, Papp JD, Jewell LD, Fedorak RN. Mucosal protective effects of vitamin E and misoprostol during acute radiation-induced enteritis in rats. Dig Dis Sci 1992;37:205.
31. Delaney JP, Bonsack M, Hall P. Intestinal radioprotection by two new agents applied topically. Ann Surg 1992;216:417.
32. Delaney JP, Bonsack ME, Felemovicius I. Lumenal route for intestinal radioprotection. Am J Surg 1993;166:492.
33. Klimberg VS, Salloum RM, Kasper M, et al. Oral glutamine accelerates healing of the small intestine and improves outcome after whole abdominal radiation. Arch Surg 1990;125:1040.
34. Klimberg S. Prevention of radiogenic side effects using glutamine-enriched elemental diets. Recent Results Cancer Res 1991;121:283.
35. Mann WJ. Surgical management of radiation enteropathy. Surg Clin North Am 1991;71:977.
36. Russell JC, Welch JP. Operative management of radiation injuries of the intestinal tract. Am J Surg 1979;137:433.
37. Galland RB, Spencer J. Surgical management of radiation enteritis. Surgery 1986;99:133.
38. Mäkelä J, Nevasaari K, Kairaluoma MI. Surgical treatment of intestinal radiation injury. J Surg Oncol 1987;36:93.
39. Miholic J, Schwarz C, Moeschi P. Surgical therapy of radiation-induced lesions of the colon and rectum. Am J Surg 1988;155:761.
40. Cross MJ, Frazee RC. Surgical treatment of radiation enteritis. Am Surg 1992;58:132.
41. DeCosse JJ, Rhodes RS, Wentz WB, et al. The natural history and management of radiation induced injury of the gastrointestinal tract. Ann Surg 1969;170:369.
42. Stein RS. Radiation-recall enteritis after actinomycin-D and adriamycin therapy. South Med J 1978;71:960.
43. Berthrong M. Pathologic changes secondary to radiation. World J Surg 1986;10:155.
44. Carr ND, Pullen BR, Haselton PS, Schofield PF. Microvascular studies in human radiation bowel disease. Gut 1984;25:448.
45. Mendelson RM, Nolan DJ. The radiological features of chronic radiation enteritis. Clin Radiol 1985;36:141.
46. Russell JC, Welch JP. Operative management of radiation injuries of the intestinal tract. Am J Surg 1979;137:433.
47. Shibata HR, Freeman CR, Roman TN. Gastrointestinal complications after radiotherapy for carcinoma of the uterine cervix. Can J Surg 1982;25:64.
48. Galland RB, Spencer J. Surgical management of radiation enteritis. Surgery 1986;99:133.
49. Hatcher PA, Thomson HJ, Ludgate SN, Small WP, Smith AN. Surgical aspects of intestinal injury due to pelvic radiotherapy. Ann Surg 1985;201:470.
50. Nussbaum ML, Campana TJ, Weese JL. Radiation-induced intestinal injury. Clin Plast Surg 1993;20:573.
51. Scott TE, Moellman JR. Intravenous glutamine fails to improve gut morphology after radiation injury. J Parenter Enteral Nutr 1992;16:440.
52. Klimberg VS, Souba WW, Dolson DJ, et al. Prophylactic glutamine protects the intestinal

mucosa from radiation injury. Cancer 1990; 66:62.
53. Delaney JP, Bonsack ME, Felemovicius I. Misoprostol in the intestinal lumen protects against radiation injury of the mucosa of the small bowel. Radiat Res 1994;137:405.
54. Baughan CA, Canney PA, Buchanan RB, Pickering RM. A randomized trial to assess the efficacy of 5-amino sacyclic acid for the prevention of radiation enteritis. Clin Oncol 1993;5:19.
55. Empey LR, Papp JD, Jewell LD, Fedorak RN. Mucosal protective effects of vitamin E and misoprostol during acute radiation-induced enteritis in rats. Dig Dis Sci 1992;37:205.
56. Rodier JF, Janser JC, Rodier D, et al. Prevention of radiation enteritis by an absorbable polyglycolic acid mesh sling. A 60-case multicentric study. Cancer 1991;68:2545.
57. Dasmahapatra KS, Swaminathan AP. The use of a biodegradable mesh to prevent radiation-associated small-bowel injury. Arch Surg 1991;126:366.
58. Williams RJ, White H. Transposition of the greater omentum in the prevention and treatment of radiation injury. Neth J Surg 1991; 43:161.
59. Covens A, Thomas G, DePetrillo A, Jamieson C, Myhr T. The prognostic importance of site and type of radiation-induced bowel injury in patients requiring surgical management. Gynecol Oncol 1991;43:270.
60. Swan RW, Fowler WC, Boronow RC. Surgical management of radiation injury to the small intestine. Surg Gynecol Obstet 1976;142:325.
61. Marks G, Mohiudden M. The surgical management of radiation-injured intestine. Surg Clin North Am 1983;63:81.
62. Hasselgren P-O, Fischer JE. Prevention of radiation enteritis. In: Nelson RL, Nyhus LM, eds. Surgery of the Small Intestine. Norwalk, CT: Appleton & Lange, 1987:217.
63. Goldstein F, Khoury J, Thornton JJ. Treatment of chronic radiation enteritis and colitis with salicylazosulfapyndine and systemic corticosteroids. A pilot study. Am J Gastroenterol 1976;65:201.
64. Bakare SC, Shafir M, McElhinney AJ. Exclusion of small bowel from pelvis for postoperative radiotherapy for rectal cancer. J Surg Oncol 1987;35:55.
65. Chen JS, ChangChien CR, Wang JY, Fan HA. Pelvic peritoneal reconstruction to prevent radiation enteritis in rectal carcinoma. Dis Colon Rectum 1992;35:897.
66. Lechner P, Cesnik H. Abdominopelvic omentopexy: Preparatory procedure for radiotherapy in rectal cancer. Dis Colon Rectum 1992;35:1157.

67. Kavanah MT, Feldman MI, Devereux DF, Kondi ES. New surgical approach to minimize radiation-associated small bowel injury in patients with pelvic malignancies requiring surgery and high-dose irradiation. A preliminary report. Cancer 1985;56:1300.
68. Rodier J-F, Janser J-C, Rodier D, et al. Prevention of radiation enteritis by an absorbable polyglycolic acid mesh sling. A 60-case multicentric study. Cancer 1991;68:2545.
69. Devereux DF, O'Connell SM, Spain DA, Robertson FM. Peritoneal leukocyte response following placement of polyglycolic acid intestinal sling in patients with rectal carcinoma. Dis Colon Rectum 1991;34:670.
70. Silvain C, Besson I, Ingrand P, et al. Long-term outcome of severe radiation enteritis treated by total parenteral nutrition. Dig Dis Sci 1992; 37:1065.
71. Zentler-Munro PL, Bessel EM. Medical management of radiation enteritis—an algorithmic guide. Clin Radiol 1987;38:291.
72. Yeoh EK, Horowitz M, Russo A, et al. Gastrointestinal function in chronic radiation enteritis—effects of loperamide-N-oxide. Gut 1993; 34:476.
73. Localio SA, Gouge TH. Surgical treatment of radiation enteritis. In: Nelson RL, Nyhus LM, eds. Surgery of the Small Intestine. Norwalk, CT: Appleton & Lange, 1987:205.
74. Poddar PK, Bauer J, Gelernt I, Salky B, Kreel I. Radiation injury to small intestine. Mt Sinai J Med (NY) 1982;49:144.
75. O'Brien PH, Jenrett JM, Garvin AJ. Radiation enteritis. Am Surg 1987;53:501.
76. Black WC, Ackerman LV. Carcinoma of the large intestine as a late complication of pelvic radiotherapy. Clin Radiol 1965;16:278.
77. Sandler RS, Sandler DP. Radiation-induced cancers of the colon and rectum: Assessing the risk. Gastroenterology 1983;84:51.
78. Gajraj H, Davies DR, Jackson BT. Synchronous small and large bowel cancer developing after pelvic irradiation. Gut 1988;29:126.
79. Marks G, Mohiudden M. The surgical management of the radiation-injured intestine. Surg Clin North Am 1983;63:81.
80. Kuroki F, Iida M, Matsui T, et al. Intraoperative endoscopy for small intestinal damage in radiation enteritis (letter). Gastrointest Endosc 1992;38:196.
81. Schofield PF, Carr ND, Holden D. Pathogenesis and treatment of radiation bowel disease: Discussion paper. J R Soc Med 1986;79:30.
82. Harling H, Balslev I. Long-term prognosis of patients with severe radiation enteritis. Am J Surg 1988;155:517.
83. Cuthbertson AM. Resection and pull-through

for rectovaginal fistula. World J Surg 1986; 10:228.
84. Varma JA, Smith AN, Busuttil A. Correlation of clinical and manometric abnormalities of rectal function following chronic radiation injury. Br J Surg 1985;72:875.
85. Varma JS, Smith AN, Busuttil A. Functional of the anal sphincters after chronic radiation injury. Gut 1986;27:528.
86. Allen-Mersh TJ, Wilson EJ, Hope-Stone HF, Mann CV. The management of late radiation-induced rectal injury after treatment of carcinoma of the uterus. Surg Gynecol Obstet 1987; 164:521.
87. Gazet JC. Parks' coloanal pull-through anastomosis for severe, complicated radiation proctitis. Dis Colon Rectum 1985;28:110.
88. Varma JS, Smith AN. Anorectal function following coloanal sleeve anastomosis for chronic radiation injury to the rectum. Br J Surg 1986;73:285.
89. Cooke SAR, Wellsted MD. The radiation-damaged rectum: Resection with coloanal anastomosis using the endoanal technique. World J Surg 1986;10:220.
90. Bricker EM, Kraybill WG, Lopez MJ. Functional results after postirradiation rectal reconstruction. World J Surg 1986;10:249.

8

Constipation and Chemotherapy-Induced Emesis

JOHN T. VETTO
HANK J. SCHNEIDER
IRENE PEREZ VETTO

The common gastrointestinal (GI) motility disorders associated with cancer and its treatment—constipation and chemotherapy-induced emesis (CIE)—are so ubiquitous that they are often overlooked by oncology care providers. In fact, these disorders are usually of great distress to the patient, producing frequent morbidity and occasional mortality. This chapter reviews the physiology and etiology of each of these common disorders as well as current recommendations for their prevention and therapy.

CONSTIPATION

Little practical literature exists on the subject of cancer-related constipation, partly because its definition is vague and often individually defined, and partly because some oncologists may consider it a trivial problem. In actuality, constipation represents an inhibition of a major bodily function and is often more discomforting to patients than their baseline cancer pain.[1,2]

Constipation affects 4.53 million Americans each year and was reported by Grosvenor et al[3] to affect 41% of cancer patients participating in Eastern Cooperative Oncology Group trials. The frequency of constipation among cancer patients is found to be even higher when oncology care providers, such as nurse clinicians, assess the patient in detail.[4] Constipation rates as high as 90% have been found among patients treated with chronic morphine in centers such as the Cleveland Clinic when in-depth surveys were conducted by specialized oncology personnel.[5]

Common symptoms that should be assessed include not only decreased frequency of stools, but also excessive straining, a sensation of incomplete emptying, abdominal fullness and crampy discomfort, increased flatus, and abdominal pain. This pain is often crampy and colicky, but also may be rectal or hemorrhoidal in nature.[2]

The symptoms of anorexia, nausea, vomiting, and pain may indicate the presence of fecal impaction, a particularly severe type of constipation common in cancer patients. Paradoxical diarrhea, incontinence and coexisting urinary problems also are common with this condition.[6] Impaction may also cause fevers as high as 39°C, dysrhythmias, and tachypnea.[7,8] In one study, 54 of 55 patients with impaction had hemorrhoids. This same study noted that 42% of patients admitted to a geriatric ward had fecal impaction.[9]

Along with a careful history, a complete physical examination is crucial to the accurate assessment of the cancer patient with possible constipation, or impaction. Rectal examination is helpful but may not always be diagnostic, as a *high* impaction may occur (particularly if the patient has a carcinoma).[6] The abdomen may be distended in such patients, whereas in other cancer patients constipation may be noted by simply observing or feeling stool in the colon through the thin, scaphoid abdomen. Because the cecum is the most distensible part of the colon and therefore is most affected by the increased intraluminal pressure present with impaction, a distended cecum with distal small bowel air-fluid levels on a plain abdominal radiograph is highly suggestive of this disorder.[10]

Physiology

Each day approximately 9 L of fluid enters the digestive tract, including 2 L from ingested liquids and the remainder from gastrointestinal secretions. One liter eventually passes across the ileocecal valve and enters the colon. The main function of the colon is to absorb approximately 90% of this fluid by passive, osmotic means.[11]

Three types of movements occur in the colon: segmental, propulsive, and mass movements. Segmental movements are involved in the churning and mixing of food, while propulsive movements (peristalsis) push the colonic contents forward. Mass movements, usually occurring once or twice per day, expel the contents of the colon and are typified by the gastrocolic reflex. Forward motion in the colon results from stimulation of parasympathetic fibers, whereas sympathetic innervation, primarily from T8 to L3 nerve roots, decreases peristaltic activity and increases anal sphincter tone.[12]

Factors that increase colonic absorption or slow colonic transit would therefore be expected to cause constipation, as outlined in the next section.

Causative Factors

Considering the myriad factors that can result in constipation in the patient with cancer (Table 8-1), it is not surprising that this problem is so common in such patients. These factors can be divided into three general categories: primary (those that cause constipation in any patient), secondary (those causes that are specific to cancer patients), and iatrogenic, especially drug effects. Because many of the causes commonly thought of as cancer related may be due to treatment side effects, there is obvious overlap between these categories.[2,6]

PRIMARY CAUSES

The same factors that cause constipation in the patient without cancer are operative in cancer patients. Often these factors are more pronounced in the latter setting. The most important such factor is a lack of dietary fiber. This may be reflective of either generally

Table 8-1. Causes of Constipation in the Patient with Cancer

PRIMARY
Lack of fiber, malnutrition, bulk laxatives given
Dehydration, diuretics, vomiting without adequate fluids
Lack of exercise, immobility

SECONDARY
Electrolyte imbalances: hypercalcemia, hypokalemia
Disturbances of bowel routines (*e.g.*, hospitalization)
Poor dentition, defects in saliva
Renal failure
Pain
Malignant neuropathy
Malignant obstruction

IATROGENIC (DRUG-INDUCED)
Narcotics
Chemotherapeutic agents
Vinca alkaloids, 10-Edam, verapamil
Ondansetron
Antidepressants
Tricyclic antidepressants
Phenothiazines
Muscle relaxants
Hormones
Sucralfate
Iron
Antacids containing aluminum or calcium

poor nutrition or a lack of adequate oral intake. Similarly, dehydration is particularly prominent in such patients for a variety of reasons, including therapy-related emesis (discussed later in this chapter), high output renal failure, and the use of diuretics.

Although only 20 to 30 minutes a day of walking may be all the exercise needed to maintain normal bowel function, this is not achieved in many cancer patients, including those who are bedridden or immobilized by therapy.[13]

SECONDARY CAUSES

Causative factors for constipation specific to the cancer patient are many. The electrolyte imbalances of hypercalcemia and hypokalemia are both very common in cancer patients. In one study, constipation decreased by 70% in a cohort of such patients who were treated for their hypercalcemia with fluids, with or without other agents (steroids, pamidronate disodium, calcitonin, mithramycin).[14] Hypokalemia is common with diuretic use and can be prevented by routine potassium administration. Potassium should be administered cautiously, however, as cancer patients commonly have coexistent renal insufficiency and may easily progress to hyperkalemia.

Poor dentition and a decrease in the quantity and quality of saliva, which may be secondary to generalized poor health or to cancer treatments such as head and neck irradiation, contribute to poor nutrition, lack of dietary fiber intake, and dehydration. Another factor often overlooked causing constipation in cancer patients is a disruption of normal bowel routines and the lack of privacy that results from chronic illness, intensive therapy, and prolonged hospitalizations.[2,6,15]

The patient's tumor itself may cause constipation through several factors. Pain from constipation and impaction may be misdiagnosed as cancer pain and treated with additional doses of narcotic, which may thus actually further worsen the patient's pain.[2] Pelvic and rectal pain may also exacerbate constipation by increasing sympathetic tone to the sphincter muscles.

The patient's tumor may act directly on constipation by causing malignant obstruction or by interfering with the neurologic innervation to the intestine through some form of malignant neuropathy. In particular, cervical or thoracic lesions can promote proximal fecal impactions, whereas lumbosacral lesions may cause rectal impactions.[16] Specific neurologic disturbances may result from certain drug therapies (see next section). Transient ischemic cerebral lesions, seen commonly during induction chemotherapy for childhood leukemias, may present with constipation as an early sign.[17]

IATROGENIC (DRUG-INDUCED) CAUSES

The drugs used to treat cancer are a frequent cause of cancer-related constipation. The more commonly offending agents are discussed in detail in the sections that follow.

Narcotics. In addition to commonly causing fecal impaction,[18,19] narcotics cause constipation almost uniformly in patients with cancer. For example, in one study 65% of patients on high-dose oral oxycodone for severe cancer pain had constipation, regardless of the specific dose used.[20] Whereas one study on morphine sulphate (Contin) use for advanced cancer in hospice patients reported only an 8% constipation rate,[21] another demonstrated that by 13 months of therapy with high doses (mean dose of 120 mg/d), 100% of patients had constipation.[22] Further, alternate routes of opioid administration may not dramatically impact on the incidence of constipation; a study by Maves and Barcellos demonstrated no change in the incidence of this problem when patients on chronic oral opioids were switched to a transdermal (Fentanyl) patch.[23] Even with newer approaches to narcotic therapy, including the addition of nonopioids and specific co-analgesics to lower the opioid dose, constipation is still a commonly seen side effect.[24]

The mechanism of constipation in opioid administration has been known for some time. Briefly, it involves both peripheral and central neurologic effects that result in a decrease in segmental and propulsive movements of the intestine. These mainly anticholinergic effects are particularly pronounced in the cecum and ascending colon.[2,25,26] Such effects are so common that the World Health Organization's recommendation for prophylactic administration of laxatives with chronic narcotics has been widely adopted.[27] The prevention and treatment of narcotic-induced constipation is discussed in a later section. It should be noted here, however, that recently published guidelines for optimal administration of narcotics to cancer patients include the following recommendations designed to reduce constipation[12]:

1. Administer on a regular schedule, not on an "as necessary basis."
2. Individually titrate the dose until pain is controlled.
3. Reduce the dose if the noxious stimulus is reduced or if renal failure occurs.
4. Administer adequate prophylactic laxatives to prevent constipation.

Chemotherapeutic Agents. Among chemotherapeutic agents, vinca alkaloids are most notable for causing constipation in cancer patients. This effect is due to a neurotoxic reaction that can occur after one high dose or prolonged lower doses.[28] Vincristine and vinblastine both have been implicated, as has the newer semisynthetic vinca alkaloid, Navelbine. Constipation rates with these agents range from 46% to 52%, with 14% of cases reported as "severe." These drugs are also associated with a 12% ileus rate.[29,30]

Another agent associated with constipation is verapamil. This calcium channel blocker is occasionally added to chemotherapeutic regimens to reduce drug resistance in B-cell neoplasms and other solid tumors that express the P-glycoproteins. In this setting, constipation is reported to be the most common noncardiovascular side effect, occurring in 27% of patients. This effect is dose-related.[31] Constipation has also been reported as a side effect of therapy with 10-EDAM, an antifolate derivative.

Ondansetron. A newly recognized class of 5-hydroxytryptamine receptors ($5HT_3$) may be involved in the induction of nausea (discussed later in this chapter). Because $5HT_3$ receptors are present on enteric neurons, $5HT_3$ blocking agents, such as ondansetron hydrochloride (Zofran), may produce constipation.[33] In practice, this side effect is mild, occurring in 7% and 8% of patients in controlled and uncontrolled trials, respectively. One trial showed a 2% to 6% constipation rate occurring in a dose-related fashion, using doses ranging from 1 to 8 mg.[34]

The constipating effect of ondansetron appears to be a real effect of the drug, occurring more frequently than in placebo.[35] Interestingly, the constipation seen in adults with ondansetron is not observed in children who receive it for bone marrow transplant preparation-related chemotherapy.[36] The incidence of constipation with ondansetron is increased in adults when the dopamine D_2 antagonist, metopimazine, is administered along with ondansetron to treat anticipatory vomiting.[37]

In general, the mild constipation caused by ondansetron in occasional patients does not offset the benefit of this drug in treating chemotherapy-induced emesis. Odansetron remains an important antiemetic for patients treated with highly emetogenic chemotherapy regimens, especially those containing cyclophosphamide (Cytoxan) and cisplatin.[34,38,39]

Antidepressant Medications. Although there is little actual controlled data to substantiate their use, coadministration of antidepressants with narcotics for treatment of cancer pain is gaining popularity. The agents often used for this purpose include amitriptyline, nortriptyline, imipramine, desipramine, doxepin, trimipramine, and trazodone. These agents probably work on alternate pathways of pain and may have efficacy in phantom limb syndromes and postherpetic neuralgia, other common components of pain in cancer patients.[40] It is well known that constipation is a side effect of several antidepressant classes including the tricyclic antidepressants, phenothiazines, and muscle relaxants.[8]

Other Medications. As indicated in Table 8-1, a number of other medications commonly administered to cancer patients can cause or promote constipation. Such agents include hormones that decrease gut motility (endorphins, prolactin, secretin, and glucagon), sucralfate, iron, and antacids containing either aluminum or calcium.[6,8] Of note, another common cause of iatrogenic constipation is the administration of bulk-forming laxatives without co-administration of sufficient amounts of fluid.[41]

SUMMARY: CAUSATIVE FACTORS

1. Primary causative factors (those that cause constipation in any patient) include: lack of fiber, poor fluid intake, and lack of exercise.
2. Secondary factors (causes specific to cancer patients) include electrolyte imbalances (especially hypercalcemia and hypokalemia), poor dentition with saliva lacking in quality and quantity, disruption in normal routine, and lack of privacy. Also important is constipation caused by the tumor itself (directly or through increased opiate use to manage tumor-related pain).
3. Iatrogenic causes (usually drug-related) include narcotics, chemotherapeutic agents, ondansetron, antidepressants, and others (see Table 8-1).

Adverse Effects of Constipation

The importance of preventing and treating constipation in a cancer patient is evidenced by the many potential complications of this problem. Constipation, in particular fecal impaction, can result in incontinence, diarrhea, decubitus ulcers (from leakage with irritation of skin), urinary tract infections, pseudo-obstruction, worsening of cancer pain, nausea and vomiting, problems with drug absorption, pneumothorax (from straining), encephalopathy, rectal prolapse, and volvulus.[6,12] Rarely, impaction can result in perforation, either due to the impaction itself or to resulting stercoral ulceration.[42] Shock can result from perforation or from massive fluid efflux into the bowel in a patient with an obstructing impaction.

ASSESSMENT TOOLS

Nursing tools used to assess the severity of constipation include the McCorkle and Young Symptom Distress Scale and the Constipation Assessment Scale. The first is a linear scale of eleven symptoms, of which constipation is one. A recent study showed no significant difference between nurse and patient scoring of the severity of this symptom, indicating that this scale is fairly accurate for quantifying the severity of constipation.[43] Even more useful is the Constipation Assessment Scale, an eight-item scale (Table 8-2), which significantly correlates with both the presence and intensity of constipation.[44]

Table 8-2. Constipation Assessment Scale*

SCALE:
Abdominal distention or bloating
Change in amount of gas passed rectally
Less frequent bowel movements
Oozing liquid stool
Rectal fullness or pressure
Rectal pain with bowel movement
Small volume of stool
Unable to pass stool

SCORING:
1. Ask patient if each item is "no problem" (score = 0); "some problem" (score = 1); or "severe problem" (score = 2).
2. Total score ranges from 0 (no problem with constipation) to 16 (severe constipation).

*Data from McMillian SC, Williams FA. Validity and reliability of the constipation assessment scale. Cancer Nurs 1989;12:183.

Table 8-3. Therapy of Constipation in Cancer Patients

PREVENTION
Adequate fluids[a] and fiber
"Bowel routine"
Prophylactic laxative, especially for patients on narcotics[b]

TREATMENT
Mild constipation
- use or escalate existing dose of mild laxative

Continued constipation
- rectal forms of mild laxatives
- osmotic laxatives
- enemas

Impaction
- low = manual disimpaction
- high = enema, rule out colon malignancy

[a] Eight glasses of water per day in patients able to take oral fluids and who are not fluid restricted.
[b] Recommendation: Senekot, 2 tablets by mouth twice daily.

Therapy

The therapy for constipation in patients with cancer includes both prevention of constipation and treatment for the condition when preventive measures were not employed or have failed. Both prevention and therapy require a thorough understanding of the various classes of laxatives available. An overall plan for the prevention and therapy of constipation is outlined in Table 8-3.

PREVENTION

Prevention of constipation is clearly the best method of treatment. Central to preventive measures is the avoidance of the many factors that contribute to constipation in the patient with cancer (see Table 8-1). Active measures to prevent constipation include providing adequate fiber and carbohydrates in the diet, making commodes accessible and usable to the patient with limited motion, providing adequate fluids, and assuring a regular bowel routine.[6,45,46]

Good sources of fiber include fruits, vegetables, dried beans, peas, and whole grain breads and cereals. Unprocessed brans should be avoided as they contain phytic acid which binds iron, calcium, and zinc to result in nutrient deficiencies in already malnourished patients. Co-administration of adequate fluids along with fiber is essential, as a high-fiber diet in dehydrated individuals may actually worsen constipation.[2] In dehydrated patients, laxatives such as Citrucel™ and Metamucil™ that add inert fiber to the colon contents are relatively contraindicated (see below). In patients who are able to take oral intake, the general recommendation for adults is eight glasses of water per day.[2]

TYPES OF LAXATIVES

Whether used for prevention or therapy, laxatives generally fall into five categories: bulk-forming agents, emollient laxatives, anthraquinone glycosides, synthetic polyphenolics, and osmotic laxatives.

Bulk-forming Agents. Agents that add inert fiber to the diet are many. The two most commonly used in this country include methylcellulose fiber (*e.g.*, Citrucel) and psyllium derivates (*e.g.*, Metamucil). Although these agents are widely prescribed to prevent narcotic-induced constipation, co-administration of fluid is essential.[6] The usual dose of methylcellulose is 1 to 1.5 gm by mouth 2 or 3 times daily, and of psyllium derivatives 1 to 2 teaspoons in water or juice by mouth 1 to 3 times daily.

Emollient Laxatives. Docusate sodium (Colace), 50 to 200 mg by mouth every day, and docusate calcium USP, 240 mg by mouth every day, are surface-active wetting and dispensing agents. These drugs cause stool softening via water and fat penetration of fecal material. Co-administration of these agents with mineral oil causes increased intestinal absorption of the latter; therefore, administering both types of laxatives together is not recommended.

Anthraquinone Glycosides. These naturally occurring laxatives act by stimulating the smooth muscle of the colon, resulting in increased peristalsis. Thus, these agents reverse the effect of narcotics on the colon without affecting their analgesic properties. This class of laxatives includes several plant-derived compounds including senna, cascara, frangula, rhubarb, and aloes. Agents in both this class of laxatives and the synthetic polyphenolics (see below) are often referred to as *stimulant cathartics*.

The senna derivatives are especially effective in patients who are taking narcotics or are bedridden.[2,47,48] Available in many forms, the most popular is a tablet (Senokot). It is estimated that one half tablet of Senokot reverses the constipating effects of 60 mg of codeine.[49] The usual dose of Senokot is two tablets twice daily. This dose can be increased to a maximum of eight tablets in 24 hours.[2]

The anthraquinone glycosides have few side effects. The most common problems with these agents include cramping and melanosis coli. The former is least frequently seen with Senokot; the latter is a harmless discoloration of the colonic mucosa that disappears when these agents are discontinued.[2,6,8]

The second most commonly used anthraquinone is cascara, available in extract or syrup form. The usual dose is 5 mg qhs with a range of between 2 and 10 mg/d.[2]

Synthetic Polyphenolics. These agents include phenolphthalein, oxyphenisatin, and bisacodyl. Bisacodyl is the most commonly used agent in this class and is available in both oral (dose: 1 to 3 tablets qhs) and rectal suppository (dose: 1 per day, as necessary) forms. Bisacodyl causes a fairly high incidence of cramping. The synthetic polyphenolics are frequent causes of melanosis coli, as many of these compounds are vital stains.[2,49]

Osmotic Laxatives. These agents include magnesium citrate (dose 200 mg by mouth), Milk of Magnesia™ (15 to 30 mL by mouth), and Lactulose™ (15 to 30 mL by mouth 2 to 4 times daily). These ionic compounds pull water osmotically into the lumen of the colon to increase the volume of stool and to stimulate peristalsis. These agents are best for bowel cleansing in patients with low levels of bulk or fluid in the stool.[47] Also included in this class are lavage solutions (*e.g.*, Golytely, Colyte™), which contain nonabsorbable sulfate and polyethylene glycol. The dosage is 4 to 6 L by mouth over a maximum of 3 to 4 hours.

PREVENTION OF NARCOTIC-INDUCED CONSTIPATION

Whereas the osmotic laxatives are not used for preventative measures, controversy exists as to which of the other classes of laxatives are best for this purpose. Although the emollient laxative Colace often is prescribed along with narcotics,[6] actual data substantiating this use are lacking, and at least one study suggests that standard doses do not provide a prophylactic benefit.[50] Further, because this agent contains a detergent, prolonged use of the drug may cause gastritis.[49] In contrast, Senokot is well tolerated with minimal side effects and is generally recommended as a preferred agent for constipation prevention in patients on narcotic therapy (see Table 8-3).

TREATMENT

If preventive therapy begins to fail, particularly in cancer patients on narcotics, the dose of the abovementioned agents can be escalated (see Table 8-3). If these measures fail and bowel clearance is needed, rectal forms of these same agents or osmotic laxatives may be used.

Enemas are usually used when these other methods have failed. Enema administration in the cancer patient should be gentle, using low volumes and low pressures. Various types of enemas can be employed including phosphate, biphosphate, oil retention, tap water, and soap suds. The use of soap suds enemas is generally discouraged as they cause electrolyte abnormalities and are harsh.[2]

The treatment of fecal impaction poses a particular problem. Whereas this condition is often refractory to gentler agents, harsh laxatives may precipitate serious complications. Osmotic agents and stimulant cathartics should be avoided. Lubricant laxatives such as mineral oil may work acutely, but prolonged administration may cause aspiration pneumonitis and may interfere with fat-soluble vitamin absorption.

The best treatment of distal impaction involves manual fragmentation. This procedure begins with application of a local anesthetic and use of lidocaine jelly with progressive dilatation of the rectum. A scissoring motion of two fingers is then used to break up and extract stool. Repeat sessions are usually necessary.[6]

SUMMARY: THERAPY OF CONSTIPATION

1. Prevention is the best therapy. Active measures include dietary fiber, adequate oral fluids, and assuring a regular bowel routine.
2. Laxatives may be used when needed. These include bulk-forming agents (*e.g.*, Metamucil), emollient laxatives (*e.g.*, Colace), anthraquinone glycosides (*e.g.*, Senekot), synthetic polyphenolics (*e.g.*, Bisacodyl), and osmotic laxatives (*e.g.*, Milk of Magnesia).
3. Enemas are used when other methods fail. Manual fragmentation is the best method to use in cases of fecal impaction.

SUMMARY: CONSTIPATION

Constipation is a common problem in cancer patients that can produce serious morbidity and occasional mortality. A disorder with many causes, constipation is best treated with preventive measures that can be incorporated into the daily routines of cancer care. When these measures fail, both over and under treatment must be avoided to prevent development of further problems.

CHEMOTHERAPY-INDUCED EMESIS

The treatment of chemotherapy-induced emesis (CIE) has undergone a revolution in the last 20 years. The widely held belief that nausea was an inevitable sequel to effective chemotherapy is reflected by the paucity of research devoted to this area until the 1980s.[51] Subsequently, an increased understanding of the role of neuroreceptors, in particular serotonin and dopamine, led to the use of high-dose metoclopramide (Reglan) in the 1980s,[52] largely developed for the severe nausea induced by cisplatin.[53] The 5-hydroxytryptamine (5-HT$_3$) receptor blockers such as ondansetron (Zofran) and granisetron (Kytril) recently have been found to be more potent and have fewer side effects than high-dose metoclopramide.[54]

Although the volume and quality of clinical trials devoted to antiemetic research has increased and improved in the last two decades, the problem of CIE has not been conquered. Thirty percent of patients undergoing chemotherapy still suffer from this complication,[55] and continued research to develop new approaches is needed.

Harmful Effects of Nausea and Vomiting

Apart from the obvious desire to avoid unpleasant symptoms, the treatment of nausea and vomiting is critical to avoiding serious physical and metabolic derangements.

Protracted vomiting causes dehydration, activating the renin-angiotensin-aldosterone pathway. The net result is that potassium and hydrogen ion secretion is increased in an effort to retain sodium ions and conserve total body water. A concomitant rise in antidiuretic hormone increases the permeability of the collecting duct system to allow water to be reabsorbed down an osmotic gradient.

The resulting hypokalemia is manifested clinically as muscle weakness, lassitude, constipation, and eventually as cardiac arrhythmias such as ventricular ectopy. If vomiting is severe enough, sodium depletion may also occur, leading to hypovolemia, hemoconcentration, oliguria, and hypotension.[56]

Malnutrition can result from chronic nausea and vomiting by a variety of mechanisms. These include calorie loss, malabsorption, and noncompliance with medications essential to the patient's cancer treatment.[57] Physical injuries may also occur. A dramatic example is Boerhaave's syndrome (see Chapter 3, *Traumatic Rupture of the Esophagus*). Mallory-Weiss tears (see Chapter 3 for a complete discussion of gastrointestinal bleeding) may also occur, leading to upper gastrointestinal bleeding. Rarely, transmural rupture of the stomach has been reported secondary to forceful emesis.[58]

Pathologic fractures may occur, especially in bones weakened by osteoporosis or metastatic deposits. Vomiting can result in rectus muscle hematomas and in subconjunctival and subdural hemorrhage, especially in patients on anticoagulant therapy. The sudden onset of facial purpura in a mask-like distribution has been described in association with forceful vomiting.[59] This phenomenon occurs in a classic pattern on the face and neck and, despite causing great concern to the patient, resolves spontaneously without need for intervention. In patients with a depressed state of consciousness or impaired gag reflex, vomiting carries the risk of aspiration pneumonia with associated high morbidity.

Psychological effects of vomiting include depression, fatigue, and anticipatory vomiting (see below). Social effects can include loss of dignity and independence, avoidance of social contact and even job loss, which can compound the adverse psychological effects. In up to 30% of cancer patients, the resulting decreased quality of life may lead to refusal of potentially curative but toxic chemotherapy regimens. Up to 20% of patients have been reported to withdraw from treatment specifically because of continued problems with nausea and vomiting.[60]

SUMMARY: HARMFUL EFFECTS OF NAUSEA AND VOMITING

1. Nausea and vomiting can lead to serious physical and metabolic derangements including dehydration, hypokalemia, malnutrition, esophageal injury, or hemorrhage.
2. Psychologic effects are also possible including depression, fatigue, and anticipatory vomiting.

Neurophysiology of Nausea and Vomiting

Vomiting is a lower brainstem reflex closely related to the control of breathing and shares some of the same efferent pathways to the respiratory musculature. The prodromal symptoms of emesis (pallor, diaphoresis, salivation, tachycardia) are autonomically mediated, but the act of vomiting itself is somatically mediated and technically requires a wakeful state to occur.[61] It is interesting to note that in certain circumstances vomiting can be a welcome or pleasant experience owing to the associated relief that follows. Examples include the vomiting associated with a migraine headache or with narcotic use. Vomiting associated with increased intracranial pressure can be effortless.

The model for the neurophysiology of vomiting is based on the research of Borison and Wang[62] (Figure 8-1), who identified two key neural centers involved in the vomiting reflex. Electrical stimulation of the dorsal portion of the lateral reticular formation near the tractus solitarius induces vomiting in animals. Ablation of this area results in dampening of the vomiting reflex. These workers proposed that this vomiting center has a central coordinating function, receiving neural input from visceral structures, cortical centers, and the chemoreceptor trigger zone, to produce a coordinated vomiting response via the medulla.

The chemoreceptor trigger zone is located in the area postrema which, if ablated, dampens or eliminates the vomiting reflex to systemically acting emetogenic agents such as intravenous apomorphine. It is hypothesized that the chemoreceptor trigger zone, located outside of the blood brain barrier, is sensitive to systemic emetogenic substances

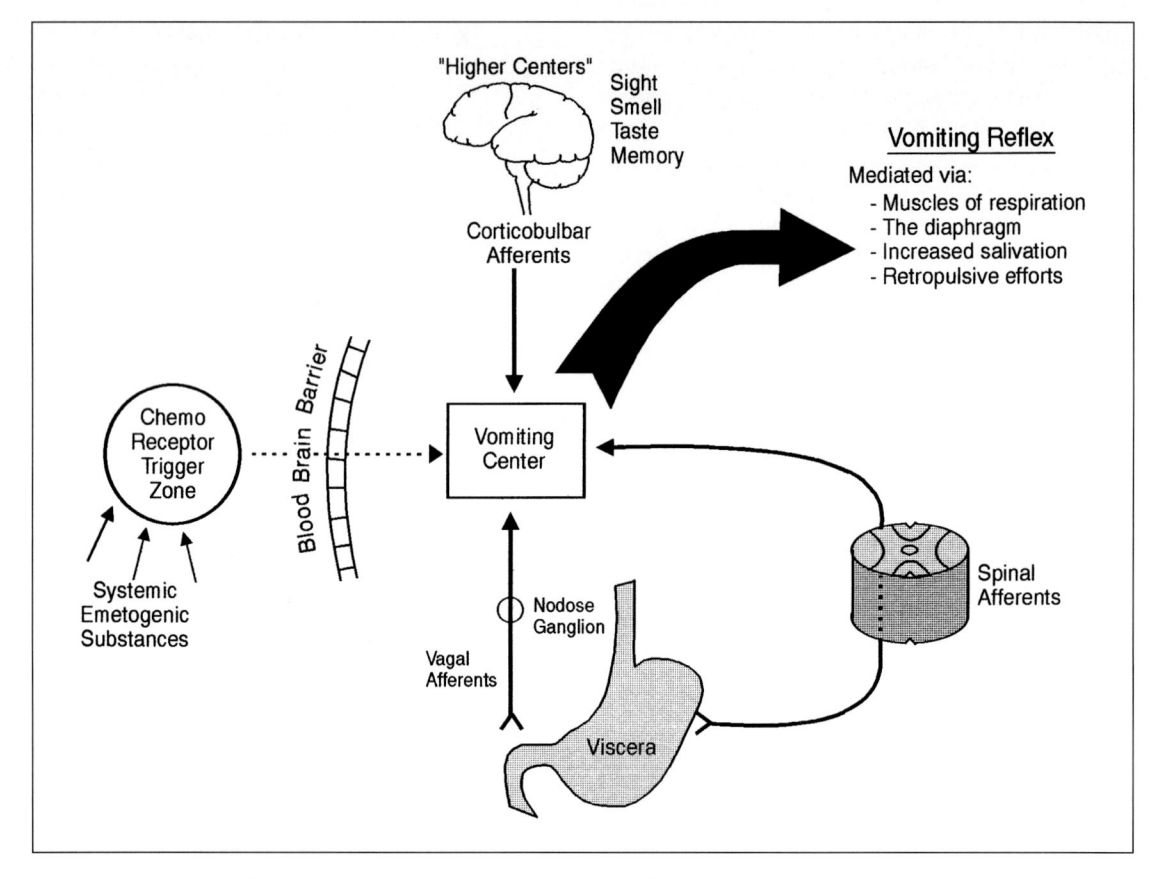

Figure 8-1. Neuropathways of Nausea and Vomiting. Data from Borison HL, Wang SC. Physiology and pharmacology of vomiting. Pharmacol Rev 1953;5:193 (see text for details).

and relays information to the vomiting center, inside the blood brain barrier, by neuronal input.

The stomach and other viscera influence vomiting via vagal and sympathetic efferents. Severing these nerves greatly dampens the vomiting response to potent emetic agents such as orally ingested copper sulphate solution. These afferent pathways are thought to relay directly to the vomiting center, bypassing the chemoreceptor trigger zone.[56]

Corticobulbar afferents can stimulate the vomiting center directly when triggered by sensory input such as smell and taste. Memory is involved in this context. However, vomiting can occur in decerebrate animals, indicating that these centers are not essential to the vomiting reflex.[63]

Efferent pathways from the vomiting center are mainly somatic, involving the vagus, phrenic, and spinal nerves, causing retrograde peristalsis, diaphragmatic contraction, and salivation, resulting in the vomiting reflex. Vestibular afferents, important in the mechanism of motion sickness, are not believed to be involved in the nausea and vomiting of chemotherapy.[61]

Temporal Patterns of Chemotherapy Induced Emesis

Effective treatment and prophylaxis of chemotherapy-induced emesis requires an appreciation of the timing of onset of side effects in relation to treatment. The three main categories observed are acute, delayed, and anticipatory nausea and vomiting.[64]

Most common is acute vomiting, beginning within 1 to 2 hours after dosing, reaching a peak at 4 to 10 hours, and usually resolving within 12 to 24 hours.[65] Agents can be categorized by their ability to produce acute emetic episodes (Table 8-4).

Delayed nausea and vomiting occurs 1 to 5 days after administration of chemotherapy, with a peak frequency between 48 and 72 hours.[57] It is usually less severe but of longer duration than the acute type.

Anticipatory emesis is a conditioned response to highly emetogenic agents (see Table 8-4), wherein nausea and vomiting actually precede a scheduled dose. This type of response has a tendency to occur when nausea is severe or poorly controlled. Anticipatory vomiting is associated with agents that have a strong taste or smell, is mediated via higher centers, and is difficult to treat once established.[56,57] Anxiolytics, especially those with amnestic properties such as lorazepam, are useful adjuncts to therapy for anticipatory vomiting. However, effective pre-emptory antiemetic therapy is of paramount importance.

It should be noted that some agents do not fit into the above categories.[68] For example, cyclophosphamide is notable for producing chemotherapy-induced emesis typically 6 to 12 hours after administration.

General Guidelines for the Treatment of Chemotherapy-Induced Emesis

Due to inter- and intrapatient variation in effectiveness of antiemetic agents, it is difficult to have rigid guidelines for therapy. However, certain general principles can be summarized:

1. The emetogenic potential of the chemotherapeutic drug must be considered (see Table 8-4). The treatment of the most highly emetic agent should guide the choice of antiemetic. For example, cisplatin will cause chemotherapy-induced emesis in greater than 90% of patients,[57] whereas vincristine rarely causes emesis. Therefore, in a vomiting patient receiving both drugs in combination, treating for cisplatin-related emesis should be sufficient.[69]

2. The timing of the onset of chemotherapy-induced emesis helps pinpoint the responsible agent when combination regimens are being used. Most drugs that cause acute chemotherapy-induced emesis manifest the onset of symptoms within 90 minutes of dosing.[65] As noted previously, common exceptions include cyclophosphamide, with an onset between 6 and 12 hours, and cisplatin, which may cause emesis up to 1 to 5 days after treatment. Anticipatory vomiting usually occurs on an average of 17 hours prior to dosing, and

Table 8-4. Emetic Potential of Chemotherapeutic Drugs*

MILDLY EMETOGENIC	MODERATELY EMETOGENIC	HIGHLY EMETOGENIC
Fluorouracil	Carmustine	Cisplatin
Methotrexate	Doxorubicin	Nitrogen mustard
Etoposide	Carboplatin	Streptozocin
Vincristine	Mitomycin	Dacarbazine
Bleomycin	Asparaginase	Dactinomycin
6 Mercaptopurine	Azacitidine	Cyclophophamide
	Procarbazine	
	Mitomycin C	

*Data from Gralla RJ, Tyson LB, Kris MG, et al. The management of chemotherapy-induced nausea and vomiting. Med Clin N Am 1987;71:2 and Graves T. Emesis as a complication of cancer chemotherapy: pathophysiology, importance and treatment. Pharmacotherapy 1992;12(4):337.

is typically associated with previous episodes of poorly controlled nausea and vomiting and with more potent emetogenic agents.
3. Chemotherapy-induced emesis is more easily prevented than treated once established. Therefore, it is generally better to use antiemetics prophylactically and treat with more aggressive therapy, decreasing their use as necessary (*e.g.*, if excessive sedation occurs).
4. Good initial response to therapy should be documented and the same drugs used again on future occasions. Patient preference should be respected, as this will usually reflect successful antiemetic control. Reassurance and attention to the patient's psychological needs are critically important. The self-limiting nature of the emetic episodes can be emphasized, as well as the benefit of sleep.
5. Dehydration should be prevented (either by oral fluids on a *little and often* basis, or by intravenous normal saline) to prevent potassium-wasting and renally propagated metabolic alkalosis, which can occur with intractable vomiting and consequent dehydration.
6. Care should be taken to remove environmental triggers to nausea and vomiting. These include poor oral hygiene, unpleasant odors, and stale food trays. A position of comfort should be sought. Care should be taken with brushing teeth or changing dentures to avoid stimulating a gag reflex.
7. Other causes of nausea and vomiting in addition to chemotherapy-induced emesis must be borne in mind and eliminated. These may include bowel obstruction and fecal impaction (see previous section), raised intracranial pressure, uremia, hypercalcemia, infective gastroenteritis, gastritis, nausea associated with alcohol abuse or withdrawal, and drug toxicities, such as those associated with digoxin, ergot alkaloids, and opiate therapy.
8. Chemotherapy-induced emesis, especially if it has an anticipatory component, may benefit from anxiety-reducing measures such as behavioral therapy and the use of an adjunctive sedative or amnestic agent such as lorazepam.
9. There are five classes of drugs used to treat chemotherapy-induced emesis including:
   - Dopamine Antagonists (*e.g.*, metaclopramide, prochlorperazine)
   - 5-HT$_3$ receptor antagonists (*e.g.*, ondansetron, granisetron)
   - Corticosteroids (*e.g.*, dexamethasone)
   - Cannabinoids
   - Benzodiazepines (*e.g.*, lorazaepam)

Combination regimens using drugs from different classes, with different mechanisms of action have given excellent results.

Single Agent Therapy for Chemotherapy-Induced Emesis

METOCLOPRAMIDE

Metoclompramide is a synthetic substituted benzamide that is thought to act by sensitizing visceral tissue to the actions of acetylcholine, which results in increased antral contractions as well as duodenal and jejunal peristalsis. Metoclopramide also relaxes the pyloric sphincter and duodenal bulb. The net effect is to increase gastric emptying and proximal small bowel transit time.

Research also has shown that in high doses metoclopramide acts as a dopamine receptor antagonist at the chemoreceptor trigger zone and is effective against cisplatin-induced nausea and vomiting.[2]

Toxicity is common but mild and includes sedation (70%) and diarrhea (45%) in patients receiving high doses (*i.e.*, 1 to 3 mg/kg). Extrapyramidal symptoms such as akathisia and dystonic reactions are reported in 3.1% of patients on high-dose therapy,[70] particularly in males under the age of 30. Diphenhydramine can be given intravenously (IV), intramuscularly (IM), or orally for these problems (50 mg), with rapid response in most cases. Tardive dyskinesias occur in the elderly, especially in women, and discontinuation of metoclopramide therapy is usually the only treatment needed.[71]

Dosing Guidelines. Effective antiemetic control is achieved in more than 75% of patients by the oral or intravenous route in the following doses:

Oral	2 mg/kg, 1 hour before and at 1, 3, 5, 8, and 11 hours postchemotherapy.
Intravenous	2 mg/kg starting 30 minutes before chemotherapy and repeated every 2 hours for three subsequent doses.
Rectal	An alternative route of administration when medications are not well tolerated orally or there are venous access problems, but the bioavailability can fluctuate greatly.[72]

Indications. Metoclopramide may be used for all moderate to severe emetic challenges caused by chemotherapeutic agents (see Table 8-1). For cisplatin-induced nausea and vomiting it should be combined with dexamethasone, 20 mg IV. Oral dosing is useful to prevent delayed nausea and vomiting and oral prednisone can then be used in combination for outpatient therapy. Prophylactic diphenhydramine may be given in patients under age 40 to prevent dystonic reactions and lorazepam may be given concurrently to prevent anticipatory vomiting.

ONDANSETRON HYDROCHLORIDE

As discussed in the previous section, ondansetron is a 5-hydroxytryptamine$_3$ receptor antagonist that is thought to act either centrally in the chemoreceptor trigger zone or peripherally on vagal nerve terminals, or possibly at both sites. Chemotherapy-induced emesis is known to be associated with release of serotonin from the enterochromaffin cells of the small intestine[73] in animals, and which also rises after cisplatin administration in parallel with the onset of emesis in humans.[74]

Side effects associated with ondansetron include headaches, constipation, abdominal pain, and xerostomia. No extrapyramidal symptoms have been reported, making it preferable to metoclopramide in this respect. There is little information available regarding use of this drug in children under the age of 4, but children from 4 to 12 years of age should receive half the adult dose. No dosing modifications have been found to be necessary in the elderly.

Dosing Guidelines.

Oral	8 mg by mouth three times daily. Start 30 minutes before chemotherapy and continue for 1 to 2 days after completion.
Children	(ages 4–12) 4 mg by mouth three times daily.
Intravenous	0.15 mg/kg infusion over 15 minutes, every 4 hours, ×3 doses.

Indications. Ondansetron is the most effective single agent available for cisplatin-induced chemotherapy-induced emesis, controlling symptoms in this setting in up to 75% of patients.[54] The drug is also effective for other potent emetogenic agents such as cyclophosphamide, doxorubicin, and methotrexate (with or without 5-fluorouracil [5-FU]). Ondansetron has been shown to be even more effective when combined with dexamethasone.[74] Oral dosing renders it suitable for outpatient therapy.[75] It may be useful in treating the side effects of radiation therapy (see Chapter 7).

Improved symptom control has led to the use of more intensive emetogenic regimens, exposing limitations to the efficacy of ondansetron. When high-dose cisplatin is combined with high-dose etoposide or carmustine (BCNU) ondansetron has been found to be ineffective in controlling chemotherapy-induced emesis.[76]

GRANISETRON

Granisetron is a 5-HT$_3$ receptor antagonist that has recently been made available in the United States. It is considered the most selective 5-HT$_3$ antagonist currently available.[77] Associated side effects described in the package insert include headache (reported in 14% of patients), somnolence, diarrhea (4%), and constipation (3%). Its main advantage over ondansetron is that it has a 9-hour half-life, and a single dose usually provides 24 hours of control of chemotherapy-induced emesis.[78]

Dosing Guidelines. Granisetron is given intravenously as a single dose 10 mg/kg over 5 minutes, 30 minutes before chemotherapy is begun.

Indications. Granisetron is very effective in the prevention of cisplatin-induced emesis and is as effective or more effective than standard metoclopramide or steroid antiemetic combinations.[78]

A recent multicenter study evaluated 184 patients receiving high-dose cisplatin chemotherapy (81 to 120 mg/m^2) to a range of doses of granisetron from 10 to 40 mg/kg given as a single intravenous dose without dexamethasone.[77] These investigators found no significant differences in efficacy among patients in the four treatment groups. The drug was well tolerated at all doses tested. Vomiting was completely prevented in 40% to 47% of patients. Headache was reported in 20% of these patients, diarrhea in 11%, constipation in 7%, and somnolence in 6%. Randomized comparative trials looking at ondansetron versus granisetron are currently in progress. Comparisons currently in the literature are difficult to analyze because of variations in dosing and schedule of administration. Preliminary data show no differences in control of emesis or nausea among patients receiving cisplatin-based chemotherapy.

DEXAMETHASONE

Dexamethasone is a corticosteroid that can be used singly or in combination with other antiemetics. The mechanism of steroids in antiemesis is thought to involve inhibition of prostaglandin formation.[79] As a single agent, the antiemetic potency of dexamethasone is superior to prochlorperazine but less effective than metoclopramide.[80] In combination therapy, this agent augments the antiemetic effects of drugs such as ondansetron and metoclopramide. Some side effects, such as increased appetite, mood elevation, and reduced metoclopramide-associated diarrhea may be of therapeutic benefit.[81] Other less useful side effects include somnolence, perineal or pharyngeal itch, and insomnia. Concerns regarding the use of an immunosuppressive agent in the presence of malignant disease are theoretical.

Dosing Guidelines. 20 mg IV 30 minutes before chemotherapy, followed by 10 mg by mouth, every 6 hours ×4 doses.

Indications. Dexamethasone is effective for a moderate emetic challenge such as the Cytoxan/methotrexate/5-fluorouracil (CMF) regimen. It is unsuitable as a single agent for highly emetogenic regimens such as high-dose cisplatin[61] but is very useful in combination therapy in such cases (see below).

DELTA 9 TETRA HYDROCANNABINOL

This major psychoactive component of marijuana and hashish is available commercially as Marinol (dronabinol). Its antiemetic properties are associated with euphoria; patients who fail to experience these feelings of elation and heightened awareness are reported also to fail to derive the antiemetic effects.[82] This agent also acts as an appetite stimulant, a beneficial side effect in most chemotherapy patients. Patients develop tachyphylaxis to the drug's side effects but not to the antiemetic effects.

The mechanism of action of Marinol is uncertain but theories have included an effect on prostaglandin synthesis[83] and on endorphins.[84] Centrally located cannabinoid receptors have also been implicated.[85]

Side effects including tachycardia, conjunctival injection, orthostatic hypotension, and syncope may occur. This drug also has a potential risk of dependency and abuse, and may exacerbate mania, depression, and schizophrenia.

Dosing Guidelines. 5 to 7.5 mg/m^2, 1 to 3 hours prior to chemotherapy, then repeat at 2 to 4 hours after for a total of 4 to 6 doses per day. In the absence of side effects the dose may be increased if necessary in increments of 2.5 mg/m² to a maximal dose of 15 mg/m².

Indications. Ineffective for highly emetogenic agents such as cisplatin therapy, Marinol is effective for moderate emetic challenges such as Nitrogen mustard/Vincristine/Procarbazine/Prednisone (MOPP) and carmustine (BCNU). Use of this agent should be reserved for patients in whom other, more conventional antiemetics have failed. It should be avoided in patients with a history of psychiatric disorders.

PROCHLORPERAZINE

This phenothiazine shares the toxic potential of other such agents, including extrapyramidal reactions, especially in children. Some preparations also contain sulphites, which may cause an allergic response in sensitized individuals. Long-term use does not result in tolerance but can be hepatotoxic.

Prochlorperazine is thought to act by blocking dopamine (D_2) receptors in the chemoreceptor trigger zone.[86] In addition, this agent increases lower esophageal sphincter pressure.[87]

Dosing Guidelines. 10 mg every 4 to 6 hours IM or by mouth.

Indications. The use of prochlorperazine as a single agent is limited by a relative lack of efficacy when compared with high-dose metoclopramide, corticosteroids, and cannabinoids.[88] It is suitable for mildly emetogenic agents such as 5-FU, leucovorin, bleomycin, and methotrexate, and is useful for outpatient therapy of delayed nausea and vomiting.

LORAZEPAM

This drug is a benzodiazepine with sedative and anxiolytic properties mediated allosterically through gamma-aminobutyric acid (GABA) receptors.[89,90] It has antiemetic properties comparable to metoclopramide.[91]

Adverse effects include arteriospasm with intra-arterial injection, and this route is strictly contraindicated. Both oral and IV dosing must be diluted according to the manufacturer's guidelines.

Dosing Guidelines. 0.025 to 0.05 mg/kg IV every 4 hours ×4 doses.

Indications. As an adjunct to therapy to provide an anxiolytic effect, particularly in the treatment of anticipatory nausea and vomiting.

Combination Therapy

Numerous studies have demonstrated the superiority of combining antiemetics for increased efficacy.[51] Examples include the use of dexamethasone with metoclopramide or with ondansetron.[75] As already noted, combination therapy may have incidental benefits, such as the reduction in metoclopramide-associated diarrhea by dexamethasone. Steroids also increase the antiemetic potency of phenothiazines[92] and of cannabinoids. Drug combinations may be used to prevent specific side effects; for example, diphenhydramine can be added to the antiemetic regimen to prevent extrapyramidal side effects associated with metoclopramide.

Some general guidelines for combination therapy are as follows:

1. Combinations should have different mechanisms of action.
2. Overlapping toxicities should be avoided.
3. Beneficial side effects should influence selection.

Dosing Guidelines. Triple drug therapy can be used combining a neuroreceptor blocker, corticosteroid, and benzodiazepine or antihistamine in the treatment of nausea and vomiting associated with high dose-cisplatin therapy, as follows (for cisplatin dose >99 mg/m²):

Metoclopramide 3 mg/kg IV 30 minutes before and 90 minutes after chemotherapy
 OR
Ondansetron 0.15 mg/kg IV 30 minutes before, then at 4 and 8 hours after the first dose
 PLUS

Dexamethasone 20 mg IV 40 minutes before chemotherapy
PLUS
Lorazepam 0.025 to 0.05 mg/kg IV 35 minutes before chemotherapy

For a lesser emetogenic challenge, these guidelines can be modified and the oral route used (for example, for cyclophosphamide plus doxorubicin):

Metoclopramide 2 to 3 mg/kg orally every 2 hours ×3 doses, then every 4 hours ×3 doses
PLUS
Dexamethasone 20 mg IV as above
PLUS
Diphenhydramine 50 mg IV or orally with the first and then every other dose of metoclopramide.

Cannabinoid use is most often limited by the incidence of side effects, in particular, dysphoric reactions. This can be prevented by combination therapy with prochlorperazine, 10 mg IM or orally every 4 to 6 hour.[93]

Therapy of Common Adverse Effects of Antiemetic Agents

SEDATION

If the patient becomes unarousable, withhold further drug administration. Monitor vital signs and provide general supportive care as indicated.

EXTRAPYRAMIDAL REACTIONS

Patients may display extrapyramidal signs, especially after receiving any of the phenothiazines. This includes such symptoms as incoordination, tremor, slurred speech, nystagmus, or ataxia. Discontinue administration of antiemetics and treat with diphenhydramine (Benadryl) 25 mg IV.

DIARRHEA

Evaluate carefully for other causes of diarrhea. Diarrhea is fairly common with many chemotherapeutic agents, and can be treated with a number of medications.

HEADACHE

This is associated with ondansetron administration and can be treated with acetaminophen with or without codeine.

SUMMARY: THERAPY OF CHEMOTHERAPY-INDUCED EMESIS

1. Consider the emetogenic potential of drugs used and treat for the most likely drug (see Table 8-4). Consider timing of chemotherapy-induced emesis.
2. Prevention is better than treating established chemotherapy-induced emesis. Remove environmental triggers to chemotherapy-induced emesis.
3. Prevent dehydration.
4. Single agents include metoclopramide, ondansetron, granisetron, dexamethasone, Delta 9 tetrahydrocannabinol, prochlorperazine, and lorazepam.
5. Antiemetics may be combined for superior efficacy. Combinations should include drugs with different mechanisms of action.

SUMMARY: CHEMOTHERAPY-INDUCED EMESIS

The antiemetic agent or agents chosen should be powerful enough to suppress the maximal emetic stimulus typical of a given chemotherapeutic agent or combination of agents. Treatment should be started before chemotherapy and continued for a duration characteristic of the emetogenic agent used. Combination *multireceptor* therapy may be necessary for more refractory chemotherapy-induced emesis, and attention should be paid to practical considerations such as dehydration, anxiety, and alternative underlying causes of nausea and vomiting.

Paradoxically, whereas the 5 HT_3 receptor antagonists represent a significant breakthrough in the therapy of chemotherapy-induced emesis, they have spawned a new generation of more intensive chemotherapeutic regimens. Chemotherapy-induced emesis therefore persists as a significant problem in clinical oncology. Continued research is necessary in this important aspect of the care of the patient with cancer.

REFERENCES

1. McGuire L. Pain management. In: Otto SE Oncology Nursing. St Louis: Mosby Year Book, 1991:388.
2. Cameron JC. Constipation related to narcotic therapy—a protocol for nurses and patients. Cancer Nurs 1992;15:372.
3. Grosvenor M, Bulcarage L, Chlebowski RT. Symptoms potentially influencing weight loss in a cancer population—correlations with primary site, nutritional status, and chemotherapy administration. Cancer 1989;63:330.
4. Addington-Hall JM, MacDonald LD, Anderson HR, et al. Randomized controlled trial of effects of coordinating care for terminally ill cancer patients. BMJ 1992;305:1317.
5. Twycross RG, Lack SA. Symptom control in far advanced cancer: pain relief. London: Pittman, 1983:43.
6. Wrenn K. Fecal impaction. N Engl J Med 1989;321:658.
7. Gurll N, Stear M. Diagnostic and therapeutic considerations for fecal impaction. Dis Colon Rectum 1975;18:507.
8. Wright BA, Staats DO. The geriatric implications of fecal impaction. Nurse Pract 1986;11:53.
9. Read NW, Abouzerkry L, Read MG, et al. Anorectal function in elderly patients with fecal impaction. Gastroenterology 1985;89:959.
10. Hughes JJ, Neuffler TH. Diagnostic imaging of postoperative fecal impaction. Ala J Med Sci 1986;23:420.
11. Goldfinger SE. Constipation and diarrhea. In: Wilson JD, Braunwald AB, Isselbacher AB, Petersdorf RG, Martin JB, Fauci AS, Rout RK. Harrison's principles of internal medicine. New York: McGraw-Hill, 1991:256.
12. Glare P, Lickiss JN. Unrecognized constipation in patients with advanced cancer: a recipe for therapeutic disaster. J Pain Symptom Manage 1992;7:369.
13. Yakabowich M. Prescribe with care: the role of laxatives in the treatment of constipation. J Geront Nurs 1990;16:4.
14. Ralston SH, Gallacher SJ, Patel U, et al. Cancer-associated hypercalcemia: morbidity and mortality. Ann Intern Med 1990;112:499.
15. Johnston IDA, Gibson JB. Megacolon and colvulus in psychotics. Br J Surg 1960;47:394.
16. Gore RM, Mintzer RA, Calenoff L. Gastrointestinal complications of spinal cord injury. Spine 1981;6:538.
17. Pihko H, Tyni T, Virkola K, et al. Transient ischemic cerebral lesions during induction chemotherapy for acute lymphoblastic leukemia. J Pediatr 1993;123:718.
18. Spira IA, Rubenstein R, Wolff D, et al. Fecal impaction following methadone ingestion simulating acute intestinal obstruction. Ann Surg 1975;181:15.
19. Fetterman LE. Colonic fecal impaction in a young drug addict. JAMA 1967;202:1056.
20. Glare PA, Walsh TD. Dose ranging study of oxycodone for chronic pain in advanced cancer. J Clin Oncol 1993;11:973.
21. Tsuneto S, Hayashi A, Miyazaki M, et al. A clinical survey of controlled-release morphine sulfate for cancer pain relief in a Japanese hospice. Postgrad Med J 1991;67(suppl 2):S79.
22. Kim BS, Chung HC. Experience with a controlled-release oral morphine for cancer pain management. Postgrad Med J 1991;67 (suppl 2):S82.
23. Maves TJ, Barcellos WA. Management of cancer pain with transdermal fentanyl: phase IV trial, University of Iowa. Journal of Pain and Symptom Management 1992;7:S58.
24. Schug SA, Zech D, Grand S, et al. A long-term survey of morphine in cancer pain patients. Journal of Pain and Symptom Management 1992;7:259.
25. Adler HT, Atkinson AJ, Ivy AC. Effect of morphine and dilaudid on the ileum and of morphine, dilaudid, and atropine on the colon of man. Arch Intern Med 1942;69:974.
26. Donatelle EP. Constipation: pathophysiology and treatment. American Family Physician 1990;42:1335.
27. Ground S, Zech D, Lynch J, et al. Validation of World Health Guidelines for pain relief in head and neck cancer: a prospective study. Ann Otol Rhinol Laryngol 1993;102:342.
28. Brown JK, Hogan CM. Chemotherapy. In: Groenwald SL, Fogge MH, Goodman M, Yarbro CH, eds. Cancer nursing: principles and practice. Boston: Jones and Bartlett, 1990:266.
29. George MJ, Heron JF, Kerbrat P, et al. Navelbine in advanced ovarian epithelial cancer: a study of the French oncology centers. Semin Oncol 1989;16(suppl 4):30.
30. Sandler SG, Tobin W, Henderson ES. Vincristine induced neuropathy. A clinical study of

fifty leukemic patients. Neurology 1969;19: 367.
31. Pennock GD, Dalton WS, Roeske WR, et al. Systemic toxic effects associated with high-dose verapamil infusion and chemotherapy administration. J Natl Cancer Inst 1993;83: 105.
32. Keueny N, Israel K, O'Hehir M. Phase II trial of 10-Edam in patients with advanced colorectal carcinoma. Am J Clin Oncol 1990;13:42.
33. Talley NJ, Phillips SF, Haddad A, et al. GR 38032F (ondansetron), a selective 5HT$_3$ receptor antagonist, slows colonic transit in healthy man. Dig Dis Sci 1990;35:477.
34. Mitchell PLR, Evan BD, Allan SG, et al. Ondansetron reduces chemotherapy induced nausea and vomiting refractory to standard antiemetics. N Z Med J 1992;105:73.
35. Markham A, Sorkin EM. Ondansetron: an update of its therapeutic use in chemotherapy-induced and postoperative nausea and vomiting. Drugs 1993;45:931.
36. Hewitt M, Cornish J, Pamphilon D, et al. Effective emetic control during conditioning in children for bone marrow transplantation using ondansetron, a 5-HT$_3$ antagonist. Bone Marrow Transplant 1991;7:431.
37. Herrstedt J, Sigsgaard T, Boesgaard M, et al. Ondansetron plus metopimazine compared with ondansetron alone in patients receiving moderately emetogenic chemotherapy. N Engl J Med 1993;328:1076.
38. Beek TM, Ciociola AA, Jones SE. Efficacy of oral ondansetron in the prevention of emesis in outpatients receiving cyclophosphamide-based chemotherapy. Ann Intern Med 1993; 118:407.
39. Smith RN. Safety of ondansetron. Eur J Cancer Clin Oncol 1989;25(supp 1):S51.
40. Egbuniko IG, Chaffee BJ. Antidepressants in the management of chronic pain syndromes. Pharmacotherapy 1990;10:262.
41. Fisher RE. Psyllium seeds: intestinal obstruction. California Western Medicine 1938;48:190.
42. Maull KI, Kinning WK, Kay S. Stercoral ulceration. Am J Surg 1982;48:20.
43. Holmes S, Eburn E. Patients' and nurses' perceptions of symptom distress in cancer. J Adv Nurs 1989;14:840.
44. McMillian SC, Williams FA. Validity and reliability of the constipation assessment scale. Cancer Nurs 1989;12:183.
45. Tasman-Jones C. Constipation: pathogenesis and management. Drugs 1973;5:220.
46. Kallman H. Constipation in the elderly. Am Fam Physician 1983;27:179.
47. Godding EW. Physiological yardsticks for bowel function and the rehabilitation of the constipated bowel. Pharmacology 1980 (suppl);1:88.
48. Maguire LC. Prevention of narcotic-induced constipation. N Engl J Med 1981;305:1651.
49. Godding EW. Therapeutics of laxative agents with special reference to anthraquinones. Pharmacology 1976;14(supp 1):78.
50. Goodman J, Pang J, Bessman AN. Diocytyl-sodium sulfosuccinate: an ineffective prophylactic laxative. J Chronic Dis 1976;29:59.
51. Gralla RJ, Tyson LB, Kris MG, et al. The management of chemotherapy-induced nausea and vomiting. Med Clin North Am 1987;71:2.
52. Gralla RJ, Itri LM, Pisko LE, et al. Antiemetic efficacy of high dose metoclopramide: randomized trials with placebo and prochlorperazine in patients with chemotherapy-induced nausea and vomiting. N Engl J Med 1981; 305:905.
53. Frustaci S, Tumolo S, Tirell U, et al. High dose metoclopramide versus dexamethasone in the prevention of cisplatin induced vomiting. Proc Am Soc Clin Oncol 1983;2:87.
54. Marty M, Pouillart P, Scholl S, et al. Comparison of the 5-Hydroxytryptamine$_3$ (serotonin) antagonist ondansetron (GR 38032F) with high dose metoclopramide in the control of cisplatin-induced emesis. N Engl J Med 1990;322: 816.
55. Craig JB, Powell BL. Review: the management of nausea and vomiting in clinical oncology. Am J Med Sci 1987;293:34.
56. Lee M, Feldman M. Nausea and vomiting. In: Sleisenger M, Fordtran JS, eds. Gastrointestinal disease: pathophysiology, diagnosis, management. 5th ed. Philadelphia: WB Saunders, 1993:509.
57. Tortorice PV, O'Connell MB. Management of chemotherapy-induced nausea and vomiting. Pharmacotherapy 1990;10(2):129.
58. Gapp GA, James EC, Iwen GW, et al. Post emetic rupture of herniated cardia of the stomach. A variant of Boerhaave's syndrome. JAMA 1982;247:811.
59. Alcalam J, Ingber A, Sandbank M. Mask phenomenon: post-emesis facial purpura. CUTIS 1986;38:28.
60. Marty M. Future trends in cancer treatment and emesis control. Oncology 1993;50:159.
61. Laszlo J, Contach PH. Nausea and vomiting of chemotherapy. In Holland JF, Frei E, Bast RC, et al, eds. Cancer medicine, 3rd ed. Philadelphia: Lea and Febiger, 1993:2261.
62. Borison HL, Wang SC. Physiology and pharmacology of vomiting. Pharmacol Rev 1953;5:193.
63. McCarthy LE, Borison HL, Spiegel PK, et al. Vomiting: radiographic and oscillographic correlates in the decerebrate cat. Gastroenterology 1974;67:1126.
64. Graves T. Emesis as a complication of cancer chemotherapy: pathophysiology, importance

and treatment. Pharmacotherapy 1992;12(4): 337.
65. Gralla RJ, Kris MG, Tyson LB. Controlling emesis in patients receiving cancer chemotherapy. Recent Results Cancer Res 1988;108:89.
66. Jacobsen PB, Redd WH. The development and management of chemotherapy-related anticipatory nausea and vomiting. Cancer Invest 1988;6:329.
67. Morrow GR. Clinical characteristics associated with the development of anticipatory nausea and vomiting in cancer patients undergoing chemotherapy treatment. J Clin Oncol 1984;2:1170.
68. Fetting JH, Grochow LB, Folstein MF, et al. The course of nausea and vomiting after high dose cyclophosphamide. Cancer Treat Rep 1982;66:1487.
69. Gralla RJ. An outline of antiemetic treatment. Eur J Cancer Clin Oncol 1989;25(suppl 1):S7.
70. Kris MG, Tyson LB, Gralla RJ, et al. Extrapyramidal reactions with high dose metoclopramide. N Engl J Med 1983;309:433.
71. Wilholm BE, Mortimer O, Boethius G, et al. Tardive dyskinesia associated with metoclopramide. Br Med J 1984;288:545.
72. Tami JA, Waite WW. Metoclopramide suppository considerations. Drug Intelligence & Clinical Pharmacy 1988;22:268.
73. Gunning SJ, Hagan RM, Tyers MB. Cisplatin induces biochemical and histological changes in the small intestine of the ferret. Br J Pharmacol 1987;90:135.
74. Rath U, Upadhyaya BK, Arechevala E, et al. Role of ondansetron plus dexamethasone in fractionated chemotherapy. Oncology 1993;50:168.
75. Beck TM. Efficacy of ondansetron tablets in the management of chemotherapy-induced emesis: review of clinical trials. Semin Oncol 1992;19:6(suppl 15)20.
76. Lazarus HM, Blumer JL, Bryson JC. Antiemetic efficacy and pharmacokinetic analysis of GR38032F during multiple day cisplatin prior to autologous bone marrow transplantation. Proc ASCO 1990;8:327.
77. Navari RM, Kaplan HG, Gralla RJ, Grunberg SM, Palmer R, Fitts D. Efficacy and safety of granisetron, a selective 5-Hydroxytryptamine-3 receptor antagonist, in the prevention of nausea and vomiting induced by high-dose cisplatin. J Clin Oncol 1994;12:2204.
78. Smith IE. A dose-finding study of granisetron, a novel antiemetic, in patients receiving cytostatic chemotherapy. J Cancer Res Clin Oncol 1993;119:350.
79. Rich MW, Abdulhayoglu G, Disaia PJ. Methylprednisolone as an antiemetic drug during cancer chemotherapy: a pilot study. Gynecol Oncol 1980;9:193.
80. Markman M, Sheidler V, Ettinger DS, et al. Antiemetic efficacy of dexamethasone. Randomized double blinded cross-over study with prochlorperazine in patients receiving cancer chemotherapy. N Engl J Med 1984;311:549.
81. Allan SG, Cornbleet MA, Warrington PS, et al. Dexamethasone and high-dose metoclopramide efficacy in controlling cisplatin-induced nausea and vomiting. Br Med J 1984;289:878.
82. Sallon SE, Zinberg NE, Frei E. Antiemetic effects of delta-9-tetrahydrocannabinol in patients receiving cancer chemotherapy. N Engl J Med 1975;293:795.
83. Vincent BJ, McQuiston, DJ, Einhorn LH, et al. Review of cannabinoids and their antiemetic effectiveness. Drugs 1983;25(1):52.
84. London SW, McCarthy LE, Borison HL. Suppression of cancer chemotherapy induced vomiting in the cat by nabilone, a synthetic cannabinoid. Proc Soc Exp Biol Med 1979;160:437.
85. Matsuda LA, Lolait SJ, Brownstein MJ, et al. Structures of a cannabinoid receptor and functional expression of the cloned DNA. Nature 1990;346:561.
86. Isaacs B, MacArthur JG. Influence of chlorpromazine and promethazine on vomiting induced with apomorphine in man. Lancet 1954;2:570.
87. Brock-Utne JG, Rubin J, Welman S, et al. The action of commonly used anti-emetus on the lower esophageal sphincter. Br J Anaesth 1978;50:295.
88. Bakowski MJ. Advances in antiemetic therapy. Cancer Treat Rep 1984;11(3):237.
89. Martin M. The benzodiazepines and their receptors: 25 years of progress. Neuropharmacology 1987;26:957.
90. Bormann J. Electrophysiology of $GABA_A$ and $GABA_B$ receptor subtypes. Trends Neurosci 1988;11:112.
91. Laszlo J, Clark RA, Hanson DC, et al. Lorazepam in cancer patients treated with cisplatin: a drug having antiemetic, amnesic, and anxiolytic effects. J Clin Oncol 1985;3:864.
92. Baker JJ, Lokey JL, Price NA, et al. Comparison of dexamethasone plus prochlorperazine to placebo plus prochlorperazine as antiemetics for cancer chemotherapy [Abstr]. Proc Am Soc Clin Oncol 1980;21:339.
93. Cunningham D, Forrest GJ, Soukoup M, et al. Nabilone and prochlorperazine: a useful combination for emesis induced by cytotoxic drugs. Br Med J 1985;291:864.

II

EXTRA-ABDOMINAL SURGICAL PROBLEMS

9

Chronic Venous Access in the Cancer Patient

BRIAN J. EASTRIDGE
ALAN T. LEFOR

Vascular access is one of the most needed and most commonly used techniques in the care of the patient with cancer. Gaining access to the vascular system is a common problem for which the surgeon is consulted to assist in the care of the patient receiving chemotherapy. It is also one which, although often treated as a routine matter, can have serious consequences and therefore must be taken seriously by physician and patient alike.

Central venous access via the subclavian vein was first described by Aubaniac in 1952 in France.[1] Subsequently, in the United States, Wilson and colleagues in 1962 routinely utilized central access devices for measurement of central venous pressure.[2]

As the technique of central venous access became more routine, an increasing number of indications arose for their placement. With time, advances in polymer science made it possible to place chronic indwelling central access devices.

As the number of protocols using intravenous chemotherapeutic agents for the primary or adjunctive treatment of various types of malignancies has steadily increased, the use of long-term indwelling venous access devices has become commonplace in the realm of clinical oncology. Initially implemented by Broviac[3] in 1973 and subsequently modified by Hickman[4] in 1979, these devices have revolutionized the care of the oncology patient. Since then, many new devices have been introduced to include implantable access systems. More recently, a peripherally inserted central catheter has been developed to provide intermediate term central access. As the field of oncology has evolved, so has the need for new and improved approaches to venous access.

INDICATIONS

For many patients, the placement of an indwelling central venous access device is indicated due to physical or psychological factors associated with repeated venipuncture necessitated by the obliteration of peripheral veins. Peripheral venous access is gradually lost in most oncology patients because of the sclerosing nature of chemotherapeutic agents.

Therefore, the utility of the indwelling venous access device rests in its provision for chronic central venous access for chemotherapy administration, total parenteral nutrition, long-term antibiotic therapy, or the administration of blood and blood products. Additionally, as many of these patients require frequent laboratory blood tests, the indwelling catheter allows a portal for access without the necessity for repeated venipuncture.

An indwelling central venous access device is not without potential for morbidity and even mortality. As such, the benefit of placing such a device needs to be carefully measured against the potential risks associated with it. Important factors contributing to this decision include access availability, type and length of therapy, patient compliance, and so forth.

VASCULAR ACCESS DEVICES

Several techniques exist for obtaining chronic central venous access in the cancer patient. Each of these methods has its own relative indication as well as advantages and disadvantages in regard to placement, care, and management of potential complications.

The overall use of these devices varies from one center to another based on individual preferences and the nature of the protocols being used. At the University of Maryland Cancer Center, 322 access devices were surgically placed in 274 cancer patients over a 30-month period.[15] A total of 209 of 322 (65%) were catheters and 113 of 322 (35%) were subcutaneous infusion ports (Table 9-1). At the time of that study, P.A.S. Ports™ and PIC lines were not utilized.

Subclavian Catheter

The nontunneled subclavian catheter is the oldest and most widely used form of indwelling central venous access. Most often, this catheter is used in an acute inpatient setting when the patient has limited peripheral access and yet does not require long-term intravenous therapy.

The advantage of this device is that it is usually inserted at the bedside and can be changed over a guidewire using a modified Seldinger technique.[5] Also, this type of catheter is available in multiple lumen capacity. A recent report from a major cancer center suggests that these catheters may be used *in lieu* of surgically placed venous access devices for long-term access.[6] Although this study should encourage others to use this less expensive method, the level of support necessary to make it successful may limit its general applicability.

Although routine changing of these catheters is often practiced, studies have failed to demonstrate the effectiveness of this to reduce infection; thus, subclavian catheters should be changed only when there is a definite clinical indication.[7] In addition, the polyvinyl chloride from which the catheter is made tends to be stiff and quite thrombogenic.

Peripherally Inserted Central Catheter

The peripherally inserted central (PIC) catheter has shown utility in the treatment of patients requiring intermediate durations of therapy with a mean of 12 to 20 days.[8,9] These PIC catheters are single lumen devices placed percutaneously through a *peel-away* introducer via the cephalic vein in the antecubital region and advanced to their central venous location. One advantage of this type of device is that it can be inserted by specially trained nursing personnel in the patient's own home; thus obviating the necessity for operative placement of a central venous access device. In addition, this device requires minimal maintenance for patency and subsequent use. However, many patients may not have adequate antecubital venous access due to previous chemotherapy, intravenous drug abuse, morbid obesity, and so forth. As such, the PIC catheter system is not a practical alternative. Yet another limitation of this catheter is its single lumen capacity and thus it may be difficult to coordinate multiple modalities of intravenous therapy. Occasionally, due to its placement in the antecubital fossa, catheters can be kinked or rendered nonfunctional by the mobility of the elbow joint.

Hickman Catheter

The subcutaneously tunneled catheter consists of a silastic catheter with a Dacron cuff,

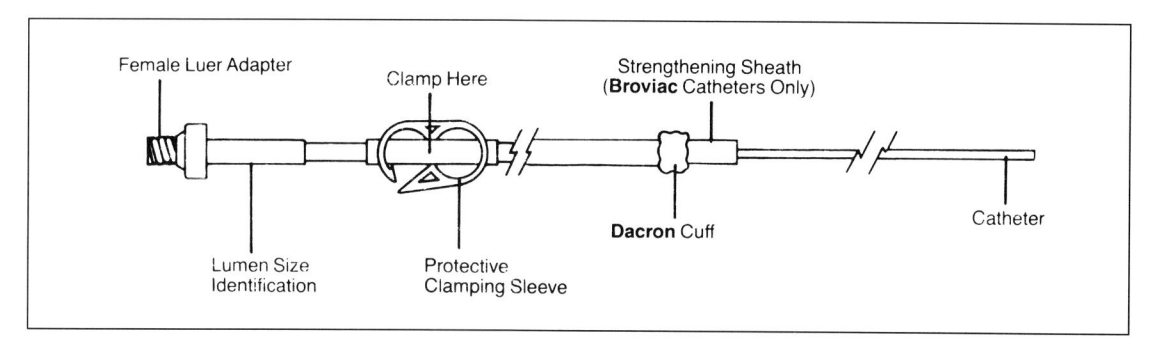

Figure 9-1. Schematic diagram of the Hickman catheter. Bard Access Systems, Salt Lake City, UT; reprinted with permission.

which is positioned within the subcutaneous tissue at the time of operation (Fig. 9-1). After its incorporation into the tissue by a fibrotic reaction, this cuff restricts the migration of skin flora along the catheter tract and provides an anchor against device migration. In addition, several manufacturers now produce this device with a second silver impregnated cuff that has been reported to decrease the incidence of device-related infection.[10,11] This finding has not been universal, however. In a carefully controlled prospective study of 200 cancer patients,[12] investigators found no significant effect of the silver impregnated cuff on the incidence of catheter-related infection. Its routine use cannot be recommended on the basis of this study.

The subclavian tunneled catheter is most useful in the treatment of patients with hematologic malignancies or those undergoing bone marrow transplantation. This type of device has merit in these circumstances as these patients may require multiple modalities of intravenous therapy as well as frequent blood sampling to evaluate their hematologic status. In addition, this device is conveniently accessed and is pain-free with respect to the delivery of therapy.

These catheters are available as one-, two- or three-lumen devices. Single-lumen catheters are most useful for the administration of antibiotics and similar situations in which frequent blood sampling is not anticipated. Double-lumen catheters are most commonly used for cancer patients, allowing fluid and drug administration at the same time that blood is withdrawn. Triple-lumen catheters are used only in particular therapeutic regimens where multiple drugs are to be administered simultaneously. Table 9-1 shows a 30-month single center experience with placement of catheters. As discussed below, a significantly higher complication rate was observed with triple-lumen catheters compared with double-lumen catheters.[15] Therefore, the number of lumens should be selected specifically for the anticipated therapy.

Due to its nature, this type of catheter does have inherent disadvantages. Because some length of the catheter protrudes from the skin, both the catheter and the site must routinely be maintained by either the patient or the patient's family. Without routine catheter care, the risk of infection increases precipitously. Also, these devices must routinely be flushed according to a regimented protocol, thus making this type of device labor intensive for the patient. Not to be underestimated are the alterations in self-image and the limitations in activities of daily living and lifestyle imposed by this type of device. Lastly, because this type of device is partially external, it is susceptible to damage and dislodgement; as such, additional attention must be given, especially in the pediatric population.

Table 9-1. Devices Placed at the University of Maryland Cancer Center: Number of Lumens

Device	Number of Lumens	Number of Devices
Hickman™ Catheter	1	1
	2	160
	3	48
Subcutaneous Port	1	101
	2	12

Adapted from Eastridge BJ and Lefor AT. Complications of indwelling venous access devices in cancer patients. J Clin Oncol 1995;13:233.

Subcutaneous Infusion Port

The subcutaneous infusion port consists of three basic parts: (1) a reservoir (0.4 mL capacity) with a superficial silicone rubber septum, (2) a silastic catheter, and (3) a locking hub to affix the catheter to the reservoir. Once again, these devices are placed surgically and are available in single or dual port varieties, with the single-lumen port being used most routinely. A single center experience is shown in Table 9-1, which demonstrates the more common use of the single-lumen variety.

This type of device is most commonly employed in the therapy of patients with solid tumors necessitating fairly infrequent access. Because this device is totally subcutaneous, it may be less susceptible to infection than the tunneled silastic catheter and, as such, imposes few restrictions on patient activities. It has been suggested that the risk of infection is more related to the frequency of access rather than the type of device placed. In addition, this device is low profile and virtually imperceptible and thus has fewer associated psychologic sequelae.

The disadvantage of the subcutaneous port is its limited luminal access and limited use in the obese patient. A relatively minor disadvantage to this type of system is that accessing the device requires a percutaneous puncture. In addition, this device probably should not be used for continuous home infusion of chemotherapy or total parenteral nutrition (TPN) due to the risk of extravasation.

P.A.S. Port™

This peripherally inserted subcutaneous port (Pharmacia-Deltec Inc.) is a relatively new addition to the central access armamentarium. To its advantage, this device is relatively easy to insert and can be inserted at the patients bedside. As such, the peripheral port is less costly than conventional centrally inserted devices.[13,14] In addition, because it is peripherally placed, operative complications such as pneumothorax, hemothorax, and major vascular injury are avoided.

The limitations of this type of access device are its limited luminal capacity, as with the centrally placed subcutaneous port, and the catheter-related problems due to the mobility of the elbow joint, as with the PIC catheter.

SUMMARY: VASCULAR ACCESS DEVICES

1. Indwelling venous access devices are placed for chronic central venous access to simplify chemotherapy administration, total parenteral nutrition, long-term antibiotic therapy, or the administration of blood and blood products.
2. Percutaneously placed nontunneled subclavian catheters may be useful for short-term therapy; longer term use has been reported.
3. A PIC line is useful in intermediate term therapy. It may not be useful in many patients because it requires good antecubital venous access. Its single-lumen capacity may also be a limiting factor in certain therapeutic programs.
4. Subcutaneous tunneled catheters (e.g., Hickman catheter) are very useful for regimens requiring frequent access, but they require considerable daily care by the patient.
5. Subcutaneous infusion ports require little care and are useful for regimens requiring relatively infrequent access.

6. The P.A.S. port™ is placed peripherally and passed centrally but is limited by its small caliber.

PREOPERATIVE CARE

The ultimate goal of surgery is the safe and successful placement of indwelling central venous access devices. This begins with the history and physical examination. The examining physician should specifically inquire about bleeding disorders, history of deep venous thrombosis, or history of prior central venous access devices.

Frequently, several chronic central access devices may be required over the treatment course of an oncology patient. If such a history is obtained, it is imperative to evaluate the patient's central venous circulation. The least invasive method of evaluation is a venous duplex scan, which can yield information regarding vascular patency. Haire et al[16] demonstrated by duplex scanning that 14% of patients with a previous subclavian central access device had persistent venous obstruction preventing subsequent central access placement. In yet another study, patients with a history of central venous access device studied by preoperative venous duplex scanning demonstrated a 40% incidence of central venous thrombosis, but in these instances, the surgeon was directed to an alternative patent central vein by the study.[17] More recently, duplex scanning has been demonstrated to be 89% to 100% sensitive and 94% to 100% specific in the evaluation of upper extremity and central venous systems relative to contrast venography.[18-21] If venous duplex scanning proves unsatisfactory, contrast venography may be useful in elucidating venous access options. However, contrast evaluation of the venous system, as it is an invasive procedure, is associated with several risks including bleeding, acute allergic reaction, renal insufficiency, and venous thrombosis. In general, patients with a history of previous central catheters should not be brought to the operating room for placement of a venous access device without obtaining an evaluation of their central veins. Once a satisfactory site for the placement of venous access has been established, the immediate preoperative planning phase may commence.

Preoperatively, consent should be obtained by a staff member with a thorough knowledge of the procedure. The patient should be thoroughly apprised of the benefits as well as the attendant risks involved in the placement, use, and maintenance of the access device. The procedure should be explained in its entirety and the surgeon should not belittle placement of the access device as a minor procedure. In addition, it is often helpful to patients to discuss possible alternatives to device placement and the advantages that chronic access will offer them. In addition, all patients should be thoroughly informed with respect to the potential risks associated with the procedure, including: bleeding, infection, pneumothorax and hemothorax, and vascular and catheter thrombosis. Patients should also be told that the device may not be placed if access cannot be obtained.

Thrombocytopenic patients with platelet counts less than $40,000/mm^3$ may require platelet transfusion immediately prior to device placement so as to minimize the potential for bleeding complications. In addition, occasionally blood products such as fresh frozen plasma or cryoprecipitate are required for similar reasons. Several authors have detailed specific approaches for patients with thrombocytopenia.[22-25]

SUMMARY: PREOPERATIVE CARE

1. Patients are assessed with a history and physical examination. Patients with a history of prior central venous access devices must be assessed for patency of the central veins, usually with a venous duplex study.

2. Patients must be carefully apprised of risks and complications including bleeding, catheter infection, catheter and venous thrombosis, and hemothorax and pneumothorax.
3. Patients with thrombocytopenia (platelet count <40,000/mm³) may require platelet transfusion prior to surgery.

OPERATIVE STRATEGIES AND TECHNIQUES

Initially, in the treatment course of the cancer patient, central venous access is obtained by accessing the superior vena cava via the internal or external jugular, subclavian, or cephalic veins (Fig. 9-2). Because the upper central circulation may gradually be obliterated due to thrombus or contraindicated by such conditions as superior vena cava (SVC) syndrome associated with tumor impingement, the inferior vena cava may be accessed through the saphenous or femoral veins when needed.[21] In rare circumstances, patients may require laparatomy to access gonadal veins or to directly access the vena cava, or thoracotomy to access the azygous vein or to directly access the right atrium.[26] It is readily apparent that the operating surgeon must be well versed in vascular anatomy.

Positioning

Traditional surgical teaching has dictated that for the placement of percutaneous central access, the patient should be positioned with an interscapular roll to elevate the shoulders and have the head turned to the contralateral side.[27,28] In addition, the Trendelenburg position has long been thought to aid in the placement of such devices. However, in a study[29] recently published, magnetic resonance imaging was used to determine the true structural relationships in the region of the subclavian vein. In this study, it was determined that the neutral anatomic position was the best position and that placement of an interscapular roll led to compression of the subclavian vein between the first rib and the clavicle, which made successful placement more difficult. In addition, by turning the head to the opposite side, the angle between the subclavian vein and internal jugular vein, which is usually 90 degrees, is actually increased, thereby increasing the chances for catheter malposition in the internal jugular vein[29] (Fig. 9-3). In a venographic study by Land,[30] it was determined that the Trendelenburg position does not produce any increased distension of the subclavian veins. Most likely, the caliber of the subclavian veins is dictated by its fibrous attachments to adjacent anatomic structures. Therefore, neutral anatomic position seems to be the most advantageous position for the placement of percutaneous central venous access. The Trendelenburg position is of no utility when accessing the subclavian system, but may be practical when accessing the jugular system as these veins dilate.

Intraoperative Preparation

After the patient has been brought to the operating room and placed in the neutral anatomic position on the operating table, anesthesia is administered. Most often, local anesthesia (1% lidocaine) with concurrent intravenous sedation is adequate for placement of a chronic central access device. Infrequently, owing to individual patient variables, local anesthesia alone or even general anesthesia may be required. In the University of Maryland Cancer Center series, general anesthesia has been required in less than 1% of patients. At this point, the site to be cannulated is prepared with sterile solution of povidone iodine or comparable solution. Perioperative antibiotics are unnecessary as a routine consideration.

Operative Approach

An important determination to be made prior to beginning the procedure is the approach

Chronic Venous Access in the Cancer Patient

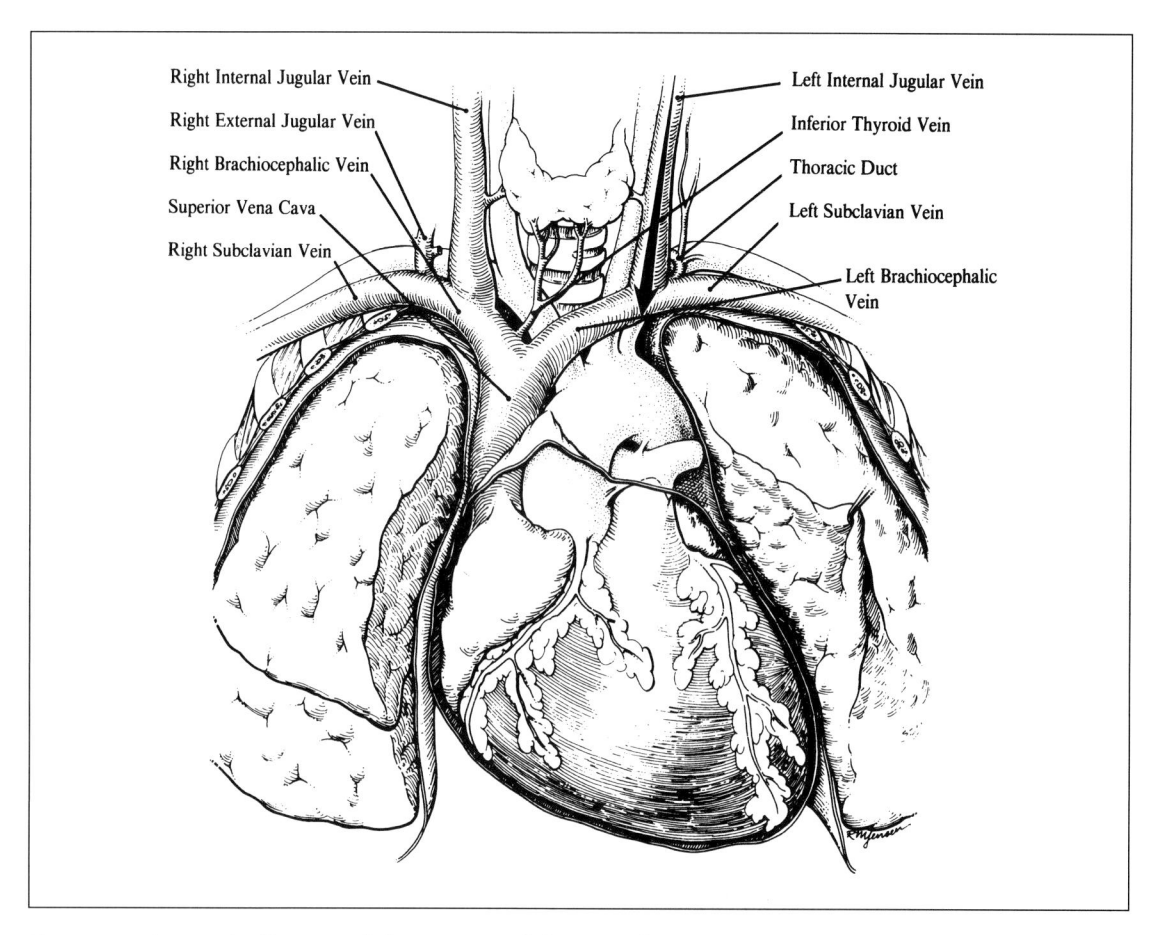

Figure 9-2. Anatomic diagram of the veins used for central venous access. Drawing by Robin M. Jensen, CMI, from Wendt JR. Surgical Rounds July 1992:639; reprinted with permission.

to be used. A summary of the approaches most commonly used is shown in Table 9-2. Percutaneous placement has been advocated as simple and rapid, made possible by the development of the peel-away introducer. However, although venous cutdown is usually somewhat more time-consuming, it is advocated by Raaf and Heil[31] as the procedure of choice. They advocate internal jugular or external jugular cutdowns as the ideal routes of access, citing certainty of placement and near 0% risk of pneumothorax as the rationale for this approach. In addition, it is cited as safe in patients with thrombocytopenia (platelet count <20,000/mm^3) and has been performed at the Maryland Cancer Center in 1000 consecutive patients without operative complications. Cephalic vein cutdowns are readily performed, but the vein is sometimes of inadequate caliber to admit the catheter. The route of access used in the University of Maryland Cancer Center series[23] in the placement of 322 devices in 274 cancer patients is shown in Table 9-3. The choice of the approach used was usually based on preference of the surgeon. In some cases, a second approach was undertaken after failure of one method.

Percutaneous Access

Employing a percutaneous technique, the central venous system can be accessed for placement of an indwelling venous access device. Accessing the subclavian veins can be achieved by inserting a 16-gauge needle

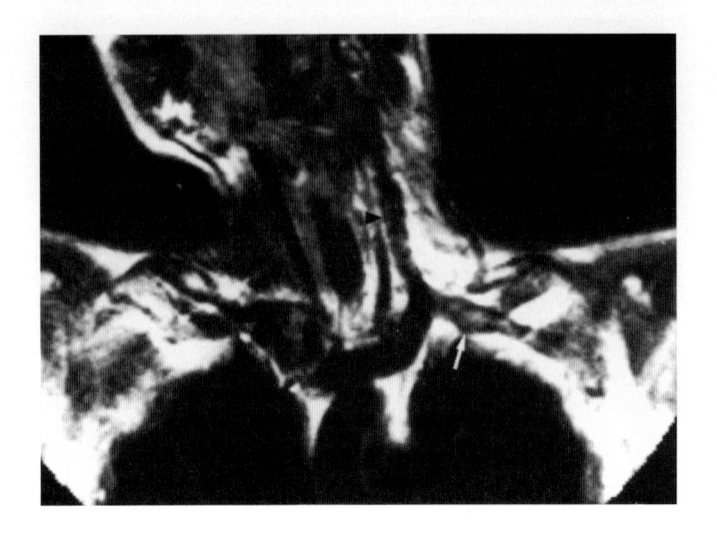

Figure 9-3. MRI scan of the veins of the neck demonstrating an increased angle between the left jugular vein (*arrowhead*) and the left subclavian vein (*arrow*), which promotes malpositioning of the catheter; this is further support for using the neutral anatomic position. Jesseph et al. Arch Surgery 1987;122:1208; reprinted with permission.

2 cm inferior to the clavicle at its midpoint and advancing it toward the sternal notch. To cannulate the internal jugular vein, the cannulation needle is introduced at the apex of the intersection of the anterior and posterior divisions of the sternocleidomastoid muscle and advanced at a 45 degree angle to the skin toward the ipsilateral nipple. Occasionally, a supraclavicular approach may be employed to gain access to the central venous circulation at the confluence of the subclavian and internal jugular veins. This method is performed by supraclavicular needle entry at the intersection of the lateral boundry of the sternocleidomastoid muscle and the clavicle with subsequent angulation of the needle toward the contralateral nipple. Finally, the inferior central venous system may also be approached percutaneously through the femoral vein. This is accomplished by palpating the femoral pulse at the inguinal ligament and percutaneously cannulating the vein approximately 2 cm medial and inferior to the arterial pulse.

One of the problems associated with percutaneous placement may be locating the subclavian vein. Aberrant anatomy and normal variability may predispose to pneumothorax, hemothorax, arterial injury, and brachial plexus injury. Investigators have attempted to improve identification of the vein with real time ultrasound guidance.[32] This novel approach may be safer, although the equipment needed is fairly expensive.

Once the vessel has been cannulated, a guidewire is passed into the central circulation. If cardiac ectopy is noted, the wire is slowly withdrawn until the baseline rhythm is restored. On occasion, it may not be readily apparent whether the central vein or the corresponding artery has been cannulated. Therefore, several techniques can be used to determine the nature of the vessel so as not to risk misplacement of a large bore access device intra-arterially. First, a small bore single-lumen catheter can be advanced over the wire and the wire removed. At this point, blood gas sampling can be performed to determine whether the vessel cannulated is venous or arterial. The disadvantage to this step is that it is time consuming and gives no indication as to position. By comparison, pressure transduction of the catheter is simple

Table 9-2. Commonly Used Approaches for the Surgical Placement of Vascular Access Devices

PERCUTANEOUS
    Subclavian Vein
    Internal Jugular Vein
CUTDOWN
    Cephalic Vein
    External Jugular Vein
    Internal Jugular Vein
    Saphenous Vein

Table 9-3. Devices Placed and Reasons for Removal by Route of Placement: University of Maryland Cancer Center Series

Route	Number Placed	Sepsis	Thrombosis	No Longer Needed	Other
Subclavian	127/95	19/5	12/5	9/3	16/2
Cephalic	31/10	3/1	5/2	1/0	2/0
Int. Jugular	15/1	3/0	0/0	0/0	1/0
Ext. Jugular	20/6	2/0	2/0	1/2	0/0
Saphenous	16/1	1/0	2/0	0/0	0/0
Total	209/113	28/6	21/7	11/5	19/2

The numerator is the number of catheters and the denominator is the number of subcutaneous ports in each element of the table. All subclavian vein devices were placed percutaneously. All cephalic vein, external jugular vein and saphenous vein devices were placed by cutdown. Internal jugular devices were placed by cutdown (8/0) and percutaneously (7/1). Adapted from Eastridge BJ and Lefor AT. Complications of indwelling venous access devices in cancer patients. J Clin Oncol 1995;13:233.

and less time consuming, but also gives no indication as to position. The best method by which to determine wire position is the intraoperative fluoroscopy (Fig. 9-4). The advantage to this technique is that it is expeditious and concurrently indicates ultimate catheter position. In a study undertaken at the University of Maryland, the use of intraoperative fluoroscopy added little to operative time and expense.[15] The use of fluoroscopy should be considered essential in the surgical placement of these devices.

Although correct positioning of the guidewire is assured by intraoperative fluoroscopy, there are four findings, in addition to radiography, that suggest correct placement and are useful if radiography is not used. First, ready backflow of blood into the syringe should be present. Second, the guidewire should advance easily into the vein. A guidewire that has to be forced is likely going into a small tributary. Third, when the guidewire is removed it should be straight or have a gentle curve.[33] A twisted, angular guidewire rarely is a result of passage into the right side of the heart. Fourth, blood should be easily aspirated from each lumen of the device.

Having confirmed guidewire position by fluoroscopy, the respective subcutaneous tunnel (when placing a tunneled catheter) or pocket (when placing a subcutaneous port) is fashioned. To create a subcutaneous tunnel, an appropriate site is chosen for catheter exit from the skin. Care should be taken in choosing this site, especially when aesthetics are an important patient concern. To minimize infection, the tunnel should be at least 10 cm long from the catheter exit site to the subclavian puncture site. At this point, a 5-mm incision is made through the dermis at both the catheter exit site and the vessel cannulation site. Having done this, a subcutaneous tunneler is used to draw the catheter through the tunnel so that the fibrous cuff lies within the

Figure 9-4. The guidewire is inserted through the needle and will pass optimally inferiorly into the inferior vena cava. Fluoroscopy is always used to ascertain correct guidewire position thus avoiding return to the operating room for catheter malposition. From Fares L. Surg Gynecol Obstet 1986; 162:277; reprinted with permission.

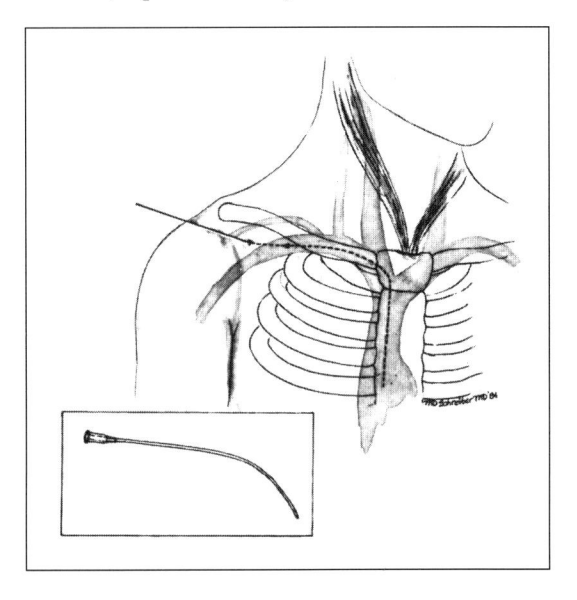

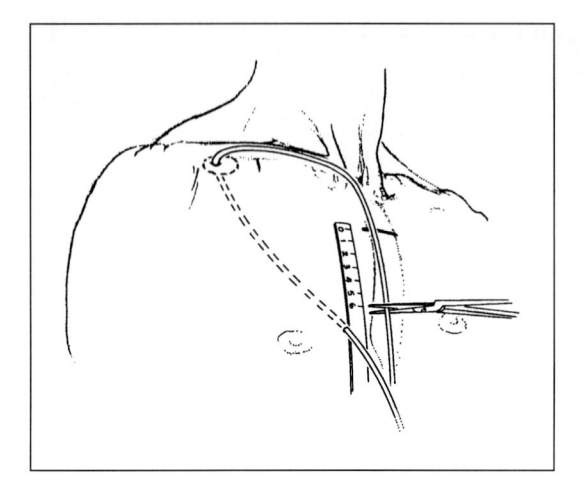

Figure 9-5. The catheter is tunneled subcutaneously and cut to length with the tip at the level of the angle of Louis. From DeVita VT, Hellman S, Rosenberg SA. Principles and practice of oncology. 4th ed. Philadelphia: JB Lippincott, 1994:559; reprinted with permission.

subcutaneous tissue (Fig. 9-5). Care should be taken with placement of the subcutaneous tunnel exit site as the patient must be able to access the device for maintenance.

With respect to the subcutaneous port, a small transverse skin incision is made and the pocket is developed inferiorly at the level of the pectoralis fascia at an appropriate site. In obese patients, it may be helpful to excise some of the subcutaneous fat leaving the device no more than 1 cm beneath the skin level. It is absolutely essential that the device is not located beneath the incision used to create the pocket because repeated puncture through the incision to access the port has been associated with an increased rate of infection. Because the device is entirely subcutaneous, the tunnel from the port to the vein puncture site (in a percutaneously placed device) need not be very long and we typically place the device 2 to 3 cm inferior to the venipuncture site. The port is then fixed to the pectoralis fascia in at least two points using nonabsorbable suture (Fig. 9-6), creating three-point fixation with the catheter as the third point. Of the more than 400 ports placed over a 5-year period at the University of Maryland Medical Center, there has not been a single instance of a flipped port because of inadequate fixation with this technique. This technique avoids the potential for flipping of the port or subsequent dislodgement of the catheter. Once the port is fixed in place, a subcutaneous tunnel is created to the guidewire insertion site using a small clamp. It is also critically important that only noncoring (Huber) needles are used to access the device. The use of a regular needle will result in degradation of the injection septum necessitating device removal.

The catheter or port is then flushed with a dilute heparin solution (100 U/mL) and cut to the appropriate length. A dilator is placed over the guidewire and removed followed by the dilator and peel-away sheath complex (Fig. 9-7). The catheter, having been cut to a length to rest at the atriocaval junction, is inserted through the sheath as the dilator and wire are removed. The sheath is then peeled away and the skin wounds are closed.

One problem with use of the peel-away sheath in percutaneous placement of either catheters or ports is kinking of the sheath in a tight subclavian tract. This is usually obviated by performing the venipuncture in a lat-

Figure 9-6. The subcutaneous infusion port is placed in a pocket and secured with at least two nonabsorbable sutures above the pectoralis major muscle, which with the catheter provide three-point fixation to prevent a "flipped port." From Harvey WH, et al. Surg Gynecol Obstet 1989;169: 495.

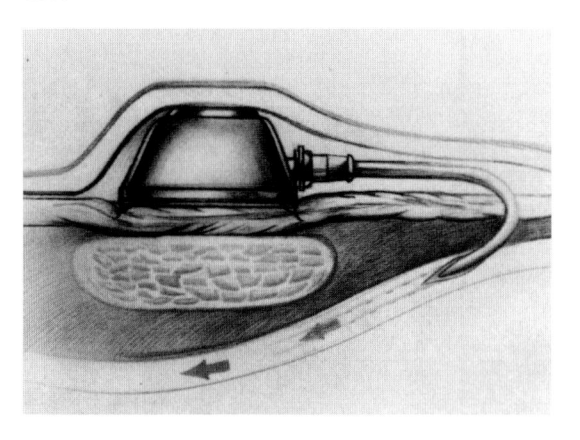

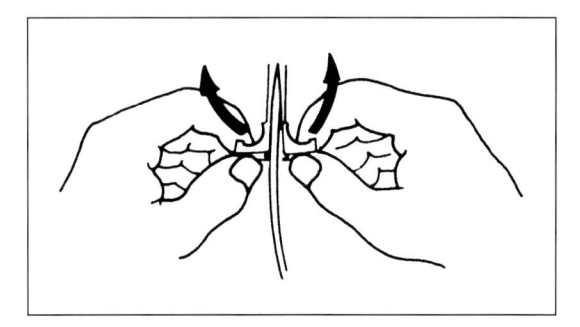

Figure 9-7. Using the peel-away introducer, the catheter is inserted in the introducer and with a peeling motion while the assistant holds the catheter, the sheath is removed. Bard Access Systems, Salt Lake City, UT; reprinted with permission.

eral and somewhat inferior position. The use of a sheath slightly larger than the catheter may also eliminate this problem. A recently described technique[34] is helpful when kinking of the sheath prevents passage of the catheter. These authors describe measuring the distance from the skin entry site to the point of kinking on a chest x-ray film obtained intraoperatively. By retracting the sheath this distance, the catheter can be inserted and usually will pass without difficulty.

Cutdown

In employing a cutdown venotomy via the cephalic, internal jugular, external jugular, saphenous, or femoral vein, the catheter is inserted under direct vision without the necessity for guidewire placement.

The internal jugular cutdown is performed by making a 3-cm incision over the body of the sternocleidomastoid muscle approximately 1 cm cephalad to the clavicle. The platysma muscle is divided and the external jugular vein is isolated (Fig. 9-8A). If the external jugular vein has already been used or is insufficient, the internal jugular vein can be isolated through the same incision. By dissecting at the posterolateral margin of the sternocleidomastoid muscle, the internal jugular vein is encountered and can subsequently be mobilized for cannulation[31] (Fig. 9-8B).

The cephalic vein also can be used to gain access to the superior central venous circulation. To mobilize the cephalic vein, a 3-cm incision is made over the deltopectoral groove. At this region, the vein is superficial and easily isolated. On occasion, the vein is small and attempts can be made to dilate the vessel over a guidewire for subsequent device insertion.[22]

The inferior central venous system can likewise be cannulated via venous cutdown techniques. To perform this procedure, a 3-cm transverse incision is made 3 cm inferior and medial to the femoral pulse at the inguinal ligament. By this technique, the saphenofemoral junction can be isolated and the saphenous vein or the femoral vein can be utilized for placement of the access device[21,35] (Fig. 9-9). Importantly, the tunnel should be at least 20 cm in length to minimize infection, with the catheter typically exiting at the level of the umbilicus.

In placing venous access devices via cutdown and venotomy, one major difference exists between small- and large-caliber vessel cannulation. Relatively small vessels can be distally ligated and the catheter fixed to the proximal vein by a circumferential ligature (see Fig. 9-8C). However, in large vessels such as the internal jugular vein and the femoral vein, a purse string of nonabsorbable monofilament suture such as polypropylene is placed in the exposed vein wall and the venotomy made through the purse string to not totally occlude the vein when the device is placed.

Intra-Abdominal Venous Access

Once relatively simple means of access have been exhausted, more invasive access portals can be obtained. Within the abdomen, several veins exist for placement of an indwelling catheter.[36] Using a right flank approach, the abdominal fascia is divided and the peritoneum is mobilized medially, and a Kocher's maneuver performed. From this operative

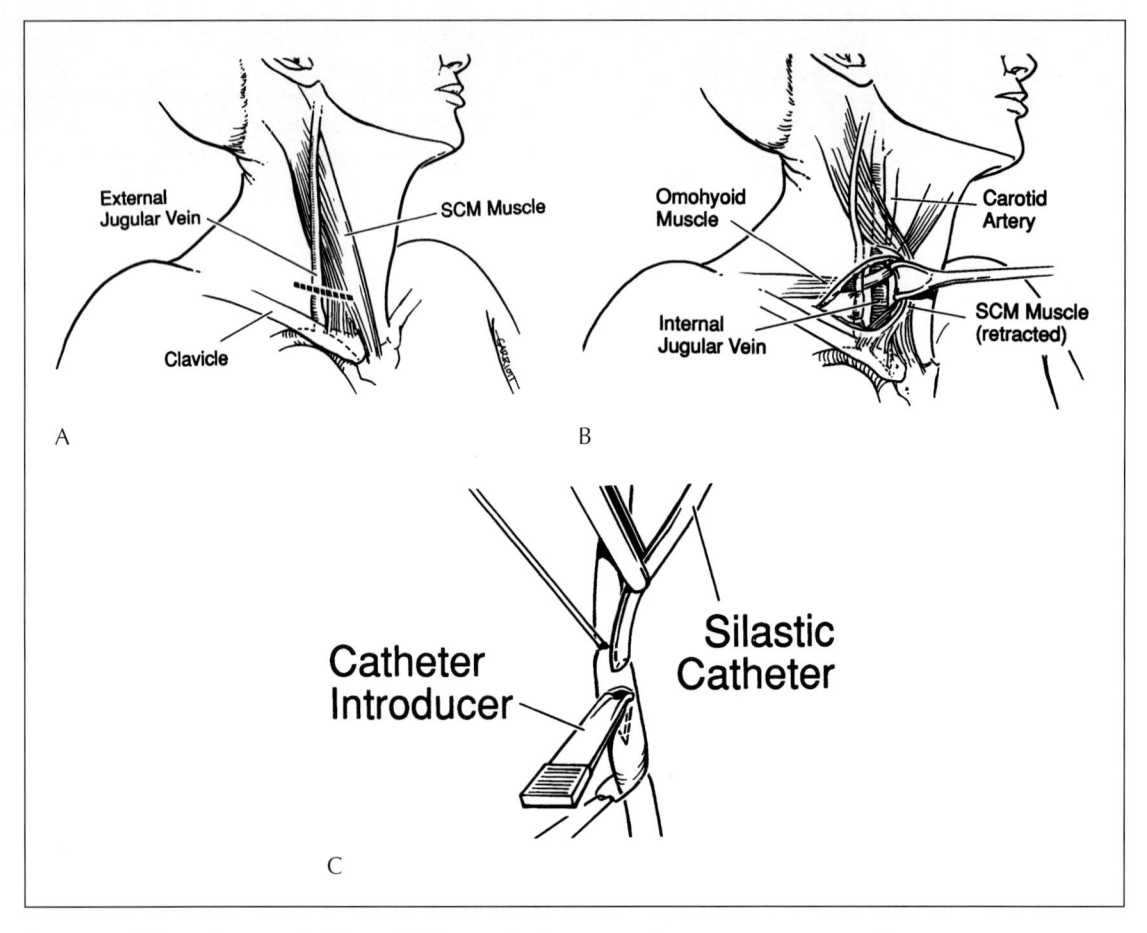

Figure 9-8. The catheters of either a Hickman device or a subcutaneous port may be placed via internal jugular vein cutdown. The patient is positioned with the head turned to the contralateral side **A**. An incision is made above the clavicle between the two heads of the sternocleidomastoid muscle. Dissection is carried deeper until the internal jugular vein is identified **B**. After obtaining proximal and distal control of the vein with vessel loops or fine silk ties, a transverse incision is made with a #11 blade **C**. Using a plastic catheter introducer, the already tunneled and trimmed to length catheter is passed into the superior vena cava. From Raaf J. Surg Gynecol Obstet 1993;177:295; reprinted with permission.

field, venous access can be gained to the right gonadal vein, the right common iliac vein, or the inferior vena cava directly. Using a left flank approach, one can access the left gonadal vein and the left common iliac vein. The disadvantage to the left-sided approach is that one cannot access the inferior vena cava directly and that placement of a device through the left gonadal vein risks thrombosis of the left renal vein.

Intrathoracic Venous Access

In very rare instances, the paucity of venous access may require directly cannulating the superior central venous system. The usual means by which to approach this situation is via a right anterolateral thoracotomy through the sixth intercostal space. The azygous vein or one of its prominent branches can be cannulated in a manner similar to that previous-

Chronic Venous Access in the Cancer Patient

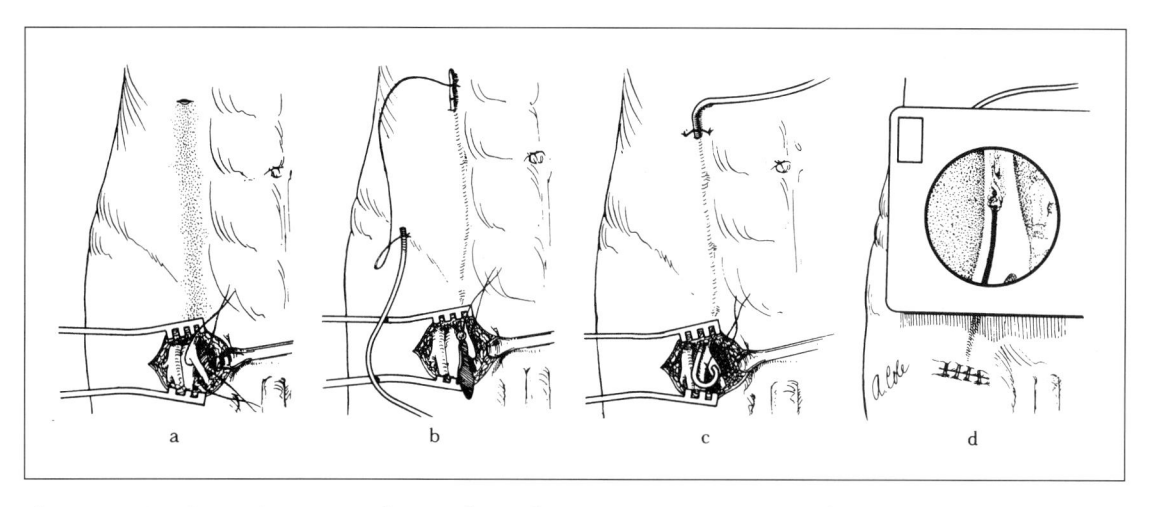

Figure 9-9. An alternative approach uses the saphenous vein in patients with inaccessible upper extremity central veins. **A.** The greater saphenous vein is exposed at its junction with the femoral vein. **B.** The catheter is tunneled at least 20 cm from the level of the umbilicus and trimmed to length so that the tip is at the level of the junction of the common iliac veins. **C.** The venotomy is made after silk ties are placed around the vessel, and the catheter placed using a catheter introducer. **D.** Fluoroscopy is used to check the position of the catheter tip. From Curtas S, Bonarentura M, Megnid MM. Surg Gynecol Obstet 1989;168.

ly discussed. Finally, as a last resort, the right atrium can be accessed directly. This is done by incising the pericardium and placing a purse string suture in the right atrial appendage. From this point, an atriotomy is performed and the access device inserted and secured in position.

Use of Fluoroscopy and Radiography

The intraoperative use of fluoroscopy is extremely helpful for optimal guidewire positioning and catheter placement. It is essential for all surgically placed vascular access devices. Postoperatively, all patients should have an appropriate radiograph (usually an erect chest x-ray film taken at end-expiration; a KUB for saphenous devices) to confirm catheter position and to exclude complications such as pneumothorax and hemothorax or catheter malposition (Fig. 9-10). It is not necessary to obtain this x-ray film in the operating room; it can be obtained in the recovery room because it is needed only to diagnose pneumothorax, as catheter position has already been assured by fluoroscopy. If necessary, a tube thoracostomy can be placed in the recovery room.

Figure 9-10. At the end of the procedure, a chest radiograph is obtained in the operating room demonstrating the catheter tip at the atrial-caval junction.

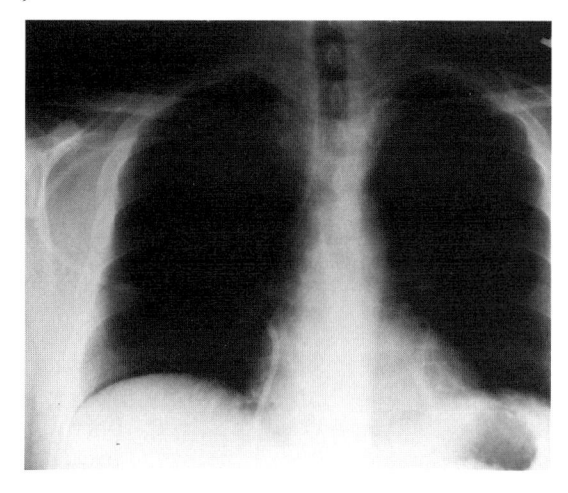

SUMMARY: OPERATIVE STRATEGIES AND TECHNIQUES

1. The ideal position on the operating table is with the patient flat and head pointing straight up. Trendelenburg's position is not useful in subclavian vein access because the vein does not dilate.
2. Most of these devices can be placed with local anesthesia and intravenous sedation; general anesthesia is rarely needed.
3. Percutaneous access is useful for the subclavian or internal jugular veins. A guidewire is advanced after the vessel is cannulated and the position of the guidewire checked fluoroscopically.
4. The internal jugular, external jugular, cephalic, or saphenous veins can be accessed *via* a cutdown.
5. After accessing the vein, the device is passed either through an introducer (percutaneous approach) or through a venotomy (cutdown approach).
6. The device is trimmed so that the tip is at the atriocaval junction (upper body) or at the confluence of the common iliac veins (saphenous vein approach).
7. Fluoroscopy is used for every procedure to identify the position of the guidewire and the catheter tip, and may be useful to correctly position a catheter that is not in the desired location.
8. At the end of the procedure, an upright chest radiograph is taken at end-expiration to evaluate for pneumothorax.

INTRAOPERATIVE MORBIDITY AND COMPLICATIONS

Complications of chronic central venous access devices can be categorized as operative or postoperative. Of interest is that the instruction manual for the percutaenous introducer kit (Bard Access Systems, Salt Lake City, UT) lists 28 potential complications including air embolism, bleeding, brachial plexus injury, cardiac arrhythmia, cardiac tamponade, device erosion, catheter embolism, device occlusion, device sepsis, device extrusion or rotation, endocarditis, extravasation, fibrin sheath formation, hematoma, hemothorax, hydrothorax, intolerance reaction, inflammation, vessel or viscus laceration, vessel or viscus perforation, pneumothorax, spontaneous tip retraction, thoracic duct injury, vascular thrombosis, vessel erosion, and usual surgical risks. As with any surgical procedure, inherent risks are incurred when undertaking the placement of any central venous access device. The most significant intraoperative complications include hemorrhage, pneumothorax or hemothorax, and an inability to gain central venous access. Patients should be specifically counseled about these potential problems.

Hemorrhage

An operative complication with significant potential for patient morbidity is hemorrhage. To exacerbate this problem is the fact that many cancer patients have pre-existing hematologic defects; thrombocytopenia being the most common. Most authors recommend preoperative platelet transfusion for patients with absolute platelet counts of less than 40,000/mm^3 to minimize the risk of significant intraoperative hemorrhage. In addition, several surgeons advocate the use of cephalic or saphenous cutdown over percutaneous placement in this situation.[15,23] By the cutdown technique, the central venous system can be accessed under direct vision wherein vascular control can be carefully maintained. Life-threatening hemorrhage is an infrequent complication of chronic central venous catheter placement and usually occurs in association with inadvertent pleurotomy leading to the development of a hemothorax. The usual scenario of this complication is persistent bleeding from the subcutaneous tunnel or pocket, which can often be controlled with direct pressure.

Pneumothorax and Hemothorax

Other intraoperative complications worthy of note are pneumothorax and hemothorax.

Most commonly, these complications result from percutaneous placement of a central venous access device via the subclavian approach and less frequently via the internal jugular approach.

The reported incidence of pneumothorax is 1% to 3% depending on the series examined.[37-40] In many instances, a small pneumothorax requires no definitive treatment and spontaneously resorbs at a rate of approximately 1% per day. Larger or symptomatic pneumothoraces generally require the placement of an intrathoracic vent (Heimlich valve) percutaneously inserted through the second intercostal space at the midclavicular line. These vents have a one-way valve mechanism, which minimizes the potential for the development of a tension pneumothorax. In rare instances, a tension pneumothorax or a pneumothorax refractory to conservative treatment may require the placement of a tube thoracostomy for the purpose of pleural decompression.

A hemothorax, which is less frequent than a pneumothorax, on the other hand, should always be treated with tube thoracostomy, both to minimize continued hemorrhage and to prevent chronic complications associated with the development of a fibrothorax due to organization of the hematoma and subsequent scar formation.

In evaluating patients for pneumothorax as a result of the percutaneous placement of these devices, one must be cognizant of the possibility of a delayed pneumothorax. This has been reported as late as 5 days after placement of a sublavian catheter.[41] This can be a serious complication, especially if the patient undergoes positive pressure ventilation subsequent to device placement.

In the series of 322 devices placed at the University of Maryland Cancer Center,[15] of 231 devices placed percutaneously, pneumothorax occurred in 4 (2%) and hemothorax in 1 (0.5%).

Failure to Place Device

In a small number of patients, vascular access cannot be obtained due to thrombus associated with previous devices, vascular aberrancies, or inability of the patient to tolerate the procedure. At the University of Maryland, the policy of "one side at a time" with respect to central venous access is followed. If access cannot be obtained on one side, even through attempts at cannulation of multiple veins on that side, the patient is rescheduled for surgery on another date. The rationale for this decision is to prevent bilateral complications such as pneumothorax, which could have catastrophic results. In the University of Maryland Medical Center series, devices were not placed in 4 of 326 patients or 1.2%.[15]

SUMMARY: INTRAOPERATIVE MORBIDITY AND COMPLICATIONS

1. In general, intraoperative complications occur relatively infrequently and, if treated appropriately, have little long-term adverse patient sequelae.
2. Hemorrhage may be exacerbated by thrombocytopenia often seen in patients receiving chemotherapy. Platelet transfusion may be indicated. Cutdown techniques are advocated by some to avoid this complication.
3. Pneumothorax occurs in about 2% of access procedures, usually as a result of a subclavian approach. Tube thoracostomy may be necessary.
4. Attempts to insert vascular access devices should be limited to one side at a single operative sitting. If it is necessary to attempt the opposite side after failing to achieve access, then a chest radiograph must be obtained to avoid the potential for a bilateral pneumothorax.

POSTOPERATIVE CARE

Once the indwelling access device has been placed, its care and maintenance are of paramount importance. This is not only for preservation of catheter function, but also to avert potentially disastrous latent complications. Adequate maintenance requires the coordinated effort of the patient, the surgeon, the oncologist, and the nursing staff. Without strict adherence to a regimented protocol of catheter care, device failure is almost certainly imminent.

Dressings

Generally thought of as insignificant, the choice of postoperative dressing can affect the long-term outcome of the access device. A number of different types of dressings are available. Most recently, the development of transparent dressing has been advocated by some physicians to avoid the inconvenience of having to change dressings to inspect the catheter exit site.[42-44] However, experimental clinical evidence suggests a higher rate of bacterial colonization with this type of dressing in contrast to a simple gauze dressing.[45-50] In addition, this higher rate of bacterial colonization has been correlated with a significant increase in the rate of device-related bacteremia.[46,51] In numerous studies, the use of a gauze dressing applied to the catheter exit site and changed using sterile technique three times per week was associated with a lower relative incidence of infection than other dressing regimens.[46,52] Therefore, only dry gauze and tape dressings are used at the University of Maryland Cancer Center.

Use of the Newly Implanted Device

Once the venous access device has been placed and its position confirmed by x-ray film, it can be immediately accessed for use if necessary. One special consideration is for the immediate use of the subcutaneous infusion port. If it is known that the access device will need to be used immediately, it can be sterilely accessed intraoperatively. The advantage to intraoperative port accession is that the degree of swelling in the immediate postoperative period makes accessing the port extremely uncomfortable to the patient as well as difficult due to a decreased ability to palpate the port precisely. Therefore, use of a newly implanted port is generally delayed for several days.

Long-Term Maintenance

To ensure longevity of the central venous access device, measures must be taken to minimize the risk of latent complications that would require device removal. To decrease the incidence of catheter thrombosis, these devices are routinely flushed with a dilute heparin solution (100 U/mL).

Tunneled devices are flushed with 3 mL per lumen per day. By comparison, subcutaneous infusion ports are flushed with 3 mL of dilute heparin solution after each use or once per month, whichever is more frequent. All devices are flushed using strict aseptic technique to minimize the risk of catheter-related infection.

Catheter Removal

Once the necessity for the central venous access device has been expended, or in the event of complication, the device can be removed. In the case of the tunnelled device, the region over the fibrous cuff is palpated and infiltrated with 1% lidocaine. A 1-cm cutdown is performed over the region of the cuff. It is often advantageous to mobilize the distal catheter initially to avoid inadvertent catheter transection and subsequent embolization. Once the distal catheter is removed, it can be cut and sent for culture if indicated. At this point, the cuff is mobilized along with the proximal catheter and the remainder of the device removed. Subcutaneous infusion ports are removed in a similar manner by infiltrating the area over the subcutaneous pocket and incising the scar. The port is mobilized using a combination of blunt and sharp dissection and the nonabsorbable sutures are identified and cut. After removing the device *in toto*, the wound can be closed or left to heal by secondary intention if the removal was necessitated by infection. It is important to examine the removed device to be sure that it has been entirely removed. If there is any doubt, then a radiograph should be obtained immediately to eliminate the possibility of a retained catheter segment or catheter embolus.

SUMMARY: POSTOPERATIVE CARE

1. Dry gauze and tape dressings provide the optimal coverage at the exit sites to decrease the incidence of infections.
2. Catheters can be used immediately after placement, but ports should not be used for a few days unless access is obtained in the operating room at the time of placement.
3. Catheters are flushed daily with heparin 100 U/mL, whereas ports are flushed monthly or after each use.
4. Care is taken at the time of device removal to avoid catheter shear and subsequent embolization.

POSTOPERATIVE COMPLICATIONS

One way to study the incidence of complications with vascular access devices is to evaluate the reasons for the removal of the devices. In the University of Maryland Medical Center series, of 209 catheters, 35% remained in place, 27% were in place at the time of the patients' death, and 38% were removed.[15] Of the 113 subcutaneous infusion ports placed, 52% remained in place, 30% were in place at the time of death, and 18% were removed (Fig. 9-11). A summary of the reasons for removal is shown in Table 9-3.

The reasons for device removal in this series are shown in Figure 9-12. Of the 79 (38% of all placed) catheters removed, 11 were removed for completion of therapy, 21 for thrombosis, 28 due to sepsis, and 19 for miscellaneous causes. Of the 20 (18% of all placed) subcutaneous ports removed, 5 were from patients who had completed therapy, 7 for thrombosis, 6 for sepsis, and 2 for miscellaneous causes.

Thrombosis

With experience, it is apparent that vascular

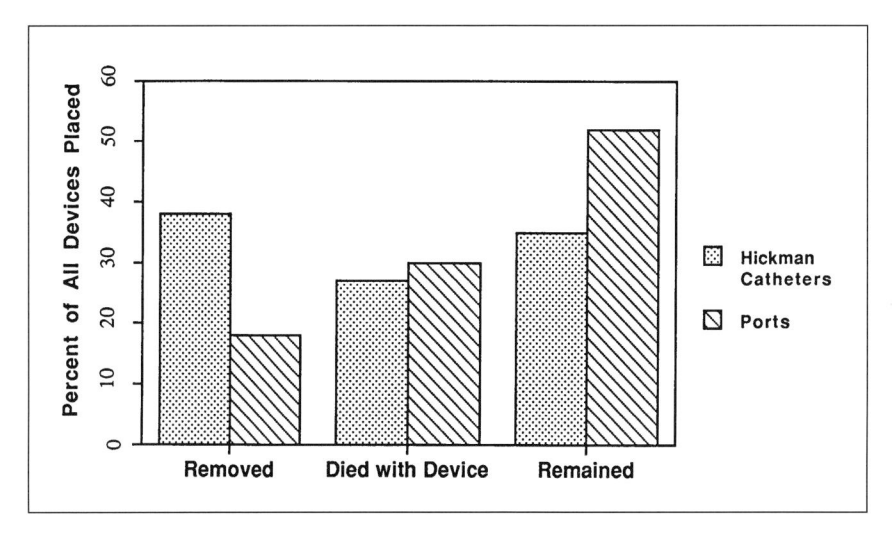

Figure 9-11. Fate of devices placed at the University of Maryland Cancer Center over a 30-month period as the percent of all devices placed. From Eastridge BJ, Lefor AT. J Clin Oncol 1995;13:233.

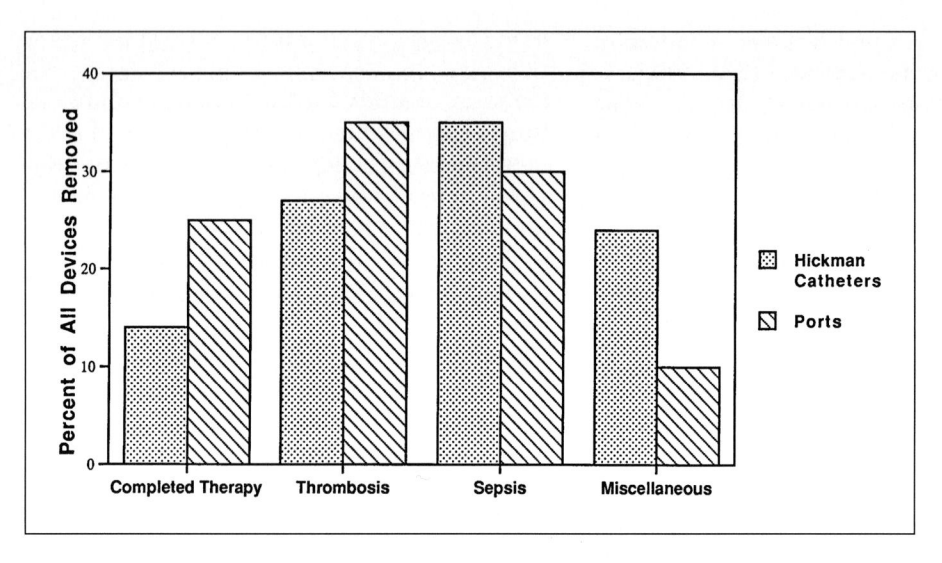

Figure 9-12. Rate of complications as a percent of all devices removed with both catheters and subcutaneous ports at the University of Maryland. From Eastridge BJ, Lefor AT. J Clin Oncology 1995;13:233.

thrombosis is a problem of major proportion with respect to the maintenance of the chronic indwelling central venous access device. In reviewing Virchow's triad, the factors that predispose a patient to vascular thrombosis are hypercoagulability, stasis, and endothelial injury.[53] Any number of these factors or a combination may effect thrombosis in the oncology patient. Several disease-related factors may induce a hypercoagulable state in select types of malignancy. Stasis can occur for several reasons, for instance, primary mediastinal tumors, mediastinal metastasis, or multiple catheters,[54] which impede cardiac return. Vascular endothelial disruption can result from actual catheter insertion through the vessel wall or continuous irritation of the endothelium by the catheter tip with stiffer materials manifesting a greater propensity for thrombosis.[55,56]

Three catheter-related variables appear to be associated with venous thrombogenicity: catheter composition, catheter diameter, and catheter tip location.[15] Indwelling venous access devices with a larger diameter tend to have a higher incidence of thrombosis and a shorter mean time until failure than do catheters with a relatively smaller diameter. The experience with double-lumen catheters (10 French diameter) and triple-lumen catheters (12.5 French) is shown in Table 9-4. These data suggest that triple-lumen catheters have a significantly ($p<0.05$) higher rate of thrombosis, probably due to increased diameter.

In addition, several investigators have implicated high catheter tip placement to be correlated with a higher incidence of venous thrombosis.[15,57–60] This increased incidence of thrombogenicity may potentially be due to chronic endothelial injury related to a greater degree of catheter tip mobility, especially when the tip is in proximity to the turbulent flow at the confluence of the innominate veins.

Venous thrombosis is present in 4% to 50% of vessels with indwelling access devices if these patients are evaluated by routine venographic studies.[59–65] However, if one were to include only patients with symptomatic venous thrombosis, the thrombosis rate would be ascertained as 0% to 4%.[59–65] It is thus apparent that the majority of thrombi associated with indwelling central venous access devices are asymptomatic. In the University of Maryland Medical Center series, thrombosis was observed in 21 of 209 (10%) catheters and 7 of 113 (6%) subcutaneous ports. Interestingly, 15 of 19 devices removed had the tip of the catheter above the level of T3.

When symptomatic, the clinical presentation is one of either catheter malfunction or pain and swelling associated with the affected venous system. Classically, the presentation of clinical symptoms is insidious and is characterized by vague pain or discomfort in the face, neck, chest, scapular region, or arm.[66,67] Extremity swelling is a relatively late sequela in the evolution of the thrombus. Thrombus-associated catheter malfunction can be secondary to gross venous thrombosis or fibrin sheath formation. With a fibrin sheath, thrombus is propogated from the actual venotomy site extending the length of the catheter and sometimes beyond, thus, creating a functional obstruction. Furthermore, this sheath can act as a one-way valve allowing infusion but not withdrawal of blood (withdrawal occlusion, see below).

When venous thrombosis is suspected, thorough evaluation is warranted to minimize patient morbidity. The patient can be studied by invasive or noninvasive means using venography or duplex scanning. Venography yields a more detailed examination to include the venous anatomy, the absolute extent of the thrombus, and the degree of venous collateralization (Fig. 9-13). The degree of collateral flow can indicate the chronicity of the venous obstruction. However, venography sometimes can be technically difficult owing to swelling of the involved extremity, and the patient does incur some risk with the administration of contrast dye. On the other hand, duplex scanning is quite effective in denoting the presence and extent of central venous thrombosis.

Having ascertained the presence of a central venous thrombus, management strategies must be addressed. Most surgeons advocate the administration of intravenous heparin to prevent propogation of the thrombus. If the venous thrombosis can be treated conservatively, the venous access device can often be spared. However, if there is involvement of the vena cava, intractable pain associated with the venous occlusion, or notable propogation of the clot while the patient is therapeutically anticoagulated, then the device must be explanted as it is undoubtedly the nidus for the venous thrombosis. In some patients in whom venous access is particularly difficult, every effort is made to salvage the catheter. Whereas several studies have concluded that no significant incidence of pulmonary embolus has ever been attributed to the presence of thrombosis of the upper central venous system,[68,69] more recent data suggests that upper central venous thrombosis can have significant implications.[66,70] Fibrinolytic agents have been used for the treatment of catheter-associated venous thrombosis but have had only limited success, being more effective in the setting of acute venous occlusion than in the chronic circumstance under which most venous thrombi develop.[71,72]

However, in the circumstance of isolated catheter obstruction secondary to thrombus, the use of fibrinolytic therapy has proved very beneficial in terms of catheter salvage rates.[73–78] By injecting a solution of urokinase (5000 U/mL) equal to the residual volume of the occluded catheter and aspirating the catheter lumen after 15 minutes, the restitution of catheter patency has been greater than 90% in most studies.[73]

Table 9-4. Incidence of Thrombosis in Indwelling Catheters: University of Maryland Cancer Center Series

Lumens	Thrombosed	Nonthrombosed
2	11	149
3	10	38

Adapted from Eastridge BJ and Lefor AT. Complications of indwelling venous access devices in cancer patients. *J Clin Oncol* 1995;13:233.

Infection

Infection is one other major threat in terms of post-operative morbidity. This factor is espe-

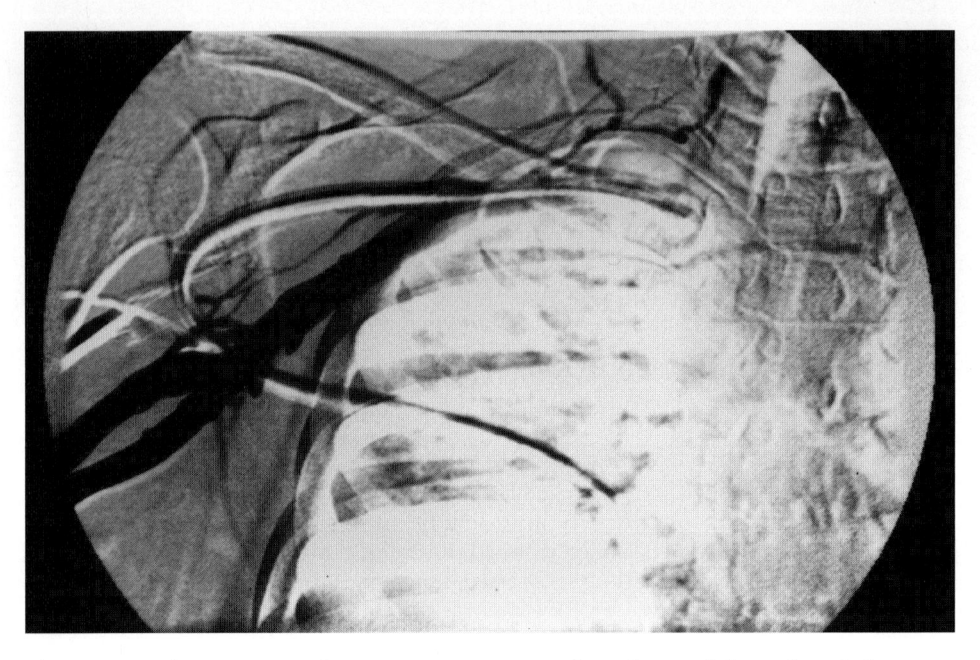

Figure 9-13. This venogram demonstrates a venous thrombosis of the right subclavian vein.

cially important as many oncology patients are either intrinsically or therapeutically immunosuppressed. Patients with catheter-related infections typically present with vague symptoms of fever with or without local inflammatory responses. Typically, patients present during a neutropenic phase of their illness whether it is primary or iatrogenic.[79-81] With such a clinical scenario, the patient should have both central and peripheral blood cultures drawn from the line. Any drainage from the catheter exit site should be cultured and the port pocket aspirated if indicated. In addition, other likely sources of infection should be evaluated. (Catheter infections are discussed further in Chapter 16.) In the University of Maryland Medical Center series,[15] 28 of 209 (13%) catheters and 6 of 113 (5%) subcutaneous ports were removed for infection.

Several potential mechanisms have been postulated as the cause of catheter-related infection. The most obvious source of infection would be poor technique, including improper irrigation or home maintenance, at the time the device is accessed.[82] As such, it is very important to implement a strictly regimented protocol of device maintenance. Secondly, it has been proposed that skin flora are able to migrate along the external surface of implanted catheters to gain access to the venous system.[83]

Conversely, several authors have also supported the notion that an intraluminal source of infection can be present. In one study, electron microscopy of catheters removed from oncology patients revealed that most of these catheters possessed intraluminal glycocalyx colonized by gram-positive organisms.[85] One final theory by which catheter-related infection can occur is through enteric bacterial translocation associated with altered mucosal integrity leading to subsequent seeding of the device.[85]

Infectious complications can be categorized as exit site infections, tunnel infections, port pocket infections, or catheter-associated bacteremias. The most common infectious complication is the exit site infection, characterized by erythema, induration, tenderness, or drainage from the device exit site. It is limited in extent to between the cuff and the skin entrance site. Exit site infections are frequently secondary to normal skin flora and occur with increased incidence during periods of neutropenia. Usually, systemic antimicrobial therapy directed against the offending organism is sufficient to clear the infection and consequently spare the device. Tunnel infections and port pocket infections are similar entities as both are essentially closed-space infections. These infections present as erythema, induration, or tenderness over the catheter between the cuff and the venous cannulation site or over the port site, respectively. In addition, these patients may even present with septicemia due to their closed space infection. Under these circumstances, it is necessary to remove the device to prevent further sequelae. Again, the most common causa-tive organisms are gram-positive skin flora which should be treated with antibiotics after device explantation. True device-related bacteremia can be associated with either gram-positive flora or gram-negative enteric organisms. Most of these infections can be treated adequately with intravenous antibiotics via the catheter itself. However, in the circumstance of fungemia, most of these catheters require removal as the mycotic organisms tend to be resistant to parenteral therapy with an indwelling foreign body.[86,87]

Another point worth noting is the fact that multiple-lumen catheters have a higher propensity for development of infection. As the luminal number increases, the mean time until catheter failure decreases significantly.[15,88,89] This may be partially explained by the number of times that the ports are accessed as well as an increased amount of colonized glycocalyx with a greater number of device lumens. Subcutaneous infusion ports are even more resistant to infection, which presumably is due to the unexposed nature of the device.[90-97]

Withdrawal Occlusion

Although it is certainly ideal to be able to use these devices for both the administration of therapeutic agents and the withdrawal of blood, thus avoiding repeated peripheral venipuncture, it sometimes is impossible to withdraw blood, although infusion continues without difficulty. After determining that the catheter cannot be used to withdraw blood, a contrast study should be obtained through the device to ascertain that the tip of the catheter is still in the vascular lumen. Migration of the device must be ruled out as a cause of the inability to withdraw blood. In one study of implanted ports, withdrawal occlusion occurred in 19% of patients and was successfully treated with urokinase.[98] Withdrawal occlusion was shown to be due to a fibrin sheath around the catheter beginning at the catheter entrance to the central vein and extending 1 to 5 cm beyond the tip of the catheter. This sheath acted as a flap-valve preventing withdrawal of blood but allowing infusion. Having determined that the tip is still inside the vessel, urokinase can be used to clear the fibrin sheath. Withdrawal occlusion is not necessarily an indication for device removal.

Catheter Shear

Catheter shear is an entity characterized by device fracture with subsequent extravasation (incomplete) or distal embolization (complete) of the retained catheter fragment. It is associated with percutaneous cannulation of the subclavian vein wherein the vein is entered medial to the intersection of the first rib and clavicle, and thus the proximal catheter is susceptible to shearing forces between thes two bony structures.[99-104] Interestingly, this entity often can be identified on the initial postoperative radiograph as a "pinched off sign."[99,100,105-107] Most authors advocate the removal of such catheters prior to 6 months to minimize the risk of device fracture and consequent embolization. Once embolized, these catheter fragments require extraction via invasive radiologic techniques.[108-110]

Unusual Complications

A number of rare complications of long-term venous access devices have been described and are worth mentioning. Hydrothorax has been described, which was believed to be the cause of death in patients receiving central hyperalimentation.[111,112] Of importance, this complication was delayed in its appearance. Thus, these patients had functioning catheters that eroded through the vessel wall allowing infusion into the thoracic cavity, which was felt to be due to osmotic injury to the wall of the vein. A similar complication was reported with erosion of the tip and resultant pericardial infusion with the chemotherapeutic agent 5-FU.[113] Of note is that this patient had symptoms of pericarditis. These cases underscore the need for regular aspiration of blood to assure that the tip is in the vascular tree. Any doubt is easily dissipated with a contrast study through the device. Although extremely uncommon, the delayed formation of an arteriovenous fistula also has been reported in patients with central venous access devices.[114] Poor fixation to the chest wall of a subcutaneous infusion port may lead to a "flipped port," which is noted when the usual configuration is not palpable at the time of access. This can be averted by careful attention to the fixation at the time of placement, and if it occurs, must be repaired operatively.

SUMMARY: POSTOPERATIVE COMPLICATIONS

1. Venous thrombosis is a significant complication of vascular access devices. There is a direct correlation between catheter diameter and the likelihood of thrombosis. A thorough evaluation using venography or duplex scanning is warranted when this complication is suspected. Thrombosis of the vein requires removal of the device, although thrombolytic agents are useful if thrombosis is limited to the catheter.
2. Infection is also a major postoperative complication, and may present as exit site infections, tunnel infections, port pocket infections, or catheter-associated bacteremias. Exit site infections may often be treated successfully with parenteral antibiotics. Tunnel and pocket infections usually require removal of the device as they are closed-space infections. Bacteremias are usually treated with antibiotics alone, whereas fungemia is difficult to treat successfully without removal of the device.
3. Catheter shear may result in embolization to the heart of a fragment of the catheter. Catheters noted to be pinched between the clavicle and first rib should be removed within 6 months to minimize the likelihood of this complication.
4. Withdrawal occlusion is usually due to a fibrin sheath at the tip acting as a flap-valve and can be treated with urokinase. A contrast study should be obtained to assure that the catheter tip is still in the vascular tree.

SUMMARY

Ever since their introduction, the indications for and use of chronic central access devices have increased in the treatment of patients with neoplastic disease. The indications for the institution of such devices is based on a number of physical and psychological factors.

Several devices are available for providing central access in the oncology patient. These devices can be placed peripherally or centrally by percutaneous or cutdown methods and can be external or totally implanted systems. The decision about which device to use is based on a number of individual patient factors.

Preoperative preparation includes history and physical examination as well as appropriate venous imaging studies as dictated by the patient's preoperative assessment. In addition, informed consent is obtained and the patient counseled with respect to potential complications.

In the operating room, the patient is placed in the neutral anatomic position and anesthesia administered. Venous access is then established according to a preoperative plan using the appropriate device and site. The use of intraoperative fluoroscopy often is beneficial with respect to device positioning.

In the postoperative period it is imperative that a protocol for device maintenance be instituted to minimize latent complications. This includes a regimen of regular dressing changes and catheter flushes.

Complications can be classified as intraoperative or postoperative. Intraoperative complications most noteworthy are hemorrhage, pneumothorax, and hemothorax. These entities are usually easily recognized and if managed appropriately, lead to very minimal chronic morbidity. On the other hand, complications such as thrombosis, infection, and catheter shear usually are latent and insidious and can have profound consequences with respect to adverse patient outcome.

In conclusion, the placement and maintenance of an indwelling central venous access device in the oncology patient require cooperative effort on the part of the patient, physicians, nurses, and ancillary health care staff. Through their efforts, device longevity is extended and patient morbidity is decreased.

REFERENCES

1. Aubaniac R. *L'injection intraveineuse sons-claviculaire.* Presse Med 1952;60:1456.
2. Wilson JN, Grow JB, et al. Central venous pressure in optimal blood volume maintenance. Arch Surg 1962;85:563.
3. Broviac JW, Cole JJ, Schribner BH. Prolonged parenteral nutrition in the home. Surg Gynecol Obstet 1974;139:24.
4. Hickman RO, Buckner CD, Clift RA, et al. A modified right atrial catheter for access to the venous system in marrow transplant recipients. Surg Gynecol Obstet 1979;148:871.
5. Seldinger S. Catheter replacement of the needle in percutaneous arteriography: new technique. Acta Radiol 1953;39:368.
6. Broadwater JR, Henderson MA, Bell JL, Edwards MJ, et al. Outpatient percutaneous central venous access in cancer patients. Am J Surg 1990;160:676.
7. Cobb DK, High KP, Sawyer RG, et al. A controlled trial of scheduled replacement of central venous and pulmonary-artery catheters. N Engl J Med 1992;327:1062.
8. Lozano H, et al. Clinical evaluation of the Percucath for both pediatric and adult home infusion therapy. Journal of Intravenous Nursing 1991;14:249.
9. Rountree D. The PIC catheter. Am J Nursing 1991;91:22.
10. Maki DG, Cobb L, Garman JK, et al. An attachable silver-impregnated cuff for prevention of infection with central venous catheters: a prospective randomized multicenter trial. Am J Med 1988;85:307.
11. Groeger JS, Lucas AB, Coit D, LaQuaglia M, Brown AE, Turnbull A, Exelby P. A prospective, randomized evaluation of the effect of silver impregnated subcutaneous cuffs for preventing tunneled chronic venous access catheter infections in cancer patients. Ann Surg 1993;218(2):206.
12. Flowers R, Schwenzer K, et al. Efficacy of an attachable subcutaneous cuff for the prevention of intravascular catheter-related infection: a randomized controlled trial. JAMA 1989;261(6):878.
13. Pearl JM, Goldstein L, Ciresi K. Improved methods in long term venous access using the P.A.S. port. Surg Gynecol Obstet 1991;173:313.
14. Finney R, Albrink MH, Hart MB, Rosemurgy AS. A cost-effective peripheral venous port system placed at the bedside. J Surg Res 1992;53:17.
15. Eastridge BJ, Lefor AT. Complications of indwelling venous access devices in cancer patients. J Clin Oncol 1995;13:233.
16. Haire WD, Lynch TG, Lieberman RP, Edney JA. Duplex scans before subclavian vein catheterization predict unsuccessful catheter placement. Arch Surg 1992;127:229.
17. Kraybill WG, Allen BT. Preoperative duplex imaging in the assessment of patients with venous access. J Surg Oncol 1993;52:244.
18. Pollak EW, Walsh J. Subclavian-axillary thrombosis: role of noninvasive diagnostic methods. South Med J 1980;73:1503.
19. Langesfeld M, Hershey FB, Thorpe l. Duplex b-mode imaging for the diagnosis of deep venous thrombosis. Arch Surg 1987;122:587.
20. Lensing WA, Prandoni P, Brandjes D. Detec-

tion of deep venous thrombosis by real time b-mode ultrasonography. N Engl J Med 1988;320:342.
21. Curtas S, Bonaventura M, Meguid MM. Cannulation of the inferior vena cava for long-term central venous access. Surg Gynecol Obstet 1989;168:121.
22. Coit DG, Turnbull AD. A safe technique for placement of implantable vascular access devices in patients with thrombocytopenia. Surg Gynecol Obstet 1988;167:429.
23. Stellato T, Gauderer W, Lazarus H, Herrzig R. Percutaneous silastic catheter insertion in patients with thrombocytopenia. Cancer 1985; 56:2691.
24. Foster PF, Moore L, Sankara HN, Hart ME, Ashmann MK, Williams JW. Central venous catheterization in patients with coagulopathy. Arch Surg 1992;127:273.
25. Ricci JL, Reiner DS. Simple technique for long-term central venous access in the patient with thrombocytopenic carcinoma. Surg Gynecol Obstet 1991;172:145.
26. Pokorny WJ, et al. Use of azygous vein for central catheter insertion. Surgery 1985;97:362.
27. Shires GT, Canizaro PC, Lowry SF. Fluid, electrolyte, and nutritional management of the surgical patient. In: Schwartz S (ed). Principles of surgery. 4th ed. New York, Mc-Graw-Hill, 1984:45.
28. Fisher JE. Metabolism in surgical patients: protein, carbohydrate, and fat utilization by oral and parenteral routes. In: Sabiston DC (ed). Textbook of surgery. 14th ed. Philadelphia, WB Saunders, 1991:116.
29. Jesseph JM, Conces DJ, Augustyn GT. Patient positioning for subclavian vein catheterization. Arch Surg 1987;122:1207.
30. Land RE. Anatomic relationships of the right subclavian vein: a radiologic study pertinent to percutaneous subclavian vein catheterization. Arch Surg 1971;102:178.
31. Raaf JH, Heil D. Open insertion of right atrial catheters through the jugular veins. Surg Gynecol Obstet 1993;177:295.
32. Sukigara M, Yamazaki T, Hatanaka M, Nagashima N, Omoto R. Ultrasonic real time guidance for subclavian venipuncture. Surg Gynecol Obstetr 1988;167:239.
33. Kern KA, Fischer JE. The geometry of the central venous catheter wire stylette as an indicator of correct catheter position. Surg Gynecol Obstet 1983;156(3):361.
34. Heyd RL, Rosser JC. Preventing kinking of the peel-away sheath during insertion of a long-term central venous catheter using percutaneous subclavicular venipuncture. Surg Gynecol Obstet 1991;172:148.
35. Fokalsrud EW, Berquist W, Burke M, Ament M. Long-term hyperalimentation in children through saphenous central venous catheterization. Am J Surg 1982;143:209.
36. Parsa MH, Tabora F, Freeman H. Vascular cannulation techniques in intravenous drug addicts and in patients with limited or difficult intravenous access. Contemp Surg 1987; 31:31.
37. Moosa HH, Julian TJ, Rosenfeld CS, Shadduck RK. Complications of indwelling central venous catheters in bone marrow transplant recipients. Surgery 1991;172:275.
38. Pessa ME, Howard RJ. Complications of Hickman-Broviac catheters. Surg Gynecol Obstet 1985;161:257.
39. Brothers TE, Niederhuber JE, Roberts JA, Ensminger WD. Experience with subcutaneous infusion ports in three hundred patients. Surg Gynecol Obstet 1988;166:295.
40. Sitzmann JV, Townsend TR, Siler MC, Bartlett JG. Septic and technical complications of central venous catheterization. Ann Surg 1985;202:766.
41. Herrman R, Weber FL. Delayed pneumothorax: a complication of subclavian vein catheterization. JPEN J Parenter Enteral Nutr 1987; 11:215.
42. Brendel V. Current concepts in the care of central line catheters. Proceedings of the National Intravenous Therapy Association 1983;6:272.
43. Lawes EG. CVP dressings [letter]. Crit Care Med 1985;13:61.
44. Vasquez RM, Jarrad MM. Care of the central venous catheterization site: the use of transparent polyurethane film. J Parenter Enteral Nutr 1984;8:181.
45. Dickerson N, Horton P, Smith S, Rose R. Clinically significant central venous catheter infections in a community hospital: association with type of dressing. J Infect Dis 1989;160:720.
46. Conly JM, Grieves K, Peters BA. A prospective randomized study comparing transparent and dry gauze dressings for central venous catheters. J Infect Dis 1989;159:310.
47. Maki DG. Study of polyantibiotic and povidone iodine ointments on central venous and arterial catheter sites dressed with gauze or a polyurethane dressing [abstract 933] In: Program and abstracts of the 24th Interscience Conference on Antimicrobial Agents and Chemotherapy. Washington, DC: American Society for Microbiology, 1986.
48. Craven DE, Lichtenberg DA, Kunches LM, et al. A randomized study comparing a transparent polyurethane dressing to dry gauze dressing on peripheral intravenous catheter

sites. Infection Control 1985;6:361.
49. Parsa MH, Lau K, Jampayas I, Tan M, Sampath A, Freeman HP, et al. Intravenous catheter related infection. Infections in Surgery 1985;4:789.
50. Marrie TJ, Costerton JW. Colonization of transparent dressings for intravenous catheters. Infections in Surgery 1987;6:475.
51. Pettigrew RA, Lang SDR, et al. Catheter related sepsis in patients on intravenous nutrition: a prospective study of quantitative catheter cultures and guidewire changes for suspected sepsis. Br J Surg 1985;72:52.
52. McCredie KB, Lawson M, Marts K, Stern RN. A comparative evaluation of transparent dressings and gauze dressings for central venous catheters. JPEN 1984;8:96.
53. Greenfield L. Complications of venous thrombosis and pulmonary embolus. In: Greenfield LJ (ed): Complications in surgery and trauma. 2nd ed. Philadelphia, JB Lippincott, 1990:430.
54. Haire WD, Lieberman RP, Edney J, et al. Hickman catheter induced thoracic vein thrombosis: frequency and sequelae in patients receiving high dose chemotherapy and marrow transplantation. Cancer 1990;66:900.
55. Ryan JA, Abel RM, Abbott WM. Catheter complications in total parenteral nutrition: a prospective study of 200 consecutive patients. N Engl J Med 1974;290:757.
56. Welch GW, McKee DW, Silverstein P, et al. The role of catheter composition in the development of thrombophlebitis. Surg Gynecol Obstet 1974;138:421.
57. Stanislav GV, Fitzgibbons RJ, et al. Reliability of implantable central venous access devices in patients with cancer. Arch Surg 1987;122:1280.
58. Puel V, Caudry M, et al. Superior vena cava thrombosis related to catheter malposition in cancer chemotherapy given through implanted ports. Cancer 1993;72:248.
59. Bozzetti, F., Scarpa, D., Terno, G., et al. Subclavian vein thrombosis due to indwelling catheters: A prospective study on 52 patients. J Parenter Enteral Nutr 1983;7:560.
60. Laidlow JM, Powell-Tuck J, Wood SR, Lennard-Jones JE, Bartram CI. The use of a skin tunnelled silicone rubber catheter for parenteral feeding to avoid central venous thrombosis. JPEN J Parenter Enteral Nutr 1980;4:604.
61. Ross AH, Griffith CD, Anderson JR, Grieve DC. Thromboembolic complications with silicone elastomer subclavian catheters. J Parenter Enteral Nutr 1982;6:61.
62. Pottecher T, Forrier M, Picardat P, et al. Thrombogenicity of central venous catheters: prospective study of polyethylene, silicone, and polyurethane catheters with phlebography or post-mortem examination. Eur J Anaesthesiol 1984;1:361.
63. Brismar B, Hardstedtt C, Jacobson S, Kager L, Malmborg A. Reduction of catheter associated thrombosis in parenteral nutrition by intravenous heparin therapy. Arch Surg 1982; 117:1196.
64. Blalock HA, Pillai MOV, Hill RS, Matthews JR, Clarke, AG, Wade JF. Use of modified subcutaneous right atrial catheter for venous access in leukemic patients. Lancet 1980;1:993.
65. Ruggiero RP, Aisenstein TJ. Central catheter fibrin sleeve-heparin effect. J Parenter Enteral Nutr. 1983;7:270.
66. Horattas MC, Wright DJ, et al. Changing concepts of deep venous thrombosis of the upper extremity—report of a series and review of the literature. Surgery 1988;104:561.
67. Puel V, Chaudry M, et al. Superior vena cava thrombosis related to catheter malposition in cancer chemotherapy given through implanted ports. Cancer 1993;72:2248.
68. Barnett T, Levitt LM. Effort thrombosis of the axillary vein with pulmonary embolism. JAMA 1951;126:1413.
69. Barrios CH, Zuke JE, Blaes B, Hirsch JD, Lyss AP. Evaluation of an implantable venous access system in a general oncology population. Oncology 1992;49:474.
70. Black MD, French GJ, Rasuli P, Bouchard AC. Upper extremity deep venous thrombosis. Underdiagnosed and potentially lethal. Chest 1993;103:1887.
71. Rubenstein M, Creeger WP. Successful streptokinase therapy for catheter-induced subclavian vein thrombosis. Arch Intern Med 1980; 140:1370.
72. Lokich JJ, Bothe A, Benotti P, Moore C. Complications and management of implanted venous access catheters. J Clin Oncol 1985;3: 710.
73. Lawson M, Bottino JC, Hurtubise MR, McCredie KB. The use of urokinase to restore the patency of occluded central venous catheters. American Journal of Intravenous Therapy and Clinical Nutrition 1982:29.
74. Hurtubise MR, Bottino JC, Lawson M, McCredie KB. Restoring patency of occluded central venous catheters. Arch Surg 1980; 115:212.
75. Glynn K, Langer B, Jeejeeboy KN. Therapy for thrombotic occlusion of long term intravenous alimentation catheters. J Parenter Enteral Nutr 1980;4:387.
76. Nakamura S. The use of urokinase for declotting. Postgrad Med 1970;8:218.
77. Cunliffe MT, Polomano RC. How to clear

catheter clots with urokinase. Nursing 1986: 16;40.
78. Haire WD, Lieberman RP, Lund GB, Edney J, Wieczorek BM. Obstructed central venous catheters. Cancer 1990:2279.
79. Larson EB, Wooding M, Hickman RO. Infectious complications of right atrial catheters used for venous access in patients receiving intensive chemotherapy. Surg Gynecol Obstet 1981;153:369.
80. Takasugi JK, O'Connell TX. Prevention of complications in permanent central venous catheters. Surg Gynecol Obstet 1988;167:6.
81. Newman KA, Reed WP, Bustamante CI, Schimpff SC, Wade JC. Venous access devices utilized in association with intensive cancer chemotherapy. Eur J Cancer 1989;25:1375.
82. Bozzetti F. Central venous catheter sepsis. Surg Gynecol Obstet 1985;161:293.
83. Maki DG. Infections associated with intravascular lines. In: Schwartz M, Remmington J, eds. Current topics in clinical infectious disease. New York: McGraw-Hill, 1982:309.
84. Tenney JH, Moody MR, Newman KA, et al. Adherent microorganisms on lumenal surfaces of long term intravenous catheters. Arch Intern Med 1986;146:1949.
85. Tancrede CH, Andremont AO. Bacterial translocation and gram negative bacteremia in patients having hematologic malignancies. J Infect Dis 1985;15:99.
86. Eppes SC, Troutman JL, Gutman LT. Outcome of treatment of candidemia in children whose central catheters were removed or retained. Pediatr Infect Dis J 1989;8:99.
87. Dato VM, Dajani AS. Candidemia in children with central venous catheters: role of catheter removal and amphotericin B therapy. Pediatr Infect Dis J 1990;5:309.
88. Early TF, Gregory RT, Wheeler JR, Snyder SO, Gayle RG. Increased infection rate in double lumen versus single lumen Hickman catheters in cancer patients. South Med J 1990;83:34.
89. Pemberton LB, Lyman B, Lander V, et al. Sepsis from triple versus single lumen catheters during total parenteral nutrition in surgically or critically ill patients. Arch Surg 1986;121:591.
90. Pegues D, Axelrod P, et al. Comparison of infections in Hickman and implanted port catheters in adult solid tumor patients. J Surg Oncol 1992;49:156.
91. May GS, Davis D. Percutaneous catheters and totally implantable access systems: a review of reported infection rates. Journal of Intravenous Nursing 1988;11:97.
92. Greene FL, Moore W, Strickland G, McFarland J. Comparison of a totally implantable access device for chemotherapy (Port-A-Cath) and long-term percutaneous catheterization (Broviac). South Med J 1988;81:580.
93. Wurzel CL, Halom K, Feldman JG, Rubin LG. Infection rates of Broviac-Hickman catheters and implantable venous devices. Am J Dis Child 1988;142:536.
94. Ross MN, Haase GM, Poole MA, Burrington JD, Odom LF. Comparison of totally implanted reservoirs with external catheters as venous access devices in pediatric oncologic patients. Surg Gynecol Obstet 1988;167:141.
95. Mirro J, Rao BN, Stokes DC, et al. A prospective study of Hickman/Broviac catheters and implantable ports in pediatric oncology patients. J Clin Oncol 1989;7:214.
96. Caldwell JW, Melendez PR, Johnson RH. Experience in seventy-six patients comparing subcutaneous infusion ports and implanted right atrial catheters. Clin Res 1990;38:113A.
97. Groeger JS, Lucas AB, Brown AE. Venous access device infections in adult cancer patients: catheters versus ports. Program and abstracts of the 28th Interscience Conference on Antimicrobial Agents and Chemotherapy. Los Angeles: American Society for Microbiology, 1988.
98. Tschirhart JM, Rao MK. Mechanism and management of persistent withdrawal occlusion. Am Surg 1988;54:326.
99. Aitken DR, Minton JP. The "pinch-off sign": a warning of impending problems with permanent subclavian catheters. Am J Surg 1984;148:633.
100. Hinke DH, Zandt-Stastny DA, et al. Pinch-off syndrome: a complication of implantable subclavian venous access devices. Radiology 1990;177:353.
101. Kirvela O, Satokari K. In situ breakage of a totally implanted venous access system. J Parenter Enteral Nutr 1989;13:99.
102. Rubenstein RB, Alberty RE, Michaels LG, et al. Hickman catheter separation. J Parenter Enteral Nutr 1985;9:754.
103. Franey T, DeMarco LC, Geiss AC, Ward RJ. Catheter fracture and embolization in a totally implanted venous access catheter. J Parenter Enteral Nutr 1988;12:528.
104. Noyen J, Hoorntje J, et al. Spontaneous fracture of the catheter of a totally implantable venous access port: case report of a rare complication. J Clin Oncol 1987;5:1295.
105. Lafreniere R. Indwelling subclavian catheters and a visit with the "pinched-off sign". J Surg Oncol 1991;47:261.
106. Carr ME. Catheter embolization from implanted venous access devices: case reports. Angiology 1989;12:319.
107. Saifi J, McDowell RT, et al. In-situ breakage of

an implantable venous access system. Eur J Surg Oncol 1987;13:159.
108. Fisher RG, Ferreyro R. Evaluation of current techniques for nonsurgical removal of intravascular foreign bobies. Am J Radiol 1978; 130:541.
109. Edwards AC, Sowton E. Management of embolized central venous catheters. BMJ 1978;2: 669.
110. Huang TY, Abaskaron M. Non-surgical removal of intravascular fragmented catheters. Am Fam Physician 1984;30:177.
111. McDonnell PJ, Qualman SJ, Hutchins GM. Bilateral hydrothorax as a life-threatening complication of central venous hyperalimentation. Surg Gynecol Obstet 1984;158:577.
112. Iberti TJ, Katz LB, Reiner MA, Brownie T, Kwun KB. Hydrothorax as a late complication of central venous indwelling catheters. Surgery 1983;94:842.
113. Cathcart-Rake WF, Mowery WE. Intrapericardial infusion of 5-fluorouracil. Cancer 1991; 67:735.
114. Sato O, Tada Y, Sudo K, Ueno A, Nobori M, Idezuki Y. Arteriovenous fistula following central venous catheterization. Arch Surg 1986;121:729.

Management of Chemotherapy Extravasation

10

STEPHEN E. ETTINGHAUSEN

Although accounting for only 2% to 5% of all adverse drug reactions, the inadvertent infiltration of vesicant chemotherapeutic agents into extravascular tissues may result in major patient morbidity and significantly alter or interrupt an active treatment regimen in the cancer patient.[1] In several series the incidence of extravasation has ranged from 0.27% to 6% for doxorubicin, an anthracycline vesicant antibiotic on which the majority of clinical experience is based.[2-4]

In recent years, there has been a heightened awareness by physicians and nurses to the seriousness of such injuries and, hence, probably a decrease in their incidence and magnitude.[5] However, two major types of clinical situations and groups of risk factors have been identified that predispose to the development of such injuries. Their recognition can alert the clinician to take preventative measures and to make the appropriate protocol changes to lower the risk of extravasation. One group of risk factors relates to technical and methodological variables including failure to release a proximal tourniquet, use of metal butterfly needles, use of continuous infusion pumps, injection under pressure or under hurried circumstances, and use of an opaque dressing over the injection site.[6-12] Other risk factors for extravasation are related to anatomic factors. These include the presence of superior vena cava syndrome, lymphatic or venous obstruction from prior radiation or surgery, infusion through small fragile mobile veins, or through veins previously punctured and in spasm or with holes in proximity to the drug infusion site.[6-12]

Infiltration injuries generally occur in subcutaneous sites related to percutaneously placed intravenous needles or catheters.[12] The most common sites are the dorsum of the hand, the wrist, and the forearm and, when considered together, account for approximately 90% of extravasation injuries.[12] Other less frequent locations include the elbow, the foot, and the inguinal region.[12] Although the use of permanent central venous access ports and catheters has probably decreased the incidence of drug extravasations, the mechanisms of such injuries are unique to these devices. They include: displacement of the Huber needle from the silicon diaphragm of subcutaneous ports; lacerations or tears in the Silastic catheter in the subcutaneous tunnel; retrograde tracking of the vesicant along the catheter outside of the central vein due to thrombosis; and separation of the port from the catheter with infusion into the subcutaneous pocket.[13-16]

Extravasation injuries can be classified by the pathophysiology of the damage in which the offending agent binds or does not bind nucleic acids (Table 10-1).[12] Extravascular infiltration of agents that bind nucleic acids produces the most severe and debilitat-

Table 10-1. Chemotherapeutic Agents Producing Significant Extravasation Injury

DRUGS THAT BIND NUCLEIC ACIDS
Anthracyclines (doxorubicin, daunorubicin, epirubicin)
Mitomycin-C
Mithramycin

DRUGS THAT DO NOT BIND NUCLEIC ACIDS
Vinca Alkaloids (vincristine, vinblastine, vindesine)
Alkylating Agents (mechlorethamine or nitrogen mustard)

Data from Rudolph R, Larson DL. Etiology and treatment of chemotherapeutic agent extravasation injuries: a review. J Clin Oncol 1987;5:1116.

ing injuries because tissue damage results not only from initial drug contact but also from continuous exposure as the drug binds to tissue DNA.[12] The most carefully characterized extravasation injury caused by these agents is that resulting from doxorubicin (Adriamycin), although similar types of injury may be inflicted by the infiltration of other anthracycline antibiotics (*e.g.*, daunorubicin, epirubicin) as well as by mitomycin-C and actinomycin-D.[1,5,12]

The mechanism of doxorubicin tissue injury is probably inhibition of DNA replication and transcription.[1,2,9] Another cause of tissue damage may be cell membrane injury mediated by the action of free radicals.[17,18]

CLINICAL CHARACTERISTICS OF EXTRAVASATION OF NUCLEIC ACID-BINDING AGENTS

Extravasation of a vesicant drug such as doxorubicin may initially be suspected by local burning and pain during the infusion.[7,12] However, the absence of symptoms does not rule out drug infiltration.[12] The pain may become severe and may vary in duration from minutes to hours, although, uncommonly, it may last several days.[12] Erythema may be visualized early after the extravasation or may be discerned several weeks after the inciting event.[7,12] Redness on the overlying skin may blanch with pressure—suggesting an inflammatory response or infectious process.[12] However, cellulitis and cutaneous abscesses usually are not associated with the extravasation injury.[10,12] In fact, histologic studies of doxorubicin extravasation in both animal models and patients do not demonstrate any significant inflammatory cell infiltrates in the early stage of injury.[10,12,19] In some cases, the erythema results from tissue deposition of red doxorubicin crystals and consequently does not blanch with pressure.[9] Further evidence for this observation is provided by the finding of red fluorescence of the affected tissues when viewed under ultraviolet light.[20-22]

The redness of doxorubicin extravasation must be differentiated from an "Adriamycin flare," which may develop along the course of the infused vein.[23] In contrast to extravasation, the flair is painless and commonly resolves within 2 hours following infusion.[12] This phenomenon may represent a local allergic response and occurs in approximately 3% of patients receiving doxorubicin.[23,24] If the drug extravasation is minor, then no significant further tissue damage occurs and the healing process results in a residual area of induration with minimal or no alteration in function.[7]

More serious infiltration of extravascular tissues causes more progressive injury with localized edema and induration followed by blistering and superficial loss of skin.[12] The exact cause of skin necrosis induced by doxorubicin is unclear. However, experimental data suggest that the injury is drug-concentration dependent and requires the injection of doxorubicin at a dose of at least 0.01 to .02 mg/mL subdermally in a rat model and of 0.5 mg/mL subcutaneously in mice.[25,26] By 2 to 4 weeks postinjury, a small necrotic ulcer may form in the center of the infiltrated tissues (Fig. 10-1).[5,22] The ulcer is usually painful and has an irregular shaggy center. Following a major extravasation, the ulcer may be significantly larger and the time course for its development may be markedly shortened.[12] At its outset, the ulcer may

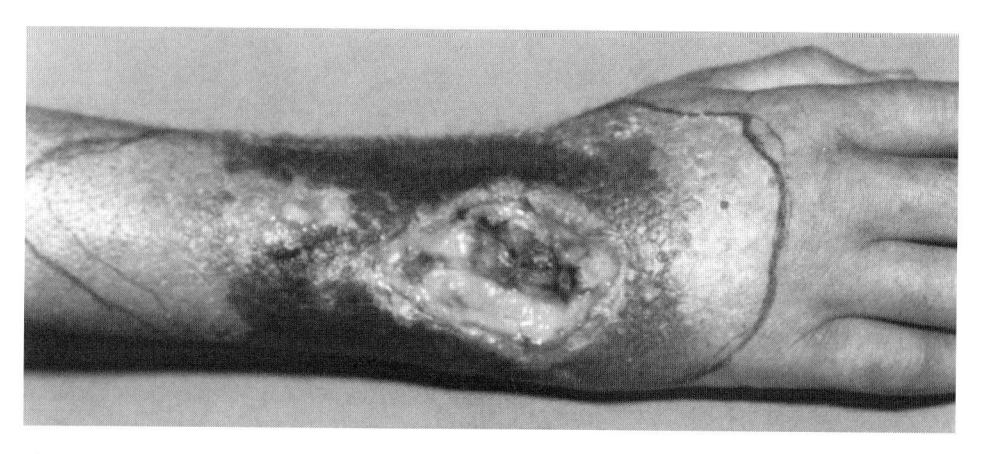

Figure 10-1. Severe doxorubicin extravasation occurring on the dorsum of the right wrist and hand. The injury shows a typical ulcer with overlying necrotic debris, surrounded by erythematous edematous skin and subcutaneous tissues. The wound required operative debridement including several extensor tendons (to the limits of the dark lines) and was closed with a split-thickness skin graft. (Photograph courtesy of David L. Larson, MD, Medical College of Wisconsin, Milwaukee, WI; with permission.)

appear rather benign, falsely lulling the physician into passive observation.[6,12,27] However, if operative intervention is not undertaken, then the tissue necrosis continues unabatedly and an eschar develops over the ulcer which will enlarge both in diameter and depth.[12] Necrosis of the extensor or flexor tendons may result from vesicant extravasation on the hand or distal forearm.[8,12,27] Unless patients are severely immunocompromised, tissue destruction caused by doxorubicin usually does not manifest any systemic signs.[10] Untreated, the damaged area may eventually display some minor degree of healing, although the ultimate outcome is chronic morbidity with continued pain, neuropathy, and decreased joint mobility due to scarring of associated tendons and muscles.[12] Very small ulcers without associated pain may be indicative of less significant extravasation and may heal on their own.[12]

Similar to the injury produced by radiation, the ulcers of doxorubicin extravasation rarely display significant spontaneous healing.[12,22] Experimental studies have shown that, possibly owing to persistent doxorubicin binding to cellular DNA, the drug interferes with fibroblast replication and organization necessary for spontaneous wound healing.[8,28] Moreover, contraction in these wounds is slower than the same process in normal healing.[25] Lastly, doxorubicin has been found to persist in extravasation wounds for up to 5 months.[29] As a result, insidiously progressive tissue loss may continue if not treated appropriately with maximal damage observed as late as 5 months after injury.[7] Although only speculative, the drug may be continually recycled in the bed of the ulcer with release from injured and dying cells and uptaken by contiguous viable tissues.[12] The effects of extravasation on wound healing are further discussed in Chapter 14.

Previously irradiated skin and subcutaneous tissues may break down and ulcerate following systemic administration of doxorubicin in a "radiation recall" phenomenon.[30-32] However, this effect is observed only rarely, and as such prior radiation therapy does not preclude the use of doxorubicin when it is otherwise indicated.[12] Moreover, repeat cycles of doxorubicin are not contraindicated if an extravasation injury has previously occurred as long as significant wound healing has taken place.[5,12]

SUMMARY: CLINICAL CHARACTERISTICS OF EXTRAVASATION

1. Suspect extravasation with burning and pain in the area of the infusion. Erythema can occur early or late and is unreliable. A flare along the course of the vein is not uncommon and must be differentiated from extravasation injuries.
2. A minor extravasation usually resolves with minimal or no alteration of function. More serious infiltrations lead to progressive injury with edema, blistering, and superficial skin loss.
3. By 2 to 4 weeks postinjury a small necrotic ulcer may form. This ulcer can appear fairly benign at first, but without operative intervention will progress.

TREATMENT: INITIAL NONOPERATIVE CARE

The first line of treatment for doxorubicin extravasation is the maintenance of a heightened awareness of the magnitude of an injury and of the earliest signs of infiltration as have been described above. When leakage of drug is suspected, the infusion should be immediately discontinued and the intravenous line aspirated. The subsequent treatment recommendations are based on the experience of Larson[5] who compiled the largest series in the world's literature of chemotherapy extravasation injuries in 175 cancer patients. Perhaps surprisingly, many protocols active in hospitals and clinics today for the treatment of vesicant extravasation and advanced by nursing specialists are based on information supplied by the drug manufacturers using *in vitro* or animal data and not large clinical experiences (Larson DL, personal communication).[33]

As suggested by Larson, the site of infiltration should be immediately elevated for 48 hours and ice applied directly to the affected area for 15-minute intervals four times a day.[5,12,34] The use of cold has been supported in experimental studies.[35] Following the intradermal injection of doxorubicin in a murine model, local cooling to 17°C for up to 60 minutes significantly reduced the extent of ulceration.[35] Similarly *in vitro* studies with human tumor cells demonstrated a reduced cytotoxic effect for doxorubicin at lower temperatures.[35]

Some authors have recommended local application of heat for these injuries.[1] Although local heat might facilitate absorption of extravascular drug and reduce local toxicity, high temperatures might also dangerously raise metabolic demands of already damaged tissues.[12] In fact, experimental studies of doxorubicin in mice have demonstrated that topical heating exacerbates the cutaneous damage produced by intradermal injection of the drug.[35] Furthermore, those animals receiving local heat suffered a significantly higher mortality rate than those which did not.[35]

A large number of topically applied or locally injected doxorubicin antidotes have been tested with variable success. Many reports are based solely on animal studies or small anecdotal clinical experiences and, consequently, the overall efficacy of these drugs has not been definitively established.[12] Based on his large clinical series, Larson has strongly recommended against the use of any of the various drug antidotes citing absence of proved efficacy in patients and a potential for exacerbation of the injury.[5,12] However, two agents, dimethyl sulfoxide (DMSO) and corticosteroids are worth describing separately.

Although studies with topical DMSO in animal models have produced conflicting results, clinical investigation in patients has suggested a beneficial effect in reducing injury.[4,17,20,36–40] In one series of 20 patients with doxorubicin or daunorubicin infiltration, topical 99% DMSO was administered every 6 hours for 14 days.[4] No patient developed ulceration or required operative treatment and minimal toxicity was associated with DMSO. Other authors have reported smaller numbers of patients with whom topical DMSO has significantly reduced the otherwise expected injury.[39,40]

As previously noted, corticosteroids have been used at the site of injury to reduce the presumed associated inflammation.[7,33,41] However, histologic studies have failed to demonstrate significant inflammatory infiltrates.[10,19] Moreover, in animal models, studies have not shown any significant therapeutic efficacy.[20,26,42–44] The local use of steroids may also produce a major risk for life-threatening infections originating at the site of ulceration and skin barrier breakdown, because these patients are immunocompromised by their cancer and cytotoxic chemotherapy.[5]

Although not evaluated in patients, another group of agents, the oxomorpholinyl radical dimers, have shown a protective effect in a swine model following intradermal injection of anthracyclines and mitomycin-C.[45]

A large number of other agents have been evaluated but have not shown efficacy or have actually worsened the local effects of doxorubicin. These substances include sodium bicarbonate, sodium thiosulfate, heparin, calcium gluconate, α-tocopherol, magnesium sulfate, lidocaine, cimetidine, diphenhydramine, propanolol, N-acetylcysteine, hyaluronidase, isoproterenol, glutathione, L-carnitine, coenzyme-Q_{10}, phentolamine, bupivicaine, cysteine, WR-2721, vitamin E, benzoic acid, and hyperbaric oxygen.[7,8,10,12,17,18,20,26,37,38,42–44,46–48]

SUMMARY: INITIAL NONOPERATIVE CARE

1. Stop infusion and aspirate intravenous line.
2. Elevate extremity and apply ice (cold compresses) for 15-minute intervals four times a day for 48 hours.
3. Do not use topical or locally injected antidotes (including corticosteroids).
4. Topical DMSO.
5. Careful observation and subsequent care (see below).

Modified from Larson DL: What is the appropriate management of tissue extravasation by antitumor agents? Plast Reconstr Surg 1985;75:397–402.

TREATMENT: OPERATIVE AND SUBSEQUENT CARE

An aggressive treatment plan has been recommended by some authors with approaches of early excision and debridement of tissues involved in all significant extravasations.[2,10,49] However, a more conservative management algorithm has shown that some lesser injuries including small painless ulcers do heal spontaneously, sparing surgery for those patients.[5,12,34] Moreover, early wound excision may not adequately allow determination of the exact area of the tissue at risk.[5,12] In his series of 175 patients, Larson did not perform any early excisions and only 34 patients subsequently required operative debridement.[5] The author found that more extensive infiltration was more likely to require surgery, which usually was performed 2 to 3 weeks after injury.[50] The indications for wound excision included painful ulceration or major blister formation or continued erythema, swelling, and pain even in the absence of ulceration.[5,12,34]

The excision should include debridement not only of the ulcer bed and any necrotic material but also of all adjacent, swollen, reddened tissues (Fig. 10-2)[5,6,8,12,27,34] These latter areas often are infiltrated with residual drugs and are the source of the patient's pain.[12] Tissues containing doxorubicin may be better delineated with the use of an ultraviolet light.[21] Under such conditions, these areas appear to have a violet glow, which is produced

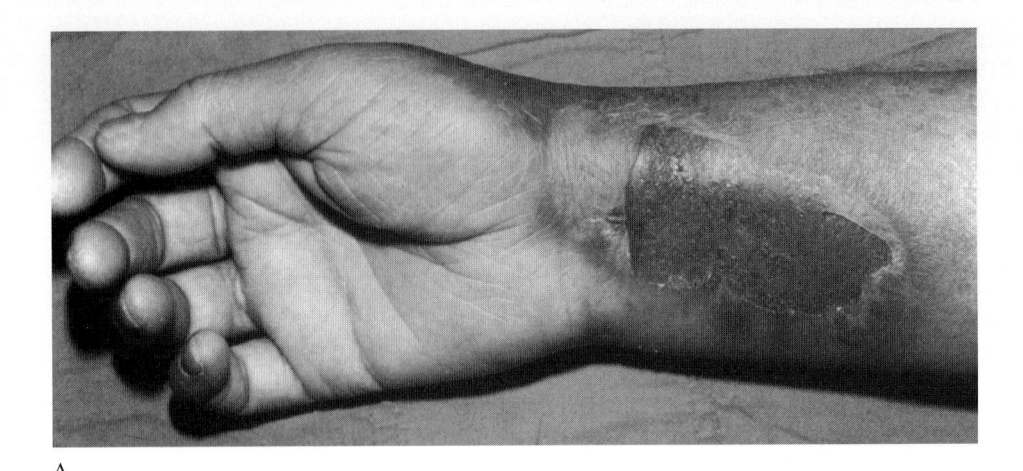

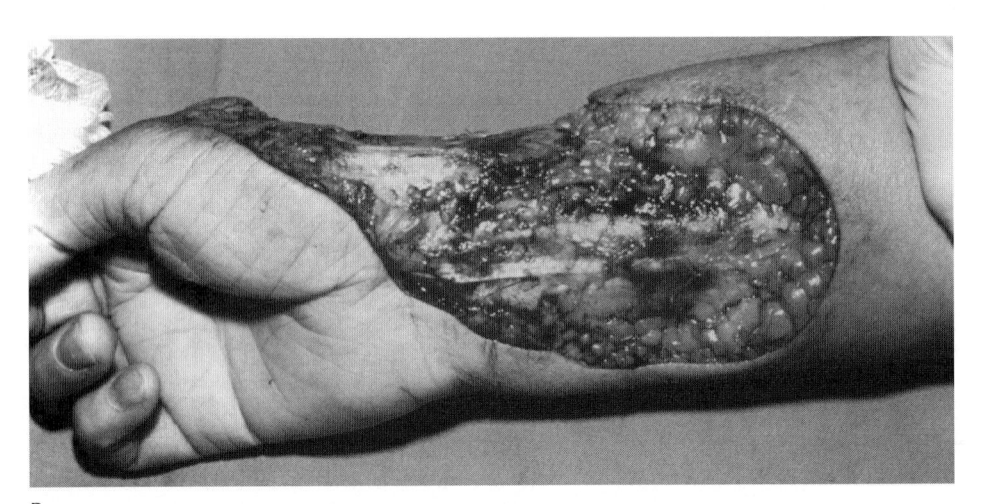

Figure 10-2. Definitive treatment of 7-day-old doxorubicin infiltration injury on the volar aspect of the right wrist extending onto the dorsum of the hand. **A.** A large central area of skin loss with surrounding infiltrated tissues. **B.** All abnormal tissues were excised leaving viable tendons at the depth of the wound. **C** and **D.** Delayed coverage of the exposed tissues was successfully achieved with a split-thickness skin graft. (Photographs courtesy of David L. Larson, MD, Medical College of Wisconsin, Milwaukee, WI; with permission.)

by the characteristic red-orange fluorescence of doxorubicin and the purple color of the ultraviolet light.[21] Another method used to identify doxorubicin-infiltrated tissues is the demonstration of autofluorescence by microscopic examination of frozen sections.[8,50] Several authors have used intravenous fluorescein (10 mg/kg) and ultraviolet light to aid in the intraoperative differentiation between viable and nonviable tissues.[20,21]

The operative management of injuries on the dorsum of the hand or distal forearm may be particularly problematic because of associated tendon involvement.[5,8,12,27] When tendons are exposed after debridement of nonviable paratenon, a difference of opinion exists as to whether the tendon should be left intact or be excised because a suboptimal function outcome is usually the result with either approach.[12] Larson believes that the

Management of Chemotherapy Extravasation

C

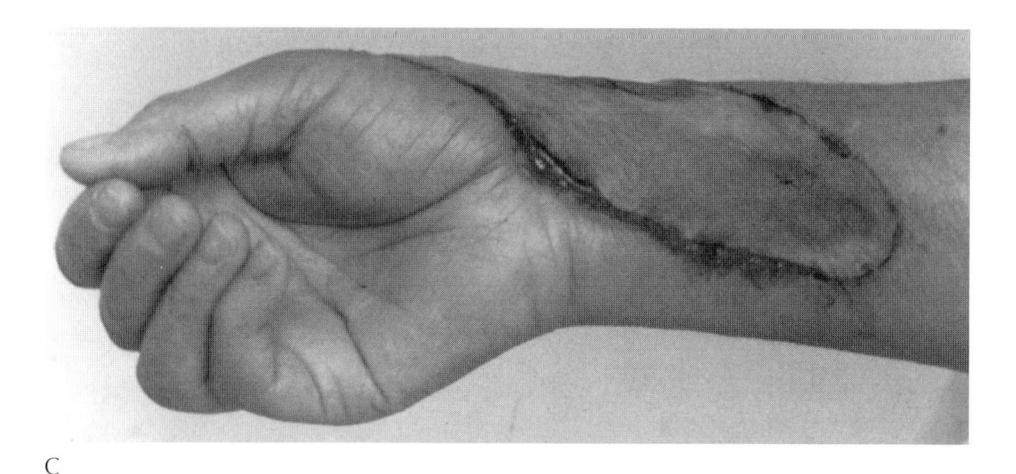

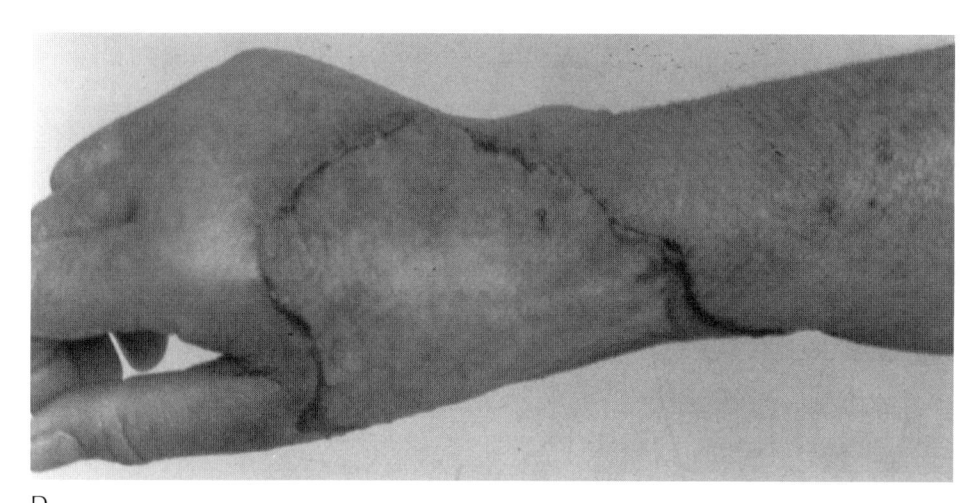

D
Figure 10-2. (*continued*)

morbidity and disadvantage of the functional debit caused by debridement of these tendons is outweighed by the benefit of an assured closure of a potentially life-threatening wound in the cancer patient.[5,12]

Following debridement, most wounds should be treated with frequent dressing changes until a satisfactory granulation base is observed.[5,12] Several authors have recommended the use of half-strength sodium hypochlorite (Dakin's solution) as it may aid in the debridement of the necrotic material and inactivate any residual doxorubicin in the wound.[2,10,11,22,46]

Delayed application of a split thickness skin graft usually 2 or 3 days later, provides the simplest approach to wound coverage (Fig. 10-2, **C** and **D**).[5,8,10,12,27,34,49] The autologous skin may be harvested at the time of the operative debridement and stored appropriately until use.[5,34] Significant graft loss may result not only from infection or shear forces but also any residual doxorubicin in the wound bed.[8,10,12,51] Xenografts of porcine origin or human allografts may be used for temporary wound coverage and for determination of the appropriate timing for placement of the autograft.[5,34] Alternatively, quantitative wound biopsies may also help in judging the optimal time for graft application.[10] Chemotherapy may be restarted usually by 1 week later and when the wound is covered and take is assured.[5]

Another approach for wound closure is the use of flap reconstruction.[2,6,10,51] However, the complexity of flaps including the associated risk of the procedures must be weighed against the clinical context of the cancer patient who may require additional chemotherapy as soon as the wound is healed.[12] Free flaps with microvascular anastomoses or myocutaneous or fasciocutaneous flaps provide the best wound coverage and are probably resistant to the deleterious effect of residual doxorubicin in the wound.[8,11,12,51] Random abdominal pedicle flaps also have been used for wound coverage.[2,8,10] However, this approach has the disadvantage of several delay procedures needed before complete transfer of the flap to the recipient site is achieved.[12]

Lastly, physical therapy plays a major role in rehabilitation of extremity extravasation injury, particularly when wounds lie adjacent to or over joints.[12] Physical therapy should be initiated after the initial 2 days of conservative therapy following the primary injury and with more severe injuries, after wound closure is achieved.[12]

SUMMARY: OPERATIVE AND SUBSEQUENT CARE

A. Resolving or absent local pain, swelling, or skin breakdown; small *painless* ulcer
  1. Resumption of normal activity
  2. Physical therapy
B. Persistent pain, swelling, and erythema; large or painful ulcer
  1. Surgical excision (debridement of all abnormal tissue)
    • Harvest split thickness skin graft (STSG) during same procedure and store appropriately until use
  2. Temporary dressings until wound ready for permanent coverage
    • Gauze with saline of one half strength Dakin's (sodium hypochlorite) solution
    • Gauze with saline of one half strength Dakin's (sodium hypochlorite) solution
    • Xenograft (porcine)
    • Human allograft
  3. Permanent wound coverage
    • STSG
    • Flap (random pedicle, myocutaneous, fasciocutaneous, free)
  4. Physical therapy

Modified from Rudolph R, Larson DL: Etiology and treatment of chemotherapeutic agent extravasation injuries: a review. J Clin Oncol 1987;5:1116 and Larson DL: What is the appropriate management of tissue extravasation by antitumor agents? Plast Reconstr Surg 1985;75:397.

EXTRAVASATION INJURIES CAUSED BY AGENTS THAT DO NOT BIND TO NUCLEIC ACIDS

Extravasation injuries caused by chemotherapeutic drugs that do not bind to nucleic acids produce less severe damage than those that do.[12] A nonbinding vesicant agent instantly destroys infiltrated tissues but is rapidly metabolized to a nontoxic form.[12,22] Normal repair mechanisms can then mediate healing of the injured tissue.[22] Chemotherapeutic drugs that cause such types of injuries are the vinca alkaloids (*e.g.*, vincristine, vinblastine, and vindesine) and certain alkylating agents (*e.g.*, mechlorethamine or nitrogen mustard).[12,22] Following the extravasation of one of the vinca alkaloids, injury evolves over the next 3 to 4 weeks.[1] Treatment recommendations have included local application of heat and infiltration of the site with hyaluronidase, or injection of saline and steroids at the injury site followed by icepacks.[1,12]

Extravasation of mechlorethamine causes pain and erythema within hours at the site of injection.[1] Ignoffo and Friedman[1] have suggested that the mainstay of therapy is local dilution with alkaline agents or sodium thiosulfate. In contrast, Larson and colleagues[5,12] have successfully treated such injuries from vinca alkaloids and nitrogen mustard with the same regimen used to treat anthracycline injuries–ice and elevation without the use of local drug antidotes.

PREVENTION

Perhaps the best treatment for extravasation injuries is prevention. Most centers have instituted strict guidelines for clinicians to use during infusion of vesicants. Clearly, active knowledge of the anatomic and methodological risk factors for drug extravasation as enumerated above allow treating personnel to avoid or mitigate such high-risk situations. As a result, vesicants are best given through flexible plastic cannulas well anchored into large veins.[12] Optimally, the drug is given through a freely flowing intravenous line over 2 to 5 minutes to minimize the time during which catheter dislodgement might occur.[6,7] The vesicant infusion should be followed by adequate saline flushing to clear the intravenous line, the cannula, and the vein of the noxious agent.[52]

Another strategy to minimize the morbidity of a potential extravasation, is selecting an infusion site away from the dorsum of the hand, distal forearm, or elbow.[2,7,12] Even a moderate infiltration injury at these locations could translate into significant disability because of the relative lack of muscle protecting underlying tendons, ligaments, joint capsule, or neurovascular structures.[6,12,22] Using veins over the proximal forearm is a safer approach as leakage there would more likely involve skin, subcutaneous fat, and muscle and would cause a comparatively less debilitating injury.[6,12,22]

In the last decade, there has been a great expansion in and enthusiasm for the use of permanent central venous catheters.[14–16] Although there are no prospective studies that directly compare the incidence of extravasation with central venous catheters and ports versus simple peripheral venous lines, the former have decreased the incidence of infiltration injuries.

SUMMARY: PREVENTION

1. Follow institutional guidelines.
2. Use flexible, well-anchored plastic catheters inserted carefully into large veins. Avoid veins away from the dorsum of the hand, distal forearm, or elbow.
3. Administer through a freely flowing intravenous line over 2 to 5 minutes.
4. Flush the line adequately when the infusion is completed.

SUMMARY

Extravasation of vesicant agents occurs rarely but may cause significant morbidity and force major delays in subsequent chemotherapy treatments.[12] Although prevention is the optimal clinical approach to this problem, the first line of therapy is a high degree of suspicion by medical personnel administering these drugs.[12,52] When extravasation occurs or is suspected, the infusion should be stopped immediately. The extremity should be elevated and cold packs applied to the site.[5,12,34] If larger or painful ulcerations or persistent pain, swelling, or redness are noted, the entire site should be debrided.[5,12,34] Delayed coverage of the wound is later performed, optimally using a split thickness skin graft which provides the best and simplest form of wound closure.[5,12,34] Lastly, intensive physical therapy for injuries involving the extremities plays a major role in the reestablishment of satisfactory joint and tendon function and consequently in reduction of long-term morbidity.[12] An algorithm for the treatment of these injuries is shown in Figure 10-3.

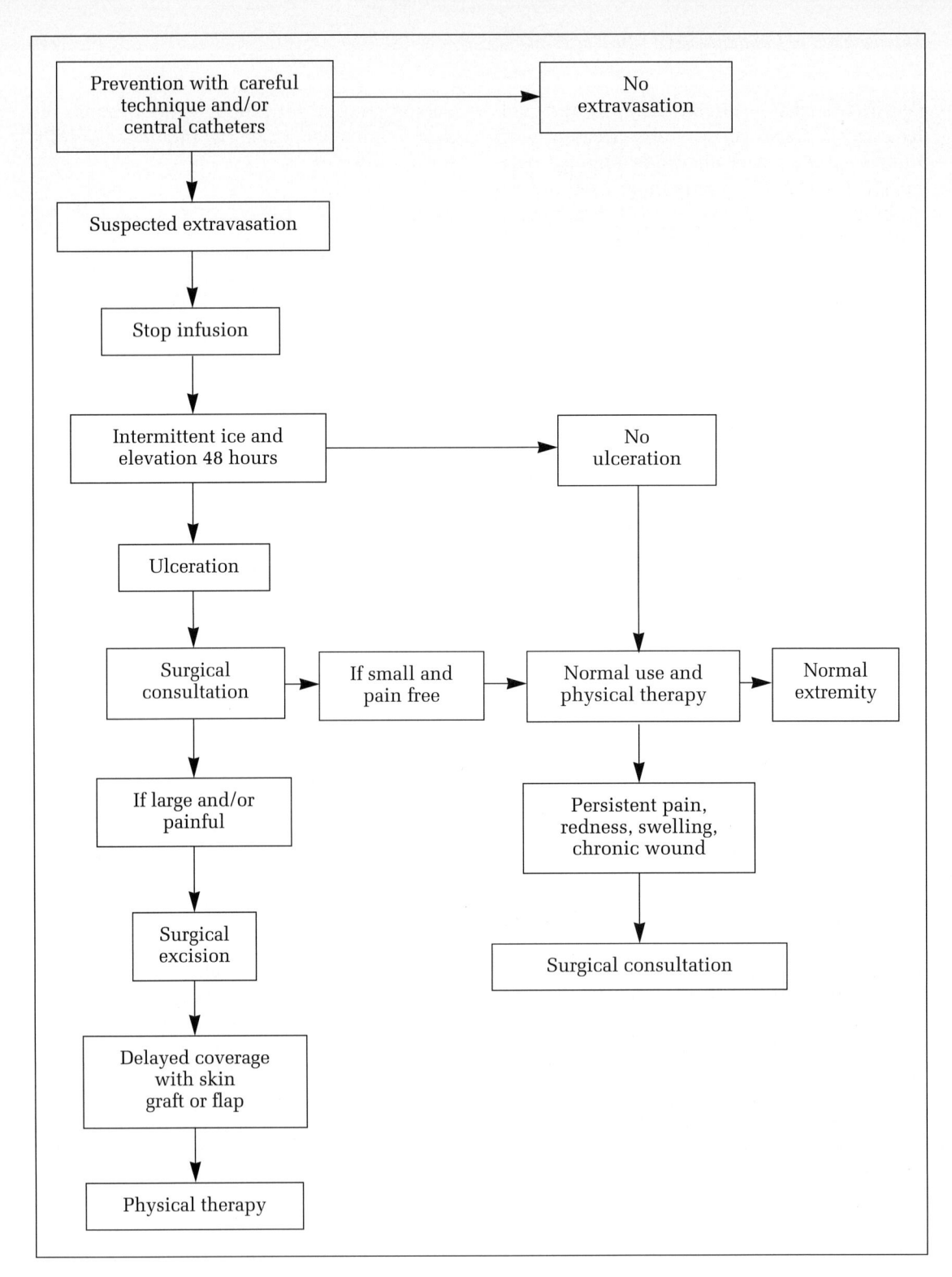

Figure 10-3. An algorithm for the treatment of extravasation injuries. (Adapted from Rudolph B, Larson DL. Etiology and treatment of chemotherapeutic agent extravasation injuries: a review. J Clin Oncol 1987;5:1116, by Schäffer M and Barbul A.)

REFERENCES

1. Ignoffo RJ, Friedman MA. Therapy of local toxicities caused by extravasation of cancer chemotherapeutic drugs. Cancer Treatment Reports 1980;7:17.
2. Laughlin RA, Landeen JM, Habal MB. The management of inadvertent subcutaneous Adriamycin infiltration. Am J Surg 1979;137:408.
3. Pitkanen J, Asko-Seljavaara S, Grohn P, et al. Adriamycin extravasation: surgical treatment and possible prevention of skin and soft-tissue injuries. J Surg Onc 1983;23:259.
4. Oliver IN, Aisner J, Hament A, et al. A prospective study of topical dimethyl sulfoxide for treating anthracycline extravasation 1988;6:1732.
5. Larson DL. What is the appropriate management of tissue extravasation by antitumor agents? Plast Reconstr Surg 1985;75:397.
6. Rudolph R, Stein RS, Pattillo RA. Skin ulcers due to Adriamycin. Cancer 1976;38:1087.
7. Reilly JJ, Neifeld JP, Rosenberg SA. Clinical course and management of accidental Adriamycin extravasation. Cancer 1977;40:2053.
8. Bowers DG, Lynch JB. Adriamycin extravasation. Plast Reconstr Surg 1978;61:86.
9. Upton J, Mulliken JB, Murray JE. Major intravenous extravasation injuries. Am J Surg 1979;137:497.
10. Linder RM, Upton J, Steen R. Management of extensive doxorubicin hydrochloride extravasation injuries. J Hand Surg 1983;8:32.
11. Snyderman RK, Krasna MJ. Adriamycin extravasation injuries. Plast Reconstr Surg 1986;77:683.
12. Rudolph B, Larson DL. Etiology and treatment of chemotherapeutic agent extravasation injuries: a review. J Clin Oncol 1987;5:1116.
13. Lokich JB, Moore C. Drug extravasation in cancer chemotherapy. Ann Intern Med 1986;104:124.
14. Lokich JJ, Bothe A, Benotti P, Moore C. Complications and management of implanted venous access catheters. J Clin Oncol 1985;3:710.
15. Watterson J, Heisel M, Cich JA, Priest JR. Intrathoracic extravasation of sclerosing agents associated with central venous catheters. Am J Pediatr Hematol Oncol 1988;10:249.
16. Brothers TE, Von Moll LK, Niederhuber JE, et al. Experience with subcutaneous infusion ports in three hundred patients. Surg Gynecol Obstetr 1988;166:295.
17. Svingen BA, Powis G, Appel PL, Scott M. Protection against Adriamycin-induced skin necrosis in the rat by dimethyl sulfoxide and α-tocopherol. Cancer Res 1981;41:3395.
18. Upton PG, Yamaguchi KT, Myers S, et al. Effects of antioxidants and hyperbaric oxygen in ameliorating experimental doxorubicin skin toxicity in the rat. Cancer Treatment Reports 1986;70:503.
19. Luedke DW, Kennedy PS, Rietschel RL. Histopathogenesis of skin and subcutaneous injury induced by Adriamycin. Plast Reconstr Surg 1979:63:463.
20. Petro JA, Graham WP III, Miller SH, et al. Experimental and clinical studies of ulcers induced with Adriamycin. Surgical Forum 1979;30:535.
21. Cohen FJ, Manganaro J, Bezozo RC. Identification of involved tissue during surgical treatment of doxorubicin-induced extravasation necrosis. J Hand Surg 1983;8:43.
22. Rudolph R. Toxic drug ulcers. In Rudolph R, Noe JM (eds). Chronic wound problems. Boston, Little Brown, 1983:95.
23. Ostrowski MJ. An unusual allergic reaction in a vein following intravenous Adriamycin. Clin Oncol 1976;2:179.
24. Vogelzang NJ. "Adriamycin flare": a skin reaction resembling extravasation. Cancer Treatment Reports 1979;63:2067.
25. Rudolph R, Suzuki M, Luce JK. Experimental skin necrosis produced by Adriamycin. Cancer Treatment Reports 1979;63:529.
26. Cohen MH. Amelioration of Adriamycin skin necrosis: an experimental study. Cancer Treatment Reports 1979;53:1003.
27. Rudolph R. Ulcers of the hand and wrist caused by doxorubicin hydrochloride. Orthopedic Review 1978;7:83.
28. Rudolph R, Woodward M, Hurn I. Ultrastructure of doxorubicin (Adriamycin)-induced skin ulcers in rats. Cancer Res 1979;39:463.
29. Garnick M, Isreal M, Khetarpal V, et al. Persistence of anthracycline levels following dermal and subcutaneous Adriamycin extravasation. Proceedings of the American Association for Cancer Research 1981;22:173.
30. Donaldson SS, Glick JM, Wilbur JR. Adriamycin activating a recall phenomenon after radiation therapy. Ann Intern Med 1974;81:407.
31. Cohen SC, Dibella NJ, Michalak JC. Recall injury from Adriamycin. Ann Intern Med 1975;83:232.
32. Cassady JR, Richter MP, Piro AJ, Jaffe N. Radiation-Adriamycin interactions: preliminary clinical observations. Cancer 1975;36:946.
33. Birdall C, Naliboff AR. How do you manage chemotherapy extravasation? Am J Nurs 1988;88:228.
34. Larson DL. Treatment of tissue extravasation by antitumor agents. Cancer 1982;49:1796.
35. Dorr RT, Alberts DS, Stone A. Cold protection

and heat enhancement of doxorubicin skin toxicity in the mouse. Cancer Treatment Reports 1985;69:431.
36. Desai MH, Teres D. Prevention of doxorubicin-induced skin ulcers in the rat and pig with dimethyl sulfoxide (DMSO) Cancer Treatment Reports 1982;66:1371.
37. Dorr RT, Alberts DS. Failure of DMSO and vitamin E to prevent doxorubicin skin ulceration in the mouse. Cancer Treatment Reports 1983;67:499.
38. Okano T, Ohnuma T, Efremidis A, Holland JF. Doxorubicin-induced skin ulcer in the piglet. Cancer Treatment Reports 1983;67:1075.
39. Oliver IN, Schwarz MA. Use of dimethyl sulfoxide in limiting tissue damage caused by extravasation of doxorubicin. Cancer Treatment Reports 1983;67:407.
40. Lawrence HJ, Walsh D, Zapotowski KA, et al. Topical dimethylsulfoxide may prevent tissue damage from anthracycline extravasation. Cancer Chemother Pharmacol 1989;23:316.
41. Zweig JI, Kabakow B. An apparently effective countermeasure of doxorubicin extravasation. JAMA 1978;239:2116.
42. Dorr RT, Alberts DS, Chen HSG. The limited role of corticosteroids in ameliorating experimental doxorubicin skin toxicity in the mouse. Cancer Chemother Pharmacol 1980;5:17.
43. Coleman JJ, Walker AP, Didolkar MS. Treatment of Adriamycin-induced skin ulcers: a prospective controlled study. J Surg Oncol 1983;22:129.
44. Loth TS, Eversmann WW. Treatment methods for extravasation of chemotherapeutic agents: a comparative study. J Hand Surg 1986;11A:388.
45. Averbuch SD, Boldt M, Gaudiano G, et al. Experimental chemotherapy-induced skin necrosis in swine: mechanistic studies of anthracycline antibiotic toxicity and protection with a radical dimer compound. J Clin Invest 1988;81:142.
46. Zweig JI, Kabakow B, Wallach RC, et al. Rational effective medical treatment of skin ulcers due to Adriamycin. Cancer Treatment Reports 1979;63:2101.
47. Bartkowski-Dodds L, Daniels JR. Use of sodium bicarbonate as a means of ameliorating doxorobucin-induced dermal necrosis in rats. Cancer Chemother Pharmacol 1980;4:179.
48. Dorr RT, Alberts DS. Pharmacologic antidotes to experimental doxorubicin skin toxicity: a suggested role for beta-adrenergic compounds. Cancer Treatment Reports 1981;65:1001.
49. Argenta LC, Manders EK. Mitomycin C extravasation injuries. Cancer 1983;51:1080.
50. Bleicher JN, Haynes W, Massop DW, Daneff RM. The delineation of Adriamycin extravasation using fluorescence microscopy. Plast Reconst Surg 1984;74:114.
51. Hodgkinson DJ. Doxorubicin extravasation injuries. J Hand Surg 1983;8:498.
52. Banerjee A, Brotherston TM, Lamberty BGH, Campbell RC. Cancer chemotherapy agent-induced perivenous extravasation injuries. Postgrad Med J 1987;63:5.

11

Vascular Problems in the Cancer Patient

MICHAEL P. LILLY

Although tumors arising from blood vessels are exceedingly uncommon, serious problems affecting the major arteries and veins frequently complicate the treatment of the patient with cancer. These problems can affect large, medium, and small arteries and veins and be a source of significant morbidity and mortality. The best known association is that of venous thrombosis and malignant tumors which was characterized by Trousseau in 1865.[1] Idiopathic thrombosis of arteries and veins remains an important presentation for patients with occult malignancy. Over recent years, our understanding of tumor cell biology, the complexity of blood coagulation and thrombolysis, and the pathophysiology of atherosclerosis has advanced dramatically and provided new insight into the association of malignant disease and vascular problems. The increasing age of the population of the United States and the success of programs designed to improve the early detection of cancer have resulted in the identification of an increasingly large population of patients with malignant tumors and concomitant peripheral vascular disease. This chapter reviews the current understanding of the effects of tumors on the coagulation system and the circulation, the effects of cancer treatment on blood vessels, and the diagnosis and treatment of specific vascular problems in cancer patients.

PATHOPHYSIOLOGY

Primary Vascular Tumors

PRIMARY TUMORS OF SMALL VESSELS

Primary tumors of blood vessels are rare and most frequently involve small caliber vessels: arterioles, capillaries, and venules. Table 11-1 lists the principal vascular tumors as classified by Enzinger and Weiss.[2] Most blood vessel neoplasms are benign and many are hamartomas that present in childhood and regress spontaneously. Because these tumors involve small blood vessels, necessary excision infrequently compromises perfusion to major organ systems and vascular reconstruction is rarely necessary. Many such tumors are congenital and arise in the skin or the subcutaneous tissues and are treated by plastic and reconstructive surgeons. Several comprehensive works are available on the treatment of such conditions (e.g. reference 3). Malignant tumors such as hemangiosarcoma or hemangiopericytoma commonly arise in the skin or solid organs and require *en bloc* resection by methods common to the treatment of other tumors of the organs involved. Kaposi's sarcoma, which arises most likely

Acknowledgment: This work was supported in part by National Institute of Diabetes and Digetive and Kidney Diseases Grant DK 02181 (Clinical Investigator Award, M.P. Lilly).

Table 11-1. Classification of Vascular Tumors

BENIGN VASCULAR TUMORS
  Localized hemangioma
    • Capillary hemangioma
    • Cavernous hemangioma
    • Venous hemangioma
    • Arteriovenous hemangioma
    • Epithelioid hemangioma
    • Hemangioma of granulation tissue type
    • Miscellaneous hemangiomas of deep soft tissues
  Angiomatosis
  Glomus tumor
  Vascular ectasia

VASCULAR TUMORS OF INTERMEDIATE MALIGNANCY
  Epithelioid hemangioendothelioma
  Spindle cell hemangioendothelioma
  Malignant endovascular papillary angioendothelioma

MALIGNANT VASCULAR TUMORS
  Angiosarcoma, lymphangiosarcoma
  Kaposi's sarcoma

Adapted with permission from Enzinger FM, Weiss SW. Soft tissue tumors. 2nd ed. St Louis, CV Mosby, 1988:489.[2]

from endothelial cells, has achieved increased attention in recent years owing to its association with HIV infection. This tumor is rarely curable and is associated with second primary malignancies, such as lymphoma, leukemia, or myeloma, in one third of cases.[4]

PRIMARY TUMORS OF LARGE VESSELS

Malignant tumors of the great vessels are exceedingly rare. Less than 200 cases of primary malignant tumors of the major arteries and veins had been reported by 1988 according to a review by Fenoglio and Virmani.[5] Most arise from smooth muscle cells or fibroblasts and thus are termed *leiomyosarcomas* (~70% of the total) or malignant fibrous histiocytomas.[5-7] Tumors of the great veins constitute about two thirds of the primary tumors of the great vessels and at least 85% are malignant.[6] Most leiomyosarcomas of the large veins arise in the inferior vena cava, and these tumors develop almost exclusively in women.[8] Venous obstruction by the tumor mass is the source of symptoms that are defined by the location of the venous blockage and can include edema, ascites, and hepatomegaly. These tumors tend to metastasize late in their course and surgical excision is the treatment of choice. Occasionally these tumors can extend intraluminally along the great veins into the heart as do certain renal cell tumors. Resection in these cases may require cardiopulmonary bypass or other approaches.[9,10] Vena cava reconstruction may be accomplished with either autogenous or prosthetic techniques. Iliac and femoral veins occasionally can be excised without replacement, particularly if the veins have been partially obstructed and collateral channels are well developed.

Primary malignancies of the great arteries occur with about 20% of the frequency of venous cancers, and these tumors arise twice as often in the pulmonary arteries as in the aorta.[5] About half of pulmonary artery malignancies are leiomyosarcomas or undifferentiated sarcomas.[11] The most frequent symptoms of pulmonary artery sarcomas are dyspnea or congestive heart failure and chest pain. Many patients show signs of right heart failure and pulmonary arteriography may make the diagnosis. The outcome of pulmonary artery malignancies is poor with or without surgery. Most sarcomas of the aorta have the histologic features of malignant fibrous histiocytomas.[5,12] These tumors are evenly distributed in the thoracic and the abdominal aorta, but are more common in men (~3:1). Aortic sarcomas produce symptoms by arterial obstruction through growth of the tumor mass or by embolization. Many patients also report constitutional symptoms such as fever, malaise, or weakness.[5] Diagnosis is made most commonly at autopsy or surgery, but imaging techniques such as computed tomographic (CT) scanning or magnetic resonance imaging (MRI) have demonstrated these tumors in some cases.[12,13] An aggressive diagnostic evaluation of patients with unusual peripheral emboli may be the key to diagnosis. Treatment of these cancers is surgical excision with appropriate vascular reconstruction using standard vascular surgical procedures and techniques.

Paraganglionoma of the Carotid Bifurcation. Paraganglionomas of the carotid bifurcation (carotid body tumors) arise from neural crest tissues that migrate to the adventitia of the carotid bifurcation and function normally as chemoreceptor tissues. Similar tumors may develop from the same precursor cells in the orbit, the jugular bulb, the middle ear, the ganglion nodosum of the vagus nerve, and in the aortic bodies along the aortic arch, the innominate, and the pulmonary arteries. Although these tumors contain neurosecretory granules, most paraganglionomas are nonfunctional. Bilateral tumors are found with metachronous presentation in about 8% of cases, and approximately 2% to 6% of these tumors are malignant based on local or distant metastasis.[14] The histologic appearance of these tumors is not helpful in grading the risk of malignancy. Although most tumors are benign, the inexorable growth of these lesions produces displacement and compression of the arteries, veins, nerves, and other structures of the neck, and excision is always recommended.

Paraganglionomas of the carotid bifurcation are highly vascular tumors with a rich blood supply from branches of the external carotid artery. Most cases present as a slowly enlarging, painless neck mass. Diagnosis has been established traditionally by arteriography, but recent reports suggest an important role for ultrasound in the evaluation of suspicious neck masses.[15–17] Carotid body tumors produce splaying of the carotid bifurcation (wine glass bifurcation), and the lesions show marked vascularity with turbulent multidirectional flow.[15] Low resistance arterial velocity patterns are seen in the external carotid artery in 80% of such cases consistent with the typical vascular supply to this tumor. Computed tomography scans or magnetic resonance imaging will define the extent of the tumor and show encroachment of surrounding structures (Fig. 11-1). Arteriography remains helpful in operative planning, and recent reports advocate preoperative embolization of these tumors as a safe and effective way to simplify surgical resection of large tumors (Fig. 11-2).[18,19] There is an association of carotid body tumor with pheochromocytoma, and measurement of plasma or urinary catecholamines in these patients is recommended.

Although these tumors are usually extra-

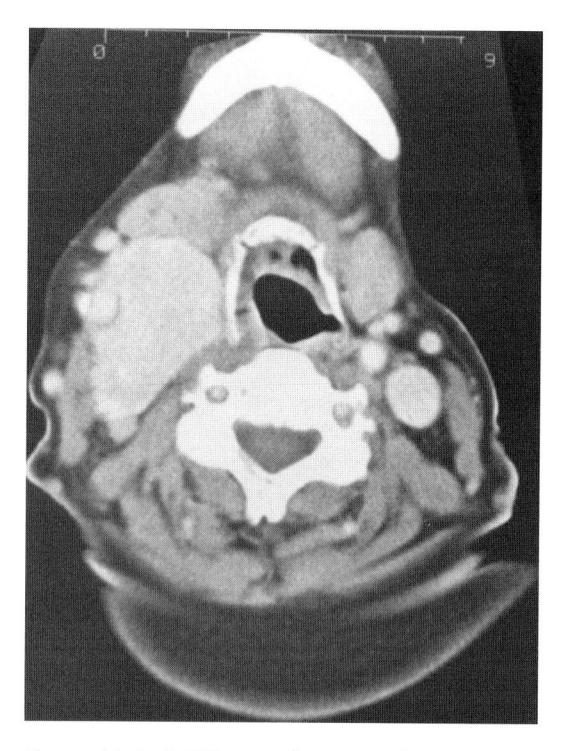

Figure 11-1. A CT scan showing a large vascular mass associated with the right carotid bifurcation and displacing the carotid arteries, the trachea, and the esophagus in a 65-year-old woman with a 15-year history of a slowly enlarging, painless neck mass. The right jugular vein is obliterated by the tumor with compensatory enlargement of the left jugular vein. Pathologic examination showed a typical carotid body paraganglioma.

arterial in their location, their excision can be quite challenging. Shamblin et al[14] classified carotid body tumors into three groups based on gross characteristics: group 1, localized tumors with minimal arterial wall involvement (26%); group 2, tumors that surround the carotid vessels and involve the arterial adventitia (46%); and group 3, adherent tumors involving the entire circumference of the arteries (28%). Treatment of large group 3 lesions may require resection of the carotid bifurcation with vascular reconstruction of the internal carotid artery. In such cases, standard techniques for the intra-operative monitoring of cerebral function and the appropriate use of intravascular shunts should be employed. Modern series indicate a perioperative mor-

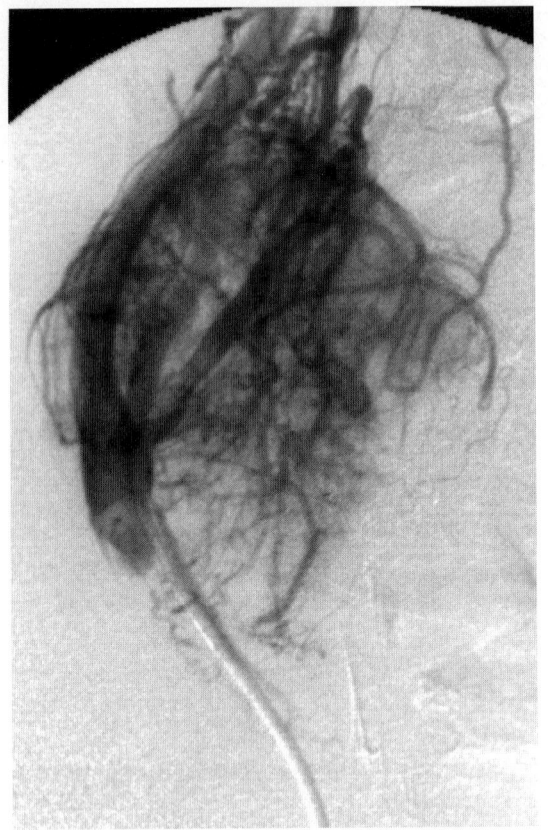

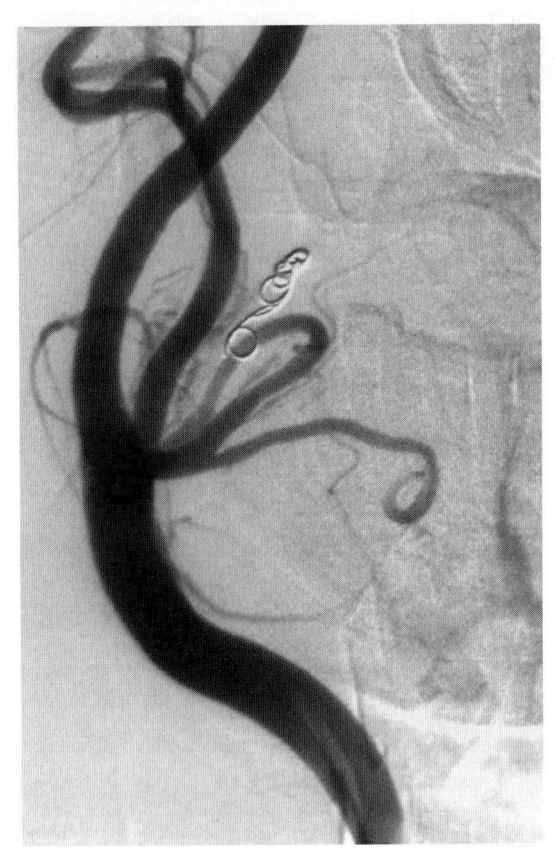

Figure 11-2. Selective digital subtraction arteriogram of the right carotid artery of the patient shown in Figure 11-1 before (**A**) and after (**B**) embolization of the tumor. In this case the major vessels to the tumor arose from the ascending cervical and the superior thyroid branches of the external carotid artery. The marked decrease in vascularity of the tumor by this technique is evident.

tality rate of less than 5% with stroke rates in the same range.[19,20] Injury to cranial nerves occurs in 16% to 30% of patients.

Atrial Myxoma. Primary malignant tumors of the heart are rare with a reported incidence of 0.002% to 0.3% at autopsy.[6,21] Benign tumors of the heart make up 75% to 90% of most series of primary cardiac tumors and 50% to 90% of benign cardiac tumors are myxomas.[6,22,23] Ninety percent of these tumors arise in the atria with a 4:1 predominance in the left atrium.[24–26] Most tumors are small, solitary, and may be pedunculated. Symptoms are produced by intermittent ball valve type obstruction leading to congestive heart failure (~70%) or by embolization of thrombus or tumor (~30%). Most emboli lodge in the cerebral circulation,[27] and this diagnosis should be considered in young patients with stroke. Peripheral tumor emboli with metastases have been reported.[28] The diagnosis of atrial myxoma often is suggested by echocardiography, but CT scanning and MRI allow more complete preoperative staging and often provide sufficient information for surgical planning (Fig. 11-3).[29] Excision is the treatment of choice and produces good intermediate term results with operative mortality of less than 5.0%.[22,24] Late recurrence may occur in 5% to 10% of cases.

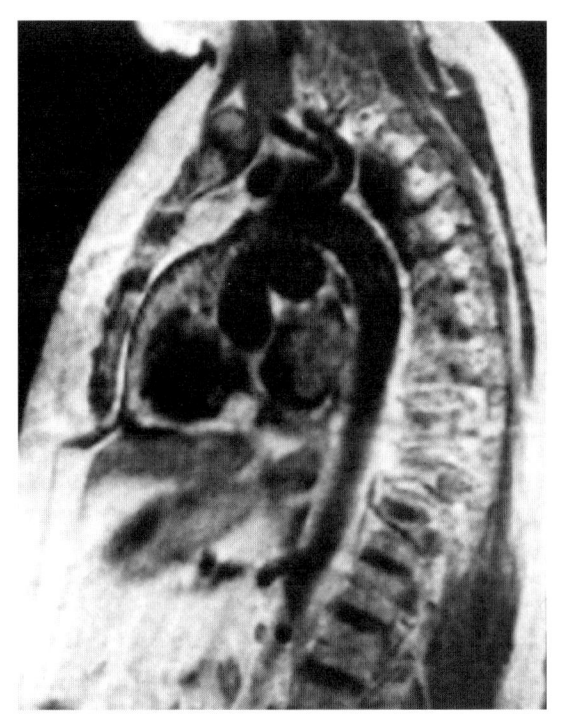

Figure 11-3. Magnetic resonance image of the heart of 25-year-old woman who presented with digital emboli. A large atrial myxoma is present in the left atrium.

SUMMARY: PRIMARY VASCULAR TUMORS

1. Most primary neoplasms of small vessels are benign and many are hamartomas that present in childhood and spontaneously regress over time. Kaposi's sarcoma, associated with HIV infection, is in this category but is malignant and is rarely curable.
2. Primary tumors of the large vessels are exceedingly rare and most arise from smooth muscle cells or fibroblasts and thus are leiomyosarcomas or malignant fibrous histiocytomas. The majority are tumors of the great veins, and at least 85% are malignant.
3. Paragangliomas of the carotid bifurcation are benign, but excision is recommended because of the mass effect of these tumors as they grow. Arteriography and other imaging modalities are important in the preoperative evaluation of these lesions. Their excision can be a technical challenge depending on their involvement with the arterial wall.
4. Atrial myxomas are rare, and usually located in the left atrium. Symptoms result from obstruction leading to congestive heart failure, or embolization, usually to the cerebral circulation. Excision is the preferred therapy.

Secondary Vascular Conditions Related to Malignancy

CELLULAR EFFECTS OF TUMORS ON THE VASCULAR SYSTEM

Recent research in the cellular biology of the development of cancer and of metastasis has revealed fundamental interactions between transformed cells and the vascular system. For tumors to grow beyond a microscopic size, malignant cells must possess the ability to recruit a new vascular supply. Malignant cells elaborate several proteins, growth factors, and mediators. They also express cell surface receptors that when released or expressed in normal cells lead to regulated growth and normal development, wound healing and tissue remodeling. When expressed by tumor cells, these factors induce angiogenesis, and permit local tumor cell invasion and the passage of tumor cells through the endothelial barrier to enter and exit the circulation.[30–32] Several proteins, enzymes, and receptors traditionally associated with the coagulation and the fibrinolytic systems are now recognized to have activities in the normal remodeling of the interstitium, in wound healing, and in metastasis.[33,34] The importance of the coagulation system in the regulation of tissue growth and the growth of tumors was illustrated by evidence that heparin and low molecular weight heparin inhibit smooth muscle proliferation after endothelial injury[35] and that angiogenesis in murine tumors could be suppressed by heparin or cortisone.[36] Fibrin deposition is a prominent feature of many solid tumors and may be important for tumor growth and invasion.[33] Green et al[37] pooled data from two large studies and suggested that patients with cancer receiving low molecular weight heparin seem to have a survival advantage over those treated with standard heparin therapy. Thus, low molecular weight heparin may have an inhibitory effect on tumor growth not seen with regular heparin. These and other observations have stimulated interest in the development of antineoplastic therapeutic approaches for tumors using anticoagulant or antiangiogenic agents.[38-41] The antiproliferative effects of heparin on vascular smooth muscle cells after injury indicate a similar relationship between coagulation proteins and arterial pathology including atherosclerosis.[42]

Secondary Effects of Tumors on the Coagulation System. Maintenance of the fluid character of blood within the circulation is the result of a delicate balance of a complex system of procoagulant, anticoagulant, and lytic zymogens and a host of activating and inhibiting factors. Although the clinical association between cancer and disorders of coagulation has been known for at least a century,[1] it is only recently that specific deficits in the coagulation system have been documented in patients with cancer. A wide range of abnormalities have been described and the synthesis of these observations into a clear picture of the pathophysiology of coagulation in cancer is yet to occur. Several recent reviews summarize current data[43-47] and a brief review is provided here.

Increased circulating levels of activated clotting factors including factors I, V, VIII, IX, and XI are one of the earliest and the most consistent coagulation abnormalities reported in patients with tumors.[48] Increased turnover of both fibrinogen and platelets has been reported in patients with advanced cancer.[49] Increased titers of circulating fibrin degradation products, D-dimer, fibrinopeptide A and B, cryofibrinogens, fibrin monomer, platelet factor 4, β-thromboglobulin, and altered fibronectin levels have been described in individual patients.[50] Other investigators have reported deficiencies in the principal inhibitors of coagulation including antithrombin-III and protein-C.[51] These findings indicate that a state of subclinical disseminated intravascular coagulation (DIC) may be common to many patients with malignancy, and that such patients may be susceptible to clinically significant thrombosis or bleeding. Thrombosis is the more likely outcome and may occur in as many as 40% of patients with cancer.[52]

The cellular mechanisms that are responsible for the measurable alterations in coagulation in cancer patients are not well known. Tissue factor is a membrane-bound glycoprotein (54 kd) that is expressed in most tissues and is the normal cellular activator of the coagulation system. Tissue factor binds factor VII allowing activation of this factor and its subsequent activation of factors IX and X which initiates coagulation. Tissue factor has been demonstrated in the extracts of tumor cells in cultured tumor cell lines in the serum and urine of patients with cancer.[53] A recent study by Callander et al[54] showed expression of tissue factor by malignant cells arising from cell types that normally express tissue factor including epithelial tumors such as lung, pancreas, breast, colon, and stomach. A second procoagulant termed *cancer procoagulant* (CP) is a 68-kd cysteine protease that directly activates factor X. This chemical is less well characterized than tissue factor.[43] The activated platelets associated with tumors may also play an important role in the procoagulant state of patients with malignancy. Normally platelets are activated by thrombin generated through the coagulation cascade, but in patients with cancer other tumor-related mechanisms have been identified including a procoagulant activity and platelet activating activity (PCA/PAA) described in an adenocarcinoma cell line by Cavanaugh and associates[55] and a second mechanism that involves tumor surface factors.[56] The binding of von Willebrand factor to cancer cells may also play a role in the activation of platelets and in the subsequent coagulation disorders of cancer.[57] There is also evidence for involvement of fibrinolytic enzymes and receptors as mediators of coagulation activation by tumors.[58]

Other tumors may elaborate factors that block the action of specific components of the coagulation system. Such inhibitors include pathologic circulating antibodies and proteins that block the activation of specific coagulation factors through protein to protein complex formation. In addition, circulating fibrin degradation products arising from the subclinical DIC state described above may have a significant impact on coagulation and possibly lead to bleeding. Specific inhibitors to factor V, factor VIII, factor X, and von Willebrand factor have been described, and the current state of this subject has been reviewed by Kunkel.[44] Some effects of tumor cells on the coagulation system may be mediated by an interaction with monocytes or macrophages, which can then elaborate procoagulant factors.[43]

Secondary Effects of Tumors on Atherosclerosis. Atherosclerosis is a chronic degenerative disease of the arterial intima and media that results in the formation of lipid-laden and calcified plaque and a gradual obliteration of the lumen of major arteries. Although this is a chronic, progressive disease, many serious, clinically recognized consequences of atherosclerosis such as myocardial infarction, stroke, and transient ischemic attack have been associated with relatively sudden changes occurring in atherosclerotic plaques.[59] These changes include fissuring of the plaque with release of atherosclerotic or thrombotic debris and intraplaque hemorrhage leading to surface disruption or a sudden increase in the hemodynamic significance of pre-existing lesions.[60,61] Rupture and intraplaque hemorrhage in atherosclerotic lesions of the carotid bifurcation are clearly associated with transient ischemia attack (TIA) and stroke.[62] Some investigators have reported an association between acute coronary or peripheral vascular events and malignant tumors.[63,64] Naschitz and associates used several indices of the activity of coronary disease to show that unstable ischemic heart disease was three times more common in the patients later found to have cancer, than in control patients.[64] These investigators also showed more rapid progression of chronic lower extremity arterial occlusive disease in patients with claudication and cancer.[63] The explanation for an association between cancer and progressive atherosclerosis is not known, but the most likely possibility seems to be the altered state of the coagulation system in patients with malignant tumors.

GROSS EFFECTS OF TUMORS

In addition to effects at a cellular level, the mass effect of the tumor may also influence vascular function. Large tumor masses in the pelvis or in the extremities can displace major arteries and veins, and may produce significant venous compression. Venous obstruction in this setting adds an additional risk factor for the development of deep venous thrombosis in these patients, and may lead to significant venous hypertension and morbidity even without frank thrombosis. Hemodynamically significant obstruction to arterial flow by extrinsic compression is uncommon without direct involvement of the artery with tumor. Direct invasion of major blood vessels by tumor occurs less often, but may lead to thrombosis or to the loss of the structural integrity of the arterial wall with pseudoaneurysm formation or arterial rupture.

SYSTEMIC EFFECTS OF TUMORS

Advanced malignancy is commonly associated with nutritional defects which may lead to weight loss and significant deficiencies in visceral protein synthesis. (See Chapter 15.) Such defects can lead to acquired deficiencies of coagulation factors and anticoagulant proteins[65] and predispose the patient to additional thrombotic or hemorrhagic complications. Reduction of hepatic synthetic capacity related to hepatic metastasis may compromise production of the circulating anticoagulant protein-C and further promote thrombosis.[51] Inanition accompanying advanced tumors can lead to significant dehydration with hemoconcentration, changes in blood viscosity, and alterations in the perfusion of certain vascular beds. These factors may predispose the patient to microvascular thrombosis. Nutritional defects related to the tumor and its therapy with radiation, surgery, or chemotherapy may also contribute to poor wound healing in these patients (the effects of cancer on wound healing is further discussed in Chapter 14). Wound breakdown and wound infection can significantly increase the morbidity of immunosuppressed patients with cancer. These problems can be compounded in patients who might require vascular surgery. Wound breakdown over a prosthetic arterial reconstruction frequently precipitates a life- or limb-threatening situation.

EFFECTS OF RADIATION THERAPY ON THE VASCULAR SYSTEM

The acute complications of radiation therapy are discussed elsewhere in this volume (see Chapter 7). Several specific effects of ionizing radiation on vascular tissues merit discussion here. Ionizing radiation has long been known to induce acute swelling and proliferation of endothelial cells and can lead to the obliteration of small arteries and veins in a radiated field. Acute radiation effects on larger arteries are similar, but the chronic morphologic changes induced by ionizing radiation are of greater clinical relevance. Lindsay et al[66,67] reported the development of changes indistinguishable from classic atherosclerosis in the aortas of dogs following radiation treatment. Accelerated progression of atherosclerosis has been described in patients receiving radiation therapy for head and neck tumors, Hodgkin's disease, or pelvic malignancies.[68-70] Ischemic symptoms have been reported from 1 to 15 years following radiation therapy and show some degree of dose dependence. The accelerated development of atherosclerosis in these patients is further exacerbated by the coexistence of other risk factors including smoking[69] and hyperlipidemia.[70,71] Radiation-induced atherosclerotic disease is characterized by the presence of typical atherosclerotic lesions in unusual locations or the more extensive involvement of arteries that commonly have localized lesions. Furthermore, Pettersson and Swedenborg[69] reported an increased risk of serious radiation-induced arterial lesions among patients who had developed other radiation-induced diseases in nearby organs, such as bowel and bladder fistulas and obstruction in patients with radiation for pelvic malignancy. Treatment approaches for radiation-induced atherosclerosis, even years after radiation, must be modified to account for both the poor vascularity and the poor healing characteristics of the radiated tissues in the operative field. Taken together, these observations have a significant impact on the treatment of arterial stenoses in radiated fields. Whereas the typical atherosclerosis of the carotid bifurcation is best handled with a localized endarterectomy, radiation-related carotid atherosclerosis often necessitates carotid bypass with careful selection of incision sites.[72] Breakdown of the wounds with exposure of the bypass, whether autogenous or prosthetic, can produce significant morbidity or mortality.[73]

EFFECTS OF SURGICAL THERAPY ON THE VASCULAR SYSTEM

Surgical therapy remains the mainstay of the treatment of many tumors and represents the most effective curative strategy for many solid tumors. Extirpation of the tumor can resolve many of the cellular and systemic effects of the tumor causing resolution of any coagulation abnormalities that might arise in such cases. However, surgery itself is associated with disorders of coagulation and may interact unfavorably with any tumor-associated coagulopathy. Although large-volume blood loss and hypothermia may lead to depletion of coagulation factors and platelets and clinical coagulopathy in the preoperative period, surgery typically produces a procoagulant state.[74] Surgery for trauma or other nonmalignant diseases is associated with a significant incidence of spontaneous deep venous thrombosis, and this risk may be further amplified in patients with underlying malignancy. These effects are most likely related to activated coagulation factors stimulated through tissue destruction in the operative field.

En bloc resection of large tumors of the extremity may require excision of major arteries or veins. Careful planning prior to surgery is critical so that prompt successful revascularization of the distal extremity is possible. Preoperative evaluation should include duplex scanning and arteriography. Surgical excision of tumors is often accompanied by lymph node dissection, which may produce significant lymphatic obstruction and swelling in the extremities. These effects are exacerbated when surgery is combined with radiation therapy and persistent lymph swelling can be a troublesome problem in such patients. Vascular surgical reconstructive options for treatment in these cases are limited.

EFFECTS OF CHEMOTHERAPY
ON THE VASCULAR SYSTEM

The local effects of chemotherapy on the vascular system as well as the details of vascular access and its complications are considered elsewhere in this volume (Chapter 9 and Chapter 10). Many chemotherapeutic agents produce significant suppression of the bone marrow leading to deficiency of circulating erythrocytes, leukocytes, and platelets (these effects are discussed extensively in Chapter 17). Of particular importance is the induction of thrombocytopenia, which may be associated with significant bleeding complications and can be a contraindication to standard anticoagulant therapy or fibrinolytic therapy in cancer patients with thrombosis. Marked granulocytopenia may also accompany chemotherapy and present an additional risk factor if vascular reconstruction is required for an acute ischemic problem. Wound breakdown and reduced ability to fight infection can significantly increase the risk of clinically important graft infection in this setting.

SUMMARY: SECONDARY VASCULAR CONDITIONS RELATED TO MALIGNANCY

1. The coagulation system is affected by tumors, as they elaborate a number of molecules with direct effects on coagulation. Several novel approaches to tumor therapy are investigating the use of antiangiogenic factors.
2. Specific deficits in the coagulation system have been identified in cancer patients. Increased circulating levels of factors I, V, VIII, IX, and XI have been consistently seen in cancer patients. These patients may have a state of subclinical DIC. Thrombosis is common in these patients.
3. Although the explanation remains unclear at this time, there is a definite association between cancer and progressive atherosclerosis.
4. Large tumors can lead to direct compression of vascular structures with resulting obstruction. In the pelvis, this can lead to deep venous thrombosis. Direct invasion of blood vessels also occurs.
5. Radiation therapy can lead to accelerated progression of atherosclerosis.
6. Surgical therapy of tumors may have effects on the vascular system with an increased risk of deep venous thrombosis. It may be necessary to resect large vessels along with a tumor, requiring careful preoperative planning.
7. Chemotherapy has a number of effects on the vascular and coagulation system. The induced neutropenia may increase the risk of infection in vascular grafts.

CLINICAL VASCULAR SYNDROMES ASSOCIATED WITH CANCER

Hemorrhage

Life-threatening hemorrhage is a result of severe clotting abnormalities observed in certain cancer patients and this subject has been reviewed recently.[44,45,47] Such bleeding is a significant cause of death among patients with acute leukemia and other malignancies. This problem is rarely treatable with surgery and successful therapy relies on appropriate treatment of the malignancy and transfusion therapy. Hemorrhage may be the principal cause of death in as many as 11% of patients with cancer and contribute to death in up to 25% of these patients.[75]

Venous Thromboembolism

Pulmonary embolism is the principal cause of death in approximately 7% of patients with cancer.[75] Autopsy studies have demonstrated an incidence of major pulmonary embolism in up to 35% of patients with advanced abdominal malignancies.[76] Large series investigating deep venous thrombosis (DVT) indicate that approximately 30% of patients with major DVT will develop pulmonary embolism. These considerations suggest that DVT is a major source of morbidity and mortality among cancer patients and that DVT may occur in up to half of patients with cancer. In addition, the development of DVT in the absence of a recognized risk factor (family history, lupus anticoagulant, deficiencies of Antithrombin III, protein C, or protein S, trauma, immobilization, surgery, or pregnancy) may be a marker for the development of subsequent symptomatic cancer. Several retrospective cohort studies comparing patients with documented thromboembolic phenomena to matched controls have supported this contention.[77-79] Recently several prospective studies have been reported that definitively show an association between idiopathic DVT and the subsequent development of overt cancer.[80-82] Monreal et al[82] prospectively compared the incidence of cancer among patients presenting with idiopathic DVT to that among patients with secondary DVT. Cancer developed in 23% of patients with idiopathic DVT compared with 6% in the secondary DVT group. Prandoni and associates[80] showed a 3.3% incidence of cancer at the time of diagnosis in 153 patients with idiopathic DVT. During subsequent follow-up, 7.6% of those with idiopathic DVT developed cancer. Fully 17% of patients with recurrent idiopathic DVT were found to have a malignancy within 2 years of initial presentation.

Based on the above considerations, all patients with known cancer are at increased risk for the development of DVT. Unfortunately, the majority of DVTs are asymptomatic and produce no reliable physical findings. Thus, a high index of suspicion combined with a low threshold for obtaining objective testing is crucial to the prompt diagnosis of DVT and the initiation of appropriate therapy. The diagnosis of DVT has traditionally been made using contrast phlebography (Fig. 11-4). Although this method is highly accurate and has formed the basis for most of our knowledge on the epidemiology and natural history of DVT, phlebography has numerous drawbacks. The test is invasive and requires cannulation of a superficial vein in the extremity, a procedure that may be impossible in some cases. The examination is performed largely with fluoroscopy and requires infusion of a significant amount of intravascular contrast medium. The test can be performed only in an appropriate radiographic suite, which severely limits the applicability of this technique in high-risk critically ill patients. Furthermore, the need for radiation and contrast make physicians reluctant to repeat contrast phlebography even if clinical circumstances should change.

These weaknesses of contrast phlebography have provided much of the impetus to the continuing development of noninvasive testing modalities, which currently provide accurate, reproducible, and repeatable evaluation of patients with suspected DVT. Impedance plethysmography was the first non-

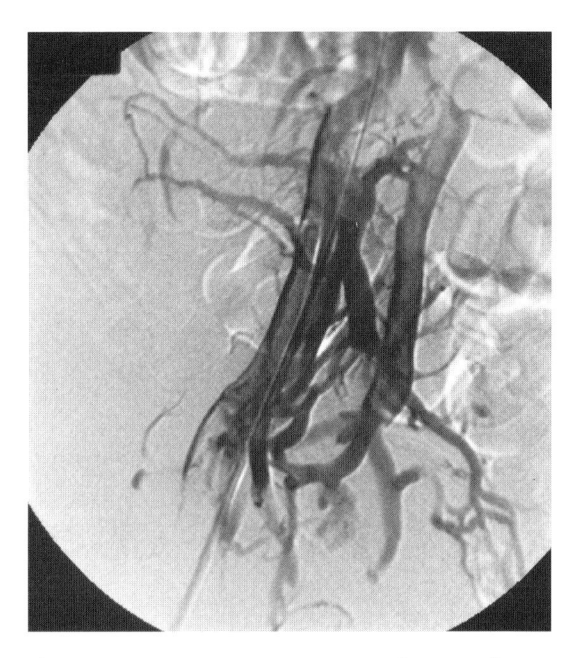

Figure 11-4. Contrast venogram of an occlusive deep venous thrombosis of the inferior vena cava and the right common iliac vein with nonocclusive thrombus visible in the external iliac and the internal iliac veins.

invasive technique to emerge with demonstrated diagnostic accuracy comparable to that of contrast phlebography for major DVT of the proximal deep veins of the lower extremity. This technique relies on sensitive measurement of the volume of the calf and diagnosis depends on the physiologic responses to brief obstruction of venous outflow by an inflatable cuff. Impedance plethysmography has several well-recognized shortcomings, including failure to detect DVT in calf veins and an inability to differentiate between venous obstruction (such as that produced by extrinsic compression from a tumor mass in the pelvis) from DVT.[83] This combination of a significant incidence of false-positive and false-negative examinations has forced clinicians to supplement impedance plethysmography with other noninvasive testing modalities or phlebography. Despite these limitations impedance plethysmography remains a valuable diagnostic test for DVT at many centers and much of the recent literature on the diagnosis and treatment of lower extremity DVT has employed impedance plethysmography.[84]

In recent years, direct ultrasound examination of the major veins of the extremities and body cavities has become possible using a combination of B-mode and Doppler techniques. Duplex ultrasound is completely portable, involves no ionizing radiation or contrast administration, and may be repeated as frequently as clinically indicated. In contrast to impedance plethysmography, duplex ultrasound can demonstrate accurately the anatomic areas of involvement of a lower extremity DVT and can show the iliac and the brachiocephalic veins as well as the inferior vena cava in most patients. Accurate detection of portal vein or hepatic vein thrombosis (this complication is also discussed in Chapter 5) is also possible with duplex ultrasonography[85,86]. Diagnosis of DVT by duplex scanning is based on three main criteria: visible thrombus in the vein, abnormalities of venous flow detected by pulsed Doppler, and inability to compress the deep veins with gentle pressure[87] (Fig. 11-5). Duplex ultrasonography of the deep veins has demonstrated excellent concordance with findings of phlebography[88,89] and has supplanted contrast phlebography and impedance plethysmography in many centers. Contrast phlebography is still of significant value for the evaluation of veins not accessible to ultrasound, in cases where duplex scanning is not definitive and in cases of calf vein DVT or suspected recurrent DVT.

As with DVT, the diagnosis of pulmonary embolism (PE) cannot be made on clinical grounds alone. Pulmonary angiography is the definitive test for pulmonary embolism. Recent refinements in technique have reduced the contrast requirements and made this test more suitable for more patients. Radioisotope ventilation or perfusion scans of the lung are useful in certain situations. Hull et al[90] have demonstrated clearly that a normal perfusion scan of the lungs combined with a normal chest radiograph effectively excludes a pulmonary embolism regardless of the clin-

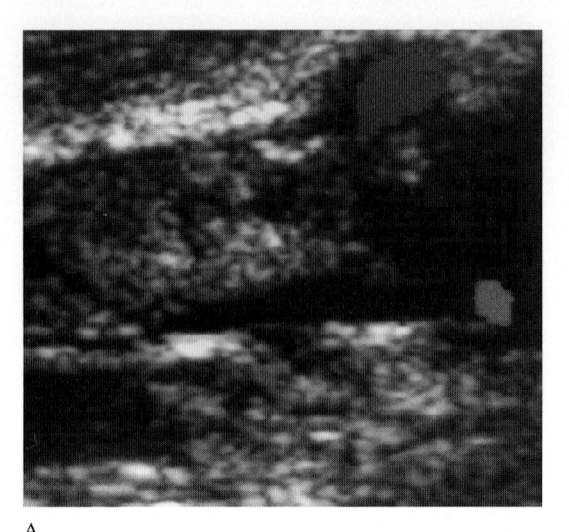

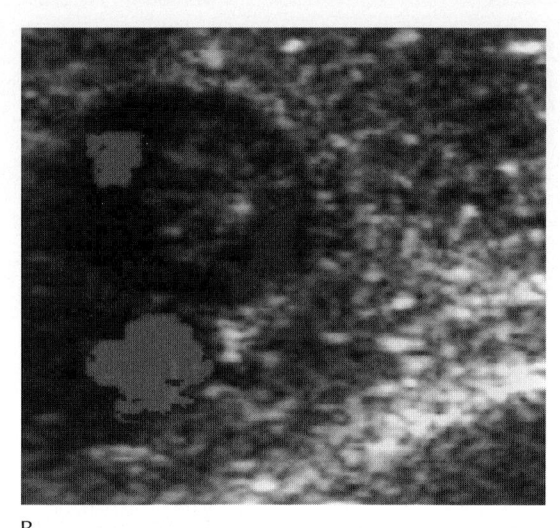

Figure 11-5. Duplex scan of the popliteal vein in a patient with occlusive deep venous thrombosis. Intraluminal echoes are visible in both the longitudinal (*left*) and the transverse view (*right*).

ical presentation. An abnormal perfusion scan, however, does not ensure the diagnosis of pulmonary embolism and may be the result of underlying pulmonary disease, which is also common in patients with malignancy. The PIOPED investigators[91] reported an 88% sensitivity for pulmonary embolism in patients with a high-probability lung scans, but only 41% of patients with arteriographic demonstration of pulmonary embolism had high-probability scans. Less than half of patients with intermediate-probability scans had pulmonary embolism in this study. Many clinicians are satisfied with this level of certainty and unless the risk of bleeding seems excessive will treat the patients with anticoagulation therapy based on a scan alone. Most practitioners will insist on angiographic confirmation of a pulmonary embolism before instituting anticoagulation therapy or other treatment for patients with marked coagulopathy and hemorrhagic risk.

TREATMENT OF DVT AND ITS COMPLICATIONS

Anticoagulation remains the standard therapy for DVT or pulmonary embolism in the cancer patient. Several recent reports indicate that anticoagulation reduces the risk of PE in patients with DVT from approximately 30% to 5% to 8%.[92–94] Anticoagulation typically is begun with heparin which is administered for 5 to 10 days to maintain the activated partial thromboplastin time (aPTT) at 1.5 to 2.0 times control. Oral warfarin therapy is started after heparinization and continued for an empiric course of 3 to 6 months. The anticoagulant level with chronic warfarin is monitored with the prothrombin time and warfarin dosage is adjusted to maintain an international normalized ratio (INR) of 2.0 to 3.0.

Significant complications may accompany the use of anticoagulants in patients with cancer and DVT. The most common undesirable effect of anticoagulation is hemorrhage.[95] The reported risk of major hemorrhage in published studies of patients treated for thromboembolic disease ranges from 4% to 17%. Careful adjustment of anticoagulant dosage is important in reducing the incidence of bleeding. Bleeding while receiving heparin therapy may be related to the dose of heparin used and several patient factors including recent surgery, age, sex, and platelet function abnormalities. Other studies show much less favorable results. Moore et al[96] reported 21 hemorrhagic complications including 8 major hemorrhages among 32 cancer patients with DVT receiving anticoagulation medication. Furthermore, 6 of the 32 patients developed a pulmonary embolism despite anticoagulation treatment.

The second major complication associated with heparin anticoagulation is thrombocytopenia. The incidence of this problem has ranged from 0% to 30%,[97] but is probably less than 10%.[97,98] Thrombocytopenia usually begins between 3 and 15 days after initiation of heparin but may develop within hours in patients who have previously received heparin. The thrombocytopenia results from the formation of immune complexes owing to antibodies to a heparin platelet complex. The incidence of major arterial and venous thrombosis in patients with heparin-associated thrombocytopenia is low (0.4%).[98] Unfortunately when such thromboses develop in this setting, the consequences can be devastating leading to unreconstructable arterial occlusions and limb loss.[99,100] The key to prevention of these serious drug-related complications is routine monitoring of the platelet count in patients receiving heparin and prompt discontinuance of all heparin administration (intravenous, subcutaneous, intra-arterial) when the platelet count drops significantly. If such patients are being treated for life-threatening thrombotic problems such as a major PE or large central DVT, anticoagulation may be continued with warfarin or other drugs, or a vena caval interruption device may need to be placed.

Several investigators have reported successful anticoagulation using heparin in patients with heparin-associated thrombocytopenia after inhibition of platelet function with aspirin and dipyridamole.[101] Others have maintained anticoagulation in patients with heparin-associated thrombocytopenia by fibrinogen depletion with snake venom (Ancrod).[102] Most authors agree that absolute thrombocytopenia (platelet count <100,000) or a decrease in platelet count by more than 50% of the pretreatment platelet count are indications withholding or discontinuing heparin administration.

Anticoagulation therapy may present some additional problems in patients with cancer. Such patients may have developed coagulation abnormalities that would contraindicate administration of anticoagulants. Spontaneous bleeding in the gastrointestinal, urinary, or respiratory tracts presents an absolute contraindication to anticoagulation. Patients with either primary or metastatic brain tumors are likewise excluded from anticoagulation therapy because of the possibility of life-threatening intracranial hemorrhage. Many patients with cancer receive cytotoxic chemotherapy and develop bone marrow suppression with temporary but profound thrombocytopenia, contraindicating the use of heparin. Certain patients may not have a contraindication at the initiation of anticoagulation therapy, but develop complications such as bleeding or thrombocytopenia during treatment. Finally, although anticoagulation is quite effective in the prevention of pulmonary embolism in patients with DVT, the protection afforded by this modality is not absolute and certain patients will have progressive thrombosis or pulmonary embolism despite adequate anticoagulation. There is also evidence that venous thrombosis in patients with certain cancers may be unresponsive to adequate anticoagulation.[103] Idiopathic venous thromboses that display similar resistance to anticoagulants can be a clue to an underlying malignancy in an otherwise healthy patient.

Thus in patients with contraindications, complications, or failure of anticoagulation therapy an alternative therapeutic approach is necessary. In such cases, mechanical interruption of the major venous channels is employed to prevent venous emboli from reaching the central circulation.[104] In recent years, the Greenfield filter has emerged as the optimal device for this purpose. The Greenfield filter is positioned in the infrarenal inferior vena cava intralumenally from either the internal jugular or the common femoral veins and may be placed percutaneously in most cases.[105,106] Several other intravena caval devices are available, including the Nitinol, Birds Nest, and VenaTech devices, but the long-term results of these appliances are less well-documented and they are generally reserved for special situations.[104,106] The Greenfield filter is extremely effective with a low incidence of major venous morbidity. The risk of a clinically significant pulmonary embolism with a Greenfield filter in place is approximately 4% and placement of the device rarely results in vena caval occlusion (caval patency rate of 98%).[107] In cases where the thrombus extends into the perirenal inferior vena cava, the Greenfield filter may be safely positioned in the suprarenal or retrohepatic vena cava.[108] Placement of intravena caval devices is not without complication. As many as 40% of patients will develop venous thrombosis at the puncture site after filter placement.[105,109] Placement of vena caval filters also can cause vena caval perforation, air embolism, and cardiac arrhythmia. Late complications include migration of the device, perforation of adjacent structures, structural failure, and caval thrombosis with recurrent pulmonary embolism.[104]

Recently, several authors have advocated use of the Greenfield filter as a primary treatment for DVT in patients with cancer to avoid the potential complications of anticoagulation in this setting.[110–112] The high efficacy of the filter in prevention of pulmonary embolism is a major advantage of this approach, and the reduced life expectancy of many cancer patients makes the risk of long-term filter-related complications low. Twenty to thirty percent of patients will develop progressive DVT after inferior vena cava filter placement[110,112] and will require later anticoagulation therapy to control extremity symptoms. Because many patients with cancer may have temporary contraindications to anticoagulation therapy for DVT, prompt insertion of a Greenfield filter to prevent life-threatening pulmonary embolism followed by later institution of anticoagulant therapy may be the best approach in many patients.

With the major improvements in the success of fibrinolytic therapy for acute arterial ischemic syndromes,[113–115] interest has increased in the potential use of fibrinolytic agents in the treatment of DVT. Several investigators have reported greater than 70% success rate in restoring patency after major iliofemoral DVT by means of direct infusion of the thrombus with urokinase or tissue plasminogen activator.[116,117] Semba and Dake[116] continued standard anticoagulation therapy for 2 to 3 months after thrombolysis and reported a 92% patency rate at 3 months. Additional studies are needed to determine whether the clinical outcome with lytic therapy is superior to that of standard anticoagulation, but lytic treatment of relatively short duration applied directly to the thrombus could have many benefits in the treatment of extensive or progressive DVT in patients with cancer. Unfortunately, use of lytic therapy does not eliminate the need for prolonged anticoagulation even if the treatment is successful. Furthermore, application of this approach to patients with cancer may be limited because the contraindications to lytic therapy are broader than those to anticoagulation.

Although many of the complications of anticoagulation treatment are common to all anticoagulant agents, some drug-specific problems may be circumvented in the near future by several new compounds. The most promising agents are several types of low molecular weight heparin (LMWH) that have a mean molecular weight of 4 to 5 kd and produce a more effective and more prolonged activation of antithrombin III than conventional, unfractionated heparin.[118] Recently, fixed dose subcutaneous administration of low molecular weight heparin was compared to standard intravenous infusion of conventional heparin in patients with proximal DVT.[119,120] These two studies demonstrated that a fixed-dose regimen of subcutaneous low molecular weight heparin was at least as effective as the standard heparin therapy for symptomatic proximal vein thrombosis. These developments indicate that anticoagulation therapy may be simplified in some patients with DVT.

Certain patients with DVT will develop extensive occlusive thrombus involving the iliofemoral system and its collaterals producing massive swelling and tissue ischemia. The mechanism of ischemia in this case is similar to that of a compartment syndrome wherein venous occlusion causes massive tissue edema, increases interstitial pressure, and causes a cessation of capillary perfusion.[121] Haimovici[122] has used the term *ischemic venous thrombosis* to describe this condition, and divided this process into two clinical patterns: (1) phlegmasia cerulea dolens (which is reversible) and (2) venous gangrene (which is not). Untreated, 80% of patients with venous gangrene die. Cancer is present in 25% to 60% of patients with ischemic venous thrombosis.[122] Early aggressive treatment of phlegmasia cerulea dolens with therapeutic anticoagulation and maximal elevation of the limb may prevent progression to frank venous gangrene. Patients with extensive iliofemoral DVT may require massive amounts of heparin (15 to 20,000 U bolus) to achieve a therapeutic effect and careful repeated monitoring of the partial thromboplastin time is mandatory. Marked elevation of the limb tends to reduce fluid accumulation and compartment pressures and minimizes permanent tissue damage produced by the venous obstruction. Thrombolytic therapy is an option in some patients with phlegmasia cerulea dolens, but in many cases of cancer with DVT active bleeding, recent surgery or intracranial disease preclude treatment with lytic agents. In some cases, direct surgical thrombectomy may be beneficial.[123,124] Historically, there is a high incidence of rethrombosis after surgical thrombectomy, but the addition of a temporary arteriovenous fistula may significantly reduce this complication and enhance long-term venous patency.[125] Most authors recommend placement of a Greenfield filter in the inferior vena cava prior to attempting venous thrombectomy to avoid the possibility of pulmonary embolism during clot manipulation. Even in the event of rethrombosis, temporary patency of the deep venous system can permit significant reduction in edema and in compartment pressures as well as provide time for institution of effective anticoagulation.

LATE COMPLICATIONS OF DVT

Most patients with advanced malignancy and DVT experience improvement of leg symptoms and swelling with or without therapy. Because the mortality in this cohort of patients is quite high, few live to develop late complications of the postphlebitic syndrome such as chronic pain, swelling, and venous ulceration. On the other hand, chronic venous scarring or occlusion in the lower extremity deep veins can produce significant morbidity in some patients by limiting mobility and requiring chronic compression therapy to control symptoms. Scarring in the superior vena cava results in the superior vena cava syndrome with swelling of the upper extremities and the head. This syndrome results most commonly from venous occlusion related to central venous catheters, large bulky tumors in the mediastinum, or scarring from central chest radiation therapy. Chronic thrombus in the inferior vena cava can produce massive lower extremity swelling and scrotal edema and occasionally the Budd-Chiari syndrome (see Chapter 5) or renal dysfunction from obstruction of the hepatic or renal veins. In the past, only symptomatic treatment was possible for these difficult conditions, but now the underlying venous blockages can be relieved in many cases with interventional techniques. Early reports of successful recanalization of venous occlusions and dilation with internal stenting of venous stenoses[126,127] have led to improved stent construction and a wider application of these techniques.[128] The durability of these procedures is not well documented, but most patients so treated have had excellent palliation of their obstructive symptoms at minimal risk.

Chemotherapy-Associated DVT. It has been shown recently that patients receiving combined chemotherapy and hormonal therapy have an increased risk of developing venous thrombosis compared with patients receiving either therapy alone. This has been studied mainly in patients with breast cancer, where the addition of tamoxifen to chemotherapy regimens has increased the incidence of thrombotic complications. This subject is thoroughly reviewed in Chapter 17.

PROPHYLAXIS AGAINST DVT

Based on the discussions above, all hospitalized patients with cancer are at increased risk for the development of DVT and this risk should be addressed with appropriate prophylactic therapy. Heparin is proved a safe and effective agent for DVT prophylaxis in high-risk medical and surgical patients providing a 60% to 70% reduction in the risk of DVT or fatal PE in treated patients.[129] Similar degrees of risk reduction have been demonstrated with the use of intermittent mechanical compression devices in other high-risk patient groups.[130,131]

Acute Arterial Occlusion:

MICROVASCULAR THROMBOSIS

Certain patients with cancer will present with cutaneous vasculitis. Greer et al[132] reported 13 patients with cutaneous vasculitis consisting of palpable purpura, maculopapular eruptions, urticarial or petechial lesions, or ulcerations. The tumors most commonly associated with cutaneous vasculitis were lymphoproliferative malignancies and hairy cell leukemia. These lesions usually showed some improvement with steroid therapy and little response to nonsteroidal and anti-inflammatory agents. Taylor et al[133] reported five cases of digital ischemia related to underlying malignancy and reviewed 23 previously reported cases in the literature. Two cases showed multiple digital artery occlusions and two showed evidence of angiitis. Several mechanisms have been proposed to explain digital ischemia in this setting. Arterial occlusion may be related to arteritis, to hyperviscosity caused by elevated levels of protein or cellular elements in the blood, or to nonspecific hypercoagulability. Four of the five cases reported by Taylor occurred in patients with solid tumors and treatment efforts were directed largely at the primary tumor with the use of symptomatic measures for the digital ischemia.

As noted above, coronary and cerebrovascular complications in patients with malignancy may be related to an effect of the tumor on pre-existing atherosclerotic lesions. Graus et al[134] reviewed pathologic material from 1970 to 1981 at the Memorial Sloan-Kettering Cancer Center (New York, NY) and found intracranial atherosclerosis with thrombosis was the most frequent cause of ischemic cerebral infarction in patients with cancer. Cerebral infarction contributed to patient death in over half of the cases. Microvascular thrombosis may be a common mechanism and may explain the increased risk of ischemic heart disease among patients with cancer[64] and the accelerated course of lower extremity claudication in similar patients.[63,135]

LARGE VESSEL THROMBOSIS.

Thrombus may develop on plaque lesions of large vessel arterial occlusive disease in patients with cancer, and produce acute limb or organ ischemia by direct arterial obstruction or by embolization. Extensive arterial thrombosis in patients with little evidence of atherosclerosis, or recurrent arterial thrombosis in the face of anticoagulation is occasionally a sign of occult malignancy (Fig. 11-6). Thrombus formation in these cases is presumed to be caused by interaction of a hypercoagulable state owing to the malignancy and plaque-related initiators of thrombosis. Systemic effects, such as changes in blood viscosity secondary to increases in protein or cellular elements, dehydration, and hemodynamic instability secondary to complications of chemotherapy, sepsis, or bleeding may also play a role. The occurrence of spontaneous large vessel thrombosis may indicate an advanced stage of carcinoma or cancer in the presence of significant comorbid conditions. In this setting, arterial thrombosis and tissue infarction may simply represent the

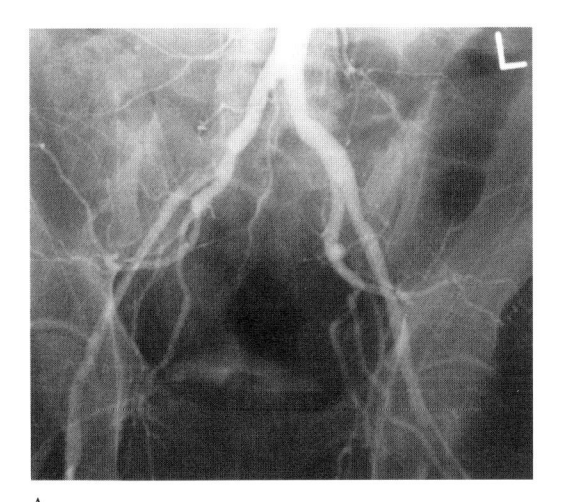

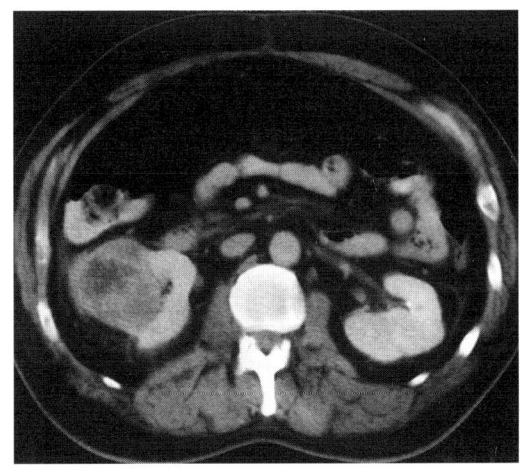

Figure 11-6. An otherwise healthy 55-year-old smoker presented with the acute onset of bilateral lower extremity ischemia. **A.** Arteriography shows mild atherosclerotic changes diffusely with thrombus in the right external iliac artery and in the left common femoral artery. **B.** An abdominal CT scan was obtained to exclude intrinsic aortic lesions as a source for emboli. This study showed an unexpected carcinoma of the right kidney. Complete echocardiography and aortography showed no abnormalities.

mechanism of death in a patient with no hope for survival. This may be the case in intestinal infarction among patients with metastatic cancer.[136] Standard vascular surgical approaches are taken in these cases and in the setting of *in situ* thrombosis vascular reconstruction is often necessary. Complete knowledge of the stage of the tumor is valuable because complex vascular reconstruction may be ill advised in patients with a short life expectancy. The use of vascular reconstruction in these cases may be limited by contraindications to anticoagulation, real or potential wound healing problems, compromised immune system, and sepsis.

EMBOLIC ARTERIAL OCCLUSION

Nonbacterial thrombotic endocarditis is frequently found in patients with malignant tumors. Emboli arising from this lesion represent the second most common cause of ischemic cerebral infarction in patients with cancer.[134] Aphasia with or without hemiparesis was the most common symptom in these patients. Others presented with diffuse, nonspecific symptoms of confusion, coma, or lethargy.[137] This condition is seen most commonly with pulmonary and gastric carcinomas.[138] The mitral valve was involved most frequently, but antecedent valvular lesions may predispose to this condition. Anticoagulation is helpful for the subset of patients with cerebral infarction related to nonbacterial thrombotic endocarditis, and this treatment did not appear to increase the risk of cerebral hemorrhage.[137] Peripheral emboli such as those producing the blue toe syndrome may also arise from nonbacterial endocarditis or from macroemboli forming on nonocclusive atherosclerotic plaque. Patients with evidence of peripheral embolization require a thorough work-up including complete arteriography, CT imaging of the aorta and its major branches, and echocardiography to identify valvular or vascular lesions that could act as sources of emboli. The identification of a single source for embolization is not always possible, and the diagnosis may be one of exclusion. When arterial plaque or aneurysm are suspected to be the source of emboli, these lesions should be treated with exclusion and bypass grafting. Patients found to have valvular heart disease and those with no obvious lesion are treated with long-term anticoagulation therapy. The development of epithelial bleeding in the gastrointestinal, the genitourinary, or the respiratory tract while on anticoagulation treatment for a an idiopathic arterial embolus may be a clue to the presence of an underlying malignancy. A thorough diagnostic evaluation of such bleeding is indicated.

Vascular Reconstruction Associated with Radical En Bloc Resections

As surgeons have struggled to expand the availability of functional and limb-sparing curative resectional approaches to more patients with advanced malignancies, it has become clear that the only remaining limitations on the extent of such procedures are the preservation of innervation, and the ability to obtain adequate soft tissue coverage. Safe and reliable major vascular, bony, and soft tissue reconstruction is possible in almost all cases. Combined major vascular reconstruction arises in two main situations: (1) resection of large head and neck tumors with possible invasion of the carotid, and (2) limb-sparing resection of large tumors of the extremities. A team approach is the key to success. Preoperative vascular evaluation should include standard noninvasive tests of arterial and venous function, duplex imaging of the arteries and veins and arteriography. In certain cases, duplex imaging of the superficial veins can identify a suitable conduit for autogenous vascular reconstruction, and transcranial Doppler examination can evaluate intracranial collateralization patterns. In cases of suspected involvement of the carotid arteries with tumor, temporary balloon occlusion of the involved vessel in the angiography suite with the patient awake can help determine whether the carotid can be ligated safely. Careful planning of the closure of the wound with well-vascularized muscle flaps will prevent wound breakdown in most situations. All arterial suture lines and the full length of any arterial conduit must be covered by healthy tissue. Carotid bypass with autogenous saphenous vein is the preferred operation if the carotid artery must be removed. The incidence of perioperative stroke in cases of carotid reconstruction after excision of bulky neck tumors with carotid involvement is 7% to 15%.[139–141] Standard arterial bypass techniques are used for revascularization of the extremity after limb-sparing resection of cancers of the extremity (Fig. 11-7) [142,143]. Autogenous saphenous vein harvested from the contralateral extremity is the preferred conduit. If the accompanying deep veins are patent venous reconstruction can be considered. In many cases the main deep vein has been occluded by the tumor for some time and alternative venous channels have developed. If venous reconstruction is not performed, the leg should be wrapped with elastic bandages and elevated to promote venous drainage and to avoid edema.

Arterial rupture is a well-known complication of the treatment of primary carcinoma in the head and neck region,[68] but may occur in other areas including the iliac and femoral arteries. The setting for this complication usually requires a combination of radiation therapy and infection or exposure of the involved artery. McCready et al[68] described the classic setting in which carotid artery rupture would be observed. The typical patient would have external beam radiation therapy to the neck followed several weeks later by primary excision of the tumor with a concomitant radical neck dissection. This would be followed by development of breakdown in the oral wound with development of an orocutaneous fistula, infection of the skin flaps, and infection or exposure of the carotid arteries. Carotid rupture is associated with exsanguinating hemorrhage and a significant risk for stroke with either prophylactic or therapeutic arterial ligation. Arterial reconstruction is compromised by the presence of an infected field and the generally poor healing of the radiated tissues. This devastating complication is reported much less frequently today owing to strategic modifications in the approach to patients with this problem. The use of immediate wound closure with well-vascularized muscle tissue obtained

Vascular Problems in the Cancer Patient 241

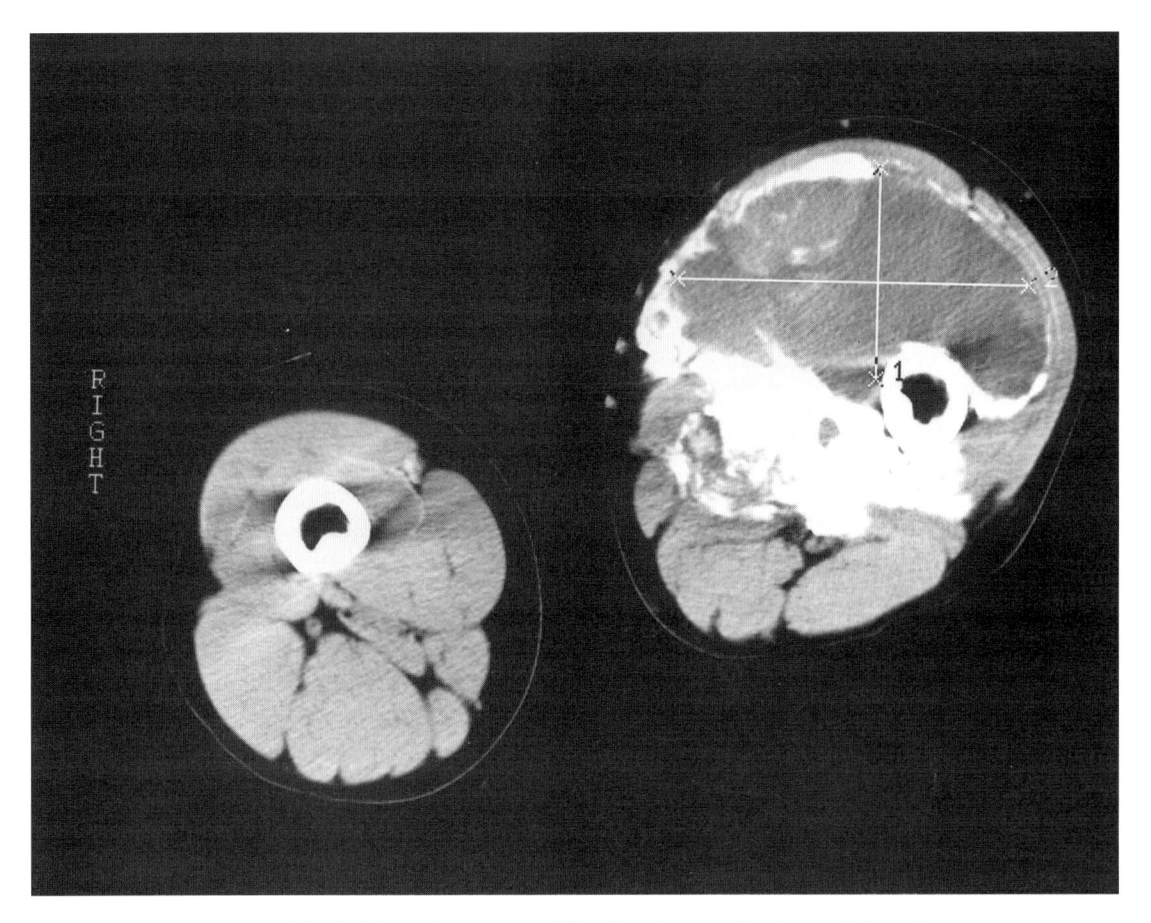

Figure 11-7. A CT scan of the left leg of a 17-year-old girl with an enlarging painless distal thigh mass. A large osteosarcoma of the femur is seen with obliteration of the superficial femoral vein and encasement of the superficial femoral artery in bony tumor.

from outside the radiated field to provide coverage to underlying critical structures has reduced the incidence of this complication dramatically.

Concomitant Vascular Conditions in Patients With Cancer

Occasionally, patients with cancer may have concomitant vascular disease. This situation will probably occur more frequently with the changing demographics of the American population and the continued high prevalence of both cancer and atherosclerosis in the population. In general, both conditions should be treated as completely as possible to obtain the best long-term survival. Additional factors may come into play when considering vascular reconstruction in patients with malignancy. These patients may have a limited life expectancy and may suffer from significant physical debility that would make extensive revascularization either impractical or ill-advised. Some patients with cancer harbor life-threatening vascular conditions, such as an abdominal aortic aneurysm (Fig. 11-8). Surgery for such concomitant conditions should be staged in almost all cases. Simultaneous surgery on an alimentary tract cancer and on the vascular system entails an unacceptably high risk of contamination of the graft with the attendant high-risk of sub-

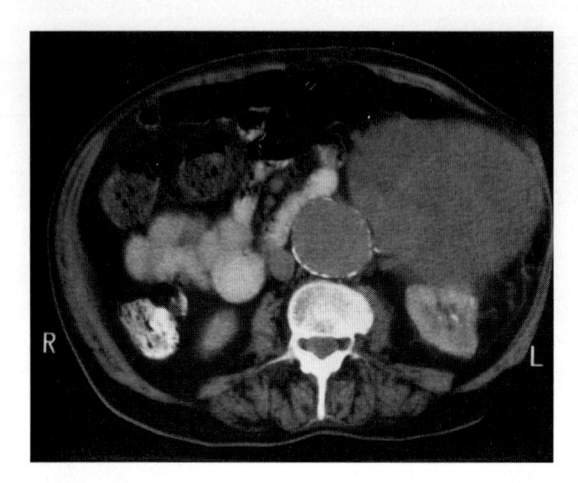

Figure 11-8. Abdominal CT scan of a 67-year-old man with a large painless left flank mass. There is a large homogeneous soft tissue mass in the retroperitoneum that displaces both the spleen and the left kidney. A 6-cm infrarenal abdominal aortic aneurysm is also noted.

sequent life-threatening graft infection. Generally, the symptomatic problem should be treated first.[144–146] Thus, cancers with obstruction or significant bleeding, or aneurysms with recent changes in caliber or with pain and tenderness are resected first. Other acute vascular conditions may occur in patients with cancer including transient ischemic attack, myocardial infarction, and lower extremity ischemia and gangrene. In each case, standard vascular reconstructions are possible but the underlying malignancy may reduce the expected gain from reconstruction. On the other hand, correction of the vascular lesions can significantly improve the patient's life expectancy and functional status and may reduce the risk of any necessary treatments for the cancer.

Accelerated Chronic Arterial Occlusive Disease

Accelerated atherosclerosis related to cancer or its treatment is managed using the same principals that guide the treatment of occlusive arterial disease in other patients. The standard indications for revascularization of peripheral vascular occlusive disease also apply to the treatment of the accelerated atherosclerotic lesions that may develop after radiation therapy for malignancy. Despite this, the technical aspects of the reconstruction in these cases may be quite different. Radiation-induced accelerated atherosclerosis is seen in two clinical areas: (1) the cervical carotid arteries after radiation therapy for cancers of the head and neck,[147,148] and (2) the iliac arteries in the pelvis after external beam or intracavitary radiation for pelvic malignancies in women. Radiation-induced changes affect the entire portion of the artery in the radiated field and thus the distribution of the occlusive disease may be more extensive. The usual inflow arteries may be involved with disease or unavailable and extra-anatomic approaches may be needed. The customary sites for vascular incisions may be in irradiated skin with little subcutaneous tissue, such as after treatment of a neck tumor with a standard radical neck dissection and radiation therapy. The arteries may be encased in dense fibrous scar tissue, thereby limiting dissection. Complications of the original treatment may further challenge the surgeon, as in the case of neck fistulas after composite resections or bowel or bladder fistulas after pelvic surgery. A complete understanding of the previous treatments and complete vascular evaluation are essential for success in these cases.

SUMMARY: CLINICAL VASCULAR SYNDROMES ASSOCIATED WITH CANCER

1. Hemorrhage may be the principal cause of death in as many as 11% of patients with cancer.
2. Venous thromboembolism is a major source of morbidity and mortality among cancer patients, with resultant pulmonary embolism as the cause of death in ap-

proximately 7% of patients with cancer. Duplex ultrasonography is an excellent diagnostic tool. The treatment is primarily anticoagulation. The Greenfield vena caval filter may be a necessary alternative in patients with contraindications to, complications of, or failure of anticoagulation therapy. All hospitalized patients with cancer are at increased risk for the development of DVT.
3. Thrombi may form in large vessels as a result of the interaction of a hypercoagulable state due to malignancy and plaque-related initiators of thrombosis, resulting in acute limb or organ ischemia.
4. Combined major vascular reconstruction with tumor resection is important in resection of large head and neck tumors and limb-sparing resection of extremity tumors.

SUMMARY

Problems affecting the vascular system are frequent complications of tumors or the treatment of tumors. The association of venous thrombosis and malignancy was noted in 1865 by Trousseau.[1] Although tumors of blood vessels are rare, they deserve consideration. Those that frequently involve small vessels are usually benign, present in childhood, and often spontaneously regress. Most tumors of large vessels arise from smooth muscle and are leiomyosarcomas or malignant fibrous histiocytomas. These tumors are much more common in veins than in arteries. Paragangliomas of the carotid bifurcation are usually benign but because of their location and growth may cause significant morbidity. Resection may require reconstruction of the internal carotid artery. Atrial myxomas are usually found in the left atrium and may present with congestive heart failure (secondary to obstruction) or embolization. Excision is the treatment of choice.

In addition to primary vascular tumors, there are a number of secondary vascular conditions related to malignancy that may complicate treatment of a tumor, or once they occur, require further therapy. Tumor cells elaborate a wide variety of vasoactive and angiogenic substances. These molecules are targets for novel therapeutic approaches. A state of subclinical DIC may be common to many patients with malignancy owing to increased circulating levels of clotting factors, with thrombosis as a likely outcome. Furthermore, there appears to be an acceleration of atherosclerosis in patients with malignancy, although there is no apparent explanation at this time. Tumors have effects on vessels by direct mechanical compression which may result in venous obstruction or hemodynamically significant obstruction to arterial flow. The nutritional depletion so often associated with malignancy may result in decreased levels of circulating coagulation factors with resultant thrombotic or hemorrhagic complications. Radiation therapy, chemotherapy, and surgery are major therapeutic modalities used in the treatment of cancer, and all may have significant effects on the vascular system.

There are a number of clinical vascular syndromes associated with cancer. Hemorrhage may be the principal cause of death in up to 11% of cancer patients. Venous thromboembolism is a significant problem in cancer patients. Pulmonary embolism is the principal cause of death in approximately 7% of patients with cancer. Interestingly, 17% of patients with recurrent idiopathic DVT were found to have a malignancy within 2 years of initial presentation. Thus, all patients with known cancer are at increased risk for the development of DVT. Duplex ultrasound is an important diagnostic modality for the identification of DVT. Anticoagulation is the standard therapy for both DVT and PE in the cancer patient. Unfortunately, there are a number of complications of anticoagulation therapy including hemorrhage and thrombocytopenia, which necessitate the use of alternative therapeutic modalities. The Greenfield vena caval filter has been widely used with good results. Prophylaxis with heparin or intermittent mechanical compression devices remains important.

The use of extensive resectional therapy in the treatment of tumors often necessitates careful consideration of the involvement of vascular structures. Combined major vascular reconstruction arises in cases of resection of large head and neck tumors and in the limb-sparing resections of large tumors of the extremities. A team approach to these situations is the key to successful resection and preservation of vascular integrity and function.

Consideration of the effects of tumors and cancer therapy on the vascular and coagulation systems is an integral part of the surgical management of the cancer patient. These problems remain a significant source of morbidity and mortality in the cancer patient, as well as a common reason for surgical consultation.

REFERENCES

1. Trousseau A. Phlegmasia alba dolens. In: Clinque Medicale de l'Hotel-Dieu de Paris. Vol 3. Paris: JB Bailliere, 1865:654.
2. Enzinger FM, Weiss SW. Soft tissue tumors. St Louis: CV Mosby, 1988:489.
3. Symposium on vascular malformations and melanotic lesions. Vol 22. St Louis: CV Mosby:1983.
4. Safai B, Miké V, Giraldo G, Beth E, Good RA. Association of Kaposi's sarcoma with second primary malignancies: possible etiopathogenic implications. Cancer 1980;45:1472.
5. Fenoglio JJ Jr, Virmani R. Primary malignant tumors of the great vessels. In: Waller BF, ed. Pathology of the heart and great vessels. New York: Churchill Livingstone, 1988:429.
6. McAllister HA, Fenoglio JJ. Tumors of the cardiovascular system. In Atlas of tumor pathology, 2nd series, fasc 15. Washington, DC: Armed Forces Institute of Pathology, 1978.
7. Raaf JH. Soft tissue sarcomas: diagnosis and treatment. St Louis: Mosby, 1993:123.
8. Kevorkian J, Cento DP. Leiomyosarcoma of large arteries and veins. Surgery 1973;73:390.
9. Novick AC, Kaye MC, Cosgrove DM, et al. Experience with cardiopulmonary bypass and deep hypothermic circulatory arrest in the management of retroperitoneal tumors with large vena caval thrombi. Ann Surg 1990;212:472.
10. Kaku K, Kawashima Y, Kitamura S, et al. Resection of leiomyosarcoma originating in internal iliac vein and extending into heart via inferior vena cava. Surgery 1981;89:604.
11. Nonomura A, Kurumaya H, Kono N, et al. Primary pulmonary artery sarcoma: report of two autopsy cases studied by immunohistochemistry and electron microscopy, and review of 110 cases reported in the literature. Acta Pathol Jpn 1988;38:883.
12. Schipper J, van Oostayen JA, den Hollander JC, van Seyen AJ. Aortic tumours: report of a case and review of the literature. Br J Radiol 1989;62:35.
13. Mason MS, Wheeler JR, Gregory RT, Gayle RG. Primary tumors of the aorta: report of a case and review of the literature. Oncology 1982;39:167.
14. Shamblin WR, ReMine WH, Sheps SG, Harrison EG Jr. Carotid body tumor (chemodectoma): clinicopathologic analysis of ninety cases. Am J Surg 1971;122:732.
15. Barry R, Pienaar A, Pienaar C, Browning NG, Nel CJC. Duplex doppler investigation of suspected lesions at the carotid bifurcation. Ann Vasc Surg 1993;7:140.
16. Worsey MJ, Laborde AL, Bower T, et al. An evaluation of color duplex scanning in the primary diagnosis and management of carotid body tumors. Ann Vasc Surg 1992;6:90.
17. Derichi LE, Serafini G, Rabbia C, et al. Carotid body tumors: US evaluation. Radiology 1992;182:457.
18. Williams MD, Phillips MJ, Nelson WR, Rainer WG. Carotid body tumor. Arch Surg 1992;127:963.
19. LaMuraglia GM, Fabian RL, Brewster DC, et al. The current surgical management of carotid body paragangliomas. J Vasc Surg 1992;15:1038.
20. Bishop GB Jr, Urist MM, El Gammal T, Peters GE, Maddox WA. Paragangliomas of the neck. Arch Surg 1992;127:1441.
21. Tillmanns H. Clinical aspects of cardiac tumors. Thorac Cardiovasc Surg 1990;38:152.
22. Blondeau P. Primary cardiac tumors–French studies of 533 cases. Thorac Cardiovasc Surg 1990;38:192.
23. Silverman NA. Primary cardiac tumors. Ann Surg 1980;191:127.
24. MacGowan SW, Sidhu P, Aherne T, et al. Atrial myxoma: national incidence, diagnosis and surgical management. Ir J Med Sci 1993;162:223.
25. St John Sutton MG, Mercier L-A, Giuliani ER,

Lie JT. Atrial myxomas: a review of clinical experience in 40 patients. Mayo Clin Proc 1980;55:371.
26. Bulkley BH, Hutchins GM. Atrial myxoma: a fifty-year review. Am Heart J 1979;97:639.
27. Desousa AL, Muller J, Campbell RL, Batnitzky S, Rankin L. Atrial myxoma: a review of the neurological complications, metastases and recurrences. J Neurol Nuerosurg Psychiatry 1978;41:1119.
28. Diflo T, Cantelmo NL, Haudenschild CC, Watkins MT. Atrial myxoma with remote metastasis: case report and review of the literature. Surgery 1992;111:352.
29. Rienmüller R, Tiling R. MR and CT for detection of cardiac tumors. Thorac Cardiovasc Surg 1990;38:168.
30. Folkman J, Shing Y. Angiogenesis. J Biol Chem 1992;267:10931.
31. Dvorak HF, Nagy JA, Berse B, et al. Vascular permeability factor, fibrin, and the pathogenesis of tumor stroma formation. Ann N Y Acad Sci 1992;667:101.
32. Liotta LA, Steeg PS, Stetler-Stevenson WG. Cancer metastasis and angiogenesis: an imbalance of positive and negative regulation. Cell 1991;64:327.
33. Costantini V, Zacharski LR. Fibrin and cancer. Thromb Haemost 1993;69:406.
34. Ellis V, Pyke C, Eriksen J, Solberg H, Danq K. The urokinase receptor: involvement in cell surface proteolysis and cancer invasion. Ann N Y Acad Sci 1992;667:13.
35. Clowes AW, Karnowsky MJ. Suppression by heparin of smooth muscle cell proliferation in injured arteries. Nature 1977;265:625.
36. Folkman J, Langer R, Linhardt RJ, Haudenschild C, Taylor S. Angiogenesis inhibition and tumor regression caused by heparin or a heparin fragment in the presence of cortisone. Science 1983;221:719.
37. Green D, Hull RD, Brant R, Pineo GF. Lower mortality in cancer patients treated with low-molecular-weight versus standard heparin. Lancet 1992;339:1476.
38. Denekamp J. Angiogenesis, neovascular proliferation and vascular pathophysiology as targets for cancer therapy. Br J Radiol 1993;66:181.
39. Zacharski LR, Costantini V, Wojtukiewicz MZ, Memoli VA, Kudryk BJ. Anticoagulants as cancer therapy. Semin Oncol 1990;17:217.
40. Fan TP. Angiosuppressive therapy for cancer. Trends Pharmacol Sci 1994;15:33.
41. Weinstat-Saslow D, Steeg PS. Angiogenesis and colonization in the tumor metastatic process: basic and applied advances. FASEB J 1994;8:401.
42. Karnowsky MJ, Wright TC Jr, Casellot JJ Jr, Choay J, Lormeau J-C, Petitou M. Heparin, heparin sulfate, smooth muscle cells and atherosclerosis. Ann N Y Acad Sci 1989;556:268.
43. Gordon SG. Cancer cell procoagulants and their role in malignant disease. Semin Thromb Hemost 1992;18:424.
44. Kunkel LA. Acquired circulating anticoagulants in malignancy. Semin Thromb Hemost 1992;18:416.
45. Bick RL. Coagulation abnormalities in malignancy: a review. Semin Thromb Hemost 1992;18:353.
46. Luzzatto G, Schafer AI. The prethrombotic state in cancer. Semin Oncol 1990;17:147.
47. Ey FS, Goodnight SH. Bleeding disorders in cancer. Semin Oncol 1990;17:187.
48. Pineo GF, Brain MC, Gallus AS. Tumors, mucus production and hypercoagulability. Ann N Y Acad Sci 1974;230:262.
49. Slickter SJ, Harker LA. Hemostasis in malignancy. Ann N Y Acad Sci 1974;230:252.
50. Sack GH Jr, Levin J, Bell WR. Trousseau's syndrome and other manifestations of chronic disseminated coagulopathy in patients with neoplasms: clinical, pathological and therapeutic features. Medicine 1977;56:1.
51. Nand S, Fisher SG, Salgia R, Fisher RI. Hemostatic abnormalities in untreated cancer: incidence and correlation with thrombotic and hemorrhagic complications. J Clin Oncol 1987;5:1998.
52. Bick RL. Alterations of hemostasis in malignancy. In: Disorders of thrombosis and hemostasis: clinical and laboratory practice. Chicago: ASCP Press, 1992;239.
53. Patrick RL, Kirshner N. Effect of stimulation on levels of TH, DA Bholase, and CA in intact and denervated rat adrenal glands. Mol Pharmacol 1970;7:87.
54. Callander NS, Varki N, Rao VM. Immunohistochemical identification of tissue factor in solid tumors. Cancer 1992;70:1194.
55. Cavanaugh PG, Sloane BF, Bajkowski AS, Taylor JD, Honn KV. Purification and characterization of platelet aggregating activity from tumor cells: copurification with procoagulant activity. Thromb Res 1985;37:309.
56. Bastida E, Ordinas A. Platelet contribution to the formation of metastatic foci: the role of cancer-induced platelet activation. Haemostasis 1988;18:29.
57. Gralnick HR. Von Willebrand factor, integrins, and platelets: their role in cancer. J Lab Clin Med 1992;119:444.
58. Zacharski LR, Wojtukiewicz MZ, Costantini V, Ornstein DL, Memoli VA. Pathways of coagulation/fibrinolysis activation in malignancy. Semin Thromb Hemost 1992;18:104.
59. Fuster V, Badimon L, Cohen M, Ambrose JA,

Badimon JJ, Chesebro J. Insights into the pathogenesis of acute ischemic syndromes. Circulation 1988;77:1213.
60. Falk E. Dynamics of thrombus formation. Ann N Y Acad Sci 1992;669:204.
61. Falk E. Unstable angina with fatal outcome: dynamic coronary thrombosis leading to infarction and/or sudden death. Autopsy evidence of recurrent mural thrombosis with peripheral embolization culminating in total vascular occlusion. Circulation 1985;71:699.
62. Lusby RJ. Lesions, dynamics and pathogenic mechanisms responsible for ischemic events in the brain. In: Moore WS, ed. Surgery for cerebrovascular disease. New York: Churchill Livingstone, 1987:51.
63. Naschitz JE, Schechter L, Chang JB. Intermittent claudication associated with cancer–case studies. Angiology 1987;9:696.
64. Naschitz JE, Yeshurun D, Abrahamson J, et al. Ischemic heart disease precipitated by occult cancer. Cancer 1992;69:2712.
65. Flinn WR, McDaniel MD, Yao JST, Fahey VA, Green D. Antithrombin III deficiency as a reflection of dynamic protein metabolism in patients undergoing vascular reconstruction. J Vasc Surg 1984;1:888.
66. Lindsay S, Kohn HI, Dakin RL, Jew J. Aortic arteriosclerosis in the dog after localized aortic X-irradiation. Circ Res 1962;10:51.
67. Lindsay S, Entenman C, Ellis EE, Geraci CL. Aortic arteriosclerosis in the dog after localized aortic irradiation with electrons. Circ Res 1962;10:61.
68. McCready RA, Hyde GL, Bivins BA, Mattingly SS, Griffen WO Jr. Radiation-induced arterial injuries. Surgery 1983;93:306.
69. Pettersson F, Swedenborg J. Atherosclerotic occlusive disease after radiation for pelvic malignancies. Acta Chir Scand 1990;156:367.
70. Silverberg GD, Britt RH, Goffinet DR. Radiation-induced carotid artery disease. Cancer 1978;41:130.
71. Gold H. Production of atherosclerosis in the rat. Effect of x-ray and a high fat diet. Arch Pathol 1961;71:268.
72. Loftus CM, Biller J, Hart MN. Management of radiation-induced accelerated carotid atherosclerosis. Arch Neurol 1987;44:711.
73. Killeen JD, Smith LL. Management of contiguous malignancy, radiation damage, and infection involving the carotid artery. Semin Vasc Surg 1991;4:123.
74. Eby CS. A review of the hypercoagulable state. Hematol Oncol Clin North Am 1993;7:1121.
75. Ambrus JL, Ambrus CM, Mink IB, Pickren JW. Causes of death in cancer patients. J Med 1975;6:61.
76. Svendsen E, Karwinski B. Prevalence of pulmonary embolism at necropsy in patients with cancer. J Clin Pathol 1989;42:805.
77. Gore JM, Appelbaum JS, Greene HL, Dexter L, Dalen JE. Occult cancer in patients with acute pulmonary embolism. Ann Intern Med 1982;96:556.
78. Goldberg RJ, Seneff M, Gore JM, et al. Occult malignant neoplasm in patients with deep venous thrombosis. Arch Intern Med 1987;147:251.
79. Griffin MR, Stanson AW, Brown ML, et al. Deep venous thrombosis and pulmonary embolism, risk of subsequent malignant neoplasms. Arch Intern Med 1987;147:1907.
80. Prandoni P, Lensing AWA, Buller HR, et al. Deep-vein thrombosis and the incidence of subsequent symptomatic cancer. N Engl J Med 1992;327:1128.
81. Aderka D, Brown A, Zelikovski A, Pinkhas J. Idiopathic deep vein thrombosis in an apparently healthy patient as a premonitory sign of occult cancer. Cancer 1986;57:1846.
82. Monreal M, Lafoz E, Casals A, et al. Occult cancer in patients with deep venous thrombosis: a systematic approach. Cancer 1991;67:541.
83. Wheeler HB, Anderson FA Jr. Impedance plethysmography. In: Kempczinski RF, Yao JST, eds. Practical noninvasive vascular diagnosis. Chicago: Year Book, 1987:407.
84. Hull RD, Hirsh J, Carter CJ, et al. Diagnostic efficacy of impedance plethysmography for clinically suspected deep-vein thrombosis: a randomized trial. Ann Intern Med 1985;102:21.
85. van Leeuwen MS. Doppler ultrasound in the evaluation of portal hypertension. In: Taylor KJW, Strandness DE Jr, eds. Duplex Doppler ultrasound. New York: Churchill Livingstone, 1990:53.
86. Lilly MP. Duplex evaluation of visceral vascular disorders. In: Strandness DE Jr, van Breda A, eds. Vascular diseases: surgical and interventional therapy. New York: Churchill Livingstone, 1994:751.
87. Killewich LA, Bedford GR, Beach KW, Strandness DE Jr. Diagnosis of deep venous thrombosis: a prospective study comparing duplex scanning to contrast venography. Circulation 1989;79:810.
88. Rose SC, Zwiebel WJ, Nelson BD, et al. Symptomatic lower extremity deep venous thrombosis: accuracy, limitations and role of color duplex flow imaging in diagnosis. Radiology 1990;175:639.
89. Comerota AJ, Katz ML, Greenwald LL, Leefmans E, Czeredarczuk M, White JV. Venous duplex imaging: should it replace hemody-

namic tests for deep venous thrombosis? J Vasc Surg 1990;11:53.
90. Hull RD, Raskob GE, Coates G, Panju AA. Clinical validity of a normal perfusion lung scan in patients with suspected pulmonary embolism. Chest 1990;97:23.
91. PIOPED Investigators. Value of the ventilation/perfusion scan in acute pulmonary embolism: results of the prospective investigation of pulmonary embolism diagnosis (PIOPED). JAMA 1990;263:2753.
92. Hull RD, Raskob GE, Hirsh J, et al. Continuous intravenous heparin compared with intermittent heparin in the initial treatment of proximal-vein thrombosis. N Engl J Med 1986;315:1109.
93. Gallus A, Jackaman J, Tillet J, Mills W, Wycherley A. Safety and efficacy of warfarin started early after submassive venous thrombosis or pulmonary embolism. Lancet 1986; II:1293.
94. Hull RD, Raskob GE, Rosenbloom D, et al. Heparin for 5 days as compared with 10 days in the initial treatment of proximal venous thrombosis. N Engl J Med 1990;322:1260.
95. Levine MN, Hirsh J. Hemorrhagic complications of anticoagulant therapy. Semin Thromb Hemost 1986;12:39.
96. Moore FD, Osteen RT, Karp DD, Steel G Jr, Wilson RE. Anticoagulants, venous thromboembolism, and the cancer patient. Arch Surg 1981;116:405.
97. Schmitt BP, Adelman B. Heparin-associated thrombocytopenia: a critical review and pooled analysis. Am J Medical Sci 1993; 305:208.
98. Warkentin TE, Kelton JG. Heparin-induced thrombocytopenia. Ann Rev Med 1989;40:31.
99. Demasi R, Bode AP, Knupp C, Bogey W, Powell S. Heparin-induced thrombocytopenia. Am Surg 1994;60:26.
100. Silver D. Heparin induced thrombocytopenia and thrombosis. Semin Vasc Surg 1988;1:228.
101. Cola C, Ansell J. Heparin-induced thrombocytopenia and arterial thrombosis: alternative therapies. Am Heart J 1990;119:368.
102. Cole CW, Fournier LM, Bormanis J. Heparin-associated thrombocytopenia and thrombosis: optimal therapy with ancrod. Can J Surg 1990;33:207.
103. Adamson DJA, Currie JM. Occult malignancy is associated with venous thrombosis unresponsive to adequate anticoagulation. Br J Clin Pract 1993;47:190.
104. Hicks ME, Dorfman GS. Vena caval filters. In: Strandness DE Jr, van Breda A, eds. Vascular diseases: surgical and interventional therapy. New York: Churchill Livingstone, 1994:1017.
105. Pais OP, Tobin KD, Austin CB, Queral LA. Percutaneous insertion of the Greenfield inferior vena cava filter: experience with ninety-six patients. J Vasc Surg 1988;8:460.
106. Dorfman GS. Percutaneous inferior vena cava filters. Radiology 1990;174:987.
107. Greenfield LJ, Michna BA. Twelve year clinical experience with the Greenfield vena cava filter. Surgery 1988;104:706.
108. Greenfield LJ, Cho KJ, Proctor MC, Sobel M, Shah S, Wingo J. Late results of suprarenal Greenfield vena cava filter placement. Arch Surg 1992;127:969.
109. Kantor A, Glanz S, Gordon DH, Sclafani SJA. Percutaneous insertion of the Kimray-Greenfield filter: incidence of femoral vein thrombosis. AJR 1987;149:1065.
110. Cohen JR, Grella L, Citron M. Greenfield filter instead of heparin as primary treatment for deep venous thrombosis or pulmonary embolism in patients with cancer. Cancer 1992; 70:1993.
111. Hubbard KP, Roehm JOF Jr, Abbruzzese JL. The bird's nest filter, an alternative to long-term oral anticoagulation in patients with advanced malignancies. Am J Clin Oncol 1994;17:115.
112. Calligaro KD, Bergen WS, Haut MJ, Savarese RP, DeLaurentis DA. Thromboembolic complications in patients with advanced cancer: anticoagulation versus Greenfield filter placement. Ann Vasc Surg 1991;5:186.
113. GUSTO Investigators. An international randomized trial comparing four thrombolytic strategies for acute myocardial infarction. N Engl J Med 1993;329:673.
114. Ouriel K, Shortell CK, DeWeese JA, et al. A comparison of thrombolytic therapy with operative revascularization in the initial treatment of acute peripheral arterial ischemia. J Vasc Surg 1994;19:1021.
115. Anderson HV, Willerson JT. Thrombolysis in acute myocardial infarction. N Engl J Med 1993;329:703.
116. Semba CP, Dake MD. Iliofemoral deep venous thrombosis: aggressive therapy with catheter-directed thrombolysis. Radiology 1994;191:487.
117. Comerota AJ, Aldridge SC, Cohen G, Ball DS, Pliskin M, White JV. A strategy of aggressive regional therapy for acute iliofemoral venous thrombosis with contemporary venous thrombectomy or catheter-directed thrombolysis. J Vasc Surg 1994;20:244.
118. Hull RD, Pineo GF. Low-molecular-weight heparins for the treatment of venous thromboembolism. Ann Med 1993;25:457.
119. Hull RD, Raskob GE, Pineo GF, et al. Subcutaneous low-molecular-weight heparin com-

pared with continuous intravenous heparin in the treatment of proximal-vein thrombosis. N Engl J Med 1992;326:975.
120. Prandoni P, Lensing AWA, Büller HR, et al. Comparison of subcutaneous low-molecular-weight heparin with intravenous standard heparin in proximal deep-vein thrombosis. Lancet 1992;339:441.
121. Brockman SK, Vasko JS. The pathologic physiology of phlegmasia cerulea dolens. Surgery 1966;59:997.
122. Haimovici H. Treatment of ischemic deep venous thrombosis. In: Bergan JJ, Yao JST, eds. Surgery of the veins. Orlando: Grune & Stratton, 1985;165.
123. Stirnemann P, Althaus U, Kirchof B, Triller J, Nachbur B, Senn S. Early phlebographic results after iliofemoral venous thrombectomy. Thorac Cardiovasc Surg 1984;32:299.
124. Rqder OC, Lorentzen JE, Hansen HJB. Venous thrombectomy for iliofemoral thrombosis. Acta Chir Scand 1984;150:31.
125. Eklof B, Einarsson E, Plate G. Role of thrombectomy and temporary arteriovenous fistula in acute iliofemoral venous thrombosis. In: Bergan JJ, Yao ST, eds. Surgery of the veins. Orlando: Grune & Stratton, 1985:131.
126. Charnsangavej C, Carrasco CH, Wallace S, et al. Stenosis of the vena cava: preliminary assessment of treatment with expandable metallic stents. Radiology 1986;161:295.
127. Zollikofer CL, Largiader I, Bruhlmann WF, Uhlschmid GK, Marty AH. Endovascular stenting of veins and grafts: preliminary clinical experience. Radiology 1988;167:707.
128. Rösch J, Keller FS, Uchida BT, Barton RE. Interventional management of large venous obstruction. In: Strandness DE Jr, van Breda A, eds. Vascular diseases: surgical and interventional therapy. New York: Churchill Livingstone, 1994:999.
129. Hirsh J. Heparin. N Engl J Med 1991;324:1565.
130. Skillman JJ, Collins REC, Coe NP, et al. Prevention of deep venous thrombosis in neurosurgical patients: a controlled, randomized trial of external pneumatic compression boots. Surgery 1978;83:354.
131. Turpie AGG, Gallus AS, Beattie WS, Hirsh J. Prevention of venous thrombosis in patients with intracranial disease by intermittent pneumatic compression of the calf. Neurology 1977;27:435.
132. Greer JM, Longley S, Edwards NL, Elfenbein GJ, Panush RS. Vasculitis associated with malignancy, experience with 13 patients and literature review. Medicine 1988;67:220.
133. Taylor LM Jr, Hauty MG, Edwards JM, Porter JM. Digital ischemia as a manifestation of malignancy. Ann Surg 1987;206:62.
134. Graus F, Rogers LR, Posner JB. Cerebrovascular complications in patients with cancer. Medicine 1985;64:16.
135. Naschitz JE, Yeshurun D, Abrahamson J. Arterial occlusive disease in occult cancer. Am Heart J 1992;124:738.
136. Bergan JJ, McCarthy WJ III, Flinn WR, Yao JST. Nontraumatic mesenteric vascular emergencies. J Vasc Surg 1987;5:903.
137. Rogers LR, Cho E-S, Kempin S, Posner JB. Cerebral infarction from non-bacterial thrombotic endocarditis, clinical and pathological study including the effects of anticoagulation. Am J Med 1987;83:746.
138. Rosen P, Armstrong D. Nonbacterial thrombotic endocarditis in patients with malignant neoplastic diseases. Am J Med 1973;54:23.
139. McCready RA, Miller SK, Hamaker RC, Singer MI, Herod GT. What is the role of carotid arterial resection in the management of advanced cervical cancer? J Vasc Surg 1989;10:277.
140. Olcott C IV, Fee WE, Enzmann DR, Mehigan JT. Planned approach to the management of malignant invasion of the carotid artery. Am J Surg 1981;142:123.
141. Biller HF, Urken M, Lawson W, Haimov M. Carotid artery resection and bypass for neck carcinoma. Laryngoscope 1988;98:181.
142. Imparato AM, Roses DF, Francis KC, Lewis MM. Major vascular reconstruction for limb salvage in patients with soft tissue and skeletal sarcomas of the extremities. Surg Gynecol Obstet 1978; 147:891.
143. Nambisan RN, Karakousis CP. Vascular reconstruction for limb salvage in soft tissue sarcomas. Surgery 1987;101:668.
144. Nora JD, Pairolero PC, Nivatvongs S, Cherry KJ, Hallett JW, Gloviczki P. Concomitant abdominal aortic aneurysm and colorectal carcinoma: priority of resection. J Vasc Surg 1989;9:630.
145. Szilagyi DE, Elliott JP, Berguer R. Coincidental malignancy and abdominal aortic aneurysm. Arch Surg 1967;95:402.
146. Morris DM, Colquitt J. Concomitant abdominal aortic aneurysm and malignant disease: a difficult management problem. J Surg Oncol 1988;39:122.
147. Elerding SC, Fernandez RN, Grotta JC, Lindberg RD, Causay LC, McMurtrey MJ. Carotid artery disease following external cervical irradiation. Ann Surg 1981;194:609.
148. Loftus CM, Biller J, Hart MN, Cornell SH, Hiratzka LF. Management of radiation-induced accelerated carotid atherosclerosis. Arch Neurol 1987;44:711.

12

Thoracic Problems in the Cancer Patient

MICHAEL FIOCCO
MARK J. KRASNA

Patients with cancer often have problems that require consultation of a thoracic surgeon. The most common of these will be discussed in detail in this chapter. These include management of malignant pleural effusions, pericardial effusions and invasion, diseases of the mediastinum, metastatic diseases to the lung, and evaluation of interstitial type lung disease in patients with malignancies. The importance of preoperative evaluation, especially in many of these patients with compromised pulmonary function, cannot be overstated; further information on preoperative considerations is found in Chapter 13. Complications associated with central venous access, which may involve a thoracic surgery consultation are discussed in Chapter 9.

MALIGNANT PLEURAL EFFUSION

Malignant pleural effusions (MPE) are a significant cause of morbidity in patients with advanced cancer. Proper treatment may improve the quality of life in these debilitated patients. The most common types of cancer to cause MPE are lung and breast carcinoma, followed by lymphoma and adenocarcinoma of unknown primary.[1,2]

Normally, the pleural space contains approximately 10 mL of fluid with a protein content of 2 gm/dL. This relatively protein-free fluid is the result of the net hydrostatic-oncotic pressure of the capillaries of the parietal pleura moving fluid into the pleural space. The pulmonary venous capillaries reabsorb 80% to 90% of this fluid. The remainder of the fluid is reabsorbed by the pleural lymphatics.

In patients with MPE, several mechanisms lead to the development of effusion including increased capillary permeability (due to inflammation or disruption of the capillary endothelium) and impaired lymphatic drainage secondary to tumor obstruction. These mechanisms are generally due to direct invasion of the pleural space by primary or metastatic tumor.

Half of all pleural effusions in adults are due to malignancy and are exudates. Transudative effusions may also occur in cancer patients. Hypoalbuminemia from malnutrition, congestive heart failure, and liver disease secondary to metastases all may cause effusions. These transudative effusions usually are small and rarely become symptomatic.

Diagnosis

Most patients with malignant pleural effusions are symptomatic. Dyspnea, cough, and chest pain are the most common symptoms. Although the physical examination is useful in determining the presence of fluid in the pleural space, a chest x-ray study remains the most valuable screening tool.

Malignant pleural effusion may often be the initial manifestation of malignancy. Chernow and Sahn[3] reported that of 96 patients with malignant pleural effusion, 44 (46%) had no prior history of cancer. Martini et al[4] reported that effusion was the initial finding in 64% of their 106 patients. Only 5% of these patients were asymptomatic. Dyspnea was the most common symptom occurring in two thirds of patients.

Thoracentesis should be the first diagnostic procedure. It has a very high diagnostic yield and may also provide some relief from pulmonary compromise. Large effusions are easily drained with little risk via thoracentesis, although re-expansion pulmonary edema may occur if fluid is removed too rapidly.[5]

The conventional fluid sample tests for evaluating pleural effusion are cell count with differential, cytology, culture, and Gram stain; lactate dehydrogenase (LDH), protein, and glucose content. Pleural fluid pH is not a reliable indictor of malignancy.[6] The evaluation of pleural fluid will determine whether the fluid is a transudate or an exudate. Transudative effusions are most commonly caused by congestive heart failure, cirrhosis, or nephrotic syndrome, whereas exudate effusions are most commonly secondary to malignancy or to postpneumonic effusion empyema.

Cytology is the best way to diagnose malignant pleural effusion. At least 250 mL of fluid should be obtained for cytology, because lesser volumes often contain too few cells for adequate evaluation.[7] More than one thoracentesis may be needed before a cytologic diagnosis of malignancy can be made. An abnormality in cytogenetics indicates with high probability that the effusion is malignant. Unfortunately, cytogenetics is not widely available; it is expensive and requires approximately 5 days to complete. Pleural fluid cytogenetics should be reserved for effusions with negative cytology and negative pleural biopsy on two occasions, in which malignancy is still suspected. If cytogenetic studies are positive, a more aggressive diagnostic approach is justified.

Pleural biopsy using a Cope-Abrams needle is another diagnostic modality that may be warranted. This technique, however, may cause pneumothorax and the diagnostic yield is still relatively low.[8]

Thoracoscopy has become a more popular and readily available diagnostic technique with the advent of improved thoracoscopic equipment. It has a lower risk than thoracotomy and carries a diagnostic yield of 93% to 96%.[9] Thoracoscopy is usually carried out after two negative thoracenteses or primarily in patients with loculated pleural effusions.

Treatment

There are numerous reports in the literature[10–17] concerning the various conservative methods for the treatment of malignant pleural effusions. These studies differ markedly in their response criteria, method of evaluation, and the extent of follow-up, which makes any comparison of the different modalities difficult.

Paramount to the success of any of these methods are drainage of the effusion (as completely as possible) and re-expansion of the collapsed lung. These goals are best accomplished by tube thoracostomy, but thoracentesis may be effective. Both thoracostomy and thoracentesis have been shown not to be effective without any sclerotherapy for treatment of malignant pleural effusions. The recurrence rate is at least 60% and reaccumulation may occur as early as 3 days after tube removal.[4,10]

Various sclerosing agents have been instilled into the pleural space to treating malignant pleural effusions. These agents differ in both their sclerosing properties and their side effects. The most commonly used agents are tetracycline, doxycycline, talc, bleomycin, nitrogen mustard, doxorubicin, and corynebacterium parvum. An effective sclerosing agent creates a chemical pleuritis, resulting in adhesion of the visceral pleura to the parietal pleura, or so-called *pleural symphysis*. This obliteration of the pleural space prevents re-accumulation of fluid.

Lung excursion allows the sclerosant to be distributed evenly throughout the pleural space and frequent position changes after instillation of the agent should be reserved for those with trapped lung. Thoracotomy is the most effective means of drainage, lung re-expansion and maintenance of the pleural surfaces in opposition, whereas the sclerosant induces pleuritis. Prior to installation, chest tube drainage should be less than 100 to 200 mL/d. This will avoid dilution of the agent within the pleural space, which would reduce the sclerosants potency. The ideal agent for sclerotherapy should be safe to handle, have minimal side effects, and be highly effective in sclerosing the pleural surfaces.[11]

Tetracycline (TCN) has been used with great success for sclerotherapy in malignant pleural effusions, with success rates of 70% to 100%.[12,13] Unfortunately, tetracycline has only historical significance because intravenous tetracycline is no longer manufactured. Doxycycline has been used as a substitute at the University of Maryland, but the success rate has been lower. Both of these drugs have minimal side effects, with pain being the most common. This can be relieved to some degree by adding 10 mL of 1% xylocaine to the sclerosant prior to instillation.

Bleomycin is a useful agent as well, with response rates of 60% to 80%.[14,15] There were two deaths in these studies which were possibly drug related. Therefore, it is recommended that the intracavitary dose not exceed 40 mg/m^2. Intrapleural bleomycin is not myelosuppressive and the incidence of pain and fever are low. It is important to remember that in this setting, bleomycin functions only as an irritant to cause pleuritis, not as a cytotoxic agent.

Nitrogen mustard was one of the first agents used for the treatment of malignant pleural effusions. Response rates were low and this agent has fallen out of vogue. Thiotepa and 5-fluorouracil also have been found to have an inadequate response rate. Quinacrine is a highly effective sclerosant whose side effects (fever, pain) are frequent, severe, and long-lasting making its use prohibitive.

Talc most likely represents the most effective sclerosing agent currently available (Fig. 12-1). It causes an intense reactive pleuritis that obliterates the pleural space. Success rates from 80% to 100% have been achieved.[16,17] The negative aspects of talc pleurodesis are the need for general anesthesia and thoracoscopy for adequate instillation. Talc is difficult to obtain in a sterile form because it must be dry sterilized. An aerosolized delivery system is now available replacing the talc poudrage system. This has been used at the University of Maryland with 100% success so far.

Two prospective randomized trials are currently underway to identify the best treatment of malignant pleural effusion. The first protocol, an intergroup study, uses talc, bleomycin, or doxycycline. The second study compares talc slurry via chest tube with talc insufflation via thoracoscopy (Fig. 12-2). The

Figure 12-1. Thoracoscopic talc poudrage showing talc sclerosis of the both the parietal and the visceral pleura.

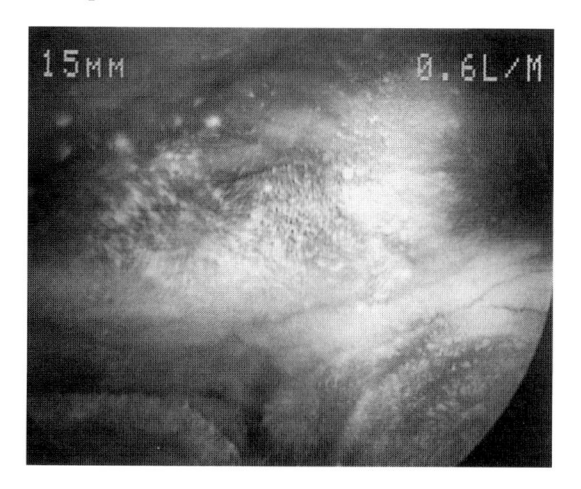

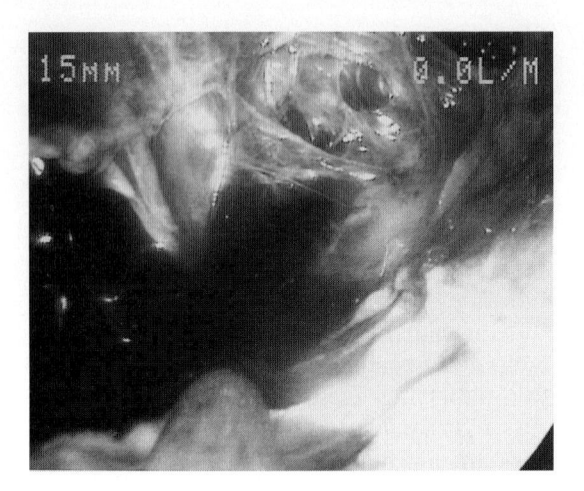

Figure 12-2. Thoracoscopic lysis of adhesions prior to draining a multiloculated effusion using an operating telescope.

results of these important studies will be available during the next few years and may identify the optimal treatment of malignant pleural effusion.

Pleurectomy should be reserved for those patients who have failed all other methods of control, can tolerate a major surgical procedure, and have a significant life expectancy. This obviously comprises a very small subset of these cancer patients. Martini et al[4] used pleurectomy in a select group of patients with 100% success (no recurrence of effusion). The mortality was 9.5% within 1 month of surgery and the complication rate was 23%. This high morbidity and mortality suggest

Figure 12-3. The Denver pleuroperitoneal shunt, which can also be used for pericardial drainage.

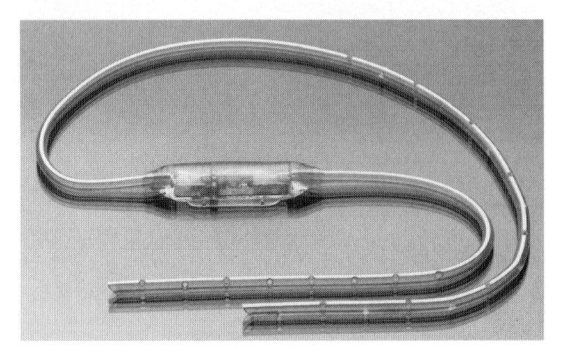

that strict patient selection be enforced if the procedure is to be performed at all.

An alternative in patients who do not respond to sclerotherapy and who are not candidates for general anesthesia or pleurectomy is the use of a pleuroperitoneal shunt (Fig. 12-3).[18] The flow of malignant cells into the peritoneum is inconsequential in these patients with limited life expectancy. Symptomatic relief is achieved if the patient is able to operate the subcutaneous pump, a simple task but not always possible for an elderly debilitated patient.

Finally, a recent report from the University of Toronto described outpatient placement of a Tenkhoff catheter into the pleural space in nine patients.[19] All patients were able to successfully drain their effusions periodically although some required the assistance of visiting nurses. Surprisingly, no infectious complications occurred and no significant pneumothoraces developed. This is certainly an alternative therapy worth further evaluation.

SUMMARY: MALIGNANT PLEURAL EFFUSION

1. Half of all pleural effusions in adults are due to malignancies and are exudates.
2. Most patients are symptomatic with dyspnea, cough, and chest pain. Chest x-ray is the best diagnostic tool. Thoracentesis should be the first procedure performed. Be sure to send the fluid for the "4 Cs": **C**ell count (with differential), **C**hemistry (LDH, protein, glucose), **C**ulture (with Gram stain) and **C**ytology.
3. The key to therapy is drainage of the effusion with re-expansion of the lung. The ideal sclerosing agent has yet to be identified, but talc may be the most effective agent currently available. Studies are currently underway to evaluate different agents.

MALIGNANT PERICARDIAL EFFUSION

Neoplasms may invade the heart by direct extension, by hematogenous spread, or most commonly, by metastasizing first to mediastinal lymph nodes and subsequently spreading retrograde to the heart via lymphatics.[20] The most common malignancies involving the heart and pericardium include carcinomas of the lung and breast, lymphoma, leukemia, and malignant melanoma.[21,22] These malignancies are usually widely metastatic by the time the heart is clinically involved.

Involvement of the pericardium by malignant neoplasm can take many forms. Pericardial effusion is the most frequently encountered manifestation.[21] The development of an effusion is insidious and the patients are therefore frequently asymptomatic. Fluid accumulation raises intrapericardial pressure, causing decreased diastolic filling of the ventricles, diminished stroke volume, and finally cardiac tamponade.

The symptoms associated with malignant pericardial effusion are nonspecific and frequently are attributed to the underlying malignancy. Nearly two thirds of these patients have no cardiovascular signs or symptoms.[23] Dyspnea occurs in 93% of symptomatic patients and is frequently associated with chest pain and cough. Signs of hemodynamic compromise include tachycardia, pulsus paradoxicus, hypotension, and elevated jugular venous pressure.[21–24]

Diagnosis

The electrocardiogram (ECG) is rarely diagnostic of malignant cardiac disease. It does, however, provide an early hint of inflammatory pericardial disease. Total electrical alternans with simultaneous alternation of both the P wave and QRS complex is considered by some to be pathognomonic of malignant pericardial effusion with tamponade; this is rarely seen.[25]

The chest roentgenogram may provide clues to the presence of a pericardial effusion, such as displacement of the pericardial fat pad or enlargement of the cardiac silhouette. A normal chest roentgenogram does not exclude the possibility of significant pericardial effusion. Fluoroscopy may show minimal pulsation of the cardiac borders with vigorous aortic pulsation suggesting tamponade.[26] Recently, computed tomography (CT) and magnetic resonance imaging (MRI) have been used more frequently to identify malignant invasion of the pericardium and differentiate these from effusions without pericardial thickening.

The echocardiogram is extremely sensitive in diagnosing pericardial effusion and should be performed on all patients with suspected malignant pericardial effusions. Other than determining the presence or absence of pericardial fluid, echocardiography also can reveal tumor masses and loculation of fluid. In addition, adhesions with evidence of a noncontracting segment can be identified. Hemodynamic compromise suggestive of tamponade is demonstrated by right atrial or right ventricular compression with decrease in left ventricular dimension, and failure of the inferior vena cava to collapse on deep inspiration.[27] Only 58% of patients with tamponade have the diagnosis made on the basis of CT scan. The pericardial fluid in these patients must then be evaluated for malignancy.

Cytologic evaluation of pericardial fluid yields a diagnosis with an 80% accuracy. Pericardial biopsy is positive in only 58% of patients with malignant pericardial effusion.[28] Lymphomas and mesothelioma are particularly prone to false-negative cytologic diagnosis.[21] For these reasons, larger pericardial biopsies often are needed independent of whether or not the patients have hemodynamic compromise.

Treatment

External beam irradiation has been advocated as the treatment of choice for malignant pericardial effusion regardless of cause. This does not relieve tamponade and offers only a 50% response rate at best.[29] As part of a long-term program to control effusions, systemic treatment with chemotherapy, hormonal therapy, or immunotherapy should be instituted as well. None of these modalities are effective in the patient with hemodynamic compromise. In these patients, surgical relief of tamponade should be undertaken.

Subxiphoid pericardiocentesis remains the mainstay of nonsurgical diagnosis and management. This procedure can be performed quickly, under local anesthesia, and it will relieve tamponade rapidly to improve cardiac performance in virtually all cases.[30] Major complications such as myocardial or coronary artery puncture, pneumothorax, and abdominal organ trauma can occur in up to 25% of patients. To decrease the morbidity, echocardiographic guidance is mandatory, proceeding with the procedure only when a significant (>1 cm) anterior effusion is present.[31] In addition, pericardiocentesis with an ECG lead hooked to the needle with an "alligator clip" detects the injury pattern as soon as the ventricle is touched.

Pericardiocentesis, however, is not a definitive treatment. Only 60% of effusions will be controlled by single or even repeated taps.[31] A multihole catheter can be inserted into the pericardium at the time of pericardiocentesis to allow drainage over several days with minimal infectious risk. One fourth of those patients treated with catheter drainage require surgical intervention to control their effusions.[32] A recent report[33] described the performance of a percutaneous balloon pericardiostomy forming a pericardiopleural window (Fig. 12-4). Numerous substances have been instilled into the pericardium as sclerosants to control effusions. Only tetracycline has demonstrated significant success, controlling effusions in 86% of cases.[34] Most of these patients require three or more treatments; 16% had significant pain despite premedication with xylocaine. Tetracycline is no longer manufactured in an intravenous form and is therefore currently unavailable in the United States. Doxycycline has been used at the University of Maryland in this setting with similar doses (500 mg to 1000 mg per instillation). Some success has been observed, but too few patients have received doxycycline to draw any conclusions. No prospective studies have been done to date.

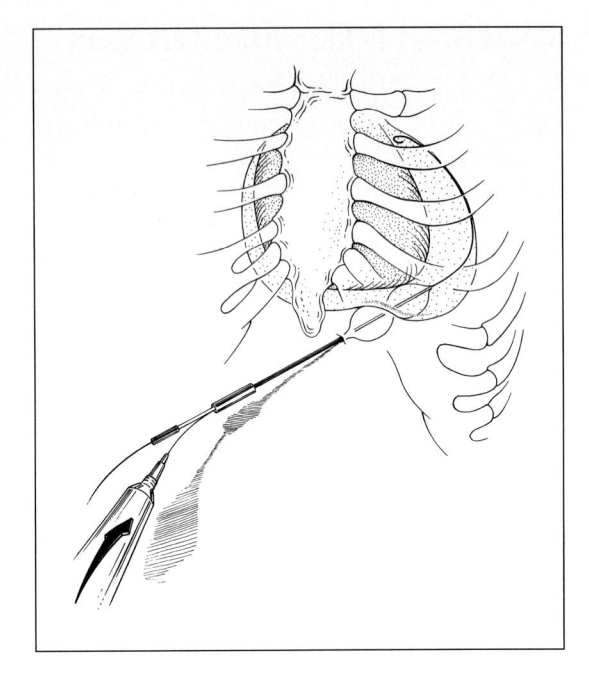

Figure 12-4. Balloon pericardiostomy using a guidewire and balloon catheter under fluoroscopic guidance. (From Ziskind AA, Pearce C, Lemmon CC, et al. Percutaneous balloon pericardiotomy for the treatment of cardiac tamponade and large pericardial effusions: description of technique and report of the first 50 cases. J Am Cardiol 1993;21:1; with permission.)

Surgical intervention with the creation of a pericardial window has been the most commonly used operative treatment for malignant pericardial effusion. An anterior thoracotomy approach for creation of a pleuropericardial window has been shown to alleviate symptoms in greater than 90% of patients.[35] Therefore, a similar procedure was recently performed at the University of Maryland using thoracoscopy instead of thoracotomy on a limited number of patients (Fig. 12-5).[36] This also allows treatment of ipsilateral pleural disease if it exists.[36]

Unfortunately, even this type of minimally invasive surgery requires general an-

Thoracic Problems in the Cancer Patient

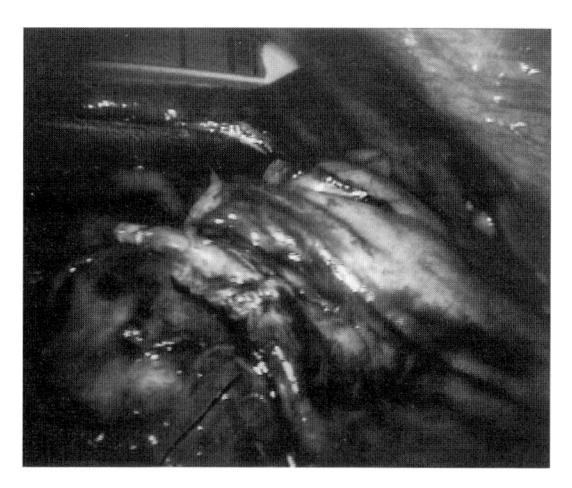

Figure 12-5. Thoracoscopic pericardiectomy using the ENDO-GIA stapler showing (*arrow*) exposed left atrium.

and pleura. This does not require retracting the ribs with all of the subsequent morbidity of a thoracotomy.

An adjunct to the subxiphoid pericardial window is the use of pericardioscopy. This has been reported to facilitate diagnosis and drain loculated areas by using a flexible bronchoscope to visualize the pericardium.[38] The procedure is probably only necessary in the patient who represents a diagnostic dilemma (Fig. 12-6).

Finally, for those patients whose malignant pericardial effusions are recalcitrant to all therapies, a pericardioperitoneal shunt can be inserted. Malignant pericardial effusions were drained in this manner in a small series of patients; the procedure was well tol-

esthesia (preferably with one-lung ventilation). This may be poorly tolerated by debilitated patients, often further compromised by their cancer and who also may be hemodynamically compromised by pericardial tamponade. For these patients, a subxiphoid approach with local anesthesia is often the safest approach.

Subxiphoid pericardiectomy has become the surgical treatment of choice for the majority of these patients. This procedure was initially described in 1829 by Larrey, a surgeon in Napoleon's army. He conducted stab wound experiments on cadavers and based the procedure on his research findings.[24] This can be performed rapidly and is well tolerated by critically ill patients. Diagnostic accuracy approaches 100% because both pericardial fluid and biopsy of the pericardium are available.[37] A small upper abdominal midline incision extended over the xiphoid process is used most often. Care is taken to identify the pericardium and a 4 × 4 cm biopsy is taken. The fluid is drained and a chest tube placed into the pericardium, which can generally be performed under local anesthesia. An alternative incision adds a subcostal extension to a midline incision. This approach allows excellent exposure for debridement decortication of the pericardium

Figure 12-6. Pericardioscopy (a flexible endoscope can also be used) used to help lyse adhesions and facilitate diagnosis of intrapericardiac disease. From Azorin J, Lamour A, Destbake MD, Morere F, de Saint Florent G. Pericardioscopy: definition, interest and result. Ann Chir 1988;42:137;reprinted with permission.

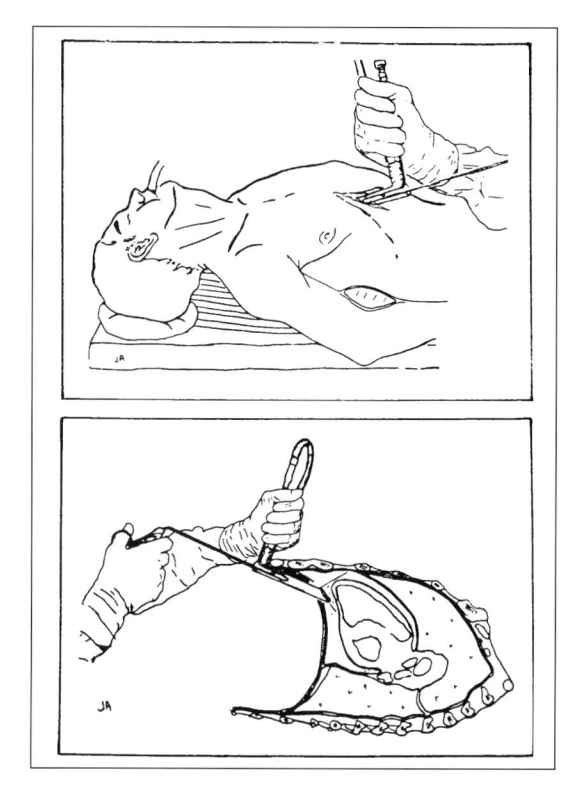

erated. It was performed under local anesthesia and the hospital stay was only 2 to 4 days with no complications.[39] This is a promising technique but requires a motivated patient to operate the subcutaneous pump. A larger prospective series of patients is needed before the advantages of this technique can be clarified.

SUMMARY: MALIGNANT PERICARDIAL EFFUSION

1. The symptoms of malignant pleural effusion are usually nonspecific. The echocardiogram is the best diagnostic test for patients with suspected malignant pleural effusion. Cytologic evaluation is usually indicated and is 80% accurate in the diagnosis of malignant pleural effusion.
2. Surgical treatment is indicated in patients with hemodynamic compromise (tamponade). Subxiphoid pericardiocentesis is easily performed, but does not represent definitive therapy. Although sclerosants have been used, the results are variable. Subxiphoid pericardiectomy is the treatment of choice and it can be performed under local anesthesia.

LYMPHOPROLITERATIVE DISEASE OF THE MEDIASTINUM

The mediastinum is divided into four distinct areas: superior, anterior, middle, and posterior. The superior mediastinum almost exclusively contains benign masses descending from the neck, the most common being retrosternal goiter.

Anterior and middle mediastinal masses were most commonly benign as described in a large series by Wychulis et al in 1971.[40] In a more recent study, the incidence of malignancy has increased to 42%, and was even higher (48%) in the last 20 years of this Duke University study.[41] Similar results were found in a series of 230 patients published by Cohen et al,[42] where the prevalence of malignancy increased from 17% to 47% from before 1970 (mainly secondary to an increase in lymphoma diagnosis from 22% to 35%). Similarly, the incidence of anterior mediastinal malignancy increased from 31% to 59%.

The anterior and middle mediastinal lymph nodes are commonly involved by lymphoproliferative diseases. This occurs in 50% to 60% of patients with Hodgkin's disease and 25% of non-Hodgkin's lymphoma patients.[43] The presence of enlarged lymph nodes or anterior mediastinal masses often is only of significance for staging or for determining therapeutic response. Therapy is altered only if the stage of Hodgkin's disease is upgraded or if the locoregional symptoms are so severe that the normal diagnostic work-up and management are disrupted. This is of little consequence to the thoracic surgeon, because the diagnosis is invariably obtained from an extrathoracic site in these cases.

When lymphoproliferative diseases are confined to the mediastinum and cannot be differentiated from other mediastinal masses, the thoracic surgeon is called on to assist in obtaining the diagnosis. As described above, this is occurring with increasing frequency.

When bulky mediastinal disease is present, defined as at least one third of the lateral chest diameter, the patient is very likely to be symptomatic. Chest pain or heaviness and cough are most common and shortness of breath may result from airway compression, lung compression, or from pleural or pericardial effusion. Superior vena cava syndrome, normally attributed to bronchogenic carcinoma, may also result from lymphoma.[44]

Differential Diagnosis

When mediastinal lymphoproliferative disease presents with involvement of the middle mediastinum, it must be differentiated from similarly presenting diseases such as histoplasmosis, sarcoidosis, and other granulomatous diseases. Skin testing, serology, bronchoscopy, and transbronchial biopsy should all be used, when appropriate, prior to referring the patient for a more invasive diagnostic approach.

More commonly, a primary lymphoproliferative disease of the mediastinum occurs in the anterior mediastinal compartment. The typical scenario is that of a large polycystic mass in the anterior mediastinum that is invading or compressing the surrounding structures. A retrosternal goiter may compress the trachea, but is usually in the superior mediastinum and should never be confused with lymphoproliferative disease except in the rare case of retrosternal thyroid carcinoma. Invasive thymoma is the most likely anterior mediastinal mass to be confused with lymphoma. Less common tumors are malignant germ cell tumors, and small cell, carcinoid, and bronchogenic carcinoma. Germ cell tumors are normally diagnosed by elevated serum tumor markers, whereas small cell, carcinoid, and bronchogenic carcinoma are differentiated from lymphoma histologically. The differentiation is imperative, because thymoma, carcinoma neurogenic tumors, and carcinoid are primarily treated with surgery as opposed to lymphomas which are treated by combined chemotherapy and radiation therapy.

Diagnostic Evaluation

A nonsurgical approach has been found to result in a diagnosis in about 60% of patients of patients with anterior mediastinal masses.[45]

Routine evaluation of anterior mediastinal masses should include physical examination, chest radiograph, and a CT scan (Fig. 12-7). Alpha fetoprotein (AFP) and β-HCG (tumor markers) should be included in the laboratory evaluation. Magnetic resonance imaging may be used as an adjunct to CT scan of the chest, but may be unnecessary (and expensive).

The goal of the thoracic surgeon in anterior and middle mediastinal tumor evaluation is to obtain an accurate diagnosis while minimizing the conduct of unnecessary diagnostic procedures, particularly major operations. In a study by Yellin et al,[46] 40 nondiagnostic procedures were performed, which included 9 major operations (thoracotomy, laparotomy, median sternotomy).

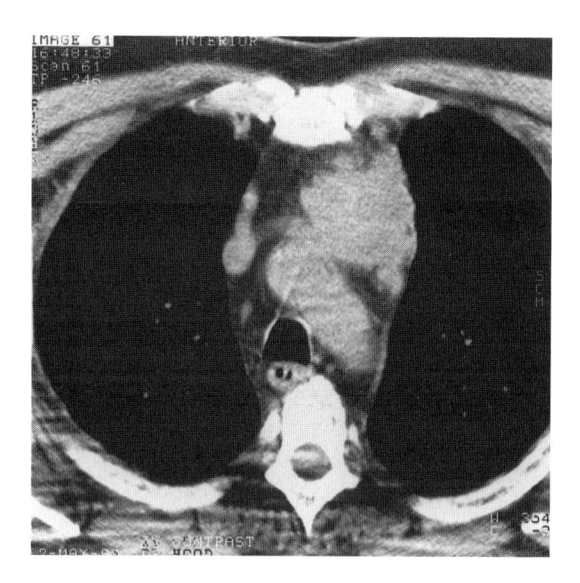

Figure 12-7. Computed tomographic scan of the chest showing an anterior mediastinal mass. Histologic examination revealed that this lesion was a thymoma.

Well-circumscribed tumors that are solitary should be excised via median sternotomy or thoracoscopy (Fig. 12-8). Benign tumors, early stage thymoma, carcinoid, and occasionally lymphoma present in this manner. Although an occasional lymphoma that is localized is unnecessarily resected in this manner, it is hard to differentiate them from the other surgically treated lesions. This helps assure a surgical cure for the other causes of tumors at the time of resection.

When a large mass is present and invading adjacent structures, it is most likely a malignancy (lymphoma, thymoma, germ cell tumors). If AFP or β-HCG levels are elevated, the diagnosis of germ cell tumor is made and a surgical diagnostic procedure is unnecessary. When other tumors are suspicious, an easily performed and safe diagnostic procedure is the first choice (bronchoscopy, thoracentesis, bone marrow aspiration, peripheral

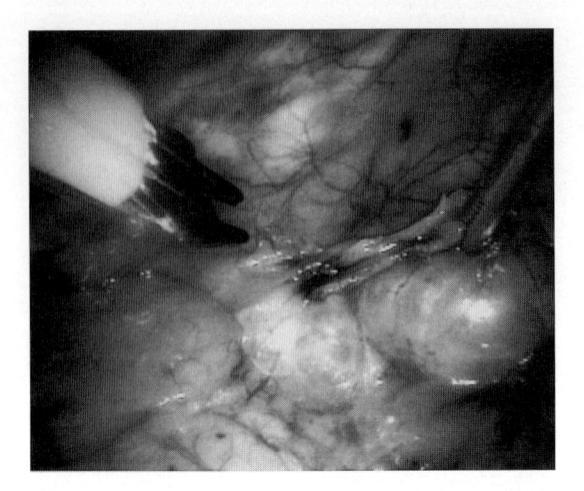

Figure 12-8. Resection of an anterior mediastinal mass using thoracoscopic techniques showing a benign 2-cm thymoma within a total thymectomy specimen.

lymph node biopsy). Only if these are noncontributory or not indicated is the anterior mediastinal mass approached directly by surgery. Although fine needle aspiration by CT-scan guidance is feasible and may be diagnostic, subtyping of lymphoma is difficult.[46] The ability to subtype lymphoma is important in determining optimal therapy and thus fine needle aspiration is not an ideal diagnostic procedure.

The choice of surgical approach (mediastinoscopy, thoracoscopy, anterior mediastinotomy, sternotomy, or thoracotomy) is determined by the location of the tumor on CT scan and the ability to perform complete resection. Frozen section at the time of surgery is used only to confirm that an adequate sample has been obtained to achieve an accurate pathologic diagnosis. Fresh specimens are also obtained for immunohistochemical and electron microscopic evaluation. "Touch preps" are particularly useful in differentiating lymphoma, carcinoid, and small cell lung cancers. Thoracoscopy is an attractive alternative to mediastinoscopy or Chamberlain procedures in patients with enlarged lymph nodes mostly on the left side[47] (Fig. 12-9).

In those patients with large mediastinal masses who present with compressive symptoms (superior vena cava syndrome, superior mediastinal syndrome, airway obstruction), it has been suggested that emergency radiotherapy be instituted prior to diagnostic evaluation. In the experience of Yellin et al,[44] this was rarely necessary. They were able to establish a diagnosis by nonsurgical means in greater than 70% of this particular subgroup of patients and the remainder underwent a surgical diagnostic procedure. Radiation treatment prior to biopsy may cloud the diagnostic picture and is preferably delayed until a diagnosis is made. Rarely, airway obstruction is severe and there is no available extrathoracic diagnostic site for biopsy. These patients may not even tolerate an anterior mediastinotomy; in this case, radiation therapy should be initiated prior to obtaining the final diagnosis.[48]

In the primary management of lymphoproliferative diseases of the mediastinum, surgery plays only a diagnostic role. When complications of therapy arise or residual or recurrent disease is present and no other *nonsurgical* treatment is warranted, then surgery may be considered. Children with recurrent or residual disease, who have been treated with chemotherapy in the past, likely have thymic hyperplasia, which is readily treated with steroids.[49]

Figure 12-9. A thoracoscopic biopsy of an anterior Hodgkin's lymphoma showing (*arrow*) the subclavian artery.

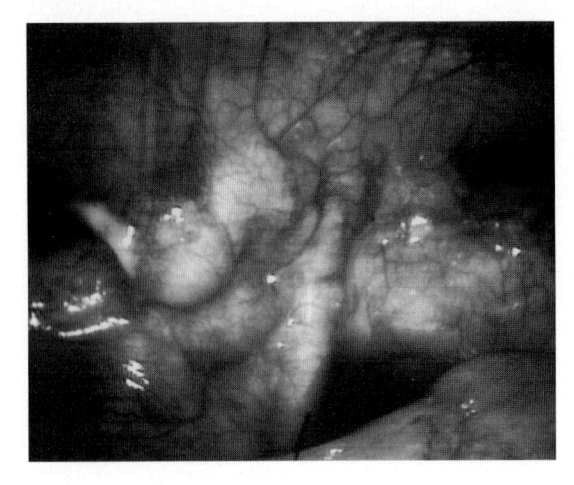

Persistent masses in the mediastinum or those with changes in size or configuration following therapy require biopsy, which is a difficult task in patients who have already received radiation. The irradiated field may even occasionally give rise to a second primary tumor. A similar approach is used, with resection rarely indicated; adequate tissue for diagnosis being the primary goal.[50-52]

Occasionally patients with airway compression require surgical resection for relief of symptoms. Likewise, debulking is often indicated for very large tumors to allow more effective chemotherapy as in the case of germ cell tumors. When a curative resection is the goal, sternotomy is the best approach. For high-risk patients, those who need only a diagnosis or those with unilateral disease, thoracoscopy is an attractive option. The role of thoracoscopy in treating thymoma is unclear and needs to be elucidated in a prospective series.

SUMMARY: LYMPHOPROLIFERATIVE DISEASE OF THE MEDIASTINUM

1. Anterior and middle mediastinal lymph nodes are most commonly involved by lymphoproliferative diseases, which when limited to the mediastinum, necessitate thoracic surgery involvement in obtaining the diagnosis.
2. Routine evaluation includes history and physical examination, chest radiography, computed tomography scan of the chest, and serum chemistries (including β-HCG and AFP).
3. A number of surgical approaches are available including: mediastinoscopy, thoracoscopy, anterior mediastinotomy, sternotomy, and thoracotomy. The procedure used is determined by tumor location and ability to completely resect it.
4. The major role of surgery in patients with lymphoproliferative diseases of the mediastinum is diagnostic.

SURGICAL APPROACH TO THE THORACIC SPINE

The vertebral column is a relatively common site for metastatic bone tumors and, occasionally, primary tumors of the bone. Neurosurgeons and orthopedic surgeons are called on to correct any instability of the bone that may arise in those patients. The role of the thoracic surgeon is to provide exposure to the affected area.

The key to the success of a stabilization procedure is adequate exposure. A well-planned approach will lead to excellent exposure to any site along the thoracic spine. However, an improperly placed or poorly planned approach often makes the procedure cumbersome and frustrating for the neurosurgeons or orthopedic surgeons.

When the vertebral bodies of T-3 through T-9 are involved, the approach is usually straight forward. A posterolateral thoracotomy is performed with the patient in the full lateral decubitus position. The standard positioning practices should be followed, including securing the patient with adhesive tape and padding any pressure points, particularly the placement of an axillary pad. The correct interspace to enter should be chosen so that the involved vertebrae are in the center of the operative field once the ribs are retracted. This will allow stabilization using the unaffected vertebral bodies above and below the one harboring tumor to secure instrumentation. Once the chest is open, the thoracic surgeon should assist in the ligation and division of any intercostal arteries that are in proximity to the involved operative site. These vessels are easily avulsed from the aorta if not handled with care. Depending on the level of thoracic spine involvement, the intercostal arteries may supply valuable collaterals to the spinal artery and therefore must be ligated lateral to the vertebral bodies to prevent compromise of the spinal blood supply.

Exposure of the upper and lower thoracic spine presents more of a challenge. A variety of procedures to expose these levels should be part of any thoracic surgeon's armamentarium. For lesions of the lower thoracic vertebrae, a low thoracoabdominal incision is used. The standard thoracoabdominal incision extends from the upper abdomen in the midline, across the costal margin, traversing the eighth or ninth intercostal spaces. This incision is often used to expose the thoracoabdominal portion of the aorta. For spinal exposure, a less extensive thoracoabdominal incision is used. We prefer to make an incision over the 11th rib extending onto the abdominal wall depending on the vertebral level involved. The 10th, 11th, or 12th rib is resected and the pleural space entered through the bed of that rib. The abdominal wall musculature is divided and the properitoneal fat exposed, leaving the peritoneum intact. The diaphragm is opened peripherally 3 to 4 cm from the costal margin in a semilunar fashion to avoid injury to the phrenic nerve where it enters the diaphragm medially. With the diaphragm open and the abdominal contents retracted within the peritoneum, the lower thoracic and upper lumber vertebrae are easily visualized. The diaphragm is reattached to the costal margin using a running polypropylene suture and a chest tube is inserted. Closure of the rib bed and abdominal musculature is performed with running suture.

Of the various spinal levels, exposure of the lower cervical and upper two thoracic vertebrae remains the most challenging. Although tumors affecting the upper thoracic vertebrae are rare, an acceptable approach to this area should be perfected by thoracic surgeons. In 1957, Cauchoix and Benet[53] described a direct approach to the cervicothoracic region via median sternotomy. Subsequent series noted an increased mortality with this approach and recommended abandoning it.[54] More recently, Standefer et al[55] have advocated median sternotomy with excision or fracture of the medial one third of the clavicle. However, this approach also has not been universally adopted.

We prefer the approach used at the Memorial Sloan-Kettering Cancer Center (New York, NY).[56] If the neck can be extended (not always possible in these patients) a subscapular roll is placed. A T-shaped collar incision is made crossing the sternocleidomastoid lateral border on each side, followed by a vertical incision onto the manubrium of the sternum (Fig. 12-10). After dividing the platysma, the clavicular head of the sternocleidomastoid muscle is dissected free and the strap muscles are divided and reflected superiorly. A flap of skin along with pectoralis major muscle is raised off of the sternum and clavicle. The periosteum is then stripped from the medial one third of the clavicle and it is divided with a Gigli's saw. Care should be taken in dividing the clavicle because the subclavian vein lies close to its inferior edge. The sternoclavicular junction is then divided and the loose areolar tissue behind the sternum is bluntly dissected. The manubrium is then partially excised using a

Figure 12-10. A schematic approach to the lower cervical and upper thoracic spine regions. We favor this approach, especially in patients with a kyphotic element. This approach can be modified and the retractor placed to the right side of the trachea rather than between the trachea and esophagus as shown here, for better visualization of primarily right sided lesions. From Charles R, Govender S. Anterior approach to upper thoracic vertebrae. J Bone Joint Surg 1989;71:81;reprinted with permission.

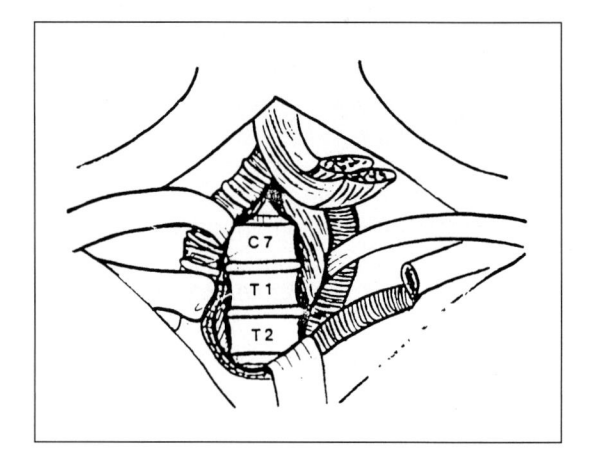

sternal saw, leaving intact the sternoclavicular junction and 1 to 2 cm of lateral sternum on the opposite side, which maintains lateral stability on that side of the chest wall. The thymic fat pad is then removed if necessary, with care taken not to injure the innominate vein that lies just beneath it. The avascular plane between the carotid sheath laterally and the trachea and esophagus medially is then developed to expose the prevertebral fascia. On the right side, the recurrent laryngeal nerve is found in this avascular plane and must be protected. On the left, the nerve runs in a more vertical plane in the tracheoesophageal groove. The resected clavicle can be used for bone grafting if needed.

Two retractors are then inserted: one is used to retract the trachea and esophagus to the left, the other to retract the innominate artery to the right. This usually affords an excellent view of C-6 through T-2. Closure is performed in layers with reapproximation of the strap muscles, anchoring of the sternocleidomastoid muscle to the remains of the clavicle, and closure of the platysma. There is no need to replace the manubrium because wound cosmetics and chest wall stability are not affected with good pectoralis muscle flaps.

In the series by Sundareson et al,[56] the only complications were a postoperative myocardial infarction in one patients and an esophageal perforation secondary to a migrating Steinmann pin, neither of which resulted in death.

We have found this to be a technically feasible procedure with low morbidity. To reduce injury to the recurrent laryngeal nerve, a left-sided approach with left clavicle resection should be used when appropriate because the course of the nerves is more consistent on the left side.

Recently we have used thoracoscopy to expose the thoracic spine, discs, and lesions along the vertebrae.[57] With thoracoscopy, one can dissect the segmental vessels safely and resect lesions of the spine without the morbidity of thoracotomy (Fig. 12-11).

Figure 12-11. A thoracoscopic view of the T-7 disc space. The disc is being removed totally thoracoscopically using standard rongeurs as well as special thoracoscopic cup biopsy forceps. (This method also can be used for removal of metastatic lesions to the vertebral body.)

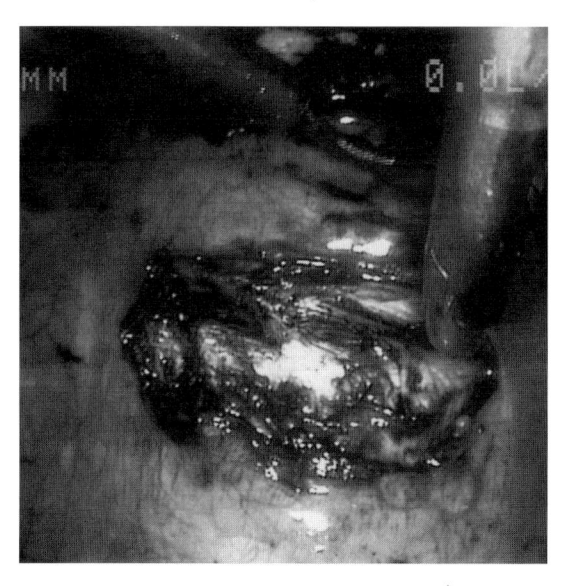

SUMMARY: SURGICAL APPROACH TO THE THORACIC SPINE

1. Thoracic surgeons are often called on to obtain exposure for procedures on the spine.
2. In T-1 and T-2, a T-shaped collar incision with a vertical incision made onto the manubrium. The clavicle is divided and dissection carried out behind the sternum. The trachea and esophagus are retracted to the left and the innominate artery to the right thus exposing C-6 through T-2.
3. For T-3 through T-9, a posterolateral thoracotomy is done.
4. For T-10 through T-12, a low thoracoabdominal incision is made.

MANAGEMENT OF PULMONARY METASTASES

Management of pulmonary nodules continues to be a challenging and often seen indication for surgery by the thoracic surgeon.[58] Although needle biopsy or bronchoscopic biopsy may be diagnostic, this is not always possible.[59] Transthoracic resection of pulmonary nodules is therefore needed to allow appropriate diagnosis to be made by obtaining a large tissue sample. In cases where the diagnosis is determined to be primary lung cancer, one should proceed with lobectomy. For lesions found to be metastatic, wedge resection is felt to be adequate.

Resection of metastases to the lung was first performed in 1939 for breast carcinoma.[60] Resection of metastases to the lung should allow the best possible local control with the least possible morbidity.[61] Chemotherapy or radiation therapy generally are not useful or are considered too morbid to accomplish a cure.

Recently, several reports have reviewed the role of pulmonary resection for metastatic soft tissue sarcomas. In one series of 93 patients with pulmonary metastases, 13 were found to be unresectable.[62] Seventeen patients underwent negative thoracotomies (no metastases found); 51 patients had resectable tumors. Five-year survival rates ranging from 10% to 35% have been reported for this disease.[62,63] When complete resection is performed, survival is significantly improved. Most patients require only a wedge resection for adequate control. Repeat metastatectomies are appropriate when complete resection is achieved and is associated with improved long-term survival. In another series, 50% of patients underwent a second or third thoracotomy for additional metastatectomy.[63] Again, the majority underwent wedge resection resulting in a survival of 25%.

Metastastecomy for colon cancer is frequently reported. McAfee et al [64] described 139 patients undergoing metastasectomy. The majority were found to be asymptomatic on routine follow-up, by x-ray study, tomography, or computed tomography scan. Six had bilateral lesions. Sixteen additional lesions were noted on the CT that were not picked up by standard chest roentgenogram. The majority of these patients underwent colectomy first. Wedge resection was performed in 68 patients; 41 had multiple metastases. In patients with colorectal cancer, very high serum carcinoembryonic antigen (CEA) level at the time of presentation is associated with a lower 5-year survival. When metastases were bilateral, the 5-year survival rate was about 15%. Another report found a 5-year survival rate of 20%.[65] The majority of patients had Dukes' C (*i.e.*, positive nodes, $T_xN_{1-3}M_0$) lesions at the time of presentation. Seventeen patients presented with simultaneous lung metastasis and colon primary tumor. Of patients found by CT scan to have pulmonary lesions, 90% were metastases. In another report of 35 patients who underwent metastastectomy for colorectal tumors, 6 presented synchronously.[66]

Resection of pulmonary metastasis for melanoma was first described by Arce in 1936.[67] Most reports agree that wedge resections represent adequate treatment.[68] Thayer and Overholt[69] described 18 patients undergoing thoracotomy wedge resection for melanoma. The 5-year survival of this group, unfortunately, was not particularly high. Because no type of chemotherapy has been useful to date in melanoma or has limited value and entails a high morbidity, a surgical approach should be appropriately aggressive. Recently, Gorenstein et al[70] found that pulmonary metastasis were the most common second site in melanoma. In 11% of the patients, metastases were isolated to the lung without metastatic spread elsewhere. Because respiratory failure is the most frequent cause of death in patients with pulmonary metastases from melanoma, resection seems appropriate. Twenty-eight patients with a first recurrence in the lung underwent routine CT scans; 25 received chemotherapy and 10 underwent sternotomy. Patients with bilateral disease were treated by staged concurrent procedures or separate thoracotomies. Ninety-seven percent underwent complete resection with a 25% overall 5-year survival obtained. The most important prognostic factor was the lung as the site of first occurrence. There was no difference in survival regarding the location of the primary tumor, its level or thickness, the disease-free interval, the tumor doubling time, unilaterality versus bilaterality, number of lesions, or type of resection performed. We recommend therefore, a very aggressive surgical approach for patients with isolated pulmonary metastasis from malignant melanoma.

In patients with breast cancer and pulmonary nodules, 50% can present with new primary adenocarcinoma in the lung.[71] Of patients with pulmonary metastasis from breast carcinoma, a wedge resection with 1- to 2-cm margins is considered adequate. Complete lymph node dissection in these patients is unnecessary unless lymph nodes are obviously enlarged The 5-year survival rate with surgical treatment is 36% to 50%[71] with isolated lung metastases.

Renal cell carcinomas also are treated aggressively when presenting with isolated metastases to the lung. Renal cell cancers presenting simultaneously with pulmonary metastases have been reported. Libby et al[73] suggest that each tumor should be treated with formal anatomic resection. Recently, interleukin 2 (IL-2) treatment prior to metastatectomy has been shown not only to decrease the size of the metastasis, but to reduce the primary tumor as well allowing complete resection to be performed.[74] Patients with renal cell cancer can achieve a 40% 5-year survival when metastases isolated to the lung were resected.

Other tumors with solitary pulmonary metastasis have been treated aggressively including carcinoma of the cervix[75] and head and neck tumors. Fifteen percent of patients with head and neck primary tumors present with additional primary tumors in the airway or upper digestive systems. New lesions in the lung are approached surgically for possible cure of a second primary tumor. In a report by Lefor et al,[76] 65 patients with pulmonary lesions after head and neck tumors were resected. All lesions should be treated with surgical resection because surgery provides the best possible cure for metastatic lesions and obviously for second (lung) primary tumors. These patients should undergo anatomic resection such as lobectomy rather than simple wedge resection.

Many different prognostic factors have been reported to help the surgeon determine operability and select those patients who would not benefit from an aggressive operative approach. Cell type, disease-free interval, tumor doubling time, tumor size, and number of tumors are the most frequently cited prognostic facts. Location of the lesion (peripheral versus central) and bilateral versus unilateral disease, the status of the local primary disease, and, finally and most importantly, the completeness of resection all are of prognostic significance.

Soft tissue sarcomas generally have better survival when the disease-free interval is longer and the tumor is unilateral. Complete resection is tantamount to achieving good survival. In colorectal carcinomas the only factors that are clearly important, are completeness of resection and original Duke's stage of the primary tumor. Regarding melanoma, only the completeness of resection has been shown as a significant prognostic indicator. Several recent reports on renal cell cancers consider lack of other metastasis or evidence of local recurrence to be the key prognostic factors.[73,74]

Adjuvant chemotherapy, immunotherapy, and radiation therapy have been advocated by oncologists but many pulmonary metastases are not responsive. Patients with testicular tumors and pulmonary metastases are treated aggressively for their primary tumor. This often results in shrinkage or complete disappearance of the pulmonary metastasis. Treatment with chemotherapy or radiation therapy may result in response of the pulmonary metastases. Follow-up pulmonary resection to eliminate residual tumors may be appropriate.

Surgical Techniques

The surgical approach to pulmonary metastasis is wedge resection. Only one report of the utility of anatomic resection in managing patients with melanoma exists.[69] Because there is always the possibility of future additional metastatic tumors arising, a lung-conserving approach should be pursued.

The type of surgical incision used varies. The role of sternotomy in managing pulmonary metastasis is not clear. Some authors advocate its use routinely to allow palpation of all of the lung tissue.[77,78] Others feel this is appropriate only for patients with anterior tumors that are few in number and bilateral in extent. It is difficult with sternotomy to palpate or resect lesions in the lower lobes. It is excellent for resecting upper lobes, middle and lingular resection, and wedges of medial basal segments of the lower lobes. It is difficult to remove lesions of the chest wall or of the diaphragm. The main advantage, however, is decreased morbidity compared with bilateral thoracotomy. Less than 10% of the patients reported in the surgical literature underwent sternotomy. Generally concomitant or staged bilateral thoracotomies are performed. The routine use of high resolution computed tomography scan with thin cuts (5-mm) may help to identify lesions in excess of 2 mm in size with an accuracy rate approaching 90%. Although sternotomy was originally advocated to palpate even the tiniest pulmonary nodules, it is unlikely that the surgeon can palpate nodules less than 1 to 2 mm preoperatively. We have used CT scan as a guide in patients with unilateral, bilateral, or transternal thoracotomy approaches.

For patients with bilateral disease, staged or simultaneous bilateral thoracotomies are an option. Although formal posterior lateral thoracotomy allows the best exposure, the morbidity may prohibit simultaneous operations at one sitting. Patients with poor pulmonary function would be better served with staged thoracotomies with at least 6 weeks separating each incision or a sternotomy. Preoperative evaluation of pulmonary function is fully discussed in Chapter 13. Small lateral thoracotomies with muscle-sparing incisions are better tolerated and when combined with epidural analgesia may allow for a concomitant approach to be performed. The use of transternal, bilateral anterior thoracotomies,[79] the so-called *clam-shell* incision, used for simultaneous bilateral lung transplants, is perfectly suited for exploring and resecting lesions in both pleural spaces. It has the advantage of the transternal approach, allowing simultaneous examination of both chests and does not require repositioning the patient.

Limited *mini-thoracotomies* for approaching pulmonary metastasis have been described using CT scan to direct the surgeon to the area immediately over the lesion.[80]

The use of thoracoscopy in performing metastatectomy (Fig. 12-12) has many possible advantages. The decreased postoperative pain, typical with thoracoscopy, is helpful especially if one is performing a bilateral approach. Patients have less postoperative pulmonary dysfunction and their overall morbidity seems to be decreased. These patients would better tolerate bilateral simultaneous resections done thoracoscopically[81] (Fig. 12-13).

Figure 12-12. Metastatic seminoma in a 30-year-old man with multiple pulmonary nodules seen thoracoscopically.

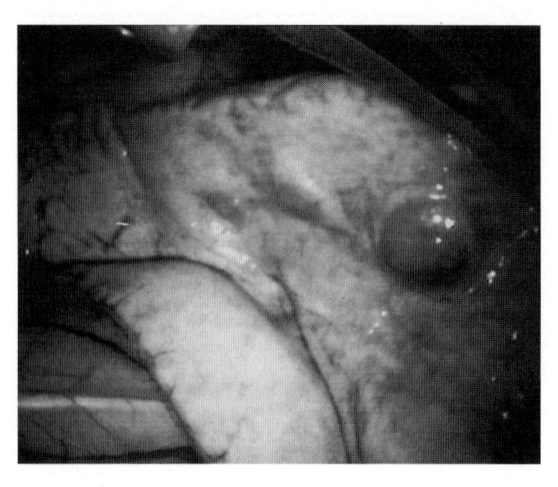

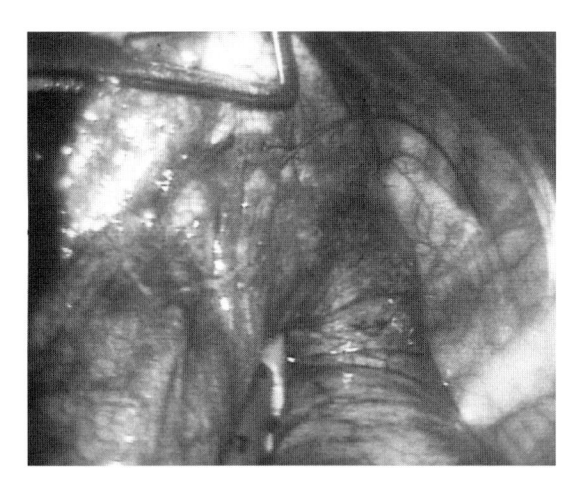

Figure 12-13. Biopsy forceps holding the superior segment of the left lower lobe for stapler application. Note the needle guide-wire entering into the left lower lobe.

SUMMARY: MANAGEMENT OF PULMONARY METASTASES

1. Pulmonary metastasectomy necessitates excision of the lesion with a wedge resection and has been described in the treatment of metastatic sarcoma, colorectal cancer, melanoma, breast cancer, and renal cell carcinoma.
2. The surgical approach to lung metastases depends on their location. Although median sternotomy remains an option, the use of bilateral thoracotomies must also be kept in mind. Thoracoscopy may be the optimal approach for excision of bilateral lesions.

EVALUATION OF PARENCHYMAL LUNG DISEASE

The primary goal of lung biopsy, in patients with infiltrate parenchymal lung disease who have underlying malignancies is to determine the cause of the lung disease. Most often this represents infection in patients who are receiving chemotherapy or radiation therapy. These patients are immunosurpressed and therefore particularly susceptible to uncommon pathogens including, but not limited to, viral infections such as cytomegalovirus (CMV), unusual fungal infections such as *aspergillosis* and *candidiasis*, and even unusual bacterial infections such as nosocomial staphylococcal, mycobacterial, and gram-negative pneumonias that are resistant to antibiotic therapy or have progressed to abscess formation. In these patients it is particularly important to make the diagnosis of an infectious process so that appropriate antimicrobial management can be initiated. If the patient is so debilitated as to preclude safe performance of an open lung biopsy to obtain a diagnosis, empiric therapy with antibiotic, antifungal, and antiviral medications is appropriate. Additionally, one wants to rule out the possibility of recurrent malignancy. This is particularly true for patients with previous lung primary tumors who now may present with either intrapulmonary metastases or lymphatic spread. Likewise, in patients with previous leukemias and lymphomas, although rare, it must be noted that intrapulmonary malignant infiltrates can occur. In these cases, patients will be placed on chemotherapy or radiation protocols reserving surgical resection only after these patients have had a complete treatment with a good response.

Finally, it must be remembered that a variety of other inflammatory diseases may occur in cancer patients unrelated to the underlying malignancy. This includes a variety of interstitial pneumonitis-type processes, sarcoidosis, eosinophilic granuloma, granulomas, allergic pneumonitis, alveolitis, sarcoidosis and, of course, the full range of vasculitides, which may occur in these patients as well. This last group of diseases is particularly important because their therapy generally utilizes anti-inflammatory medications and steroids. These diseases must be differentiated from infectious causes because treating patients with viral, fungal, or bacterial diseases with steroids would only lead to superinfection in these patients. As noted above, if the patient is so sick as to preclude the performance of an open lung biopsy, then empiric steroid therapy may be started provided it is felt safe not to give antibiotic concurrently or an antibiotic is given concomitantly empirically.

Diagnostic Evaluation

Interstitial lung disease is a general description of different pathologic entities with the chest roentgenogram and appearance on CT scan of interstitial pneumonitis or fibrosis. Although noninvasive modalities can be used to differentiate the cause, often a formal pathologic tissue diagnosis is needed to designate specific therapy. Steroids can then be used if the specific diagnosis is inflammatory disease of sarcoidosis. The decision not to use steroids may be equally important in the management of a particular patient.

The initial step in evaluating these patients should be high-resolution computerized tomographic (HRCT) scan with thin (5 mm) cuts. Following this, bronchoscopy with brushings and washings should be performed as the next diagnostic test. If this does not yield the diagnosis, lung biopsy directed to the most area most suggestive of tumor on chest x-ray film or computed tomography scan, is the next appropriate step.

In patients with nodular type densities, percutaneous needle biopsy (PNB) is an appropriate alternative to bronchoscopy. The diagnostic yield with PNB for malignant tumors is greater than 95% and for benign diseases approximately 80%.[59]

In the event that a diagnosis has not been made following the initial evaluation, open lung biopsy is the next appropriate diagnostic step. Especially in patients who are ventilator-dependent or who are very sick, requiring relatively high oxygen concentrations, lung biopsy can be accomplished through a small anterior thoracotomy incision. This is generally achieved with single lumen endotracheal tube intubation, and using an inframammary incision entering the chest through the fifth or sixth intercostal space.[82] Generally, a rib-spreading retractor is not necessary and the middle lobe on the right or the lingula on the left can be delivered into the wound. Occasionally a rib-spreading retractor is needed to obtain a specimen from one of the lobes and allows pleural fluid to be aspirated and sent for cytology and culture at the time of lung biopsy.

Alternatively, specific antibiotics or surgical therapies may be indicated. Patients with interstitial lung disease obviously present a high pulmonary risk because they have poor pulmonary function to begin with. Any operation that may put the patient at a higher postoperative risk carries a significant danger in terms of increased morbidity and mortality. These patients often have good results with thoracoscopy because the procedure can be performed safely, and, when done on an outpatient basis, patients can be sent

Figure 12-14. Schematic setup for thoracoscopic lung resection. (Reprinted with permission from Krasna MJ, Mack MJ. Atlas of thoracoscopic surgery. St. Louis, Quality Medical Publishing, Inc. 1994, p. 98.)

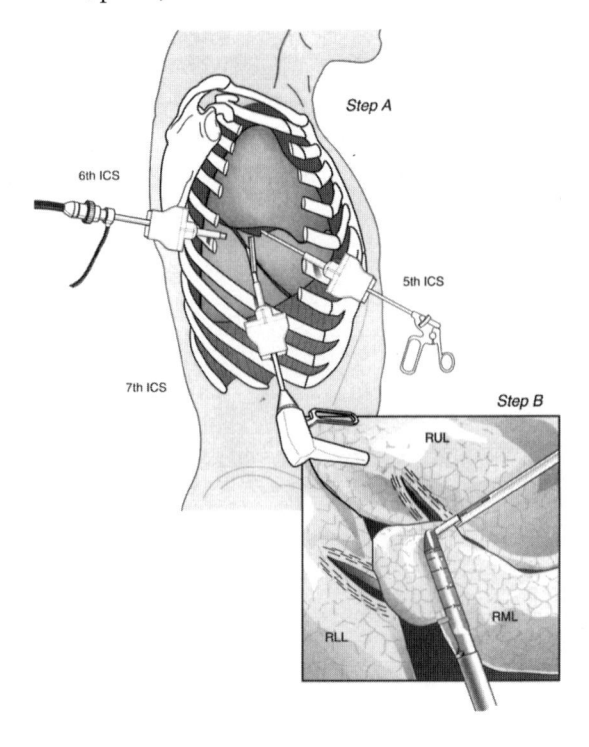

home quickly with little postoperative morbidity.[83] Open lung biopsy has been replaced with thoracoscopic lung resection for stable patients at the University of Maryland (Fig. 12-14).[84]

One additional issue deserves mention. Many reports recommend using chest x-ray to guide open lung biopsies to the worst area of suspicion.[85] Although one study claims these regions would give the highest diagnostic yield, other reports claim the opposite.[86] We have studied the role thoracoscopy has played in allowing us to sample the abnormal portion of the lung appropriately. Using thoracoscopy, we have noted that direct visualization, combined with biopsy of three segments (one from of each of the lobes), gives 100% success in obtaining a specific diagnosis. This is superior even to directed biopsy using a computed tomography scan.

A lung biopsy using either a stapler or laser usually can be performed thoracoscopically to a specific area suggestive of tumor or as directed by the computed tomography scan or chest x-ray film. Alternatively, random biopsy of each of the segments can be performed. The easiest segments to biopsy are the superior segment of the lower lobe as it lies along the fissure and the lateral segment of the middle lobe and inferior edge of the anterior segment of the upper lobe. Each of these segments lies along the major or minor fissures or at the confluence of these fissures and therefore can easily be retracted and stapled across for diagnosis. If a specific area other than these segments is not suggestive of tumor on the basis of noninvasive testing, other lung biopsies should be done as indicated provided that the suggestive lesions are relatively superficial. It is very important to keep in mind that stapling lung parenchyma may incur hemorrhage or air leak if too large a segment of tissue is biopsied. Peripheral biopsies of the lung parenchyma assures that these complications will not occur. A combination of laser to thin the tissue followed by stapling has proved useful for more central lesions with good results.

SUMMARY: EVALUATION OF PARENCHYMAL LUNG DISEASE

1. Parenchymal lung disease in patients with malignancies may represent infectious complications in this immunocompromised population. Recurrent malignancy must be ruled out.
2. Evaluation usually includes high-resolution computed tomography scan followed by bronchoscopy. Lung biopsy is performed if necessary. Percutaneous needle biopsy may be used in patients with nodular densities.
3. Thoracoscopy is an excellent method for obtaining tissue in these patients.

SUMMARY

The thoracic surgeon faces many therapeutic challenges in the cancer patient, especially those with metastatic disease. The surgeon must find a way to relieve symptoms or even prolong life, yet preferably use a minimally invasive approach. Outlined in this chapter are what we feel are the most efficient and effective ways to approach these problems, based on our experience as well as that of others. The management of these cases should be based on the individual patient and on the surgeon's own experience because what is recommended here may not be appropriate for all cases.

When the thoracic surgeon is called on to assist in making the diagnosis of cancer in patients with mediastinal masses or pulmonary infiltrates, a carefully planned approach is required. Again, the least invasive procedure likely needed to make the diagnosis is called for. The fact that a thoracic surgeon has been consulted does not mean a thoracic procedure must be performed. Many of these diagnostic dilemmas are solved by peripheral lymph node biopsy or bronchoscope. We must be familiar with the usefulness and limitations of thoracic procedures.

Exposure to the thoracic spine for stabilization procedures can be as simple as a thoracotomy or as difficult and challenging as any major thoracic procedure. Planning a strategy with our orthopedic or neurosurgical colleagues allows a rational approach for both the patient and the surgeon.

REFERENCES

1. Hausher FH, Rarbro JW. Diagnosis and treatment of malignant pleural effusions. Semin Oncol 1985:12(1)54.
2. Prakush UB, Deiman HM, Comparison of needle biopsy with cytologic analysis for evaluation of pleural effusion: analysis of 44 cases. Mayo Clin Proc 1985;60(3):158.
3. Chernow B, Sahn SA. Carcinomatous involvement of the pleura: an analysis of 96 patients. Am J Med 1977;63:695.
4. Martini N, Bains MS, Beattie EJ. Indications for pleurectomy in malignant effusion. Cancer 1975;35:734.
5. Yamuzaki S, Ogawa J, Shohzu A, et al. Pulmonary blood flow to rapidly expanding lung in spontaneous pneumothorax. Chest 1982;81:118.
6. Potts DE, Taryle DA, Sahn SA. The glucose pH relationship in parapneumonic effusions. Arch Intern Med 1978;138:1378.
7. Leff A, Hopewell PC, Costello J. Pleural effusion from malignancy. Ann Intern Med 1978;88:532.
8. Winkelman M, Pfitzer P. Blind pleural biopsy in combination with cytology of pleural effusions. Acta Cytol 1981;25:373.
9. Weisberg D, Daufman M. Diagnostic and therapeutic pleuroscopy; experience with 127 patients. Chest 1980;78:732.
10. Izbicki R, Weyhing BT III, Baker L, et al: Pleural effusion in cancer patients: a prospective randomized study of pleural drainage with the addition of radioactive phosphorous to the pleural space vs. pleural drainage alone. Cancer 1975;36:1511.
11. Anderson CB, Philpott GW, Ferguson TB. The treatment of malignant pleural effusions. Cancer 1974;33:916.
12. Austin EH, Fly MW. The treatment of recurrent malignant pleural effusions. Ann Thorac Surg 1979;28:190.
13. Wallach HW. Intrapleural tetracycline for malignant pleural effusions. Chest 1975;68:510.
14. Bitran JD, Brown C, Desser RK, et al. Intacavitory bleomycin for the control of malignant pleural effusions. J Surg Oncol 1981;16:273.
15. Paladine W, Cunningham TJ, Sponzo R, et al. Intracavitary bleomycin in the management of malignant pleural effusions. Cancer 1976;38:1903.
16. Hurley HR. Malignant pleural effusions and their treatment by talc pleurodesis. British Journal of Diseases of the Chest 1979;73:173.
17. Adler RH, Sayek I. Treatment of malignant pleural effusion: A method using tube thoracostomy and talc. Ann Thorac Surg 1976;22:8.
18. Ponn RB, Blancaflor J, D'Agostino RS, et al. Pleuroperitoneal shunting for intractable pleural effusions. Ann Thorac Surgery 1991;51:605.
19. Robinson BS, Fullerton PA, Albert JD, Sorenson J, Johnson MR. Use of pleural Tenckoff catheter to palliate malignant pleural effusion. Ann Thorac Surg 1994; 57:286.
20. Fraser RS, Viloria JB, Wong N. Cardiac tamponade as a presentation of extra cardiac malignancy. Cancer 1980;45:1697.
21. Thusther DC, Edwards JE. Secondary malignant tumors of the pericardium. Circulation 1962;26:228.
22. Pieler JM, Pluth JR, Schaff HV, et al. Surgical management of effusive pericardial disease. J Thorac Cardiovasc Surg 1985;90:506.
23. Bisel HF, Wroblewski F, Ladue IS. Incidence and clinical manifestation of cardiac metastases. JAMA 1953;153:712.
24. Alcan RE, Zubetakis PM, Marino ND, et al. Management of acute cardiac tamponade by subxiphoid pericardial window. JAMA 1982; 247:1143.
25. Theologodes A. Neoplastic cardiac tamponade. Semin Oncol 1978;5:181.
26. Markiewicz W, Borovik R, Ecker S. Cardiac tamponade in medical patients: treatment and prognosis in the echocardiographic era. Am Heart J 1986;111:1138.
27. Himeleun RB, Kircher B, Rockey DC, Schiller NB. Inferior vena cava plethora with blunted respiratory response: a sensitive echocardiographic sign of cardiac tamponade. J Am Cardiol 1988;12:1470.
28. Osuch JR, Klundedar JD, Fry WA. Emergency subxiphoid pericardial decompression for malignant pericardial effusion. Am Surg 1985; 51:298.
29. Gregory JR, McCurty MJ, Mountain CF. A surgical approach to the treatment of pericardial effusion in cancer patients. Am J Clin Oncol 1985;8:319.
30. Wong B, Murphy J, Chonge CJ. The risk of pericardiocentesis. Am J Cardiol 1979;44:1110.

31. Krikoriun JL, Hancock EW: Pericardiocenthesis. Am J Med 1978;65:808.
32. Kopecky SL, Callahan JA, Takik AJ, Seward JB, et al. Percutaneous pericardial catheter drainage: report of 42 patients consecutive cases. Am J Cardiol 1986;58:633.
33. Ziskind AA, Pearce C, Lemmon CC, et al. Percutaneous balloon pericardiotomy for the treatment of cardiac tamponade and large pericardial effusions: description of technique and report of the first 50 cases. J Am Cardiol 1993; 21:1.
34. Shepard FA, Morgan C, Evans WK, et al. Medical management of malignant pericardial effusions by tetracycline sclerosis. Am J Cardiol 1987;60:1160.
35. Gregory JR, McMurtry MJ, Mountain CF. A surgical approach to the treatment of pericardial effusion in cancer patients. Am J Clin Oncol 1985;8:319.
36. Fiocco M, Krasna MJ. Thoracoscopic pericardiectomy. Surgical Laparoscopy & Endoscopy 1992;2:258.
37. Little AG, Kremser PC, Wade JL, et al. Operation for diagnosis and treatment of pericardial effusions. Surgery 1986;89:53.
38. Millaire A, Wurtz A, deFoote P, et al. Malignant pericardial effusions: usefulness of pericardioscopy. Am Heart J 1992;124:1030.
39. Wang N, Feikes R, Morgensen T, Vymeister EE, Bailey LL. Pericardioperitoneal shunt: an alternative treatment for malignant pericardial effusions. Ann Thoac Surg 1994;57:289.
40. Wychulis AR, Payne WS, Clagett OT, et al. Surgical treatment of mediastinal tumors. J Thorac Cardiovasc Surg 1971;62:379.
41. Davis RD, Oldham HN, Sabiston DC. Primary cysts and neoplasms of the mediastinum: recent changes in clinical presentation, methods of diagnosis, management and results. Ann Thorac Surg 1987;44:229.
42. Cohen AJ, Thompson L, Edwards FH, et al. Primary cysts and tumors of the mediastinum. Ann Thorac Surg 1991;51:378.
43. Schomberg DJ, Evans RG, O'Connell MJ, et al. Prognostic significance of mediastinal mass in adult Hodgkin's disease. Cancer 1984;53:324.
44. Yellin A, Rosen A, Reichert N, et al. Superior vena cava syndrome: the myth - the facts. Am Rev Respir Dis 1990;141:1114.
45. Ferguson MK, Lee E, Skinner DB, et al. Selective operative approach for diagnosis and treatment of anterior mediastinal masses. Ann Thorac Surg 1987;44:883.
46. Yellin A, Pak HY, Burke JS, et al. Surgical treatment of lymphomas involving the chest. Ann Thorac Surg 1987;41:363.
47. Fiocco M, Krasna MJ. Thoracoscopic lymph node dissection. J Laparoendosc Surg 1992;2: 111.
48. Jeffrey GM, Mead GM, Whitehouse JM. Life threatening airway obstruction as the presentation of Hodgkin's disease. Cancer 1991;57: 506.
49. Ford EG, Lockhart SK, Sullivan MP, et al. Mediastinal mass following chemotherapy treatment of Hodgkin's disease, recurrent disease or thymic hyperplasia. J Pediatr Surg 1982;22: 455.
50. Pak HJ, Yokota SB, Friedberg HA. Thymoma diagnosed by transthoracic fine needle aspiration. Acta Cytol 1982;26:210.
51. Bonfiglio TA, Dvoretsky PM, Riscioli F, et al. Fine needle aspiration of lymphoreticular tumors of the thorax. Acta Cytol 1985;29:548.
52. Janin Y, Becker L, Wise K, et al. Superior vena syndrome in childhood and adolescence. J Pediatr Surg 1982;17:290.
53. Cauchoix J, Benet JP. Anterior surgical approaches to the spine. Ann R Coll Surg Engl 1957;21:234.
54. Hodgson AR, Stock FE, Fong HSY, et al. Anterior spinal fusion: the operative approach and pathological findings in 412 patients with Potts disease of the spine. Br J Surg 1960;48: 172.
55. Standefer M, Hardy RW Jr, Marks R, et al. Chondromyxoid fibroma of the cervical spine. Neurosurgery 1982;11:298.
56. Sundareson N, Shah J, Foley K, Rosen G. An anterior surgical approach to the upper thoracic vertebrae. J Neurosurg 1984;61:686.
57. Krasna MJ, Mack MJ. Thoracoscopic approach to the spine. In: Krasna MJ, Mack J, eds. Atlas of thoracoscopic surgery. St Louis, Quality Medical Publishing, Inc. 1994.
58. Mountain CF, McMuntrey MJ, Hermes KH. Surgery for pulmonary metastasis: a 20-year experience. Ann Thorac Surg 1984;38:323.
59. Templeton PA, Krasna MJ. The role of needle biopsy and thoracoscopy in the diagnosis of pulmonary nodules [Abstract]. Proceedings of the Society of Thoracic Surgery, 1993.
60. Barney JD, Churchill EJ. Adenocarcinoma of the kidney with metastasis to the lung cured by nephrectomy and lobectomy. J Urol 1939; 42:269.
61. Blalock A. Recent advantages in surgery. N England J Med 1944;231:261.
62. Casson AG, Putnam JB, Natarajan G, Johnston DA, Mountain C, McMurtery M, Roth JA. Five-year survival after pulmonary metastasectomy for adult soft tissue sarcoma. Cancer 1992;69: 662.

63. Verazin GT, Warneke JA, Driscoll DL, Karakousis C, Petrelli NJ, Takita H. Resection of lung Metastases from soft tissue sarcomas. Arch Surg 1992;127:1403.
64. McAfee MK, Allen MS, Trastek VF, Ilstrup DM, Deschamps C, Pairolero PC. Colorectal lung metastases: result of surgical excision. Ann Thorac Surg 1992;53:780.
65. McCormack PM, Burt ME, Bains MS, Martini N, Rusch VW, Ginsberg RJ. Lung resections for colorectal metastases: 10-year result. Arch Surg 1992;127:1403.
66. Chang AE, Schaner EG, Conkle DM, Flye MW, Doppman JL, Rosenberg SA. Evaluation of computed tomography in the detection of pulmonary metastases: a prospective study. Cancer 1979;43:913.
67. Arce MJ. Pneumonectomie totale (le tampon-drainage enchirgugie endothoracique). Mem Acad de Chir 1936;62:1412.
68. Mathisen DJ, Flye MW, Peabody J. The role of thoracotomy in the management of pulmonary metastases from malignant melanoma. Ann Thorac Surg 1979;27:295.
69. Thayer JO, Overholt RH. Metastatic melanoma to the lung: long results of surgical excision. Am J Surg 1985;149:558.
70. Gorenstein LA, Putnam JB, Natarajan G, Balch CA, Roth JA. Improved survival after resection of pulmonary metastases from malignant melanoma. Ann Thorac Surgery 1991;52:204.
71. Staren ED, Salerno C, Rongione A, Witt TR, Faber LP: Pulmonary resection for metastatic breast cancer. Arch Surg 1992;127:1282.
72. Goya T, Tsuchiya R. Surgical resection of metastatic neoplasms of the lung. Gan To Kagaku Ryoho 1990;17:771.
73. Libby DM, Altorki NK, Gold J, Pitts Jr WR, Bander NH, Frankel SS. Simultaneous pulmonary and renal malignancy. Chest 1990;98:153.
74. Kim B, Louie AC. Surgical resection following interleukin 2 therapy for metastatic renal cell carcinoma prolongs remission. Arch Sur 1992; 127:1343.
75. Matsukuma K, Miyake M, Iino H, et al. Surgical management of pulmonary metastasis from carcinoma of the uterine cervix. Acta Obstetrica Et Gynaecologica Haponica 1989;41(12):1911.
76. Lefor AT, Bredenberg CE, Kellman RM, Aust JC. Multiple malignancies of the lung and head and neck second primary tumor or metastasis? Arch Surg 1986;121:265.
77. Cooper JD, Nelems JM, Pearson FG. Extended indications for median sternotomy in patients requiring pulmonary resection. Ann Thoracic Surg 1978;26:413.
78. Johnston MR. Median sternotomy for resection of pulmonary metastases. J Thorac Cardiovasc Surg 1983;85:518.
79. Pasque MK, Cooper JD, Kaiser LR, et al: Improved technique for bilateral lung transplantation: rationale and initial clinical experience. Ann Thorac Surg 1990;49:785.
80. Daly BDT, Faling LJ, Diehl JT, Gankoff MS, Gale ME. Computed tomography-guided minithoracotomy for resection of small peripheral pulmonary nodules. Ann Thorac Surg 1991; 51:465.
81. Templeton PA, Krasna MJ. Localization of pulmonary nodules for thoracoscopic resection: use of needle/wire breast-biopsy system. AJR 1993; 160:761.
82. Gaensler EA, Carrington CB. Open biopsy for chronic diffuse infiltrative lung disease: clinical, roentgenographic, and physiological correlations in 502 patients. Ann Thorac Surg 1980;30:411.
83. Bensard DD, McIntyre RC Jr, Waring BJ, Simon JS. Comparison of video thoracoscopic lung biopsy to open lung biopsy in the diagnosis on interstitial lung disease. Chest 1993;103:765.
84. Krasna MJ, White CS, Aisner SC, et al. The role of thoracoscopy in the diagnosis of interstitial lung disease. Ann Thorac Surg 1995;59:348.
85. Miller RR, Nelems B, Muller NL, Evans KG, Ostrow DN. Lingular and right middle lobe biopsy in the assessment of diffuse lung disease. Ann Thorac Surg 1987;44:269.
86. Chechani V, Landreneau RJ, Shaikh SS. Open lung biopsy for diffuse infiltrative lung disease. Ann Thorac Surg 1992;54:296.

III

SYSTEMIC CONSIDERATIONS IN THE SURGICAL TREATMENT OF THE CANCER PATIENT

Preoperative Evaluation of the Cancer Patient

DONALD D. MATHES
DAVID L. BOGDONOFF

The oncology patient undergoing surgery may at times represent a significant challenge with respect to preoperative evaluation and preparation. Both the anatomic and physiologic alterations resulting from the presence of a malignancy as well as the consequences of previous and concurrent therapy may have profound effects on the perioperative management of the patient. In addition, the advanced age of many oncology patients results in a myriad of other medical conditions, all needing to be considered simultaneously. This chapter focuses on many of the special problems the surgeon and anesthesiologist face in the preoperative evaluation of the oncology patient including the specific areas as listed above.

AIRWAY CONSIDERATIONS IN PATIENTS WITH HEAD AND NECK CANCER

The patient with head and neck cancer can represent a particular challenge for the surgeon and anesthesiologist with respect to airway management. Large and bulky tumors that present with airway obstructive symptoms are an obvious source of difficulty. Furthermore, airway management of small, asymptomatic tumors can be difficult and necessitate emergent tracheostomy with induction of general anesthesia. Distortion of airway anatomy can occur insidiously and be subclinical until attempts at intubation reveal the extent of the airway compromise. Tumors can invade laryngeal structures and surrounding tissues without being palpable on external physical examination. The cautious clinician should always seek to rule out airway involvement prior to surgical intervention using appropriate investigational techniques as well as appropriate consultations.

In addition to the anatomic implications of the tumor itself are the potential problems introduced by adjuvant radiation therapy treatment. Radiation causes both acute and chronic changes in the treatment area and unfortunately has an unpredictable effect. Edema and swelling of tissues may occur as a result of the initial radiation treatments but they usually subside when the treatments terminate. Edema of airway structures detected at a later date almost always represents recurrent malignancy rather than postradiation changes. The chronic changes induced by radiation therapy represent greater potential problems. Fibrosis of soft tissues in the neck occurs commonly due to the progressive microvascular changes caused by radiation injury. A lack of mobility and displaceability of these tissues may prevent airway visualization during laryngoscopy and thereby complicate or prevent tracheal intubation. Often such changes are apparent on a careful clinical examination of the neck. Appropriate back-up techniques such as awake intubation with fiberoptic intubation or tracheostomy need to be considered ahead of time, and preparations made to assure that appropriate personnel and equipment are on hand. Rarely, high doses of radiation may cause laryngeal necrosis with resultant fibrosis and stenosis of the airway. Additionally, one must be aware of the potential obliteration of lymphatic and venous channels that follows radiation treatments. These changes can lead to significant postoperative swelling with airway obstruction after a surgical procedure in the neck. Thus, the physician must approach airway management in the patient with head and neck cancer with the utmost caution.

SUMMARY: AIRWAY CONSIDERATIONS

1. Assess the patient carefully *before* intervention to evaluate for possible airway involvement.
2. Obtain a careful history, especially for details of prior radiation therapy.
3. Consider awake intubation or fiberoptic intubation in the problematic patient.

PREOPERATIVE ASSESSMENT FOR LUNG RESECTION

Evaluation prior to lung resection for malignancy requires preparation, appropriate education of the patient, and the determination of resectability of the lung tumor. After determining that resection of the lung tumor is indicated to attempt to cure the patient, risk stratification through a series of pulmonary tests must be performed to identify the patient at high risk for postoperative respiratory failure. The surgical approach to lung resection for a variety of tumors is further outlined in Chapter 12.

Pulmonary function tests should be performed through three stages as described by Benumof.[1] The first stage should include spirometry, lung volumes, and arterial blood gas. Several authors[1-4] have recommended the following parameters as predictive of high risk for lung resection:

1. Forced expiratory volume in 1 second (FEV_1) less than 50% of predicted or 2.0 L/sec.
2. Maximal volume ventilation (MVV) less than 50% of predicted.
3. Residual volume (RV) per total lung capacity (TLC) greater than 50%.
4. PCO_2 greater than 46 mm Hg on room air blood gas.

If any of the above initial pulmonary function tests qualify as high risk then a ventilation-perfusion scan using such radioisotopes as ^{133}Xe or ^{99}Tc should be performed.[1] By estimating the percent of function of each lobe remaining after the planned resection, the actual postoperative FVC and FEV_1 can be predicted. A predicted postoperative FEV_1 less than 0.8 L/sec is considered high risk for the development of postoperative respiratory failure.[3,4] Gass and Olsen[3] stated that using a predicted FEV_1 of less than 30% would be a better assessment for respiratory failure because an arbitrary number of 0.8 L/sec does not take into account the size or age of the person. Also, a postoperative predicted FEV_1 greater than 0.8 L/sec does not exclude the patient from the risk of chronic respiratory failure, but it makes the risk "acceptable."[3] For a lobectomy, a postoperative predicted FEV_1 should be evaluated as a functional pneumonectomy during the initial postoperative period.[1] The remainder of the resected lung often is initially nonfunctional secondary to such conditions as atelectasis, infection, and pulmonary edema. Also, the lung tumor may be more extensive at surgery than it appeared on preoperative evaluation, and it may require a pneumonectomy.

If the second stage evaluation suggests inoperability, temporary unilateral pulmonary artery occlusion is performed isolating all the pulmonary blood flow to the nonresected lung. This creates a functional pneumonectomy except for increased dead space ventilation to the nonperfused lung. If pulmonary artery pressures (PAP) reveal pulmonary hypertension with mean PAP greater than 35 mm Hg or PaO$_2$ less than 45 mm Hg or PaCO$_2$ greater than 60, the patient should be considered inoperable.[1,4,5]

Two other studies may be useful in predicting the risk of postoperative respiratory failure: (1) the measurement of pulmonary vascular resistance (PVR) and (2) maximal oxygen consumption (VO$_2$). Fee et al[6] found a significantly higher mortality in patients with a PVR with exercise greater than 190 dyne/sec/cm^5 undergoing lung resection.[6] An elevated PVR, especially with exercise, is a key marker depicting little or no ability for the remaining pulmonary vasculature to compensate for the increase in pulmonary blood flow after lung resection.

A simpler noninvasive test is the measurement of maximal oxygen consumption with exercise (VO$_2$). Eugene et al[7] found a 75% mortality in patients with VO$_2$ less than 1 L/min and no deaths in patients with a VO$_2$ greater than 1 L/min undergoing pulmonary resection. Smith et al[8] found, in patients undergoing a thoracotomy, that five of six patients had respiratory complications with VO$_2$ less than 15 mL/kg/min and only 1 of 10 patients had respiratory complications with VO$_2$ greater than 20 mL/kg/min. At this point, measurements of both PVR and VO$_2$ should be considered helpful guides of lung resectability but not as a standard. The significance of the measurements of PVR and VO$_2$ still needs further verification (Table 13-1). The use of thoracoscopic techniques (see Chapter 12) may allow resection of lesions in some patients who otherwise would be unresectable because of operative risk.

Table 13-1. Stages for Determination of Lung Resection

STAGE I	Spirometry, lung volumes, arterial blood gas, maximum oxygen consumption
	FEV$_1$ < 50% or < 2.0 L/sec
	MVV < 50%
	RV/TLC > 50%
	PCO$_2$ > 46 mm Hg
	VO$_2$ < 15–20 ml/kg
STAGE II	Radionuclide ventilation-perfusion scan
	Postoperative predicted FEV$_1$ < 0.8 L/sec or < 30%
STAGE III	Temporary unilateral pulmonary artery occlusion mean PAP >35 mmHg
	PaO$_2$ <45 mm Hg
	PaCO$_2$ >60 mm Hg
	PVR >190 dynes•sec•cm^5 (without pulmonary artery occlusion)

FEV$_1$ = forced expiratory volume in 1 second; MVV = maximal volume ventilation; RV = residual volume; TLC = total lung capacity; VO$_2$ = maximal oxygen consumption; PAP = pulmonary artery pressure; PVR = pulmonary vascular resistance

In conclusion, there is no single pulmonary test that can accurately predict the risk of postoperative respiratory complications and failure. Instead, the physician must evaluate a series of pulmonary tests for risk stratification and then weigh these findings against the very high mortality of unresected bronchogenic carcinoma.

SUMMARY: PREOPERATIVE ASSESSMENT FOR LUNG RESECTION

1. Obtain spirometry, lung volumes, and arterial blood gas.
2. If these demonstrate a high risk, then obtain an isotope ventilation-perfusion scan to quantify function in each lobe allowing prediction of postoperative lung function.
3. If the quantitative V/Q scan suggests inoperability, then temporary unilateral pulmonary artery occlusion is indicated to assess operability.
4. Measurement of pulmonary vascular re-

sistance and maximal oxygen consumption may be useful.
5. No single test accurately predicts the risk of postoperative pulmonary problems.

PREOPERATIVE EVALUATION OF ANTERIOR AND MIDDLE MEDIASTINAL MASSES

Anterior and middle mediastinal masses are associated with a significant risk of serious complications occurring in the operating room. These masses are in the same region as the tracheobronchial tree, pulmonary artery, superior vena cava, and the heart. However, other mediastinal masses still deserve the same cautious preoperative evaluation. In adults, most anterior and middle mediastinal masses are lymphomas or metastatic carcinomas, but teratomas, thymomas, bronchogenic or pericardial cysts, and aortic aneurysms also are among the possibilities.[9] Definitive treatment is dependent on an exact tissue diagnosis of the mediastinal mass. Thus, the surgeon will be consulted to obtain a specimen before any radiation therapy or chemotherapy has been administered in order not to interfere in any way with the pathologist's ability to make a tissue diagnosis. The surgical approach to many of these lesions is described in Chapter 12.

A complete preoperative evaluation of the patient with a mediastinal mass is essential. These patients may be at high risk for complete airway obstruction or cardiopulmonary arrest if general anesthesia is induced. Under general anesthesia, extrinsic tracheobronchial compression distal to the tip of the endotracheal tube from the mediastinal mass can occur especially with muscle relaxation and positive pressure ventilation. These patients should spontaneously ventilate under general anesthesia to maintain negative intrathoracic pressure. Positive pressure ventilation can collapse an already narrowed airway and increase turbulent flow.[10,11] Compression of the pulmonary artery, heart, and superior vena cava from a mediastinal mass can lead to cardiopulmonary arrest under general anesthesia.[11] Compression of these vital structures is often exacerbated with the patient in the supine position and can be relieved in an upright, lateral, or prone position.

A history of dyspnea, stridor, wheezing, or orthopnea should warn the physician of potential airway obstruction. Postural cyanosis or syncope are findings compatible with pulmonary artery or cardiac compression. Upper extremity and facial swelling with jugular venous distention are findings suggestive of superior vena caval obstruction. If on history and physical examination there are findings of possible mediastinal compression of vital structures, general anesthesia should be avoided and biopsies obtained under local anesthesia.[12]

In the asymptomatic patient, computed tomography (CT) of the chest, inspiratory and expiratory flow volume loops from pulmonary function tests, and echocardiography

Figure 13-1. Flow volume loop before radiation therapy in upright and supine positions with marked reduction in vital capacity and expiratory flow rates. The expiratory flow rate plateau is indicative of intrathoracic airway obstruction. From Neuman GG, Weingarten AE, Abramowitz RM, et al. The anesthetic management of the patient with an anterior mediastinal mass. Anesthesiology 1984;60:144; reprinted with permission.

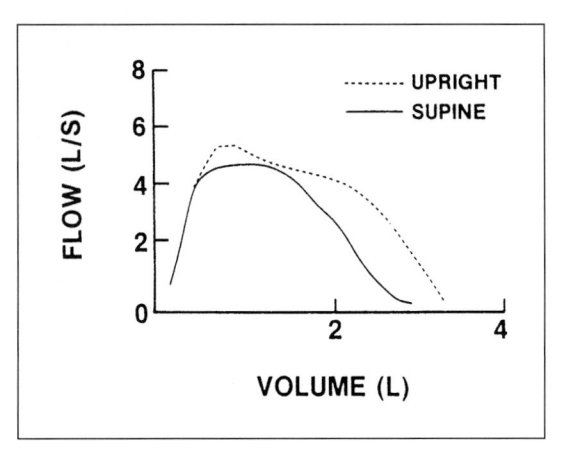

Preoperative Evaluation of the Cancer Patient

Figure 13-2. **A.** Chest x-ray showing widening of the mediastinum. **B.** CT scan of chest at the third thoracic vertebra level showing tracheal compression by the anterior mediastinal mass. **C.** CT scan of chest at fifth thoracic vertebra level showing bronchial compression. From Akhtar TM, Ridley S, Best CJ. Unusual presentation of acute upper airway obstruction caused by an anterior mediastinal mass. Br J Anaesth 1991;67:632; reprinted with permission.

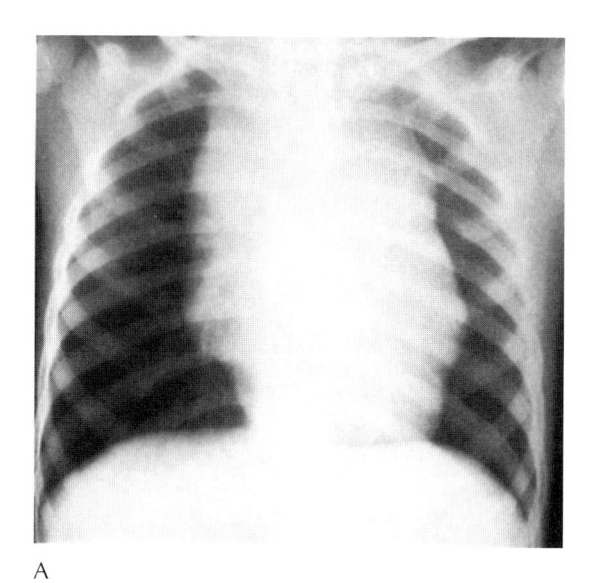

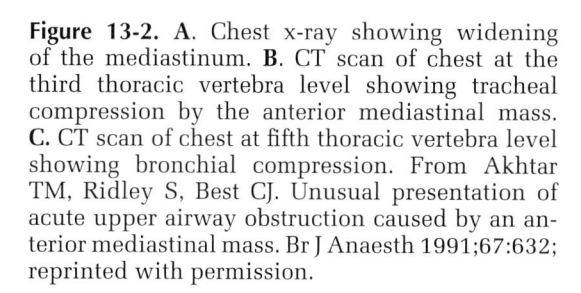

should be performed to rule out tracheobronchial, pulmonary artery, or cardiac compression. Expiratory and inspiratory flow volume loops are considered the most sensitive test for diagnosing airway impingement.[12] This test should be done in both the upright and supine positions. Most often with airway impingement, a prolonged expiratory plateau is found with the patient in the supine position, which improves in the upright position (Fig. 13-1).[12]

Computed tomography scan of the mediastinum should be reviewed closely for tracheobronchial compression or involvement of the pulmonary artery (Fig. 13-2).[13] Echocardiography should be performed in both upright and supine positions examining for decreased cardiac filling and function from encroachment of the pericardium and heart by the mediastinal mass. If there are any positive findings of these noninvasive tests, biopsy should be done under local anesthesia. If local anesthesia cannot be performed, then the patient should begin treatment in an attempt to decrease compression by the mediastinal mass. Radiation to the thorax can be used sparingly leaving a small window of unradiated tumor mass for biopsy.[9] Again before undergoing general anesthesia, the above-mentioned noninvasive tests should be performed (Fig. 13-3).

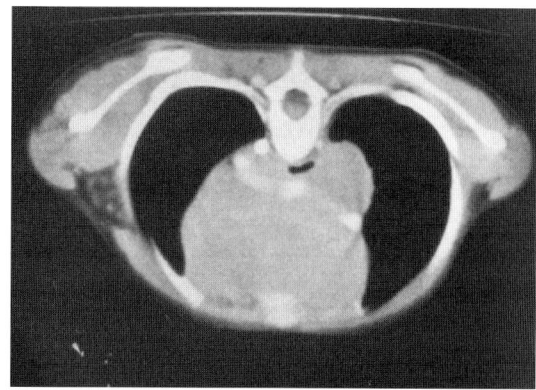

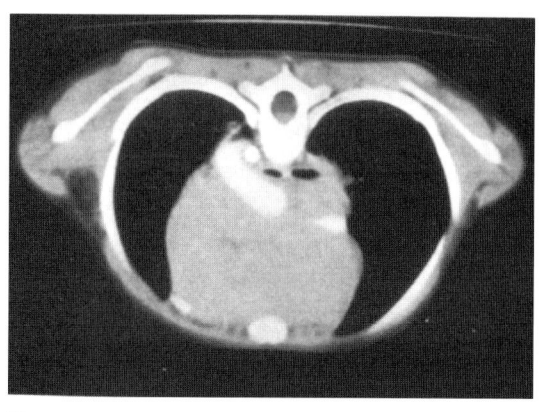

If general anesthesia is indicated despite continued positive symptoms or findings after treatment of the mediastinal mass, then the following should be implemented: (1) an awake fiberoptic intubation; (2) continuous spontaneous ventilation throughout the general anesthetic; (3) rigid bronchoscope im-

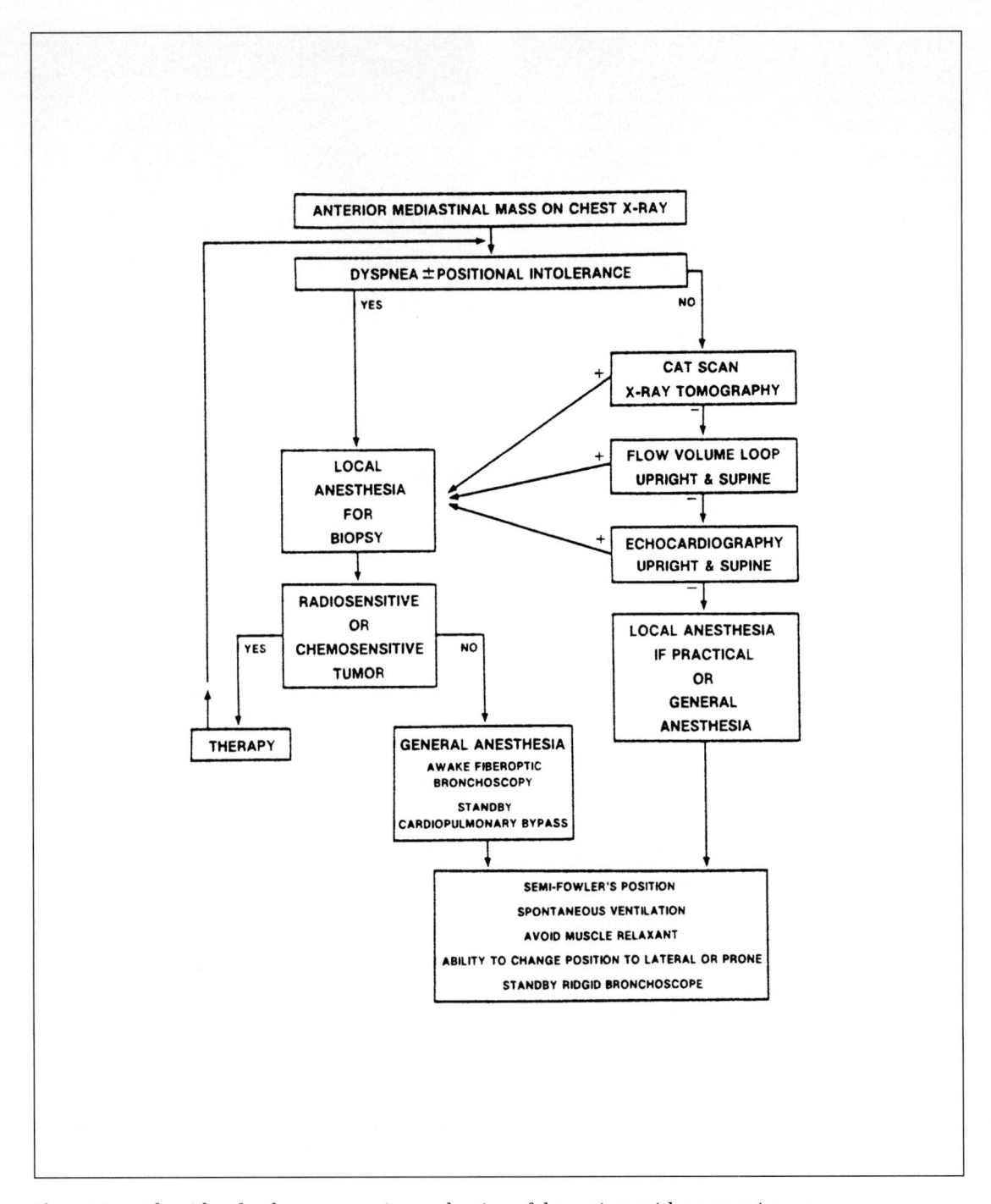

Figure 13-3. Algorithm for the preoperative evaluation of the patient with an anterior mediastinal mass. + = indicates positive finding; − = indicates negative work-up. From Neuman GG, Weingarten AE, Abramowitz RM, et al. The anesthetic management of the patient with an anterior mediastinal mass. Anesthesiology 1984;60:144; reprinted with permission.

mediately available for placement to stent open a collapsed airway; (4) ability to quickly change the patient to a lateral, prone, or sitting position if airway obstruction or cardiovascular collapse occurs; (5) femoral to femoral cardiopulmonary bypass on standby in the operating room in the event of cardiovascular collapse.

SUMMARY: PREOPERATIVE EVALUATION OF ANTERIOR AND MIDDLE MEDIASTINAL MASSES

1. Potential for airway obstruction may be suggested by a history of dyspnea, stridor, wheezing, or orthopnea.
2. In the asymptomatic patient, CT scan of the chest, pulmonary function tests, and echocardiography should be obtained.
3. Those patients with positive findings who must undergo general anesthesia should have awake fiberoptic intubation, continuous spontaneous ventilation, rapid availability of a rigid bronchoscope, and the ability to put the patient in a lateral or prone position rapidly and to apply femoral-femoral cardiopulmonary bypass.

PREOPERATIVE EVALUATION OF PERICARDIAL EFFUSIONS AND CARDIAC TAMPONADE

Pericardial effusions and cardiac tamponade, when present in the oncology patient, are most often secondary to metastasis of the malignancy to the pericardium. Furthermore, encasement of the pericardium can occur with tumors such as mesotheliomas and sarcomas.[14] Also, cardiac tamponade can occur from constrictive pericarditis from radiation therapy or an inflammatory process.[14]

The normal volume of pericardial fluid is 20 to 25 mL in humans.[15] As little as 100 to 250 mL of pericardial fluid can cause tamponade if pericardial fluid accumulates quickly.[15,16] However, as much as 1000 mL of pericardial fluid can accumulate without compromising cardiac filling if the pericardium has an opportunity to stretch slowly.[16] Cardiac tamponade occurs when the increased intrapericardial pressure prevents adequate diastolic filling, hence causing a diminished stroke volume and cardiac output. Tachycardia and an increase in systemic vascular resistance occur from increased plasma catecholamines in an attempt to maintain adequate blood perfusion. This compensation will fail if intrapericardial pressure continues to rise.[15]

A history of progressive dyspnea, retrosternal chest pain relieved with leaning forward, and abdominal discomfort from hepatic engorgement are findings compatible with pericardial tamponade. Physical examination will reveal jugular venous distention, muffled heart sounds, narrow pulse pressure, and hepatic engorgement. Pulsus paradoxus with a decrease ≥ 10 mm Hg of systolic blood pressure with inspiration is classic for pericardial tamponade but is in no way pathognomonic of pericardial tamponade, nor does the absence of pulsus paradoxus exclude the possibility of pericardial tamponade.[14] With pericardial effusions, an electrocardiogram (ECG) often will have decreased voltage and may have electrical alternans (shifting of the QRS axis). A minimum of 250 mL of pericardial effusion is needed before the cardiac silhouette begins to show evidence of a pericardial effusion.[15] The classic chest x-ray picture for a large pericardial effusion is a water bottle or globular shaped heart.

Pulmonary artery catheterization in cardiac tamponade will reveal elevation of right atrial pressure with a large x descent and a decreased or absent y descent waveform. Equalization of pressures may occur with right atrial and ventricular pressure equaling pulmonary diastolic and wedge pressure. However, patients with prior left ventricular dysfunction may continue to have higher left-sided pressures over right-sided pressures despite significant cardiac tamponade.[17]

Echocardiography can detect as little as 15 mL of pericardial fluid.[15] Furthermore, echocardiography can determine if the pericardial fluid is causing right ventricle diastolic collapse and impaired diastolic filling. Thus, echocardiography is an important guide in enabling the physician to determine the need and location for pericardial drainage.

Management of a large pericardial effusion depends on the degree of hemodynamic compromise and likely reaccumulation of the effusion. Subxiphoid pericardiocentesis under local anesthesia is most commonly done in an emergent situation. If general anesthesia is indicated, arterial line cannulation and pulmonary artery catheterization should be placed before induction and the patient placed in a semi-Fowler's position to help improve venous return.[18] The detailed management of pericardial effusions can be found in Chapter 12. The usual approach is subxiphoid pericardiectomy. In some patients, pericardiperitoneal shunt placement may be necessary.

The goals of managing pericardial tamponade are the same preoperatively and in the operating room. Maintaining a high cardiac filling pressure is essential to overcome the increase in intrapericardial pressure and to allow for adequate diastolic filling. A relative tachycardia and vasoconstriction is needed to allow for adequate cardiac output and arterial perfusion. If positive pressure ventilation is needed, then small tidal volumes and avoidance of positive end expiratory pressure (PEEP) should be implemented to minimize any decrease in right ventricular filling.

SUMMARY: PREOPERATIVE EVALUATION OF PERICARDIAL EFFUSIONS AND CARDIAC TAMPONADE

1. A history of progressive dyspnea, retrosternal chest pain relieved with leaning forward, and abdominal discomfort from hepatic engorgement are consistent with pericardial tamponade.
2. Physical examination reveals jugular venous distention, muffled heart sounds, narrow pulse pressure, and hepatic engorgement.
3. Obtain an echocardiogram.
4. For patients requiring general anesthesia, both arterial and pulmonary artery catheterization are indicated. A relative tachycardia and vasoconstriction help to improve cardiac output.

PREOPERATIVE EVALUATION OF CARCINOID SYNDROME AND PHEOCHROMOCYTOMA

The patient with carcinoid syndrome may require special preoperative preparation, particularly with respect to the choice of pharmacologic agents which must be available intraoperatively. Most patients with carcinoid tumors presenting for curative resection are diagnosed early, as in the case of a bronchial carcinoid, or postoperatively by the pathologist, as in the case of an ileal or appendiceal tumor. Such tumors are small and do not carry much of a risk of carcinoid crisis from release of humoral substances and therefore do not present a major challenge to the anesthesiologist. Most patients with the carcinoid syndrome already have tissue diagnoses of carcinoid and have elements of the various described clinical syndromes. Although rarely presenting for a curative operation, it is not uncommon for patients with advanced carcinoid disease to require either a palliative or therapeutic surgical procedure. These patients need to be adequately prepared for surgery.

Patients with carcinoid syndrome may have many symptoms and often do not manifest the classically described syndrome. Multiple hormonal substances may be released by the tumor and it is the varying amounts of the different substances that result in the varying clinical presentations. Release of 5-hydroxytryptamine (serotonin) will result in symptoms of diarrhea with abdominal cramping, respiratory distress, bronchospasm, and hypertension. Secretion of bradykinin and histamine leads to other symptoms of cutaneous flushing and hypotension as well as contributing to bronchospasm.

Preparing the patient with carcinoid syndrome for surgery requires adequate preoperative hydration. Additionally, it is important to rule out the presence of any right-sided valvular heart disease, which can result from long-standing carcinoid syndrome. Usually this would be manifested by right-sided heart failure. Echocardiography will effectively and noninvasively demonstrate any hemodynamically significant heart disease. All other measures taken are pharmacologic and involve administration of drugs to block the effects of released hormones at the end organ level as well as administration of drugs that block secretion by the carcinoid cells.

Antihistamines (both H_1 and H_2) are obvious choices for blockade of the effects of released histamine. Ketanserin may be used to block the effects of serotonin.[19] Steroids have been suggested as adjuncts, although the mechanisms behind their beneficial action are speculative. The centrally acting alpha-2 agonist (clonidine) as well as alpha- and beta-blocking drugs are possibly effective in decreasing hormonal secretion. The most effective approach probably is to administer somatostatin or its analog (octreotide) in an effort to prevent hormonal release in the first place. We use a protocol of preoperative and intraoperative administration of octreotide in moderately large doses (Table 13-2). There have been reports of catastrophic cardiovascular collapse associated with the induction of anesthesia in patients with carcinoid syndrome. Carcinoid crisis may also be precipitated by preparation of the abdomen or manipulation of any tumor mass. Most reports of problems and solutions with carcinoid crises are anecdotal and can only serve as a guide in the absence of large controlled trials. Successful resuscitation resulted from the use of large doses of octreotide during adverse events and is our recommended first line therapy.[20]

Table 13-2. Preoperative Prophylaxis in Carcinoid Patients

1. Octreotide 250 µg subcut every 8 h for 48–72 h preoperatively
2. Octreotide 250 µg subcut not more than 1–2 h preoperatively
3. Octreotide 500 µg in OR available for IV push in case of carcinoid crisis

The anesthetic approach to these patients has been reviewed by Longnecker and Roizen.[21] The anesthesiologist must avoid drugs that result in histamine release. Hypotension must be treated with fluids and an effort made to refrain from the use of catecholamines, which may result in further hormonal release by the tumor. Angiotensin may be effective if it is available. Hypertension may be treated with conventional drugs such as nitroprusside. Bronchospasm may be problematic, but it can be treated with steroids, potent inhalational anesthetics, and blocking drugs such as ketanserin.

Pheochromocytoma

Pheochromocytoma is a rare disorder that is responsible for only a small percentage of cases of hypertension. It is particularly dangerous when undiagnosed and has been responsible for deaths during the induction of anesthesia.[22] Pheochromocytomas are much less dangerous when one is aware of their existence and, in fact, large series of such cases have been recently reported with rare or no mortality.[23–25]

Common signs and symptoms of pheochromocytoma include headache, sweating, hypertension, and tachycardia. Although most patients do have symptoms from their disease, there is a great deal of variability in the symptom complexes. A number of asymptomatic patients are identified by screening tests after disease is found in a family member. The mainstay of preparation for surgery is pharmacologic manipulation with the use of alpha and possibly beta blockers or the use of metyrosine, which blocks catecholamine synthesis.[26] Other drugs and even protocols without the use of drugs have been proposed.[24,27] The management of the patient with pheochromocytoma is best handled by an approach coordinating the efforts of various involved clinical services. Symptom reduction and correction of underlying abnormalities may be achieved but demands meticulous patient monitoring during the preoperative preparatory phase. Unfortunately, there are no controlled studies of preoperative and intraoperative management, making definitive conclusions difficult.

The greatest experience and probably the most conservative approach is with the preoperative use of alpha blocking drugs.[28,29] Mortality has definitely decreased since the introduction of these drugs, leading some to assume a causative role for them in this reduction. Whether or not this is true or the result of parallel improvements in pharmacologic manipulations and physiological monitoring remains unclear. Phenoxybenzamine is a long-acting alpha blocking drug that is started at doses of 20 to 30 mg (per 70 kg) orally once or twice a day. It is gradually increased as tolerated, and as guided by diminution of symptoms, to a final dose usually between 60 and 250 mg/d. One should eliminate sweating and headaches and stabilize blood pressure in patients. Complaints of nasal stuffiness are not uncommon. Orthostatic hypotension of a moderate degree is to be tolerated. Additionally, one may see a drop in fasting blood sugar from the blockade of the inhibitory effects of catecholamines on insulin secretion. The duration of alpha blockade has also been the subject of debate, with some authors suggesting a minimum of 10 to 14 days whereas others suggest even longer durations.[29] Whereas there have been suggestions of eliminating alpha blockade due to an apparent lack of effect on mortality,[24] others have shown additional beneficial effects. Higher than usual doses of phenoxybenzamine resulted in fewer hemodynamic side effects in one recent small, controlled study.[30] An increase in intraoperative tissue oxygen delivery was demonstrated when phenoxybenzamine was used and served a protective role against the adverse effects of intraoperative catechol excesses.[31] Prazosin is a selective alpha-1 blocking drug that also has been used for preoperative preparation. Its advantages over phenoxybenzamine are theoretic owing to selective alpha-1 blockade and probably depend on the experience of the clinicians following the patient.

Beta blockade should be instituted only following the use of alpha blockers. Tachyarrhythmias or symptomatic tachycardia is the only indication for these drugs and, in fact, most patients may be prepared for surgery without them. Reports of heart failure due to unopposed alpha adrenergic stimulation have followed the institution of beta blockade without prior alpha blockade.[32]

Cardiomyopathy secondary to catechol excess may be present in this patient population and must be treated if present.[33] It is diagnosed by history and ECG and further elucidated with the aid of echocardiography. ECG changes and cardiac function may improve over time with alpha blockade or with another form of afterload reduction.[32,34] It is likely that when cardiomyopathy is present, a longer duration of preoperative pharmacologic preparation may prove useful.

Intraoperative management of the pheochromocytoma patient requires adequate hemodynamic monitoring of arterial blood pressure as well as central venous pressures. Central access is also necessary for the rapid administration of hemodynamically active drugs. Phenoxybenzamine should generally be continued and given the morning of surgery or at least in the evening prior to operation. No large trials of anesthetic administration have been undertaken and reports of virtually all possible drugs and techniques have been published. It is important to minimize anxiety and other stresses of the anesthetic induction as hypertensive responses are common despite the lack of direct tumor manipulation at these times. All adrenergic nerve endings have increased catechol levels and therefore exaggerated responses may occur secondary to any intervention. This represents the best argument for the preoperative use of metyrosine, which actually depletes the total catechol pool available by blocking synthesis.

The major challenge occurs intraoperatively during the inevitable manipulation of the tumor. Tenfold or more increases in circulating catecholamine levels have been measured during such surgical manipulation.[35] Such increases clearly lead to hypertensive crises at times and require a rapid response if blood pressures exceed 200 mm HG. Nitroprusside is a short-lasting and rapidly acting agent that is most helpful intraoperatively. Phentolamine, a short-acting alpha blocker, also is useful, particularly when high doses of nitroprusside are required. Tachycardia and ventricular ectopy are treated with esmolol, a rapidly acting beta blocker with a half-life of only 9 minutes. It is important to stop or decrease the rates of infusion of these drugs prior to ligation of adrenal veins and removal of the tumor. At this time, drastic decreases in serum catecholamines occur and the patient is susceptible to hypotension and hypovolemia secondary to vasodilation. Administering large amounts of fluid usually suffices but occasionally direct-acting vasopressors are required.

SUMMARY: PREOPERATIVE EVALUATION OF CARCINOID SYNDROME AND PHEOCHROMOCYTOMA

Carcinoid Syndrome

1. Preoperative hydration is an important element in the management of patients with carcinoid syndrome. Echocardiography is indicated to rule out right-sided heart disease.
2. Antihistamines and ketanserin (serotonin blockade) are helpful. Octreotide (a somatostatin analogue; see Table 13–2) is helpful to prevent hormonal release.
3. Intraoperatively, hypotension is treated with fluid administration and octreotide and hypertension is treated with nitroprusside and octreotide.

Pheochromocytoma

1. Alpha blockade (phenoxybenzamine) is begun preoperatively and titrated to diminish symptoms, usually a dose of 60 to 250 mg/d.
2. Beta blockade is used only after adequate alpha blockade.
3. Central access is essential intraoperatively. Nitroprusside is used to acutely manage intraoperative hypertension. Phentolamine may also be useful. Hypotension usually is managed with fluids, but short-term use of vasopressors may be needed.

HEMATOLOGIC CONSIDERATIONS IN PREOPERATIVE EVALUATION

The oncology patient can have multiple hematologic abnormalities ranging from anemia and thrombocytopenia to hypercoagulable states. The physician performing a thorough preoperative evaluation often will be required to make decisions about the need for preoperative blood products or other hematologic interventions. The specific hematologic effects of many types of cancer therapy are further discussed in Chapter 17.

Anemia

Until the 1980s, the majority of physicians thought patients should have a minimal hemoglobin of 10 gm/dL preoperatively. This thinking has now changed with the known risk of transmitting viral diseases through transfusions becoming prominent. Physicians have re-evaluated the lower limits of acceptable preoperative hemoglobin.

The first conclusion drawn was that the only indication for transfusion of red blood cells was to increase the oxygen carrying capacity of blood.[36] Second, healthy patients with good cardiopulmonary reserve can tolerate hemoglobin levels of 7 gm/dL or lower as long as they are normovolemic. Third, patients with increased oxygen demands, pulmonary or cardiac insufficiency, myocardial ischemia, and cerebrovascular disease need hemoglobin levels of 9 to 10 gm/dL or higher, depending on the extent of disease.[36,37] Fourth, chronic anemia states, such as that seen in renal failure, are much better tolerated intraoperatively compared with the acute onset of anemia. Fifth, for lower levels of hemoglobin to be tolerated, it is essential that the patient be normovolemic.[38] Hypovolemic states will decrease tissue perfusion of blood and thus directly decrease oxygen delivery to the tissue beds. Thus, every oncology patient has to be assessed individually.

Bone marrow suppression from chemotherapy or bone marrow failure from infiltration of malignancy often requires the patient to be already transfusion-dependent with little capability of compensating for any further blood loss in the operating room. The effects of chemotherapy on bone marrow are further discussed in Chapter 17. One should have a lower threshold for transfusing these patients preoperatively because they have little bone marrow reserve.

Several studies suggest that blood transfusions may increase cancer recurrence rates. Schriemer et al[39] in their review found several studies showing a higher recurrence rate of colon, rectal, breast, cervical carcinomas, and soft tissue sarcomas in surgically treated oncology patients who had received blood products. Blumberg et al[40] found a significant higher recurrence rate of surgically treated prostate, colonic, rectal, and cervical cancers in patients receiving transfusions of whole blood or greater than 3 U of homologous packed red blood cells (PRBC). Blumberg et al[40] and Gascon et al[41] concluded that an unknown mediator in the plasma of blood transfusions causes immunosuppression especially decreasing natural killer cell activity. If enough plasma was transfused (such as in a single unit of whole blood or several units of PRBCs), the immunosuppressive effects of the plasma caused a higher recurrence rate of cancer.[40] Indeed, if blood is needed in the surgical oncology patient, it should be limited to packed red blood cells to limit the amount of plasma transfused to the patient. Data supporting the clinical relevance of immunosuppression, while suggestive, is not definitive and in view of the fact that the increased risk of tumor recurrence from the transfusion of homologous blood is unproven, one should not advocate the use of autologous blood to reduce these risks (refer to Chapter 17).

Other strategies to decrease the amount of homologous blood transfused include the use of prior donated autologous blood. There is no evidence that giving autologous blood increases the risk of metastatic disease.[39] However, the patient must have normal bone marrow function for this to be effective. The use of cell saver blood in the oncology patient is debatable. At most, the risk of recurrent cancer from cell saver blood is small.[42] Karczewski et al[43] found that filtration of cell saver blood from leiomyosarcoma resection and radical cystectomy filtered 94% of carcinoma cells. Of the remaining filtered cancer cells in the cell saver blood, none of these cancer cells was able to be recultured.

No definite conclusion about the use of cell-saver blood in the surgical oncology patient can be made at this time. However, the risk of hematogenous spread of cancer cells from cell saver blood appears to be small and may be only a theoretic concern. Salsbury,[44] in the review of the literature, found that circulating cancer cells in the blood had little or no prognostic significance. Indeed, the risk of hematogenous spread of cancer from cell saver blood is most likely less than the incidence of local or hematogenous seeding from tumor resection.[43] Therefore, the surgeon and anesthesiologist must weigh the known risk of immunosuppression and the possible increased recurrence rates of certain cancers from giving several units of homologous blood versus the small and possibly only theoretic risk of recurrence of giving cell saver blood. To date, however, there have been no randomized trials of cell saver blood in operative procedures for cancer. Application of the cell saver in oncologic surgical procedures should await the results of carefully controlled trials.

Thrombocytopenia

In the oncology patient, there are multiple possible causes of thrombocytopenia including bone marrow suppression or failure, portal hypertension, hypersplenism, and idiopathic thrombocytopenia.[45] On preoperative evaluation, no absolute minimal platelet number can be recommended as required for safe conduct of surgery. Patients with chronic thrombocytopenia, such as in myelodysplastic disorders or those with rapid destruction but increased production of platelets such as with idiopathic thrombocytopenia, have less bleeding than patients with other platelet disorders.[46]

The National Institutes of Health Consensus Conference in 1987 recommended that in the presence of active bleeding, patients with platelet counts greater than 50,000/mm^3 probably will not benefit from platelet transfusions if actual platelet function is normal.[46] This conference also recommended that a bleeding time less than twice the upper limit of reference usually is not an indication for transfusion of platelets in the face of active bleeding unless there are other conditions interfering with hemostasis.[46] Schwartz recommended that asymptomatic patients with platelet counts greater than 50,000/mm^3 do not require platelet transfusion for elective surgery.[47] However, Gravlee[48] stated that platelet transfusions may be needed preoperatively in patients with platelet dysfunction from such conditions as aspirin use or uremia even with platelet counts greater than 100,000/mm^3. Also, most anesthesiologists will not place epidural catheters in patients with platelet counts less than 100,000/mm^3 because of the possible increased risk of an epidural hematoma. Hence, the thrombocytopenic patient most likely will not be eligible for the proved benefits of postoperative epidural analgesia. The use of preoperative platelet administration in the thrombocytopenic patient is discussed in Chapter 17.

Thrombocytosis

Thrombocytosis with platelet counts greater than 1,000,000/mm^3 can be seen with myeloproliferative syndromes and in solid tumors. In the myeloproliferative syndromes, thromboembolic events do occur with thrombocytosis but are rare, possibly secondary to these platelets being dysfunctional.[49] These patients' platelet counts should be lowered preoperatively for elective procedures either by chemotherapy or platelet pheresis.[49] Thrombocytosis from solid tumors has an increased incidence of thromboembolic events. These patients' platelet counts usually decrease with treatment of the solid tumor.[49]

Coagulation Abnormalities

The oncology patient may have multiple coagulation abnormalities with a strong association of malignancy with hypercoagulable states. Trousseau, in 1865, reported a strong association between thrombosis and malignancy. Increased coagulation factors, including fibrinogen with an accelerated rate of fibrinogen turnover and increased fibrin split products, are commonly found in the oncology patient.[50] Also, increased factors V, VIII, IX, and XI have been reported with malignancy (see Chapter 11).[50] Subclinical disseminated intravascular coagulopathy (DIC) is often found with malignancies. Clinically significant DIC is associated with mucin-secreting adenocarcinomas especially pancreas, stomach, and prostate. Acute promyelocytic leukemia is often associated with DIC especially during treatment from the release of thromboplastin.[51]

During the perioperative period, the

oncology patient is at increased risk of developing DIC secondary to surgical manipulation of tumor with release of tissue thromboplastin. Also, the oncology patient is at particularly high risk for venous thrombosis formation during the postoperative period, which may occur from a decreased antithrombin III level.[49] Thus, appropriate measures to prevent venous thrombosis and monitoring for the development of DIC are essential in the postoperative period. The most important factor in the therapy of DIC is the identification and treatment of the underlying cause.

Except for thrombocytopenia, hypocoagulable states are less often seen in patients with malignancy. Elevation of prothrombin time (PT) and partial thromboplastin time (PTT) can be caused by multiple factors. Direct liver damage from cancer or chemotherapy, malabsorption of vitamin K, and a consumptive coagulopathy from DIC all are common reasons for elevated PT and PTT. Certain malignancies are associated with decreased coagulation factors such as decreased factor V with chronic myelocytic leukemia.[49] Also, paraproteins from malignancy can function as anticoagulants by surrounding coagulation factors and preventing their normal function.[49] A lupus anticoagulant factor can be associated with malignancy. This factor causes a prolonged PT, but paradoxically it is more often associated with thrombosis.

In conclusion, a complete blood count, including platelets and white blood cells, and coagulation studies with PT and PTT should be obtained at the time of preoperative evaluation. Decisions to transfuse blood products should be made on an individual basis but general guidelines can be followed. If thrombocytopenia or an elevation in PT or PTT is found, then clinical or subclinical DIC should be sought after by obtaining fibrinogen and fibrin split products. Lastly, appropriate preoperative and postoperative measures to prevent thromboembolic events should be implemented secondary to the increased incidence of hypercoagulable state found in the cancer patient. These considerations are further discussed in Chapter 17.

SUMMARY: HEMATOLOGIC CONSIDERATIONS IN PREOPERATIVE EVALUATION

1. Healthy patients with good cardiopulmonary reserve can tolerate hemoglobin levels of 7 gm/dL or lower as long as they are normovolemic.
2. Patients with platelet counts of 50,000/mm^3 or greater probably will not benefit from platelet transfusions if platelet function is normal.
3. Measures must be taken to prevent venous thrombosis.
4. Oncology patients should have a complete blood count and coagulation studies as part of the preoperative evaluation.

RENAL AND ELECTROLYTE DISORDERS IN THE ONCOLOGY PATIENT

In the oncology patient, there are multiple causes for renal and electrolyte abnormalities. However, only rarely do these problems occur acutely during the preoperative period. Thus, the physician has the benefit of many of these abnormalities being thoroughly evaluated in advance. This section discusses the common problems and considerations of renal and electrolyte abnormalities that the surgeon may be presented with at the time of preoperative evaluation.

Hyponatremia

There are many causes for hyponatremia in oncology patients. Severe metastatic liver disease with ascites and hypoalbuminemia, malignant ascites, nephrotic syndrome, and congestive heart failure cause an increase in total body sodium and even greater water retention, resulting in hyponatremia. These patients should be treated with water restriction and diuretics such as spironolactone to block aldosterone effects on renal tubules and thus increase sodium and free water loss.

The syndrome of inappropriate antidiuretic hormone (SIADH) is associated with paraneoplastic syndromes commonly seen with small cell carcinoma of the lung, central nervous system disorders, and with drugs such as cyclophosphamide or vincristine. These patients clinically appear euvolemic. Diagnosis is best made with an inappropriately elevated urine osmolality compared with serum osmolality. For SIADH, fluid restriction is the primary treatment. In patients with serum sodium levels less than 120 meq/L with seizures or mental status changes, 3% normal saline plus furosemide can be used to bring the sodium to 120 meq/L over a few hours. Yet one must be careful to elevate the serum sodium slowly beyond 120 meq/L to prevent neurologic damage from central pontine myelinolysis.

The least common cause of hyponatremia is from gastrointestinal (GI) losses occurring from vomiting and diarrhea caused by chemotherapy. This can easily be corrected by giving isotonic saline. Also, artificial hyponatremia can occur from severe hyperglycemia, hyperlipidemia, or hyperproteinemia such as seen in multiple myeloma. Sodium will artificially lower 1.6 meq/L for every 100 mg/dL plasma glucose is above normal.[52] Elective surgery should be postponed with sodium less than 125 mg/L, especially if the cause of hyponatremia is unclear.

Hypernatremia

Hypernatremia in the oncology patient is most often caused by hypovolemia from a free water deficit. The cause of the free water deficit can be an inability of the kidney to concentrate urine from neurogenic or nephrogenic diabetes insipidus. Other causes include lack of replacement of GI fluid losses or an osmotic diuresis from hyperglycemia or mannitol. Replacement should initially consist of isotonic saline to expand the decreased plasma volume followed by hypotonic solutions. Again, rapid correction can lead to neurologic damage.

Hypokalemia

Hypokalemia is commonly seen in the preoperative evaluation of the oncology patient. The reasons for the hypokalemia may be multifactorial. GI losses from nasogastric suction and vomiting cause increased renal potassium loss. This occurs from increased aldosterone levels and an elevated potassium concentration in the renal tubular cells and subsequent secretion into the urine. Diarrhea has high concentrations of potassium and can lead to hypokalemia. Osmotic diuresis from mannitol or hyperglycemia, magnesium depletion, diuretics, amphotericin B, and cisplatinum all can cause renal potassium wasting. Respiratory and metabolic alkalosis also can cause hypokalemia. A decrease of $PaCO_2$ of 10 mm Hg will decrease serum potassium approximately 0.5 meq/L.[53]

Serum potassium levels less than 2.6 meq/L are associated with a large total body potassium deficit of 300 to 400 meq or more.[54] This potassium deficit should be corrected over several days with no more than 10 to 20 meq kcl/h being administered intravenously. There has been no proved benefit in trying to correct potassium in the preoperative period in an asymptomatic patient with a serum potassium of 2.6 to 3.5 meq/L.[55,56] Indeed, elective surgery does not need to be postponed for serum potassium levels between 2.6 and 3.5 meq/L unless the patient is in one of the following categories: (1) a recent acute decrease in potassium; (2) high risk of intraoperative or postoperative arrhythmias; (3) at risk for digoxin toxicity.[55,56]

Hyperkalemia

The most common cause of hyperkalemia in the oncology patient is decreased renal excretion of potassium due to renal failure. Also, a markedly increased release of intracellular potassium from cell breakdown in tumor lysis syndrome can occur from chemotherapy. Other causes of hyperkalemia include potassium-sparing diuretics, adrenal insufficiency, and metabolic and respiratory acidosis. A decrease in the pH of 0.1 U will cause an increase of 0.4 to 1.5 meq/L of serum potassium.[57]

The earliest markers of symptomatic hyperkalemia are peaked T waves on the ECG, which generally occurs with potassium levels greater than 7 meq/L but can occur at lower levels with more acute changes.[57] Peaked T waves are followed by prolongation of the PR interval, widening of the QRS complex, and eventually a sine wave pattern. Acutely, treatment for severe hyperkalemia consists of giving calcium gluconate or calcium chloride to stabilize the cardiac cell membranes followed by giving sodium bicarbonate, glucose, and insulin to lower serum potassium by driving potassium into the cell. This should be followed by more definitive treatment by administering sodium polystyrene sulfonate (Kayexalate) orally or in enemas and by giving loop diuretics. If the patient has renal failure, then peritoneal or hemodialysis with a hypokalemic bath should be performed. Elective surgery should not be performed in any patient with a serum potassium greater than 5.5 meq/L.

Hypercalcemia

The cause of hypercalcemia in the oncology patient is most often from the malignancy itself, which causes direct bone reabsorption or a paraneoplastic syndrome. However, other reasons, especially primary hyperparathyroidism, sarcoidosis, vitamin A or D intoxication, thiazide diuretics, or lithium use, should be excluded.[58] A full consultation with an oncologist or endocrinologist should be obtained to evaluate the many possible causes.

In actually determining the level of calcium, one should look at both the free ionized and serum levels. The serum level of calcium drops approximately 0.8 mg/dL for every 1 gm/dL decrease of albumin below 4.0 gm/dL.[59] It is especially important to note that the hypoalbuminemic patient may be actually hypercalcemic while appearing normocalcemic.

The symptoms of hypercalcemia are often nonspecific with anorexia, nausea, constipation, muscle weakness, mental status change, lethargy, polydipsia, and polyuria.[58] Corrected serum calcium levels greater than 13 mg/dL should be treated emergently. However, more moderate levels of hypercalcemia need not cause delay in elective surgery if the patient is asymptomatic. The electrocardiogram should be examined for evidence of shortened PR or QT intervals.[57] Renal function also should be examined because hypercalcemia can cause renal tubular damage with an inability to concentrate urine or renal calculi causing outflow obstruction.

The mainstay for the treatment of hypercalcemia is intravenous hydration with isotonic solutions plus loop diuretics to promote calcium excretion together with oral phosphate repletion. Glucocorticoids, which inhibit GI absorption of calcium, and calcitonin, which inhibits direct bone reabsorption, both are commonly used to treat hypercalcemia. Mithramycin is used only for the most refractory or critical hypercalcemic patients because of its many toxic effects as discussed under the chemotherapy section. Also, the use of intravenous phosphate is a very effective treatment for hypercalcemia, but its use can lead to ectopic calcification, renal failure, and rapid hypocalcemia.[60] Hence, intravenous phosphate should be used only under the direction of an endocrinologist or oncologist.

Hypocalcemia

Hypocalcemia in the oncology patient is most commonly due to hypomagnesemia. Hypomagnesemia causes decreased secretion of parathyroid hormone (PTH) and resistance of bone response to PTH.[54] Hypocalcemia will not easily correct until serum magnesium levels are repleted.[54] Another common cause of apparent low serum calcium levels is hypoalbuminemia. Serum calcium levels will decrease 0.8 mg/dL for every decrease of 1.0 gm/dL of albumin below 4.0 gm/dL.[59] However, ionized calcium levels will remain unchanged.

Other less common causes of hypocalcemia in oncology patients include decreased PTH secretion, decreased vitamin D metabolism or production, and hyperphosphatemia. Elevated levels of phosphate can be seen from cell breakdown from chemotherapy for lymphomas and leukemias. The elevated level of phosphate can combine with existing calcium and cause hypocalcemia.

Hypomagnesemia

The causes of hypomagnesemia in the oncology patient can be multifactorial. Reduced food intake, malabsorption, increased GI losses from vomiting or diarrhea, and increased renal loss of magnesium can all combine to cause hypomagnesemia. Magnesium depletion commonly occurs from renal wasting secondary to diuretics, amphotericin, and cis-platinum. Depletion of magnesium can cause both hypocalcemia and hypokalemia, which are both not easily correctable until magnesium levels are replenished. Severe hypomagnesemia (levels <1.0 mg/L) can cause symptoms such as hypocalcemia with muscle weakness, fasciculations, seizures, and paresthesias.[54] Also, hypomagnesemia can increase the incidence of cardiac arrhythmias. Thus, at the time of preoperative evaluation, magnesium levels should be checked for patients at risk of developing hypomagnesemia and especially for those patients at risk for developing cardiac dysrhythmias or taking digoxin.

Acute Renal Failure

Acute renal failure (ARF) in the oncology patient can be multifactorial and complex in its etiology. It is not the purpose of this section to discuss all the possible causes of acute renal failure but rather to provide the surgeon with a basic approach in the evaluation of ARF and an awareness of the common causes. ARF can be divided into three basic categories: prerenal, postrenal, and intrinsic renal failure.

PRERENAL FAILURE

Prerenal causes of ARF occur from insufficient renal perfusion. This can be caused from actual hypovolemia or from a relative decrease in effective blood volume perfusing the kidney.[54] Hypotension, congestive heart failure, and hepatic failure with ascites can all create a prerenal picture of ARF secondary to insufficient plasma volume perfusing the kidney. With renal hypoperfusion, the renal tubules reabsorb large amounts of sodium and water, hence making the urine concentrated and low in sodium. Ultimately, the use of a pulmonary artery catheter may be the best guide in improving renal perfusion through accurate intravascular repletion along with assuring adequate cardiac output.

POSTRENAL FAILURE

In ARF, postrenal failure should be excluded initially through the placement of a Foley catheter and renal ultrasound evaluating for any evidence of urinary tract obstruction. Retroperitoneal and pelvic tumors can obstruct both ureters. Prostate cancer or a pelvic tumor can cause bladder outlet obstruction and a neurogenic bladder. Evaluation of the urine can give variable results with early postobstructive failure having urine indices compatible with prerenal failure and long-standing postobstructive failure urine indices compatible with acute tubular necrosis.[54,61] Once obstruction is corrected, a postobstruction diuresis can occur leading to potential electrolyte disorders and hypovolemia if not managed carefully.

INTRINSIC RENAL FAILURE

Acute tubular necrosis (ATN) is the most common cause of acute renal failure. ATN is caused most commonly from either hypotension or nephrotoxins. Common nephrotoxins include aminoglycosides, amphotericin, cis-platinum, methotrexate, mithramycin, methyl-CCNU, streptozocin, myoglobin, and radiographic contrast media. ATN is often reversible after 2 to 3 weeks of supportive care.[54] Examination of the urine usually reveals large amounts of sediment with brownish pigmented cellular casts and renal tubular cells. Urine indices show a high urine sodium and low urine osmolality with inability to concentrate the urine.

Other causes of intrinsic renal failure include: (1) glomerulonephritis, interstitial nephritis, and vasculitis; (2) systemic diseases such as multiple myeloma, hypercalcemia, and uric acid nephropathy from tumor lysis syndrome.[54] Certain malignancies have been found to be directly associated with parenchymal renal disease. Membranous glomerulonephritis is associated with melanoma, and with lung and colon cancer.[62] Multiple myeloma can cause light chain precipitation in the renal tubules or amyloid deposition. The lymphoproliferative disorders are associated with glomerulonephritis or vasculitis of the kidney.[54]

MANAGEMENT OF ACUTE RENAL FAILURE

The first step in the initial management of ARF is diagnosing the likely cause of ARF and classifying it as prerenal, renal, or postrenal. This is best done through examination of the urine sediment and obtaining urine sodium, creatinine, and osmolality levels. It is essential that a urine sample be checked before the use of any diuretics. Diuretics will cause an increased loss of urine sodium. Hence, diuretics often cause urine electrolytes to be compatible with ATN when in actuality the patient has ARF of prerenal origin. Also, acute glomerulonephritis and vasculitis often have prerenal urine indices.[61]

Findings of brownish pigmented casts plus renal tubular cells on urine examination are compatible with ATN. Red blood cell casts are pathognomonic of glomerulonephritis. Waxy broad casts depict a more chronic renal failure that may not have been previously appreciated. Hematuria can depict vasculitis or interstitial nephritis. Myoglobinuria is compatible with rhabdomyolysis.

Bladder catheterization and renal ultrasound should be obtained to rule out any evidence of urinary tract obstruction. If small shrunken kidneys are found on ultrasound then the patient likely has had long-standing renal disease. A thorough review of the records should be done to exclude the use of any nephrotoxins such as aminoglycosides or nonsteroidal anti-inflammatory drugs. If the patient is not on hemodialysis, then a low-protein diet of approximately 30 to 40 gm/d plus fluid, sodium, and potassium restrictions should be implemented.

Elective surgery should not be done in light of ARF of unclear cause until the patient has had an appropriate renal work-up and treatment. Furthermore, if the patient is on dialysis then elective surgery should be done within 24 hours of the last dialysis treatment in order to decrease the incidence of electrolyte abnormalities and the patient's being fluid overloaded (Table 13-3).

SUMMARY: RENAL AND ELECTROLYTE DISORDERS IN THE ONCOLOGY PATIENT

1. Hyponatremia is treated with water restriction. SIADH may be associated with paraneoplastic syndromes.
2. Hypernatremia is usually due to hypovolemia and should be slowly corrected initially with isotonic saline, followed by hypotonic solutions.
3. Hypokalemia is usually due to GI tract losses, but elective surgery need not be postponed if serum potassium levels are between 2.6 and 3.5 mEq/L.
4. Hyperkalemia requires treatment. It is demonstrated by peaked T waves on ECG. Severe hyperkalemia is treated first with

Table 13-3. Urine Indices in Acute Renal Failure

	Prerenal Azotemia	Acute Tubular Necrosis
Serum BUN/creatinine	≥20	≤10
Urine sodium meq/L	<20	>40
Urine osm mosm/kg H$_2$O	>500	<350
Urine/plasma creatinine	>40	<20
Fractional excretion of sodium (FENa)*	<1	>2

*Fractional excretion of sodium: $\dfrac{\text{urine sodium}}{\text{plasma sodium}} \div \dfrac{\text{urine creatinine}}{\text{plasma creatinine}} \times 100$

calcium, followed by sodium bicarbonate and glucose, and insulin to force the potassium into the cells. The excess potassium must then be removed from the patient, usually by using sodium polystyrene sulfonate and loop diuretics. Elective surgery should not be performed with a serum potassium greater than 5.5 mEq/L.

5. Hypercalcemia is treated with intravenous hydration plus loop diuretics.
6. Hypocalcemia must be verified by considering the serum albumin. Serum calcium levels decrease 0.8 mg/dL for every decrease of 1.0 g/dL of albumin below 4.0 g/dL.
7. Acute renal failure is categorized into prerenal causes (hypovolemia), renal causes, and postrenal causes (*e.g.*, ureteral obstruction by tumor). Work-up includes urinalysis with examination of the sediment, urine electrolytes (sodium, creatinine), and osmolality. Renal ultrasound is useful to evaluate possible obstruction.

PREOPERATIVE EVALUATION OF THE CHEMOTHERAPY PATIENT

Most oncology patients who have undergone chemotherapy have received multiple cytotoxic agents. These patients are subject to multiple end organ sites of damage. The preoperative evaluation for the surgeon and anesthesiologist should always begin with a complete history and physical examination obtaining the exact cytotoxic agents the patient has received, the total amount of certain key cytotoxic agents (such as adriamycin, daunorubicin, and bleomycin), and the timing of the last cycle of any chemotherapy agents. The laboratory investigation should include a complete blood count, sodium, potassium, chloride, bicarbonate, magnesium, calcium, phosphorous, blood urea nitrogen (BUN), creatinine, liver function tests, and coagulation profile. A chest x-ray and 12-lead ECG should be obtained if one has not recently been obtained.

A history of dyspnea or dry nonproductive cough along with bibasilar crepitant rales should alert one to possible pulmonary fibrosis from such cytotoxic agents as bleomycin. These findings may be subtle and often precede radiographic changes.[63] At this point, with positive findings on history or physical examination, a chest radiograph and pulmonary function tests should be obtained. Radiographic changes most often show bibasilar interstitial changes. Pulmonary function tests should include arterial blood gas, spirometry, and diffusing capacity of carbon monoxide (DLCO). Findings compatible with interstitial fibrosis include increased A-a gradient, restrictive lung disease, and decreased DLCO. Of interest, a decreased DLCO is used often as the earliest marker of potential pulmonary toxicity from such cytotoxic agents as bleomycin.[64] These findings will help the surgeon and anesthesiologist anticipate pulmonary complications and the need for postoperative mechanical ventilation.

A history of decreasing exercise tolerance, orthopnea, paroxysmal nocturnal dyspnea, or peripheral edema should alert the physician to the possible development of congestive heart failure and cardiomyopathy from such cytotoxic agents as adriamycin and daunorubicin. A physical examination should be done looking for an S_3 gallop, fine rales on lung auscultation, jugular venous distention or hepatojugular reflux, an enlarged and tender liver, and pitting edema. A thorough review of the chest roentgenogram film should be made looking for evidence of cardiomegaly, pulmonary edema, or pleural effusions. If there are any findings on history, physical examination, or chest roentgenogram compatible with congestive heart failure and the patient has received a known cardiotoxic agent, then either transthoracic echocardiography or radionuclide scintigraphy should be obtained.

Burrows et al[65] concluded, however, that transthoracic echocardiography did not help predict intraoperative and postoperative cardiovascular events in patients without a history of congestive heart failure. Thus, echocardiography or radionuclide scintigraphy is not always needed with the use of cardiotoxic agents unless symptoms and signs of congestive heart failure are obtained on history and physical examination (Tables 13-4 and 13-5).

Bone marrow suppression, hepatic damage, coagulation dysfunction, renal and electrolyte abnormalities, and neurologic dysfunction all can occur secondary to chemotherapy. The majority of chemotherapeutic agents cause bone marrow suppression with the nadir of blood counts usually occurring within 7 to 14 days and starting to return to normal within 21 to 28 days. Also, coagulopathies can develop with such agents as L-asparaginase and mithramycin. Thus, many oncology patients require multiple blood products preoperatively.

Multiple gastrointestinal disturbances occur from chemotherapy agents, most notably the antimetabolites. Severe nausea, vomiting, stomatitis, and diarrhea can develop causing the patient to be hypovolemic, with poor nutritional status, and with multiple electrolyte abnormalities on preoperative assessment.

Drugs such as cis-platinum and methotrexate can lead to renal tubular damage along with electrolyte disorders. Also, the alkylating agents given for rapidly growing tumors such as lymphomas can cause tumor lysis syndrome with the release of multiple breakdown products causing hyperkalemia, hyperphosphatemia, hypocalcemia, and uric acid nephropathy. These patients need to be pretreated with allopurinol along with aggressive intravenous hydration, mannitol, lasix, and bicarbonate to prevent uric acid nephropathy.

Neuropathies and paresthesias have been reported to occur with vincristine, vinblastine, procarbazine, and cis-platinum.[66] Thus, neurologic examination should be performed preoperatively while looking for evidence of spinal or brain metastases and such paraneoplastic syndromes as Eaton-Lambert.

Table 13-4. Clinical Symptoms and Signs of Pulmonary Toxicity

1. Dyspnea
2. Nonproductive cough
3. Tachypnea
4. Fever
5. Bibasilar rales

Table 13-5. Clinical Symptoms and Signs of Cardiac Toxicity

1. Dyspnea
2. Orthopnea
3. Paroxysmal nocturnal dyspnea
4. Tachycardia
5. S3 gallop
6. Peripheral pitting edema
7. Right upper quadrant abdominal fullness
8. Hepatomegaly
9. Jugular venous distension or hepatojugular reflex
10. Bibasilar rales

Specific Chemotherapy Agents

ANTIBIOTICS

Antibiotic chemotherapy drugs include the anthracyclines (adriamycin, daunorubicin, and mitoxantrone), bleomycin, mitomycin C, and mithramycin. These drugs form stable complexes to DNA and thus inhibit synthesis of DNA and RNA.[67] The antibiotic agents are often of most concern to the surgeon and anesthesiologist at the preoperative assessment secondary to the known cardiac and pulmonary toxicity of these drugs.

Adriamycin (doxorubicin) and daunorubicin (daunomycin) are well-known cardiac toxic agents. Endomyocardial biopsies of adriamycin-treated patients show myocyte necrosis with mitochondria and nuclear degeneration.[68] The myocyte necrosis can continue to occur for several months after adriamycin has been discontinued.[68]

Adriamycin and daunorubicin have two different cardiotoxic effects: acutely, these drugs can cause electrocardiographic changes, and chronically a cumulative dose-dependent cardiomyopathy.[69] Common electrocardiographic changes include nonspecific ST and T wave changes, premature atrial and ventricular contractions, sinus tachycardia, and low voltage of the QRS complex.[69] Most of the electrocardiographic changes are reversible within 2 months and may be only transient during intravenous administration.[69] Only a decreased voltage of the QRS complex ($\geq$ 30%) is felt to be a possible harbinger of the development of a cardiomyopathy.[70]

Anthracycline-induced cardiomyopathy is dose-dependent. For adriamycin, a total dose equal to or greater than 550 mg/m^2 and for daunorubicin a total dose $\geq$ 600 mg/m^2 increases the risk of the development of a cardiomyopathy (Figs. 13-4 and 13-5).[71,72]

Other risk factors for adriamycin causing cardiomyopathy and at lower total cumulative dose include prior or concurrent radiation therapy of the mediastinum, pre-existing heart disease, concurrent chemotherapy with cyclophosphamide or mito-

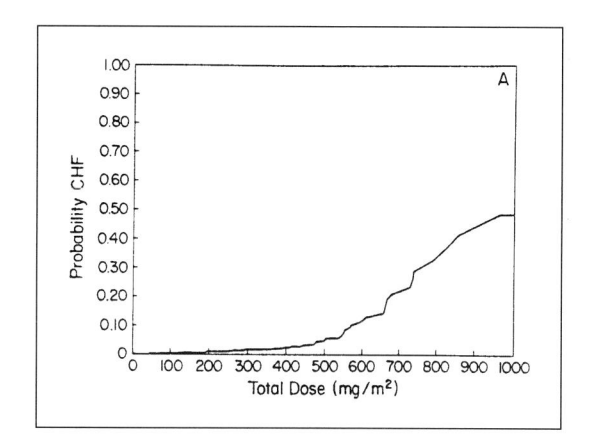

Figure 13-4. Probability of developing adriamycin-induced congestive heart failure (CHF) versus total cumulative dose of adriamycin. From Von Hoff DD, Layard MW, Basa P, et al. Risk factors for doxorubicin-induced congestive heart failure. Ann Intern Med 1979;91:710; reprinted with permission.

Figure 13-5. The percent incidence of congestive heart failure (CHF) versus total dose of daunorubicin. From Von Hoff DD, Rozencweig M, Layard M, et al. Daunomycin-induced cardiotoxicity in children and adults. A review of 110 cases. Am J Med 1977;62:200; reprinted with permission.

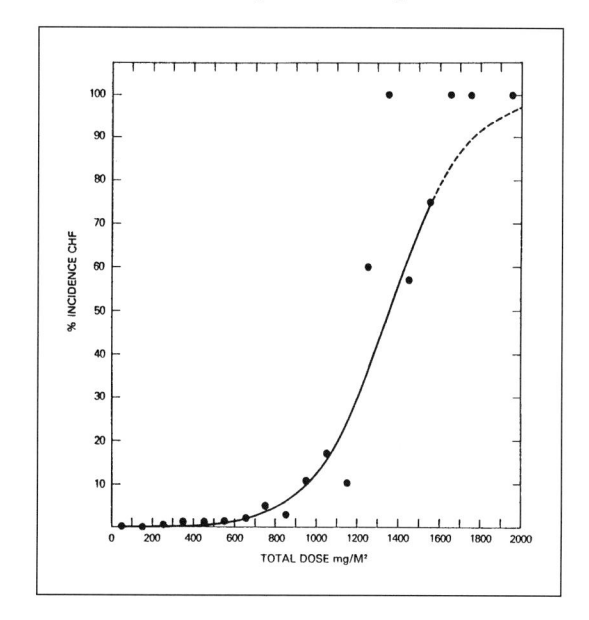

mycin C, and age greater than 70 years or 4 years or younger.[69,73–75] For daunorubicin, only total dosage and older and younger age have been shown as risk factors for cardiomyopathy.[69,72] Other risk factors have not been verified.

Mitoxantrone is a newer anthracycline developed with the hope of decreasing cardiotoxicity. Mitoxantrone has been used primarily to treat acute leukemias. Myelosuppression is the dose-limiting toxicity. However, congestive heart failure and decreasing cardiac ejection fraction have been reported with the use of mitoxantrone. Mather et al[76] reported a 15% incidence of cardiotoxicity with doses of 120 mg/m^2 versus 6% with 60 mg/m^2 and 4% with 24 mg/m^2. There appears to be increased risk of mitoxantrone cardiotoxicity with prior adriamycin use and mediastinal radiation therapy.[77] Thus, the normal precautions taken at the time of preoperative evaluation of patients on other anthracyclines should be the same for mitoxantrone (Table 13-6).

BLEOMYCIN

Bleomycin is a cytotoxic agent commonly used to treat testicular cancers and lymphomas. Bleomycin effects cause the formation of oxygen free radicals. The lung is particularly susceptible to damage from free radicals secondary to bleomycin being concentrated in the lung and having higher oxygen exposure.[78]

Lung damage from bleomycin results in the development of pulmonary fibrosis. The incidence of bleomycin-induced pulmonary fibrosis has been reported in 3% to 11% of patients.[79] Pulmonary fibrosis may develop insidiously several months after the last bleomycin dosing.[79]

Clinical symptoms of pulmonary fibrosis often precede radiographic changes. A decrease in the diffusing capacity is the earliest change seen in pulmonary function tests followed by restrictive changes on spirometry and an increase in the A-a gradient on arterial blood gas. Several authors have concluded that changes in history and physical examination may be an earlier and better indicator of the degree of pulmonary damage over radiographic and pulmonary function test finding.[67,79,80]

Several factors increase the risk of bleomycin pulmonary toxicity. A total cumulative dose of 500 U or greater in adults greatly increases the incidence of bleomycin pulmonary toxicity.[79] Prior or concurrent radiation therapy to the chest enhances the pulmonary toxicity of bleomycin with a reported incidence of 35% to 55%.[79] Patients over 70 years of age also have a higher incidence of bleomycin-induced pulmonary toxicity.[78] Other risk factors include concurrent chemotherapy with cyclophosphamide and renal dysfunction decreasing the elimination of bleomycin.[78]

The use of elevated oxygen concentrations in the bleomycin-treated patient may increase the risk of pulmonary toxicity. At present, this is a controversial topic. In 1978, Goldiner[80] et al reported a high incidence of acute postoperative pulmonary complica-

Table 13-6. Risk Factors for Anthracycline-Induced Cardiomyopathy

Adriamycin	Daunorubicin	Mitoxantrone
1. Total dose ≥550 mg/m^2	1. Total dose ≥600 mg/m^2	1. Total dose ≥100 mg/m^2
2. Radiation therapy to mediastinum	2. Age ≥65 and ≤15	2. Radiation therapy to mediastinum
3. Pre-existing heart disease		3. Prior use of adriamycin
4. Concurrent use of cyclophosphamide or mitomycin C		
5. Age ≥70 or ≤4		

tions in a subgroup of patients given greater than 28% FIO_2 and large amounts of crystalloid.[80a] This along with other case reports led to the recommendation that an FIO_2 less than 30% and a higher amount of colloid be used. However, there now have been several studies showing little pulmonary toxicity in using higher FIO_2 concentrations in the operating room.[81–83]

All the studies looking at oxygen use and bleomycin have been with small samples thus making any definite conclusion difficult. At present, the lowest FIO_2 concentration necessary to provide adequate oxygenation should be used until a larger more statistically significant study has been performed. The use of such measures as PEEP in the operating room and chest physiotherapy postoperatively allows lower oxygen concentrations to be used safely. However, one should not hesitate to use higher oxygen concentrations to prevent hypoxemia.

MITOMYCIN C

Mitomycin C is a newer chemotherapy agent used commonly in lung, breast, and gastrointestinal cancers. Myelosuppression is the dose-limiting toxicity. Other toxicities include nausea, vomiting, stomatitis, and pulmonary fibrosis.

The development of interstitial pneumonitis and pulmonary fibrosis is estimated to occur in 2.8% to 12% of mitomycin C-treated patients.[79] Risk factors for the development of pulmonary fibrosis do not appear related to total dosage or patient age.[79,84] Radiation therapy to the lungs or concomitant use of other chemotherapy drugs such as 5-fluorouracil (5-FU) may increase the risk of pulmonary toxicity, but this has not been definitely proved.[85,86] FIO_2 use greater than 30% also may contribute to pulmonary toxicity, but, again, this has not definitely been proved. As with bleomycin, FIO_2 less than 30% is recommended unless higher concentrations are needed to provide adequate oxygenation.

MITHRAMYCIN

Mithramycin is used in the treatment of testicular cancer and hypercalcemia. It is rarely used today but deserves mention because its toxic effects can have a major impact on the surgical care of the patient. Besides causing myelosuppression with thrombocytopenia and platelet dysfunction, mithramycin can cause hepatic dysfunction and a severe hemorrhagic diathesis.[87,88]

ALKYLATING AGENTS

The alkylating agents are among the most commonly used chemotherapy agents. Cyclophosphamide (cytoxan), mechlorethamine (nitrogen mustard), melphalan, busulfan, chlorambucil, and ifosfamide are common alkylating agents in use today. All these agents cause myelosuppression, which is the dose-limiting toxicity, and varying degrees of nausea and vomiting.

Cyclophosphamide has many adverse effects that have direct bearing on the preoperative assessment. The breakdown products of cyclophosphamide can cause hemorrhagic cystitis. It is important during cyclophosphamide use to maintain a high urine output with good hydration. However, cyclophosphamide is also reported to exert an antidiuretic hormone (ADH)-like effect on the kidney in which severe hyponatremia and seizures can develop with aggressive hydration.[84,88,89]

Although cyclophosphamide is rarely reported to cause interstitial pneumonitis, most often it is in association with bleomycin and carmustine (BCNU).[90,91] Cyclophosphamide also is reported to cause fulminant acute heart failure with very high doses such as 200 mg/m² used for bone marrow transplantation.[92] Of interest, cyclophosphamide inhibits plasma cholinesterase activity and can lead to prolonged effects of succinylcholine in the operating room.[93]

Ifosfamide is an isomer of cyclophosphamide used in the treatment of testicular cancers and sarcomas. Besides myelosuppression, ifosfamide side effects include hemorrhagic cystitis and neurotoxicity.[92]

Busulfan, chlorambucil, and melphalan are most often used to treat the hematologic malignancies. All three agents cause myelosuppression and interstitial pneumonitis. Busulfan is the most common of the three implicated in the development of pulmonary toxicity. Busulfan pulmonary toxicity may be enhanced with radiation therapy to the chest prior to or following busulfan therapy.[79,90] Total dosage of busulfan does not appear to contribute to pulmonary toxicity, but there are no reported cases below total dosages of 500 mg.[79] Melphalan and chlorambucil only rarely are reported to cause pulmonary toxicity.[90]

NITROSOUREAS

Nitrosourea agents include carmustine (BCNU), lomustine (CCNU), and semustine (methyl-CCNU). All these agents cause myelosuppression, which is the dose-limiting toxicity. BCNU, in high doses, causes a significant incidence of interstitial pneumonitis. There are several factors associated with BCNU pulmonary toxicity. There is a direct correlation of pulmonary toxicity with doses greater than 1000 mg/m^2 and a reported incidence of approximately 50% at doses of 1500 mg/m^2.[79,94] Also, a history of prior lung disease, tobacco use, radiation therapy, and concurrent cyclophosphamide use increase the risk of BCNU pulmonary toxicity. Renal damage has been reported with chronic use of BCNU or methyl-CCNU.[87]

Streptozocin is a nitrosourea agent used in the treatment of pancreatic islet cell carcinoma and malignant carcinoid. Streptozocin can cause hypoglycemia following infusion.[88] Other side effects include myelosuppression, transient hepatotoxicity, and renal tubular damage.[87]

ANTIMETABOLITES

The common antimetabolites in use today include methotrexate, 5-FU, cytosine arabinoside (ARA-C), 6-mercaptopurine, and thioguanine. These agents are commonly used in gastrointestinal tumors, lung cancers, and various leukemias. Major toxicities of the antimetabolites are myelosuppression and gastrointestinal disturbances often leading to severe stomatitis, diarrhea, nausea, and vomiting.

Methotrexate inhibits the enzyme dihydrofolate reductase, which causes the conversion of dihydrofolate to tetrahydrofolate. The toxic bone marrow effects can quickly be reversed with leucovorin (folinic acid).[88] Methotrexate can cause renal tubular damage, hepatic damage and, uncommonly, a reversible hypersensitivity interstitial pneumonitis.[79,84,87] Other antimetabolites reported to cause liver dysfunction include 6-mercaptopurine, which causes reversible cholestatic jaundice, and ARA-C, which causes elevated liver enzymes in up to 25% of patients.[87,88]

MITOTIC INHIBITORS

Vincristine, vinblastine, and etoposide (VP-16) are mitotic inhibitors commonly used in the treatment of testicular cancers, lymphomas, and leukemias. The major dose-limiting toxicity of vinblastine and VP-16 is myelosuppression. Vincristine's major toxicity is neurologic. Vincristine can cause severe sensory paresthesias, loss of deep tendon reflexes, abdominal pain, ileus, and constipation. Vincristine also can potentiate the release of antidiuretic hormone leading to the development of hyponatremia.[85,95]

CIS-PLATINUM

Cis-platinum is a heavy metal compound often used in the treatment of testicular, ovarian, bladder, and head and neck cancers. Dose-limiting toxicity is secondary to nephrotoxicity and myelosuppression. Cis-platinum can cause renal tubular necrosis with a decrease in the renal blood flow and glomerular filtration.[96] The extent of renal damage can be decreased greatly with a brisk, continuous diuresis with normal saline hydration, furosemide, and mannitol. Patients treated with cis-platinum may have prolonged problems with severe hypokalemia and hypomagnesemia from potassium and magnesium wasting in the urine.[84,97] Thus, it is essential that electrolyte and renal function be checked preoperatively. Neuropathies also are reported to occur with cis-platinum.[66]

PROCARBAZINE

Procarbazine is a chemotherapeutic agent used to treat lymphomas, brain tumors, melanomas, and oat cell carcinoma.[98] Myelosuppression is the dose-limiting toxicity. Peripheral neuropathies and central nervous system excitability with convulsion can occur rarely.[67] More commonly, lethargy and drowsiness occurs, which can be potentiated by such drugs as phenothiazines and barbiturates.[67] An antabuse-like reaction can occur with ethanol use. Procarbazine is a weak monoamine oxidase inhibitor.[67] Thus, sympathomimetic drugs, especially indirect acting agents such as ephedrine, should be used cautiously.

L-ASPARAGINASE

L-asparaginase is used commonly in acute lymphoblastic leukemia. Hypersensitivity reactions ranging from erythema and urticaria to bronchospasm and anaphylaxis are common on drug administration.[99] L-asparaginase inhibits protein synthesis in the liver and pancreas leading to decreased albumin, insulin, and coagulation factors.[99] Acute pancreatitis is reported to occur in 1% to 2% of patients.[99] Thus, patients should be monitored for hyperglycemia, liver function abnormalities, elevated amylase, and coagulopathy on preoperative evaluation (Table 13-7).

SUMMARY: PREOPERATIVE EVALUATION OF THE CHEMOTHERAPY PATIENT

1. Obtain a complete history including the exact agents administered and the timing of the course(s) of treatment.
2. Laboratory studies should include serum electrolytes, complete blood cell count, liver function tests, and a coagulation profile.
3. Patients who received bleomycin must be evaluated for pulmonary fibrosis.
4. Decreased exercise tolerance may indicate cardiomyopathy secondary to adriamycin or daunorubicin. Work-up includes transthoracic echocardiography or radionuclide scintigraphy.
5. Alkylating agents cause myelosuppression.
6. The use of cyclophosphamide is associated with hemorrhagic cystitis.
7. Cis-platinum is associated with nephrotoxicity.

USE OF STRESS STEROIDS

The oncology patient often has a history of exogenous glucocorticoid administration as part of a chemotherapy regimen. The physician at the time of preoperative evaluation has to decide on the use and the amount of stress steroid coverage. The patient who has received 2 weeks or more of glucocorticoids within the past year is considered at risk for adrenal suppression. However, many of these patients are capable of a normal stress response. The Adrenocorticotropic hormone (ACTH) stimulation test is the definitive test to determine adrenal suppression. Cosyntropin (250 mg) is given intravenously, and plasma cortisol levels are measured at 30 and 60 minutes after infusion along with a baseline level. A rise of 7 to 20 μg/dL of cortisol is considered normal.[100] The ACTH stimulation test is often impractical to perform the evening before surgery. Thus, all of these patients should be assumed to be at risk for perioperative adrenal insufficiency until adrenal response has been proved normal.

The normal physiologic production of cortisol is 30 mg/d. Kehlet,[101] on reviewing the literature, estimated that the adrenal cortex excreted between 75 to 150 mg of cortisol

Table 13-7. Toxicities of Chemotherapy Agents

Chemotherapy Agents	Major Toxicity
ANTIBIOTICS	
Adriamycin	Cardiomyopathy; myelosuppression
Bleomycin	Pulmonary fibrosis
Daunorubicin	Cardiomyopathy; myelosuppression
Mithramycin	Myelosuppression; hepatic dysfunction, hemorrhagic diathesis
Mitomycin C	Myelosuppression; pulmonary fibrosis
Mitoxantrone	Cardiomyopathy; myelosuppression
ALKYLATING AGENTS	
Busulfan	Pulmonary fibrosis; myelosuppression
Chlorambucil	Myelosuppression
Cyclophosphamide	Myelosuppression; hemorrhagic cystitis; SIADH
Ifosfamide	Myelosuppression; hemorrhagic cystitis
Mechlorethamine (nitrogen mustard)	Myelosuppression
Melphalan	Myelosuppression
NITROSOUREAS	
Carmustine (BCNU)	Myelosuppression; pulmonary fibrosis; renal toxicity
Lomustine (CCNU)	Myelosuppression
Semustine (methyl-CCNU)	Myelosuppression; renal toxicity
Streptozocin	Myelosuppression; hepatotoxicity; renal tubular toxicity
ANTIMETABOLITES	
Cytosine arabinoside (ARA-C)	Myelosuppression; elevated liver enzymes
Fluorouracil (5-FU)	Myelosuppression; stomatitis
6-Mercaptopurine	Myelosuppression; cholestatic jaundice
Methotrexate	Myelosuppression; hepatic and renal tubular damage
Thioguanine	Myelosuppression
MITOTIC INHIBITORS	
Vinblastine	Myelosuppression
Vincristine	Neurotoxicity; SIADH
VP-16	Myelosuppression
MISCELLANEOUS AGENTS	
Cis-platinum	Renal tubular damage; neuropathies; myelosuppression
L-Asparaginase	Hypersensitivity reaction; liver function abnormalities; coagulopathy

in the first 24-hour postoperative period and maximal adrenal cortex production was 200 mg/d of cortisol with constant ACTH stimulation. At present, many physicians administer 300 mg of hydrocortisone as stress steroid coverage over the first 24-hour perioperative period and then taper over a 2- to 3-day period. Several authors now feel that 300 mg of hydrocortisone over the first 24-hour period is excessive and may have disadvantages such as hyperglycemia, hypertension, and inhibition of wound healing.[100–104]

Chernow et al[102] evaluated cortisol response in patients with no prior glucocorticoid use undergoing surgery. They divided the patients into three groups: (1) minor surgery (inguinal hernia repair or laparoscopy), (2) moderate surgery (cholecystectomy, appendectomy or hysterectomy), and (3) severe surgery (major abdominal or vascular). They found negligible cortisol increases with minor surgery, but significant increases at 1 hour and 24 hours after moderate or severe surgery, which returned to normal at 5 days. Thus, for minor surgery, only physiologic doses of glucocorticoids are needed for adequate stress coverage. For minor surgery, Kehlet[101] recommended giving 25 mg of hydrocortisone with induction of anesthesia and then resuming normal oral glucocorticoid dose when fluid intake begins. If the patient is unable to take fluids by mouth, then Kehlet recommended 100 mg of hydrocortisone over the first perioperative 24-hour period.[101]

Udelsman et al[103] studied previously adrenalectomized primates, placing them on 1/10 physiologic, physiologic, and supraphysiologic (10 × physiologic) glucocorticoid doses for 4 days prior to performing a cholecystectomy. The subphysiologic-dosed primates had a 38% mortality rate and a high incidence of hypotension. However, Udelsman et al found no difference between the physiologic, supraphysiologic, and control group of primates in hemodynamic monitoring and surgical outcome. They also found no difference in wound healing or other deleterious effects within the supraphysiologic group. This is in contrast to prior studies on rats that showed delayed wound healing with brief glucocorticoid administration.[105,106] Udelsman et al[103] concluded that there was no clear advantage of giving supraphysiologic glucocorticoids over physiologic replacement.

In 1981 Symreng et al[104] gave known adrenally suppressed patients undergoing major surgery 25 mg of hydrocortisone intravenously followed by a continuous 24-hour infusion of 100 mg hydrocortisone. They then measured subsequent cortisol levels over 24 hours and compared these levels with those in control patients and prior glucocorticoid-treated patients with proved normal adrenal responsiveness. The hydrocortisone replaced patients had higher cortisol levels for the first 4 hours after induction of anesthesia and equivalent or higher cortisol levels for the remainder of the 24 hours. Furthermore, the glucocorticoid-treated patients with preserved adrenal function had cortisol levels nearly equal to the control group without any supplementation (Fig. 13-6). None of these patients had any episodes of hemodynamic instability or any other evidence of adrenal insufficiency.

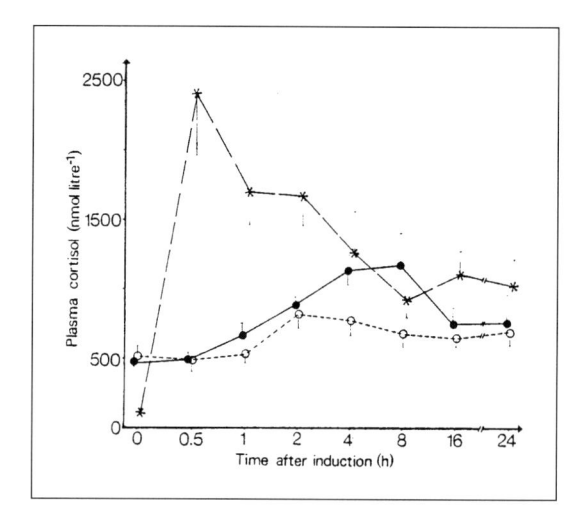

Figure 13-6. Plasma cortisol response to the stress of anesthesia and surgery. ●—● = controls; ○—○ = patients receiving long-term corticosteroid treatment with normal response to the corticotropic stimulation test and no stress steroid use during surgery; *—* = patients receiving long-term corticosteroids with subnormal response to the corticotropin test and given low-dose cortisol substitution. From Symreng T, Karlberg BE, Kagedal B, Schildt B. Physiological cortisol substitution of long-term steroid-treated patients undergoing major surgery. Br J Anaesth 1981;53:949; reprinted with permission.

Based on available data, the previous standard of giving 300 mg of hydrocortisone over the first 24-hour perioperative period is excessive. A dosage of 200 mg of hydrocortisone given over two to three divided doses during the first 24-hour perioperative period as recommended by Lampe and Roizen[100] may be used for major surgery until a larger prospective randomized study has been done. Smaller doses such as recommended by Symreng et al and Kehlet should be more than adequate for lesser procedures (*e.g.*, cholecystectomy or hysterectomy).[101,104] For minor procedures (*e.g.*, inguinal hernia repair), doses above 30 to 50 mg during the first 24-hour perioperative period are most likely not needed unless the patient is already on higher doses of glucocorticoids.[101,102]

Salem et al[107] have emphasized that perioperative glucocorticoid administration should be based on the magnitude of the stress and the known endogenous glucocorticoid production rate associated with it. For **minor surgical stress** (*e.g.*, inguinal herniorrhaphy) they recommend 25 mg of hydrocortisone equivalent. Patients with an uncomplicated postoperative course may return to their usual dose of glucocorticoids on postoperative day 1. For **moderate surgical stress** (*e.g.*, open cholecystectomy, lower extremity revascularization, colon resection), they recommend 50 to 75 mg/d of hydrocortisone equivalent. A patient receiving prednisone 10 mg should receive prednisone 10 mg preoperatively and hydrocortisone 50 mg intravenously administered intraoperatively. It is recommended that this patient receive hydrocortisone 60 mg (in three divided intravenous doses) on postoperative day 1 and return to the preoperative dose on day 2. For **major surgical stress** (esophagectomy, pancreaticoduodenectomy, cardiac surgery) the target dose is 100 to 150 mg of hydrocortisone per day for 2 to 3 days. The provision of perioperative glucocorticoid coverage must account for the patient's preoperative glucocorticoid dose as well as the duration and severity of surgery or other stress.

One must carefully monitor the patient and have a low threshold for giving further hydrocortisone if any evidence of adrenal insufficiency such as hypotension occurs. The risks associated with higher doses of corticosteroids aggravating such conditions as diabetes mellitus or hypertension must also be considered when administering perioperative glucocorticoids.

SUMMARY: USE OF STRESS STEROIDS IN PATIENTS AT RISK FOR ADRENAL INSUFFICIENCY

1. Minor Surgical Stress (*e.g.*, inguinal herniorrhaphy): 25 mg of hydrocortisone equivalent.
2. Moderate Surgical Stress (*e.g.*, open cholecystectomy, colon resection): 50 to 75 mg/day of hydrocortisone equivalent through postoperative day 1.
3. Major Surgical Stress (*e.g.*, esophagectomy): 100 to 150 mg hydrocortisone equivalent per day for 2 to 3 days.

SUMMARY

The preoperative management of the cancer patient can be a challenge for both anesthesiologist and surgeon. Clearly, there are considerations in many of these patients that are not usually necessary and call for exceptionally close cooperation in preoperative and intraoperative management.

In all of the considerations discussed in this chapter, an essential element is a complete history of prior cancer therapy (chemotherapy, radiation therapy, and prior surgery) to allow assessment of its impact on patient management. Most importantly, a full knowledge of these therapies allows complete evaluation before the next surgical intervention is undertaken.

The above discussion was intended to provide practical guidelines for the preoperative management of a number of problems that are found uniquely, or most commonly, in the cancer patient.

REFERENCES

1. Benumof JL. Preoperative cardiopulmonary evaluation. In: Benumof JL, ed. Anesthesia for thoracic surgery. Philadelphia: WB Saunders, 1987:140.
2. Boysen PG. Evaluation of pulmonary function tests and arterial blood gases. In: Kaplan JA, ed. Thoracic anesthesia, 2nd ed. New York: Churchill Livingstone, 1991:1.
3. Gass DD, Olsen GN. Preoperative pulmonary function testing to predict postoperative morbidity and mortality. Chest 1986;89:127.
4. Olsen GN, Block AJ, Swenson EW, Castle JR, Wynne JW. Pulmonary function evaluation of

the lung resection candidate: a prospective study. Am Rev Respir Dis 1975;111:379.
5. Tisi GM. Preoperative evaluation of pulmonary function. Validity, indications, and benefits. Am Rev Respir Dis 1979;119:293.
6. Fee HJ, Holmes EC, Gewirtz HS, Ramming KP, Alexander JM. Role of pulmonary vascular resistance measurements in preoperative evaluation of candidates for pulmonary resection. J Thorac Cardiovasc Surg 1978;75:519.
7. Eugene J, Brown SE, Light RW, et al. Maximum oxygen consumption: a physiologic guide to pulmonary resection. Surgical Forum 1982;33:260.
8. Smith TP, Kinasewitz GT, Tucker WY, Spillers WP, George RB. Exercise capacity as a predictor of post-thoracotomy morbidity. Am Rev Respir Dis 1984;129:730.
9. Pullerits J, Holzman R. Anaesthesia for patients with mediastinal masses. Can J Anaesth 1989;36:681.
10. Sibert KS, Biondi JW, Hirsch NP. Spontaneous respiration during thoracotomy in a patient with a mediastinal mass. Anesth Analg 1987;66:904.
11. Sperry RJ, Lake CL, Mentzer AM, Woods AM. Case 1 1987. 57-year-old man with dyspnea dsyphagia and a mediastinal mass. J Cardiothorac Vasc Anesth 1987;1:71.
12. Neuman GG, Weingarten AE, Abramowitz RM, Kushins LG, Abramson AL, Ladner W. The anesthetic management of the patient with an anterior mediastinal mass. Anesthesiology 1984;60:144.
13. Akhtar TM, Ridley S, Best CJ. Unusual presentation of acute upper airway obstruction caused by an anterior mediastinal mass. Br J Anaesth 1991;67:632.
14. Groeger JS. Shock states and cancer. In: Howland WS, Carlon GC, eds. Critical care of the cancer patient. Chicago: Year Book Medical Publishers, 1985:296.
15. Lake CL. Anesthesia and pericardial disease. Anesth Analg 1983;62:431.
16. Braunwald E. Pericardial disease. In: Braunwald E, Isselbacher KJ, Petersdorf RG, eds. Harrison's principle of internal medicine, 11th ed. New York: McGraw Hill, 1987:1008.
17. Reddy PS, Curtiss EI, O'Toole JD, Shaver JA. Cardiac tamponade: hemodynamic observations in man. Circulation 1978;58:265.
18. Desiderio DP, Kross RA, Bedford RF. Evaluation of the patient with oncologic disease. In: Rogers MC, Tinker JH, Covino BG, eds. Principles and practice of anesthesiology. St Louis: Mosby-Year Book, 1993:377.
19. Casthely PA, Jablons M, Griepp RB, Ergin MA, Goodman K. Ketanserin in the preoperative and intraoperative management of a patient with carcinoid tumor undergoing tricuspid valve replacement. Anesth Analg 1986;65:809.
20. Marsh HM, Martin JK, Kvols LK, et al. Carcinoid crisis during anesthesia: successful treatment with a somatostatin analogue. Anesthesiology 1987;66:89
21. Longnecker M, Roizen MF. Patients with carcinoid syndrome. Anesthiology Clinics of North America 1987;5(2):313.
22. St John Sutton M, Sheps SG, Lie JT. Prevalence of clinically unsuspected pheochromocytoma. Review of a 50-year autopsy series. Mayo Clin Proc 1981;56:354.
23. Roizen MF, Horrigan RW, Koike M, et al. A prospective randomized trial of four anesthetic techniques for resection of pheochromocytoma. Anesthesiology 1982;57:A43.
24. Boutros AR, Bravo EL, Zanettin G, Straffon RA. Perioperative management of 63 patients with pheochromocytoma. Cleve Clin J Med 1990;57:613.
25. Sheps SG, Jiang NS, Klee GG, van Heerden JA. Recent developments in the diagnosis and treatment of pheochromocytoma. Mayo Clin Proc 1990;65:88.
26. Perry RR, Keiser HR, Norton JA, et al. Surgical management of pheochromocytoma with the use of metyrosine. Ann Surg 1990;212:621.
27. Arai T, Hatano Y, Ishida H, Mori K. Use of nicardipine in the anesthetic management of pheochromocytoma. Anesth Analg 1986;65:706.
28. Desmonts JM, Marty J. Anaesthetic management of patients with phaeochromocytoma. Br J Anaesth 1984;56:781.
29. Roizen MF, Schreider BD, Hassan SZ. Anesthesia for patients with pheochromocytoma. Anesthesiology Clinics of North America 1987;5(2):269.
30. Grosse H, Schroder D, Schober O, Hausen B, Dralle H. The importance of high-dose alpha-receptor blockade for blood volume and hemodynamics in pheochromocytoma. Anaesthesist 1990;39:313.
31. Roizen MF, Hunt TK, Beaupre PN, et al. The effect of alpha-adrenergic blockade on cardiac performance and tissue oxygen delivery during excision of pheochromocytoma. Surgery 1983;94:941.
32. Salathe M, Weiss P, Ritz R. Rapid reversal of heart failure in a patient with phaeochromocytoma and catecholamine-induced cardiomyopathy who was treated with captopril. Br Heart J 1992;68:527.
33. Schaffer MS, Zuberbuhler P, Wilson G, Rose V, Duncan WJ, Rowe RD. Catecholamine cardiomyopathy: an unusual presentation of

pheochromocytoma in children. J Pediatr 1981;99:276.
34. Sadowski D, Cujec B, McMeekin JD, Wilson TW. Reversibility of catecholamine-induced cardiomyopathy in a woman with pheochromocytoma. Can Med Assoc J 1989;141:823.
35. Newell KA, Prinz RA, Brooks MH, Glisson SN, Barbato AL, Freeark RJ. Plasma catecholamine changes during excision of pheochromocytoma. Surgery 1988;104:1064.
36. Zauder HL. Preoperative hemoglobin requirements. Anesthesiology Clinics of North America 1990;8(3):471.
37. NIH Consensus Conference. Perioperative red blood cell transfusion. JAMA 1988;260:2700.
38. Messmer KFW. Acceptable hematocrit levels in surgical patients. World J Surg 1987;11:41.
39. Schriemer PA, Longnecker DE, Mintz PD. The possible immunosuppressive effects of perioperative blood transfusion in cancer patients. Anesthesiology 1988;68:422.
40. Blumberg N, Heal JM, Murphy P, Agarwal MM, Chuang C. Association between transfusion of whole blood and recurrence of cancer. BMJ 1986;293:530.
41. Gascon P, Zoumbos NC, Young NS. Immunologic abnormalities in patients receiving multiple blood transfusions. Ann Intern Med 1984;100:173.
42. Klimberg I, Sirois R, Wajsman Z, Baker J. Intraoperative autotransfusion in urologic oncology. Arch Surg 1986;121:1326.
43. Karczewski DM, Lema MJ, Glaves-Rapp D. The efficacy of using an autotransfusion system for removal of tumor cells from blood harvested during cancer surgery. Anesthesiology 1989;71:A87.
44. Salsbury AJ. The significance of the circulating cancer cell. Canc Treat Rev 1975;2:55.
45. Bogdonoff DL, Williams ME, Stone DJ. Thrombocytopenia in the critically ill patient. J Crit Care 1990;5:186.
46. NIH Consensus Conference. Platelet transfusion therapy. JAMA 1987;257:1777.
47. Schwartz SI. Hemostasis, surgical bleeding and transfusion. In: Schwartz SI, Shires GT, Spencer FC, eds. Principles of surgery, 5th ed. New York: McGraw-Hill, 1989:105.
48. Gravelee GP. Blood transfusion and component therapy. ASA Refresher Course Lectures. 1990;215.
49. Kempin S, Gould-Rossbach P, Howland WS. Disorders of hemostasis in the critically ill cancer patient. In: Howland WS, Carlon GC, eds. Critical care of the cancer patient. Chicago: Year Book Medical Publishers, 1985:211.
50. Jennis AA, Bauer KA. Coagulopathic complications of cancer. In: Holland JF, Frei E, Bast RC, eds. Cancer medicine, 3rd ed. Philadelphia: Lea and Febiger, 1993:2314.
51. Mendelsohn J. Principles of neoplasia. In: Braunwald E, Isselbacher KJ, Petersdorf RG, eds. Harrison's principles of internal medicine, 11th ed. New York: McGraw-Hill, 1987:421.
52. Levinsky NG. Fluid and electrolytes. In: Braunwald E, Isselbacher KJ, Petersdorf RG, eds: Harrison's principles of internal medicine, 11th ed. New York: McGraw-Hill, 1987:198.
53. Edwards R, Winnie AP, Ramamurthy S. Acute hypocapneic hypokalemia: an iatrogenic anesthetic complication. Anesth Analg 1977;56:786.
54. Flombaum C. Electrolyte and renal abnormalities in the cancer patient. In: Howland WS, Carlon GC, eds. Critical care of the cancer patient. Chicago: Year Book Medical Publishers, 1985:114.
55. Vitez TS, Soper LE, Wong KC, Soper P. Chronic hypokalemia and intraoperative dysrythmias. Anesthesiology 1985;63:130.
56. Hirsch IA, Tomlinson DL, Slogoff S, Keats AS. The overstated risk of preoperative hypokalemia. Anesth Analg 1988;67:131.
57. Roizen MF. Anesthetic implications of concurrent diseases. In: Miller RD, ed. Anesthesia, 3rd ed. New York: Churchill Livingstone, 1990:793.
58. Bajorunas DR. Disorders of endocrine function in the critically ill cancer patient. In: Howland WS, Carlon GC, eds. Critical care of the cancer patient. Chicago: Year Book Medical Publishers, 1985:143.
59. Agus ZS, Wasserstein A, Goldfarb S. Disorders of calcium and magnesium homeostasis. Am J Med 1982;72:473.
60. Mazzaferri EL, O'Dorisio TM, LoBuglio AF. Treatment of hypercalcemia associated with malignancy. Semin Oncol 1978;5:141.
61. Miller TR, Anderson RJ, Linas SL, et al. Urinary diagnostic indices in acute renal failure: a prospective study. Ann Intern Med 1978;89:47.
62. Glassock RJ, Brenner BM. The major glomerulopathies. In: Braunwald E, Isselbacher KJ, Petersdorf RG, eds. Harrison's principles of internal medicine, 11th ed. New York: McGraw-Hill, 1987:1173.
63. Klein DS, Wilds PR. Pulmonary toxicity of antineoplastic agents: anaesthetic and postoperative implications. Can Anaesth Soc J 1983;30:399.
64. Sorensen PG, Rossing N, Rorth M. Carbon monoxide diffusing capacity: a reliable indi-

cator of bleomycin-induced pulmonary toxicity. Eur J Respir Dis 1985;66:333.
65. Burrows FA, Hickey PR, Colan S. Perioperative complications in patients with anthracycline chemotherapeutic agents. Can Anaesth Soc J 1985;32:149.
66. Chung F. Cancer, chemotherapy and anaesthesia. Can Anaesth Soc J 1982;29:364.
67. Selvin BL. Cancer chemotherapy: implications for the anesthesiologist. Anesth Analg 1981;60:425.
68. Billingham ME, Mason JW, Bristow MR, Daniels JR. Anthracycline cardiomyopathy monitored by morphologic changes. Cancer Treatment Reports 1978;62:865.
69. Von Hoff DD, Rozencweig M, Piccart M. The cardiotoxicity of anticancer agents. Semin Oncol 1982;9:23.
70. Minow RA, Benjamin RS, Lee ET, Gottlieb JA. QRS voltage change with adriamycin administration. Cancer Treatment Reports 1978;62:931.
71. Von Hoff DD, Layard MW, Basa P, et al. Risk factors for doxorubicin-induced congestive heart failure. Ann Intern Med 1979;91:710.
72. Von Hoff DD, Rozencweig M, Layard M, et al. Daunomycin-induced cardiotoxicity in children and adults. A review of 110 cases. Am J Med 1977;62:200.
73. Minow RA, Benjamin RS, Lee ET, Gottlieb JA. Adriamycin cardiomyopathy risk factors. Cancer 1977;39:1397.
74. Buzdar AU, Legha SS, Tashima CK, et al. Adriamycin and mitomycin C: possible synergistic cardiotoxicity. Cancer Treatment Reports 1978;62:1005.
75. Lipshultz SE, Colan SD, Gelber RD, Perez-Atayde AR, Sallan SE, Sanders SP. Late cardiac effects of doxorubicin therapy for acute lymphoblastic leukemia in childhood. N Engl J Med 1991;324:808.
76. Mather FJ, Simon RM, Clark GM, Von Hoff DD. Cardiotoxicity in patients treated with mitoxantrone: Southwest Oncology Group phase II studies. Cancer Treatment Reports 1987;71:609.
77. Clark GM, Tokaz LK, Von Hoff DD, et al. Cardiotoxicity in patients treated with mitoxantrone on Southwest Oncology Group phase II protocols. Cancer Treatment Symposium 1984;3:25.
78. Waid-Jones MI, Coursin DB. Perioperative considerations for patients treated with bleomycin. Chest 1991;99:993.
79. Ginsberg SJ, Comis RL. The pulmonary toxicity of antineoplastic agents. Semin Oncol 1982;9:34.
80. Lewis BM, Izbicki R. Routine pulmonary function tests during bleomycin therapy. Test may be ineffective and potentially misleading. JAMA 1980;243:347.
80a. Goldiner PL, Carlon GC, Cvitkovic E, et al. Factors influencing postoperative morbidity and mortality in patients treated with bleomycin. Br Med J 1978a(1)6128:1664.
81. LaMantia KR, Glick JH, Marshall BE. Supplemental oxygen does not cause respiratory failure in bleomycin-treated surgical patients. Anesthesiology 1984;60:65.
82. Douglas MJ, Coppin CM. Bleomycin and subsequent anaesthesia: a retrospective study at Vancouver General Hospital. Can Anaesth Soc J 1980;27:449.
83. Blom-Muilwijk MC, Vriesendorp R, Veninga TS, et al. Pulmonary toxicity after treatment with bleomycin alone or in combination with hyperoxia. Br J Anaesth 1988;60:91.
84. Desiderio DP. Cancer chemotherapy: complications and interactions with anesthesia. Hospital Formulary 1990;25:176.
85. Buzdar AU, Legha SS, Luna MA, Tashima CK, Hortobagyi GN, Blumenschein GR. Pulmonary toxicity of mitomycin. Cancer 1980;45:236.
86. Chang AY, Kuebler JP, Pandya KJ, Israel RH, Marshall BC, Tormey DC. Pulmonary toxicity induced by mitomycin C is highly responsive to glucocorticoids. Cancer 1986;57:2285.
87. Riggs CE, Bennett JP. Clinical pharmacology of individual antineoplastic agents. In: Moossa AR, Schimpff SC, Robson MC, eds. Comprehensive textbook of oncology, 2nd ed. Baltimore: William and Wilkins, 1991:536.
88. Stewart FM. Cancer chemotherapy. (unpublished notes) University of Virginia 1989.
89. Green TP, Mirkin BL. Prevention of cyclophosphamide-induced antidiuresis by furosemide infusion. Clin Pharmacol Ther 1981;29:634.
90. Batist G, Andrews JL Jr. Pulmonary toxicity of antineoplastic drugs. JAMA 1981;246:1449.
91. Patel AR, Shah PC, Rhee HL, et al. Cyclophosphamide therapy and interstitial pulmonary fibrosis. Cancer 1976;38:1542.
92. Colvin M. Alkylating agents and platinum antitumor compounds. In: Holland JF, Frei E, Bast RC, eds. Cancer medicine, 3rd ed. Philadelphia: Lea and Febiger, 1993:733.
93. Dillman JB. Safe use of succinylcholine during repeated anesthetics in a patient treated with cyclophosphamide. Anesth Analg 1987;66:351.
94. Aronin PA, Mahaley MS Jr, Rudnick SA, et al. Prediction of BCNU pulmonary toxicity in patients with malignant gliomas: an assessment of risk factors. N Engl J Med 1980;303:183.

95. Robertson GL, Bhoopalam N, Zelkowitz LJ. Vincristine neurotoxicity and abnormal secretion of antidiuretic hormone. Arch Intern Med 1973;132:717.
96. Madias NE, Harrington JT. Platinum nephrotoxicity. Am J Med 1978;65:307.
97. Schilsky RL, Anderson T. Hypomagnesemia and renal magnesium wasting in patients receiving cisplatinum. Ann Intern Med 1979;90:929.
98. Carlon GC, Goldiner PL. Complications of cancer therapy. In: Howland WS, Carlon GC, eds. Critical care of the cancer patient. Chicago: Year Book Medical Publishers, 1985:9.
99. Capizzi RL, Holcenberg JJ. Asparaginase. In: Holland JF, Frei E, Bast RC, eds. Cancer medicine, 3rd ed. Philadelphia: Lea and Febiger, 1993:796.
100. Lampe GH, Roizen MF. Anesthesia for patients with abnormal function at the adrenal cortex. Anesthesiology Clinics of North America 1987;5(2):245.
101. Kehlet H. A rational approach to dosage and preparation of parenteral glucocorticoid substitution therapy during surgical procedures. A short review. Acta Anaesthesiol Scand 1975;19:260.
102. Chernow B, Alexander HR, Smallridge RC. Hormonal responses to graded surgical stress. Arch Intern Med 1987;147:1273.
103. Udelsman R, Ramp J, Gallucci WT, et al. Adaptation during surgical stress. A reevaluation of the role of glucocorticoids. J Clin Invest 1986;77:1377.
104. Symreng T, Karlberg BE, Kagedal B, Schildt B. Physiological cortisol substitution of long-term steroid-treated patients undergoing major surgery. Br J Anaesth 1981;53:949.
105. Ehrlich HP, Hunt TK. Effects of cortisone and vitamin A on wound healing. Ann Surg 1968;167:324.
106. Sandberg N. Time relationship between administration of cortisone and wound healing in rats. Acta Chir Scand 1964;127:446.
107. Salem M, Tainsh RE, Bromberg J, Loriaux DL, Chernow B. Perioperative glucocorticoid coverage: a reassessment 42 years after emergence of a problem. Ann Surg 1994;219:416.

14

Chemotherapy and Wound Healing

MICHAEL SCHÄFFER
ADRIAN BARBUL

The increasing experience using adjuvant and neoadjuvant chemotherapy has extended the limits of surgical oncology. After cytoreductive surgery, the reduced tumor burden may stimulate the host's immune system by removing circulating immune complexes and other tumor-associated immunosuppressants.[1] Because these changes are short-lived,[2] there is a biologic rationale for the onset of adjuvant therapy in the immediate perioperative period. Both experimental and clinical studies support these findings.[3–5] In other situations, tumors may not even be excised before being treated with chemotherapy, radiation, or both. Due to their accelerated cell turnover, fresh wounds are susceptible to growth inhibition by antineoplastic agents. The outcome of surgical procedures may be affected by the wound impairment caused by antineoplastic agents used to treat the underlying condition.

WOUND HEALING: BASIC PRINCIPLES

Knowledge of the processes of wound repair is basic to the understanding of changes that may be brought about by antineoplastic agents. Wound healing is a complex cascade of biochemical and cellular events designed to achieve restoration of tissue integrity following injury. Much has been learned about the individual events that comprise this cascade. However, we know little about the spatial and temporal interweaving of these events and how one biologic step sets the stage for subsequent observed phenomena. During the past decade it has become evident that the cellular immune system, growth factors and cytokines play a key role in the regulation of various phases of wound healing.

The **inflammatory phase** (day 0 to 5) (Fig. 14-1) is characterized by the interplay of platelets, acute inflammatory cells, growth factors, and cytokines. The exposure of collagen to blood products initiates the coagulation cascade and platelet degranulation with consecutive release of growth factors. Kinins and prostaglandins lead to vasodilatation and increased capillary permeability. Within a few hours, circulating immune cells appear in the wound. Polymorphonuclear cells (PMN) are the first leukocytes to enter the wound site, peaking at 24 to 48 hours.[6] Their main function seems to be the phagocytosis of bacteria to control wound infection. The presence of PMNs does not appear to be essential for normal healing of uncontaminated wounds. Macrophages appear at the site of injury within 48 to 96 hours. Initially, they participate in the inflammatory process and debridement[7]; later, they play a pivotal role in regulating the proliferative phase through the release of growth factors and cytokines.

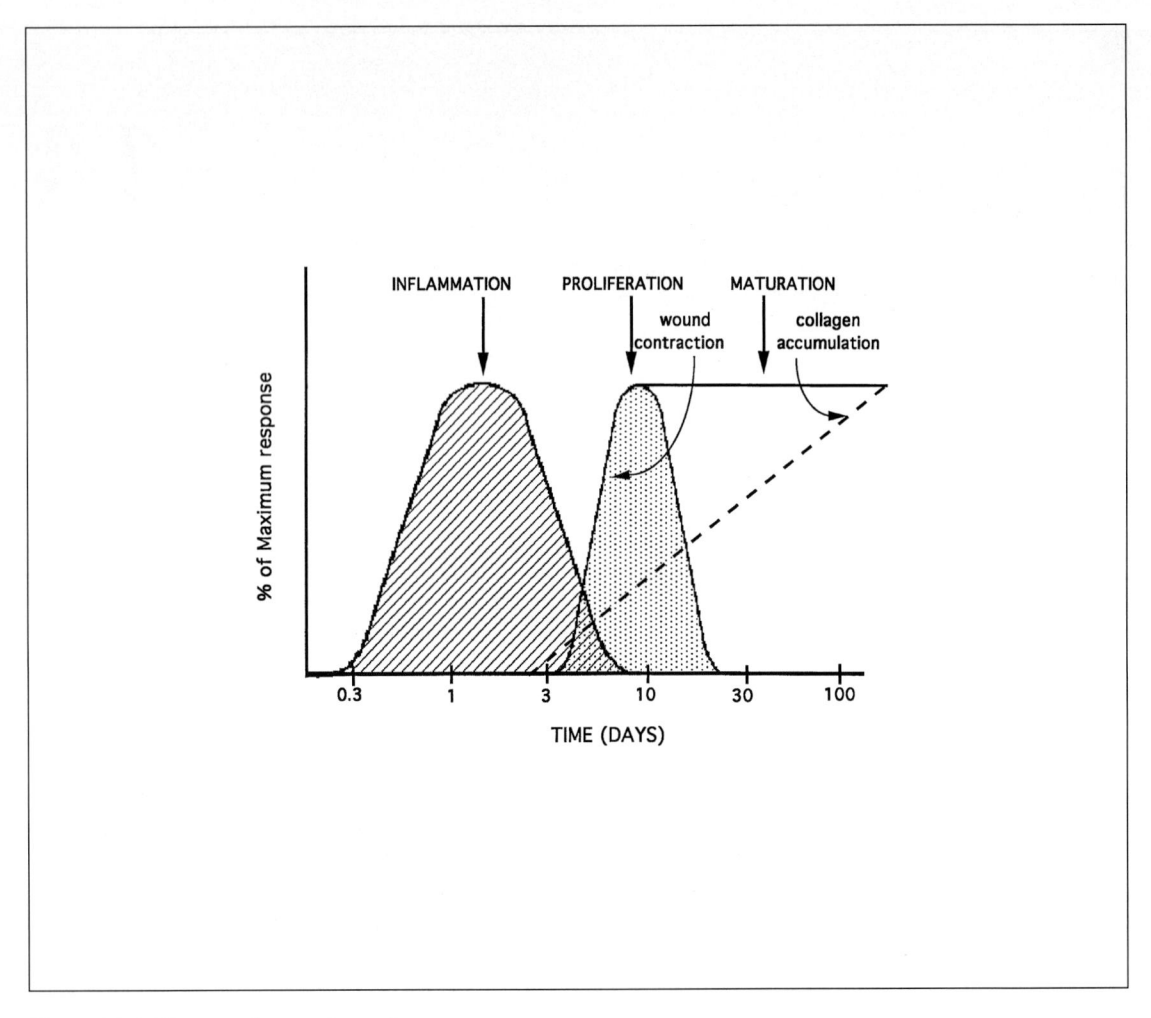

Figure 14-1. Phases of wound repair.

T-lymphocytes, the second arm of the cellular immune system, appear in significant numbers at about the fifth day postwounding[6] and have been shown to greatly influence wound healing. Global depletion of all T-cells or of T-suppressor cells only prior to, or in the early phase after, wounding leads to impaired healing.[8] Lymphotrophic agents, such as growth hormone,[9] vitamin A,[10] or arginine[11] increase wound breaking strength (WBS) and collagen deposition. Thus, in contrast to PMNs, the presence of macrophages and lymphocytes is critical to normal wound repair. During the first few days, the tensile strength of the wound is less than 5% of normal.[12]

The **proliferation phase**, characterized by the formation of granulation tissue, begins on day 3 and lasts at least 3 weeks. Granulation tissue consists of a combination of cellular elements, mainly fibroblasts and inflammatory cells, along with a few capillaries embedded in a loose extracellular matrix of collagen, fibronectin, and hyaluronic acid. Fibroblasts achieve peak numbers at about the seventh day.[6] They are the predominant synthetic cell and produce the majority of structural proteins used during tissue reconstruction. The accelerated production of collagen with subsequent cross-linking provides the principal strength characteristic of the wound. Revascularization proceeds in parallel with fibroplasia. It is initiated by cytokines, released by activated macrophages, platelets, and local conditions such as tissue hypoxia and lactic acid accumulation. The stimulus for the process of re-epithelialization is mediated by a combination of loss of contact inhibition, exposure of constituents of the extracellular matrix, particularly fibronectin,[13] and by cytokines produced by immunonuclear cells.[14] At this time, the tensile strength of the wound has not gained more than 20% of its final strength.[12]

The **remodeling stage (maturation phase)** begins around the seventh day following injury and continues for at least 1 year. The initial randomly distributed collagen fibers become cross-linked and aggregated into fibrillar bundles. As the collagen matures and the cross-links increase, the tensile strength of the wound increases to about 50% after 5 weeks and finally to 80% of normal skin. Due to a gradual reduction in cellularity and vascularity, a relatively avascular and acellular collagen scar is formed. Wound contraction, distinguished from contracture, is predominantly seen in wounds that heal by secondary intention. It usually begins around the fifth day postwounding[15,16] and appears to be a result of an interaction between fibroblast locomotion and collagen reorganization.

SYSTEMIC EFFECTS OF CHEMOTHERAPY

Because wound healing occurs within the context of the host metabolism and physiology, systemic effects of antineoplastic agents may alter wound repair. Some of the adverse effects of chemotherapy are listed in Table 14-1. Neutropenia is normally seen 7 to 10 days after initiating chemotherapy and, thus, might interfere with the early phase of healing when administered preoperatively. On the other hand, as mentioned above, the presence of leukopenia has no, or only little, effect on healing in the uncontaminated wound. Usually, in patients with a neutrophil count of 500/mm³ or greater, surgical

Table 14-1. Adverse Reactions to Chemotherapy

BONE MARROW
 Leukopenia
 Thrombocytopenia
 Anemia

CARDIOVASCULAR
 Myocardial ischemia
 Myocarditis
 Thrombophlebitis
 Other CV side effects

CUTANEOUS
 Rash
 Hyperpigmentation
 Alopecia
 Other cutaneous side effects

GASTROINTESTINAL
 Vomiting
 Nausea
 Anorexia
 Other GI side effects

HEPATIC
 Hepatic enzyme elevation
 Jaundice
 Hepatic necrosis
 Other hepatic side effects

NEUROLOGIC
 Ataxia
 Dysarthria
 Peripheral neuropathies
 Other neurologic side effects

PSYCHIATRIC
 Disorientation
 Confusion
 Other psychiatric side effects

UROGENITAL
 Nephropathy
 Renal failure
 Other urogenital side effects

OTHER SIDE EFFECTS
 Carcinogenesis
 Teratogenesis
 Mutagenesis
 Pain
 Allergic

wounds heal without difficulty and do not have an increased risk of infection. Chronic anemia, frequently associated with chemotherapy, also has been shown not to adversely affect wound repair.[17] Vomiting, nausea, diarrhea or constipation, and anorexia are common gastrointestinal side effects. Poor nutritional intake or lack of individual nutrients are well known to impair wound healing and need not be long-standing.[18–20] Importantly, even brief nutritional intervention that may not meet all nutrient requirements can reverse some of these effects (see Chapter 15).[21,22]

EFFECTS OF CHEMOTHERAPY ON WOUNDS

The majority of antineoplastic agents interfere with DNA or RNA replication, protein synthesis, or cell division and, in this way, directly affect the proliferative phase by inhibition of fibroplasia, angiogenesis, and epithelialization. Some of these specific effects on wound healing are listed in Table 14-2. Only few agents affect wound strength during the remodeling phase.

Our knowledge of the interference of chemotherapy with wound healing is mainly based on animal studies. Usually, doses of chemotherapeutic agents in different animal species and man are comparable when the dose is measured in mg/m² (surface area).[23] Assuming that these findings are applicable to humans, the results vary according to drug, the time of administration relative to wounding, the dose of drug, and the time period between surgery and subsequent investigation of wound parameters. Most antineoplastic agents have systemic effects, including weight loss, leukopenia, and anemia. To distinguish between direct impairment of wound healing and impairment secondary to one of the systemic effects, appropriate controls must be chosen. Common wound parameters are wound breaking strength of the skin, wound bursting strength of the gut, content of hydroxyproline as an index of collagen formation, ³H-thymidine uptake as an index of cellularity (new DNA formation), and histologic investigations.

Because no typical impairment patterns have been found according to drug class, including alkylating agents, antimetabolites, antibiotics, plant alkaloids, hormones, and others, the different agents will be discussed in alphabetical order.

Adriamycin (doxorubicin-hydrochloride)

Adriamyicin is a cytotoxic anthracycline antibiotic that binds to nucleic acids.[24] Decreased WBS during the entire healing period was reported when high dose Adriamycin was injected on the day of wounding.[25] The significance of time of administration relative to surgery was demonstrated by Devereux et al.[26,27] Decreased WBS was seen with a single dose injection (LD_{10}) preoperatively, on the day of surgery, or 3 days postoperatively, but no effect was observed when it was administered 7 days after wounding. In another study, only preoperative treatment resulted in impaired wound healing, whereas treatment on the day of surgery had no effect.[28] Lawrence et al[29,30] investigated the effect of Adriamycin in rats between 6 weeks prior to operation and 4 weeks postoperatively. Preoperative administration decreased WBS for at least 4 weeks in all cases. It is remarkable that no improved healing was seen by lengthening the interval between chemotherapy and wounding. Postoperative administration up to 3 weeks after wounding led to impaired WBS 1 to 2 weeks later; this might explain the findings of others[29,30] who could not demonstrate much effect by postoperative treatment. No effect was seen by treatment beyond the proliferation phase (4 weeks postoperatively) when assessed 1 or 2 weeks later. Adriamycin never decreased

Table 14-2. Effects of Chemotherapy on Wound Healing

Alteration of nitrogen balance (suppressed protein synthesis)
Impeded aggregation of platelets and deposition of fibrin
Inhibition of inflammatory cells
Inhibition of fibroplasia
Decreased production of hydroxyproline and collagen
Delayed vasodilatation and neovascularization
Impaired wound contraction
Slowed epithelialization
Impairment of collagen cross-linking
Promotion of wound infection

the wound breaking strength after a certain degree of strength had been obtained.[29,30] In another study, decreased WBS was reported 3 weeks after Adriamycin injection; this emphasizes the delayed effect on healing after intra- or postoperative application.[31] Greenhalgh and Gamelli[32] could demonstrate that early wound impairment is partially due to weight loss. Decreased skin graft take and adherence has been described by others.[33] Impaired bursting strength of intestinal anastomoses was reported after Adriamycin injection 3 days prior to operation[34] or on the day of wounding.[35]

Histologic investigations showed reduced cellularity, diminished fibroblast proliferation, decreased synthesis of hydroxyproline, and a lesser degree of capillary ingrowth.[36,37] Impaired wound healing seemed to be due to a reduction in newly synthesized collagen and not to reduced maturation.[38]

Growth factors have been shown to reverse some of the effects induced by Adriamycin. This was documented after local administration of transforming growth factor (TGF-β) alone or in combination with platelet derived growth factor (PDGF) and epidermal growth factor (EGF).[39,40] Decreased mRNA for TGF-β and collagen suggested diminished gene expression for TGF-β.[41] DeCunzo et al[36] reported increased WBS after intraperitone-al injection of interleukin-2 (IL-2) in treated but not in control animals. Allopurinol, a xanthine oxidase inhibitor and major enzyme for superoxide radical formation, prevented wound impairment and weight loss in another study.[34] Because Adriamycin is partially metabolized by xanthine oxidase, superoxide radicals may play a role in mediating Adriamycin toxicity on wound repair.[34] No reversal of Adriamycin-induced impairment was seen with vitamin E or N-acetylcysteine.[42]

In one controlled clinical trial including 7 patients with breast cancer, increased wound complications were reported when Adriamycin was given 2 to 3 weeks prior to operation.[43] Chemotherapy in combination with Adriamycin, plus two or more common antineoplastic agents within 3 or 4 weeks of operation has been documented not to increase wound morbidity.[44–47] However, a high incidence of postoperative wound complications (38%) was found in patients with advanced breast cancer who had been treated with combined preoperative irradiation and chemotherapy.[48]

Bleomycin

Bleomycin is a mixture of cytotoxic glycopeptide antibiotics that inhibit DNA, RNA, and protein synthesis.[24] Cohen et al[49] demonstrated a transient decrease of wound-breaking strength on day 7 when high-dose bleomycin was administered on the day of wounding. In another study, decreased wound breaking strength was reported during the entire healing period when bleomycin was given alone or in combination with etoposide and cisplatin on the day of surgery. However, interpretation of results is difficult because treated animals exhibited impaired weight gain.[50] Impaired intestinal WBS was seen when combined perioperative chemotherapy (bleomycin, 5-fluorouracil, and cisplatinum) was administered perioperatively, but no effect was seen by pre- or postoperative treatment alone.[51,52]

Clinical trials with combined chemotherapy, including bleomycin, cisplatin, and vindesine or methotrexate, have not shown increased wound complications.[53–55] Intracavitary administration to control malignant effusions and low-dose intralesional injection in the treatment of condyloma acuminatum were also assessed to be safe.[56,57]

Cisplatin

Cisplatin is a heavy metal complex producing intrastrand and interstrand cross-links in DNA.[24] A self-limited impairment of intestinal and skin wounds has been reported after a single preoperative injection of cisplatin.[58,59] Wile et al[60] studied the effect of intraoperative cisplatin (LD_{10}), alone or in combination with cisplatin (intraperitoneally [IP] or intravenously [IV]) and sodium-thiosulfate [IV] on bursting strength of intestinal anastomoses. All animals that received only cisplatin died, presumably from renal failure secondary to nephrotoxicity. Cisplatin (IV, but not IP) in combination with sodiumthiosulfate resulted in decreased WBS, suggesting the safe combination of cisplatin IP and sodiumthiosulfate IV (two-route chemotherapy). Cisplatin in combination with etoposide and bleomycin has been shown to impair wound healing during the entire healing period, but animals receiving cisplatin alone showed normal wound healing. Because etoposide alone had some effect 3 weeks postoperatively, only bleomycin appeared to be responsible for the reduced WBS seen by the combination treatment group.[50] In another study, no effect was seen on WBS by combined preoperative treatment with cisplatin plus 5-fluorouracil (5-FU). There also was no effect on the closing rate of artificial orocutaneous fistulae; however, severe facial cellulitis occurred in 40% of the treated animals (0% of controls) indicating increased host susceptibility to infection.[61] Combined perioperative chemotherapy (cisplatin, 5-fluorouracil, and bleomycin) caused decreased intestinal WBS, but no effect was seen by pre- or postoperative treatment alone.[51,52] Clinical trials have not shown increased wound morbidity in patients undergoing combined chemotherapy including cisplatin, bleomycin, Adriamycin, and methotrexate or 5-FU.[47,53–55,62,63] Kolb et al[62] found no increased wound morbidity in patients undergoing early postoperative cisplatin-based chemotherapy for ovarian cancer when compared with patients with other gynecological malignancies who did not receive chemotherapy. However low postoperative albumin or hemoglobin levels and advanced stage of disease were shown to be risk factors for increased wound complications. Schaefer et al[64] reported some delay in wound healing in patients subjected to multimodal treatment of advanced carcinoma of the head and neck but chemotherapy was combined with radiotherapy and administered 11 or more weeks prior to surgery.

Corticosteroids

Corticosteroids have been shown to impair wound healing in many animal and clinical trials. Animal studies demonstrated a decreased wound breaking strength at various times when steroids were administered perioperatively or during the early phase of wound healing at different dosages.[10,65–70] Treatment started 2 days or later after wounding, or pretreatment followed by a free interval of 3 days before surgery had no effect.[69] Dosage seems to be important because dose-related wound impairment has been described.[68] In another study, Vogel[70] demonstrated that low dosage even increased WBS when corticosteroids were given daily postoperatively for 20 days, whereas high dosage caused decreased WBS at any time point when treatment started at the day of wounding. Treatment on day 19 and 20 or from day 11 to day 20 increased WBS at any dose thereafter. Debility or inadequate protein intake were shown to augment wound impairment.[67,68]

Corticosteroids inhibit open wounds at any time[71] and have been shown to decrease wound contraction, to delay formation of granulation tissue, and to slow epithelialization.[72–74] Cortisone acetate appears to inhibit healing of open wounds more than methylprednisolone or medroxyprogesterone, which emphasizes the difference between various steroid compounds.[74]

Histologic examinations have shown prolonged monocytopenia and reduced wound debridement.[7] During the inflammatory stage of healing, inhibition of formation of granulation tissue and suppression of all cellular elements were demonstrated.[65,75] DNA, hydroxyproline, or protein content as an index of cellularity and collagen formation, have been shown to be reduced in wounds of steroid-treated animals.[69,76] Steroid-induced cell death seems to be mediated by a glucocorticoid receptor inducing the expression of an intracellular nuclease.[77]

Vitamin A and anabolic steroids such as testosterone and synthetics (Durabolin or Bolmantalate) have been shown to reverse the effects of steroids on wound healing. An antagonistic effect mediated through influence on lysosomal membranes was postulated.[10,66,78]

Clinical trials have supported these findings. Green[70] found increased wound complications in patients undergoing a variety of different operations when compared with literature data. The duration of preoperative steroid therapy did not influence the incidence of postoperative morbidity. Mileski et al[80,81] reported increased anastomotic leakage following colon resection and an increased morbidity and mortality after closure of a colostomy in patients with steroid treatment. In another study with patients undergoing infrainguinal arterial bypass surgery, steroid therapy was identified to be a significant risk factor for postoperative wound complications.[82]

Cyclophosphamide

Cyclophosphamide is biotransformed in the liver to an active alkylating metabolite. It cross-links tumor cell DNA[24] and is known to cause immunosuppression.[83]

Impaired wound breaking strength has been shown during the entire healing period after treatment with cyclophosphamide as a single injection on the day of surgery.[84] A delayed decrease of WBS 3 weeks postoperatively has been reported by others when high-dose chemotherapy was applied during the perioperative period.[25] Combination treatment with cyclophosphamide plus Adriamycin impairs wound healing to a greater extent than either agent alone.[25] Low-dose cyclophosphamide has been shown to have no effect.[85] Also, no effect was observed when a therapeutic dose was applied over a period of 5 days, as assessed by mechanical tests, autoradiography, and electron microscopy.[86]

Open wounds have been shown to have reduced proliferation of granulation tissue cells.[87] Müller et al[88] demonstrated decreased metabolism of extracellular matrix in wound granulomas when pretreated with cyclophosphamide; also, impaired collagen synthesis in unwounded skin was shown by van Husen et al.[89] However, no decrease in total collagen content in wound granulomas was found by others.[90] Delayed vasodilatation and neovascularization was described in abdominal wounds after a single injection of cyclophosphamide.[91,92] Anabolic steroids and vitamin C failed to reverse cyclophosphamide-induced wound impairment.[93,94]

Controlled clinical trials showed no increased wound complications in patients with breast cancer when cyclophosphamide was administered perioperatively or immediately postoperatively at a low-dose schedule.[95,96] Preoperative treatment in combination with Adriamycin, 5-FU, and tamoxifen was found not to increase postoperative morbidity.[97] High rates of impaired wound healing were reported by others when combined preoperative chemotherapy and radiation was administered.[48,98]

Dacarbazine

The mechanism of action of dacarbazine is not well known. Three hypotheses include (1) inhibition of DNA synthesis by acting as a purine analog; (2) action as an alkylating agent; and, (3) interaction with sulfhydryl groups.[24]

Robinson et al[99] reported a transient decrease of WBS on days 7 and 14 when dacarbazine was given early postoperatively, but no effect was seen by preoperative administration.

Dactinomycin (actinomycin D)

Dactinomycin is an antibiotic that forms a complex with DNA inhibiting RNA synthesis.[24] Impaired wound breaking strength during the early period of healing has been found when dactinomycin was injected as a single dose on the day of wounding.[49] Decreased WBS after topical application was reported by others.[100]

Etoposide (VePesid, VP-16)

Etoposide is a semisynthetic derivate of podophyllotoxin that inhibits DNA synthesis and causes mitotic arrest and lysis of those cells entering mitosis.[24] Smith et al showed a transient decrease of WBS 3 weeks postoperatively when etoposide was given on the day of wounding.[50] When administered in combination with cisplatin and bleomycin, decreased WBS was found at 1- and 5-week intervals. However, impaired weight gain of treated animals limits its interpretation.

No increased wound morbidity was found in an uncontrolled trial involving a small number of patients with isolated limb perfusion.[63]

5-Fluorouracil

5-Fluorouracil is an antineoplastic metabolite that interferes with the synthesis of DNA and RNA.[24] Impaired healing of the abdominal wall has been shown for the first 10 postoperative days after daily postoperative treatment.[101] A single injection of high-dose 5-FU alone or in combination with methotrexate and cyclophosphamide was reported to cause a self-limited decrease of wound breaking strength 3 weeks postoperatively.[84] Malnutrition amplifies 5-FU–induced wound impairment (wound-breaking strength decreases 2.6 times when weight loss is 20% to 25%).[102] However, no effect was seen by others.[49,85] Preoperative treatment in combination with cisplatin had no effect on WBS or on closing rate of artificial orocutaneous fistula, but severe facial cellulitis occurred in 40% of the treated animals (0% of controls) indicating increased host susceptibility to infection.[61] Delayed epithelialization and inhibition of mitosis after topical application of 5-FU in humans was described by others.[103]

5-Fluorouracil is frequently used in adjuvant chemotherapy of colorectal carcinoma. Perioperative and immediate postoperative chemotherapy has been shown to impair intestinal bursting strength when tested within the first 10 days following operation,[51,52,104] but no effect was seen by preoperative treatment alone.[51,52] In contrast, Goldmann et al[105] found a dose-related increase in leakage of intestinal anastomoses in rats when 5-FU was administered preoperatively. Noteworthy in this article, is the leakage rate of 19% among control animals, raising questions about the technique used. No impairment of colonic anastomoses was reported when chemotherapy was given early postoperatively for 5 days.[106] Intramural infiltration of 5-FU had no effect either on intestinal bursting strength or on histologic findings.[107]

Controlled clinical trials showed increased wound complications when chemotherapy was started within 7 to 10 days postoperatively, but not when withheld until the 14th day.[108,109] Rousselot et al[110] reported no increase in postoperative morbidity (compared to historical controls) when intraluminal chemotherapy was combined with systemic administration. Combined preoperative chemotherapy and radiation in patients with advanced breast cancer was reported to result in a high incidence of postoperative wound complications.[48,98]

6-Mercaptopurine

6-Mercaptopurine is a purine analog that interferes with nucleic acid biosynthesis.[24] Daily postoperative administration has been shown to cause a dose-related retardation in connective tissue organization and revascularization. Decreased DNA content, suggesting reduced cellularity, was found in wound granulomas. No change in hydroxyproline (index of collagen formation) levels was observed.[111]

Methotrexate

Methotrexate is an antimetabolite that interferes with DNA synthesis by inhibiting dihydrofolic acid reductase.[24] Calnan and Davies demonstrated dose-related wound impairment when methotrexate was administered for 5 days beginning on the day of wounding.[85] Leucovorin (folic acid) reversed this effect completely and, when given alone, even showed a transient enhancement of WBS on day 3. Preoperative treatment with methotrexate had no effect on WBS. Self-limiting wound impairment on day 14 was described when methotrexate was injected every 4 days.[43] In another study, a transient decrease of WBS during the early stage of healing was seen when it was applied as a single dose on the day of wounding[49]; however, no effect was reported by others after a single dose treatment.[84] Combined application with cyclophosphamide and 5-FU has been shown to impair wound healing 3 weeks postoperatively.[84]

In clinical studies, no or only limited wound morbidity has been found after neoadjuvant chemotherapy with methotrexate and leucovorin,[54,55,112] but a high incidence of postoperative wound morbidity was seen after combined chemotherapy and radiation.[48,98]

Mitomycin (Mitomycin C)

Mitomycin is an antibiotic that inhibits DNA, RNA, and protein synthesis.[24] No impairment in the healing of intestinal anastomoses was reported after perioperative mitomycin injection as assessed by histology, tensile strength, and hydroxyproline content.[113] Decreased wound breaking strength (laparotomy wounds and intestinal anastomoses) was seen in the early phase of wound healing when high-dose chemotherapy, in combination with 5-FU and Adriamycin, was applied on the day of wounding. However, no effect was seen when chemotherapy was administered on day 4. Both Adriamycin and 5-FU have been shown to impair wound healing. This and significant weight loss of treated animals makes interpretation difficult.[35]

Mitoxantrone

Mitoxantrone is a synthetic anthracenedione that inhibits both DNA and RNA synthesis.[24] No impaired wound breaking strength of the skin has been shown in rats 3 weeks postoperatively when mitoxantrone was administered on the day of wounding.[31]

Vinblastine

Vinblastine is a plant alkaloid that interferes with nucleic acid synthesis and with the metabolic pathway of amino acids. It affects cell enzyme production required for mitosis and produces various atypical mitotic figures.[24]

A delayed decrease in wound breaking strength 5 weeks postwounding was seen after vinblastine was administered on the day of surgery, but no effect was reported 1 and 3 weeks postoperatively.[50]

Vincristine

Vincristine is a plant alkaloid that interferes with intracellular tubulin function that causes mitotic arrest.[24] Decreased WBS during the early phase of healing was documented after vincristine injection on the day of surgery.[49]

No increased wound morbidity was reported after preoperative chemotherapy in an uncontrolled clinical trial including a small number of patients with Wilms' tumor.[114]

SUMMARY

Animal studies have demonstrated wound impairment of all investigated chemotherapeutic agents (Table 14-3). Depending on the drug, only high dosages or a therapeutic dosage affected normal wound healing. The immediate preoperative and early postoperative phases seem to be most vulnerable. However, once a certain degree of wound breaking strength had been obtained, no decrease of strength was reported. Impairment of WBS documented during the inflammatory phase of healing has little significance because no collagen has been produced yet and only the coagulum contributes to wound strength at that time. Although it might indicate a prolonged cellular phase and a delayed onset of fibroplasia.

Except with the use of corticosteroids, most clinical trials have failed to prove increased wound complications with chemotherapy (Table 14-4). In one study where Adriamycin was administered 2 to 3 weeks prior to mastectomy in patients with locally advanced breast cancer, increased wound morbidity was observed in comparison with

Table 14-3. Effects of Single Chemotherapeutic Agents on Experimental Wound Healing

Drug	Species	Type of Wound	Impairment	Reference
Adriamycin	mouse, rat	skin	yes	25–32, 36, 38–41, 43
	rat	intestine	yes	34
Bleomycin	mouse, rat	skin	yes	49, 50
Cisplatin	mouse, rat	skin	yes	59, 60
	rat	skin	no	50
	rat	intestine	yes	58
Cyclophosphamide	mouse, rat	skin	yes	25, 84, 88
	rat	skin	no	85, 86
	mouse, rat	abdominal wall	yes	91–94
	rat	open wound	yes	87
Dacarbazine	rat	skin	yes	99
Dactinomycin	mouse, rabbit	skin	yes	49, 100
Etoposide	rat	skin	yes	50
5-Fluorouracil	rat	skin	yes	84
	mouse, rat	skin	no	49, 85
	rat	abdominal wall	yes	101, 102
	human	open wound	yes	103
	rat	intestinal	yes	104, 105
	rat	intestinal	no	106, 107
6-Mercaptopurine	guinea pig	skin	yes	111
Methotrexate	rat	skin	yes	43, 85
	mouse, rat	skin	no	49, 84
Mitomycin	rat	intestinal	no	113
Mitoxantrone	rat	skin	no	31
Vinblastine	rat	skin	yes	50
Vincristine	mouse	skin	yes	49

surgery alone. However, one has to take into account the small number of patients who underwent chemotherapy. Also the fact that, in treated patients, control of local disease was felt to be "primarily unachievable by radiotherapy or surgery alone"[43] suggests a more advanced size or infiltration of surrounding tissue. The only other study showing increased wound complications in a controlled clinical trial was a multicenter study

Table 14-4. Effects of Chemotherapy on Wound Healing in Patients (controlled clinical studies)

Drug	Tumor	Time of Therapy	Effect on Wound Healing	Reference
Adriamycin	Breast	2–3 weeks preoperatively	increased complications	43
Cisplatin	Ovarian	4–42 days postoperatively	none	62
Cyclophosphamide	Breast	perioperatively	none	95
Cyclophosphamide	Breast	0–5 days postoperatively	none	96
5-Fluorouracil	Breast	7–10 days postoperatively	increased complications	108
5-Fluorouracil	Colon	14 days postoperatively	none	109
5-Fluorouracil	Colon	0–2 days postoperatively	none	110

including 1328 patients with locally advanced breast cancer at 36 institutions. The patients received either 5-FU or thiotepa or placebo. 5-Fluorouracil administered for 4 successive days beginning between postoperative day 7 and 10 was associated with a significant increase in local and systemic complications.[108] However, the high incidence of wound complications in all groups (placebo: 43%, 5-FU: 52%, thiotepa: 47%) is remarkable. Premenopausal patients undergoing 5-FU treatment were affected most. A controlled clinical trial with 5-FU treatment started after the 14th postoperative day showed no increased wound morbidity.[109]

Assessment of the high incidence of postoperative morbidity is difficult for many reasons. Patients undergoing surgery for tumor treatment often receive combined irradiation and chemotherapy. Radiotherapy, itself, is well known to impair wound healing when administered preoperatively or during the early postoperative phase[116–120] and has been shown to amplify the effect of chemotherapy on wound healing.[27] Patients with malignant diseases are already predisposed to increased postoperative morbidity[121,122] and locally advanced stage may directly affect wound healing by tumor cells present in the wound area. Malnutrition and higher age[123] of patients also are known to affect wound repair.

The increasing incidence of patients with compromised immune systems, including transplant patients with immunosuppressive treatment, or patients with AIDS will affect the day-to-day practice of modern surgeons. Chemotherapy, alone, may not increase wound morbidity in a young patient with an early stage of malignant disease, but, combined with radiation, it might accelerate wound impairment and host susceptibility to infection[61,124–126] in an elderly cachectic patient, in a young patient with AIDS, or in a patient following organ transplantation. Concomitant antibiotic therapy and nonabsorbable suture, left for an extended period of time, is recommended. Topical application of growth factors on chronic nonhealing wounds has been shown to stimulate the wound closing rate and may become available for use in patients with impaired healing after cancer surgery in the management of these problems.

REFERENCES

1. Fisher B, Gunduz N, Saffer EA. Influence of the interval between primary tumor removal and chemotherapy on kinetics and growth of metastases. Cancer Res 1983;43:1488.
2. Gunduz N, Fisher B, Saffer EA. Effect of surgical removal on the growth and kinetics of residual tumor. Cancer Res 1984;39:3861.
3. Cruz EP, McDonald GO, Cole WH. Prophylactic treatment of cancer: the use of chemotherapeutic agents to prevent tumor metastasis. Surgery 1956;40:291.
4. Ragaz J, Baird R, Rebbeck R, et al. Preoperative adjuvant chemotherapy (neoadjuvant) for carcinoma of the breast: rationale and safety report. Recent Results Cancer Res 1985;98:99.
5. Schabel FM Jr: Rationale for perioperative anticancer treatment. Recent Results Cancer Res 1985;98:1.
6. Ross R, Benditt EP. Wound healing and collagen formation. I. Sequential changes in components of guinea pig skin wounds observed in the electron microscope. J Biophysiol Biochem Cytol 1961;11:677.
7. Leibovich SJ, Ross R. The role of the macrophage in wound repair. Am J Pathol 1975;78:71.
8. Barbul A, Breslin RJ, Woodyard JP, et al. The effect of in vivo T helper and T suppressor lymphocyte depletion on wound healing. Ann Surg 1989;209:479.
9. Prudden JF, Nishihara G, Ocamp I. Studies on growth hormone. III. The effect on wound tensile strength of marked postoperative anabolism induced with growth hormone. Surg Gynecol Obstet 1958;107:481.
10. Ehrlich HP, Hunt TK. Effects of cortisone and vitamin A on wound healing. Ann Surg 1968;167:324.
11. Barbul A, Rettura G, Levenson SM. Arginine: a thymotrophic and wound promoting agent. Surgical Forum 1977;28:101.
12. Levenson SM, Geever EF, Crowley LV, et al. The healing of rat skin wounds. Ann Surg 1965;161:293.
13. Woodley DT, Bachmann PM, O'Keefe EJ. The role of matrix components in human keratinocyte re-epithelialization. In: Barbul A, Caldwell MD, Eaglstein WH, Hunt TK,

Marshall D, Pines E, Skover G, eds. Clinical and experimental approaches to dermal and epidermal repair. Normal and chronical wounds. New York: Wiley-Liss, 1991:129.
14. Lynch SE. Interaction of growth factors and tissue repair. In: Barbul A, Caldwell MD, Eaglstein WH, Hunt TK, Marshall D, Pines E, Skover G, eds. Clinical and experimental approaches to dermal and epidermal repair. Normal and chronical wounds. New York: Wiley-Liss, 1991:341.
15. Luccioli G, Robertson HR, Kahn DS. The pattern of contraction during healing of excised wounds in the rabbit. Can J Surg 1963;6:499.
16. Van Winkle W Jr: Wound contraction. Surg Gynecol Obstet 1967;125:131.
17. Hugo NE, Thompson LW, Zook EG, et al. Effect of chronic anemia on the tensile strength of healing wounds. Surgery 1969;66:741.
18. Barbul A, Purtill WA. Nutrition in wound healing. Clin Dermatol 1994;12:133.
19. Greenhalgh DG, Gamelli RL. Is impaired wound healing caused by infection or nutritional depletion? Surgery 1987;102:306.
20. Irvin TT. Effects of malnutrition and hyperalimentation on wound healing. Surg Gynecol Obstet 1978;146:33.
21. Haydock DA, Hill GL. Improved wound healing response in surgical patients receiving intra-venous nutrition. Br J Surg 1987;74:320.
22. Schroeder D, Gillanders L, Mahr K, et al. Effects of immediate postoperative enteral nutrition on body composition, muscle function and wound healing. Parenter Enteral Nutr 1991;15:376.
23. Freireich EJ, Gehan EA, Rall DP, Schmidt LH, et al. Quantitative comparison of toxicity of anticancer agents in mouse, rat, hamster, dog, monkey, and man. Cancer Chemother Rep 1966;50:219.
24. Physicians' Desk Reference, 48th ed. Montvale: Medical Economics Data Production Company, 1994.
25. Cohen SC, Gabelnick HL, Johnson RK, et al. Effects of cyclophosphamide and Adriamycin on the healing of surgical wounds in mice. Cancer 1975;36:1277.
26. Devereux DF, Thibault L, Boretos J, et al. The quantitative and qualitative impairment of wound healing by Adriamycin. Cancer 1979;43:932.
27. Devereux DF, Kent H, Brennan MF. Time dependent effects of Adriamycin and x-ray therapy on wound healing in the rat. Cancer 1980;45:2805.
28. Mullen BM, Mattox DE, Von Hoff DD, et al. The effect of preoperative Adriamycin and dihydroxyanthracenedione on wound healing. Laryngoscope 1981;91:1436.
29. Lawrence WT, Norton JA, Harvey AK, et al. Doxorubicin-induced impairment of wound healing in rats. JNCI 1986;76:119.
30. Lawrence WT, Talbot TL, Noton JA. Preoperative or postoperative doxorubicin hydrochloride (Adriamycin): Which is better for wound healing? Surgery 1986;100:9.
31. Noh R, Karp GI, Devereux DF. The effects of doxorubicin and mitoxantrone on wound healing. Cancer Chemother Pharmacol 1991;29:141.
32. Greenhalgh DG, Gamelli RL. Do nutritional alterations contribute to Adriamycin-induced impaired wound healing? J Surg Res 1988;45:261.
33. Falcone RE, Nappi JF. Chemotherapy and wound healing. Surg Clin N Am 1984;64:779.
34. Johnson H Jr, Zelnick R, Davis E, et al. Effect of allopurinol on Adriamycin-induced impairment of wound healing. J Invest Surg 1991;4:323.
35. Salm R, Wullich B, Kiefer G, et al. Effects of a three-drug antineoplastic protocol of wound healing in rats: a biomechanical and histologic study on gastrointestinal anastomoses and laparotomy wounds. J Surg Oncol 1991;47:5.
36. DeCunzo LP Jr, Mackenzie JW, Marafino BJ Jr, et al. The effect of interleukin-2 administration on wound healing in Adriamycin-treated rats. J Surg Res 1990;49:419.
37. Sasaki T, Holeyfield C, Uitto J. Doxorubicin-induced inhibition of propyl hydroxylation during collagen biosynthesis in human skin fibroblast cultures. J Clin Invest 1987;80:1735.
38. Devereux DF, Triche TJ, Webber BL, et al. A study of Adriamycin-reduced wound breaking strength in rats. Cancer 1980;45:2811.
39. Curtsinger LJ, Pietsch JD, Brown GL, et al. Reversal of Adriamycin-impaired wound healing by transforming growth factor-beta. Surg Gynecol Obstet 1989;168:517.
40. Lawrence WT, Sporn MB, Gorschboth C, et al. The reversal of an Adriamycin induced healing impairment with chemoattractants and growth factors. Ann Surg 1986;203:142.
41. Salomon GD, Kasid A, Bernstein E, et al. Gene expression in normal and doxorubicin-impaired wounds: importance of transforming growth factor-beta. Surgery 1990;108:318.
42. Shamberger RC, Devereux DF, Brennan MF. The effect of chemotherapeutic agents on wound healing. International Advances in Surgical Oncology 1981;4:15.
43. Bland KI, Palin WE, von Frauenhofer JA, et al.

Experimental and clinical observations of the effects of cytotoxic chemotherapeutic drugs on wound healing. Ann Surg 1984;199:782.
44. Bujko K, Suit HD, Springfield DS, et al. Wound healing after preoperative radiation for sarcoma of soft tissues. Surg Gynecol Obstet 1993;176:124.
45. Finn D, Steele G Jr, Osteen RT, et al. Morbidity and mortality after surgery in patients with disseminated or locally advanced cancer receiving systemic chemotherapy. J Surg Oncol 1980;13:237.
46. Morrow M, Bravermann A, Thelmo W, et al. Multimodal therapy for locally advanced breast cancer. Arch Surg 1986;121:1291.
47. Wilke H, Preusser P, Fink U, et al. Preoperative chemotherapy in locally advanced and nonresectable gastric cancer: a phase II study with etoposide, doxorubicin, and cisplatin. J Clin Oncol 1989;7:1318.
48. Badr El Din A, Coibion M, Guenier C, et al. Local postoperative morbidity following preoperative irradiation in locally advanced breast cancer. Eur J Surg Oncol 1989;15:486.
49. Cohen SC, Gabelnick HL, Johnson RK, et al. Effects of antineoplastic agents on wound healing in mice. Surgery 1975;78:238.
50. Smith RW, Sampson MK, Lucas CE, et al. Effects of vinblastine, etoposide, cisplatin and bleomycin on rodent wound healing. Surg Gynecol Obstet 1985;161:323.
51. De Roy Van Zuidewijn DBW, Hendriks T, Wobbes T, et al. Healing of experimental colonic anastomoses: effect of antineoplastic agents. Eur J Surg Oncol 1987;13:27.
52. De Roy Van Zuidewijn DBW, Wobbes T, Hendriks T, et al. The effect of antineoplastic agents on the healing of small intestinal anastomoses in the rat. Cancer 1986;58:62.
53. Bains MS, Kelsen DP, Beattie EJ Jr, et al. Treatment of esophageal carcinoma by combined preoperative chemotherapy. Ann Thorac Surg 1982;34:521.
54. Benedetti-Panici P, Greggi S, Scambia G, et al. Cisplatin, bleomycin, and methotrexate preoperative chemotherapy in locally advanced vulvar carcinoma. Gynecol Oncol 1993;50:49.
55. Benedetti-Panici P, Scambia G, Greggi S, et al. Neoadjuvant chemotherapy and radical surgery in locally advanced cervical carcinoma: a pilot study. Obstet Gynecol 1988;71:344.
56. Figueroa S, Gennaro AR. Intralesional bleomycin injection in treatment of condyloma acuminatum. Dis Colon Rectum 1980;23:550.
57. Ostrowski MJ, Halsall GM. Intracavitary bleomycin in the management of malignant effusions: a multicenter study. Cancer Treatment Reports 1982;66:1903.
58. Engelmann U, Grimm K, Grönniger J, et al. Influence of cis-platinum on healing of enterostomies in the rat. Eur Urol 1983;9:45.
59. Stiernberg CM, Williams RM, Hokanson JA. Influence of cisplatin on wound healing—an experimental model. Otolaryngol Head Neck Surg 1986;95:210.
60. Wile AG, Dileo SK, Gossett DA, et al. Intraperitoneal cisplatin with sodium thiosulfate protection in rats with intestinal anastomoses. J Surg Oncol 1993;52:265.
61. Whittle T, Lucas CE, Ledgerwood AM, et al. The effects of chemotherapy on murine wound healing and orocutaneous fistula closure. Am Surg 1990;56:407.
62. Kolb BA, Buller RE, Connor JP, et al. Effects of early postoperative chemotherapy on wound healing. Obstet Gynecol 1992;79:988.
63. Roseman JM. Effective management of extremity cancers using cisplatin and etoposide in isolated limb perfusions. J Surg Oncol 1987;35:170.
64. Schaefer SD, Middleton R, Reisch J, et al. Cisplatinum induction chemotherapy in the multi-modality initial treatment of advanced stage IV carcinoma of the head and neck. Cancer 1983;51:2168.
65. Alrich EM, Carter JP, Lehman EP. The effect of ACTH and cortisone on wound healing. Ann Surg 1951;133:783.
66. Ehrlich HP, Hunt TK. The effects of cortisone and anabolic steroids on the tensile strength of healing wounds. Ann Surg 1969;170:203.
67. Findlay CW Jr, Howes EL. The combined effect of cortisone and partial protein depletion on wound healing. N Engl J Med 1952;246:597.
68. Meadows EC, Prudden JF. A study of the influence of adrenal steroids on the strength of healing wounds. Surgery 1953;33:841.
69. Sandberg N. Time relationship between administration of cortisone and wound healing in rats. Acta Chir Scand 1964;127:446.
70. Vogel HG. Tensile strength of skin wounds in rats after treatment with corticosteroids. Acta Endocrinol 1970;64:295.
71. Hunt TK. Disorders of wound healing. World J Surg 1980;4:271.
72. Howes EL, Plotz CM, Blunt JW, et al. Retardation of wound healing by cortisone. Surgery 1950;28:177.
73. Hunt TK, Ehrlich HP, Garcia JA, et al. Effect of vitamin A on reversing the inhibitory effect of cortisone on healing of open wounds in animals and man. Ann Surg 1969;170:633.
74. Lenco W, McKnight M, MacDonald AS. Effects of cortisone acetate, methylprednisolone and medroxyprogesterone on wound

contracture and epithelization in rabbits. Ann Surg 1975;181:67.
75. Spain DM, Molomut N, Haber A. Biological studies on cortisone in mice. Science 1950; 112: 335.
76. Wehr RF, Smith JG, Counts DF, et al. Vitamin A prevention of triamcinolone acetonide effects on granuloma growth: lack of effect on propyl hydroxylase. Proc Soc Exp Biol Med 1976;152:411.
77. Compton MM, Caron LAM, Cidlowski JA. Glucocorticoid action on the immune system. J Steroid Biochem Mol Biol 1987;27:201.
78. Hunt TK. Vitamin A and wound healing. J Am Acad Dermatol 1986;15:817.
79. Green JP. Steroid therapy and wound healing in surgical patients. Br J Surg 1965;52:523.
80. Mileski WJ, Joehl RJ, Rege RV, et al. Treatment of anastomotic leakage following low anterior colon resection. Arch Surg 1988;123:968.
81. Mileski WJ, Rege RV, Joehl RJ, et al. Rates of morbidity and mortality after closure of loop and end colostomy. Surg Gynecol Obstet 1990;171:17.
82. Wengrovitz M, Atnip RG, Gifford RRM, et al. Wound complications of autogenous subcutaneous infrainguinal arterial bypass surgery: predisposing factors and management. J Vasc Surg 1990;11:156.
83. Ferguson MK. The effect of antineoplastic agents on wound healing. Surg Gynecol Obstet 1982;154:421.
84. McGonigal MD, Martin DM, Lucas CL, et al. The effects of breast cancer chemotherapy on wound healing in the rat. J Surg Res 1987;42: 560.
85. Calnan J, Davies A. The effect of methotrexate (amethopterin) on wound healing. An experimental study. Br J Cancer 1965;19:505.
86. Mann M, Bednar B, Feit J. Effect of cyclophosphamide on the course of cutaneous wound healing. Neoplasma 1977;24:487.
87. Wie H, Bruaset I, Eckersberg T. Effects of cyclophosphamide on open granulation skin wounds in rats. APMIS Sect A 1979;87:185.
88. Müller US, Wirth W, Thöne F, et al. Tierexperimentelle Untersuchungen über die antiinflammatorische und immunsuppressive Wirkung von Zytostatika. Arzneimittelforschung 1973;23:487.
89. Van Husen N, Fegeler K, Gerlach U. Zur Pathophysiologie der zytostatischen Therapie von Mesenchymerkrankungen. Z Rheumaforschung 1971;30:156.
90. Hansen TM, Lorenzen I. The effects of cyclophosphamide and azathioprine on collagen in skin and granulation tissue in rats, and the effects of cyclophosphamide on collagen in human skin. Acta Pharmacol Et Toxicol 1975; 36:448.
91. Karppinen V, Myllärniemi H. Vascular reactions in the healing laparotomy wound under cytostatic treatment. Acta Chir Scand 1970; 136:675.
92. Myllärniemi H, Peltokallio P. The effect of high dose cyclophosphamide therapy in the abdominal cavity of the rat: Adhesions and their vascular pattern. Ann Chir Gynaecol 1974;63:238.
93. Desprez JD, Kiehn CL. The effects of Cytoxan (cyclophosphamide) on wound healing. Plast Reconstr Surg 1960;26:301.
94. Gupta RC, Singh LM, Udupa KN. Effect of cyclophosphamide (Endoxan) on the process of wound healing. Indian J Surg 1970;32:127.
95. Finney R. Adjuvant chemotherapy in the radical treatment of carcinoma of the breast—a clinical trial. Am J Roentgenol Radium Ther Nucl Med 1971;111:137.
96. Nissen-Meyer R, Kjellgren K, Malmio K, et al. Surgical adjuvant chemotherapy—results with one short course with cyclophosphamide after mastectomy for breast cancer. Cancer 1978;41:2088.
97. Morrow M, Bravermann A, Thelmo W, et al. Multimodal therapy for locally advanced breast cancer. Arch Surg 1986;121:1291.
98. Sauter ER, Eisenber BL, Hoffmann JP, et al. Postmastectomy morbidity after combination preoperative irradiation and chemotherapy for locally advanced breast cancer. World J Surg 1993;17:237.
99. Robinson SJ, Nappi JF, Falcone RE. The effect of dacarbazine on wound healing. J Dermatol Surg Oncol 1988;14:975.
100. Hatiboglu I, Moore GE, Wilkens HJ, Hoffmeister F. Effects of chemotherapeutic agents on wounds contaminated with tumor cells. Ann Surg 1960;152:559.
101. Morris T, Lincoln F, Lee A. The effect of 5-fluorouracil on abdominal wound healing in rats. Aust NZ J Surg 1978;48:219.
102. Staley CJ, Trippel OH, Preston FW. Influence of 5-fluorouracil on wound healing. Surgery 1961;49:450.
103. Waldorf DS, Engel ML, Van Scott EJ. Inhibition of wound epithelialization by topical 5-Fluorouracil. Arch Dermatol 1966;94:786.
104. Morris T. Retardation of healing of large-bowel anastomoses by 5-fluorouracil. Aust NZ J Surg 1979;49:743.
105. Goldmann LI, Lowe S, Al-Saleem T. Effect of fluorouracil on intestinal anastomoses in the rat. Arch Surg 1969;98:303.
106. Hillan K, Nordlinger B, Ballet F, et al. The healing of colonic anastomoses after early in-

traperitoneal chemotherapy: an experimental study in rats. J Surg Res 1988;44:166.
107. Aszodi A, Ponsky JL. Effects of 5-fluorouracil on the healing of bowel anastomoses in rats. Am Surg 1985;51:671.
108. Cohn I Jr, Slack NH, Fisher B. Complications and toxic manifestations of surgical adjuvant chemotherapy for breast cancer. Surg Gynecol Obstet 1968;127:1201.
109. Higgins GA, Dwight RW, Smith JV, et al. Fluorouracil as an adjuvant to surgery in carcinoma of the colon. Arch Surg 1971;102:339.
110. Rousselot LM, Cole DR, Grossi CE, et al. Intraluminal chemotherapy (HN2 or 5-FU) adjuvant to operation for cancer of the colon and rectum. Cancer 1967;20:829.
111. Bole GG, Heath LE. The effect of 6-mercaptopurine on the inflammatory response stimulated by subcutaneous implantation of polyvinyl sponge. Arthritis Rheum 1967;10:377.
112. Tayler SG, Bytell DE, DeWys WD, et al. Adjuvant methotrexate and Leukoverin in head and neck squamous cancer. Arch Otolaryngol 1978;104:647.
113. Wiznitzer T, Orda R, Bawnik JB, et al. Mitomycin and the healing of intestinal anastomosis. Arch Surg 1973;106:314.
114. Bracken RB, Sutow WW, Jaffe N, et al. Preoperative chemotherapy for Wilms tumor. Urology 1982;19:55.
115. Rudolph R, Larson DL. Etiology and treatment of chemotherapeutic agent extravasation injuries: a review. J Clin Oncol 1987;5:1116.
116. Larson DL. Alteration in wound healing secondary to infusion injury. Clin Plast Surg 1990;17:509.
117. Gorodetsky R, McBridge WH, Withers HR. Assay of radiation effects in mouse skin as expressed in wound healing. Radiat Res 1988;116:135.
118. Levenson SM, Gruber CA, Rettura G, et al. Supplemental vitamin A prevents the acute radiation-induced defect in wound healing. Ann Surg 1984;200:494.
119. Mansfield C. Effects of radiation therapy on wound healing after mastectomy. Clin Plast Surg 1979;6:19.
120. Orminston MCE. A study of rat intestinal wound healing in the presence of radiation injury. Br J Surg 1985;72:56.
121. Schmidtler F, Schildberg FW, Schramm W, et al. Zur Pathogenese der postoperativen Bauchwandruptur. Münch med Wschr 1977;119:685.
122. White H, Cook J, Ward M. Abdominal wound dehiscence. Ann R Coll Surg Engl 1977;59:337.
123. Holt DR, Kirk SJ, Regan MC, et al. Effect of age on wound healing in healthy human beings. Surgery 1992;112:293.
124. Ariyan S, Kraft RL, Goldberg NH. An experimental model to determine the effects of adjuvant therapy on the incidence of postoperative wound infection. II. Evaluation preoperative chemotherapy. Plast Reconstr Surg 1980;65:338.
125. Brothers JR, Olson G, Polk HC. Enhancement of infection by corticosteroids: experimental clarifications. Surg Forum 1973;24:30.
126. Fuenfer MM, Olson GE, Polk HC. Effect of various corticosteroids upon the phagocytic bactericidal activity of neutrophils. Surgery 1975;78:27.

Nutritional Support in the Cancer Patient

JAMES L. PEACOCK

Surgeons who care for patients with cancer frequently encounter conditions of malnutrition. Nearly all forms of cancer therapy potentially impact on the nutritional status and metabolism of the cancer patient. In addition, regardless of treatment, tumor growth has nutritional consequences by the syndrome of cancer cachexia. Autopsy studies have shown that more than 20% of cancer patients die from inanition and malnutrition with no other demonstrable cause of death.[1]

Intuitive as well as scientific evidence substantiates the conclusion that weight loss and conditions of cachexia diminish the longevity of survival and the options for therapy.[2,3] For example, complications from cancer surgery are markedly increased in advanced stages of cachexia. Increased incidence of postoperative sepsis, wound dehiscence, and ileus all have been observed in malnourished surgical patients. Impairments of pulmonary function and immune status also affect the outcome of surgery.

Frequently, chemotherapy and radiation therapy must be curtailed due to poor nutritional and performance status of the patient. Surgeons are commonly called on to intervene to improve a patient's nutritional status. Therefore, this chapter focuses on the indications and risk-to-benefit analysis of nutritional support in cancer patients as well as the techniques employed to provide such support.

ASSESSMENT OF NUTRITIONAL STATUS

Recognition of malnutrition is the first step toward proper intervention on behalf of the cancer patient. The overt signs of muscle wasting are late evidence of cachexia; attention to more subtle evidence of this syndrome may allow the clinician to intervene earlier and more effectively.

Aspects of the clinical history that should alert one to potential or impending malnutrition are complaints of early satiety and the sense that "food just doesn't taste the same anymore." Sweet foods typically have less taste, whereas bitter foods taste stronger. Protein-rich foods such as red meats especially have a bitter taste. Alterations in taste are a well-documented component of cancer cachexia and have been ascribed to circulating tumor products.[4] Pancreatic cancer patients are especially prone to alterations in taste perception and in fact may even present with this complaint before a definitive diagnosis is made.

Other symptoms that identify the cachexia syndrome are weight loss and fatigue. Weight loss is measured over the previous 6 months compared with *usual* body weight, not *ideal* body weight. Weight loss less than 5% is considered small, whereas greater than 10% weight loss is definitely considered significant. Patients who are unaware of their weight may report other signs such as a change in clothing size. Symptoms of gastrointestinal dysfunction such as diarrhea or vomiting also are important predictors of weight loss. Symptoms of body protein depletion would include extremity edema or abdominal ascites.

Physical examination with respect to malnutrition in cancer patients begins with measuring and recording the total body weight. Patients should be encouraged to measure and record their weight at home. However, there is no substitute for accurate and consistent scales in the clinic.

Loss of skeletal muscle is most notable in the temporal area, the forearms and lower legs. Loss of muscle tone in the deltoid and quadriceps regions are later signs of muscle wasting. Loss of body fat is measurable in the subcutaneous tissues especially in the triceps region, the supraclavicular fossa, and the interosseous region of the hand. Dry scaly skin may be a sign of fatty acid insufficiency or zinc deficiency. Cheilosis is formation of fissures and maceration at the angles of the mouth as a result of riboflavin deficiency.

Signs of intravascular fluid leak into extravascular spaces are also evidence of poor nutrition. Sacral edema, ankle edema, and ascites occur as protein stores are depleted and capillary oncotic pressure is reduced.

Anthropometric measurement of triceps skin fold is an indicator of the body-fat compartment. This measurement is more useful as a research tool for objective measurement of nutritional status than as a clinical tool for determining who should receive nutritional intervention.

Laboratory studies can help define nutritional status as well. Total lymphocyte count and levels of albumin, transferrin, and pre-albumin are indicators of protein synthesis (see Table 15-1). Pre-albumin has the shortest half-life of these proteins and is therefore the most useful for monitoring the short-term progress of patients on nutritional support. Measurement of the 24-hour excretion of creatinine allows calculation of the creatinine-height index, which is another overall indicator of nutritional status. Delayed cutaneous hypersensitivity also indicates poor nutrition. The prognostic nutritional index (PNI) was constructed by Buzby and Muller to provide a mathematical formula for deciding which patients would benefit from nutritional support.[5] The formula is the following:

$$PNI (\%) = 158 - 16.6 [albumin(g/dL)] \\ - 0.78 [triceps\ skin\ fold\ thickness\ (mm)] - 0.20 [transferrin\ (mg/dL)] \\ - 5.8 [delayed\ hypersensitivity \\ (0 = no\ reaction, 1 = <5\ mm\ reaction, \\ 2 = >5\ mm)].$$

A score less than 30% is considered low risk for nutritional-related complications. A score greater than 60% is considered severe malnutrition and high risk for operative complications. There is general agreement that prognostic nutritional index parameters are very accurate at defining the malnourished patient. However, the data are variable as to which prognostic nutritional index thresholds predict a benefit from nutritional support.

More precise measurement of the body compartments is feasible but requires increasingly sophisticated technology, expense, and patient discomfort. The lean body mass can be predicted by neutron activation techniques. The body cell mass is measurable by potassium-40 analysis with a whole-body counter. These techniques are used primarily in research projects to quantify the metabolic status of cancer patients.

Despite the technology available to assess

Table 15-1. Laboratory Measurements of Nutritional Status

Total lymphocyte count
Serum albumin, pre-albumin
Retinol binding protein
Serum transferrin
Creatinine–height index
Triceps skin-fold thickness
Delayed cutaneous hypersensitivity
Potassium-40 analysis
Gamma-neutron activation

nutritional status, a careful history and physical examination is probably just as accurate for prediction of malnutrition. Baker et al[6] reported a prospective trial comparing the reproducibility and variability of diagnosing protein-calorie malnutrition by objective measurements with clinical examination only. Patients admitted for elective operations underwent measurement of hepatic secretory proteins (serum albumin and serum transferrin), total lymphocyte count, anthropometric evaluation, creatinine-height index, and determination of cell-mediated immunity. Total body potassium and total body nitrogen were also measured. Two independent clinical examiners used history and physical examination to classify each patient as normal nutritional status, mild malnutrition, or severe malnutrition. These clinical classifications correlated with results of objective tests to a significant degree in all categories except total lymphocyte count. The authors concluded that a general clinical assessment is a valid and sufficient technique for evaluating nutritional status before surgery.

SUMMARY: ASSESSMENT OF NUTRITIONAL STATUS

1. Weight loss greater than 10% of the pre-disease weight is considered significant. A careful physical examination is important with attention to signs of weight loss and edema, which indicate protein loss.

$$\% \text{ weight loss} = \frac{\text{usual weight} - \text{present weight}}{\text{usual weight}} \times 100$$

2. Laboratory studies including total lymphocyte count, albumin, pre-albumin, and transferrin levels are followed as indicators of protein synthesis. A 24-hour urinary urea nitrogen is also measured.

PREVALENCE OF MALNUTRITION IN CANCER PATIENTS

Weight loss is widely observed in patients with all types of cancer. The largest study that attempted to measure the prevalence of weight loss and its impact on cancer patients was conducted by DeWys et al[2] through the Eastern Cooperative Oncology Group. More than 3000 patients with various diagnoses were stratified by weight loss. Fifty-four percent had lost at least 5% of their pre-illness weight and 22% had lost greater than 10% of total body weight during the previous 6 months. This data is illustrated in Table 15-2. More importantly, this study was able to correlate the presentation of weight loss with subsequent response to chemotherapy. In nearly all types of cancer, weight loss predicted worse survival compared with patients with no weight loss and a similar site and stage of disease. Data from this study is shown in Table 15-3. Similar findings were reported by Nixon et al.[7] In this study, protein calorie malnutrition was identified by using creatinine-to-height ratios, serum albumin, and triceps skin-fold thickness. The degree of malnutrition correlated to survival. Moreover, a large proportion of deaths were secondary to cachexia. These results suggest that cachexia affected the ability of patients to respond to anticancer treatment.

Cancer patients who are facing major surgery are quite likely to have suffered malnutrition preoperatively. In one study, 92 of 159 cancer patients facing surgery had evidence of severe malnutrition based on the Prognostic Nutritional Index.[8] As described above, the PNI is based on serum albumin and transferrin levels, triceps skin-fold thickness, and evidence of delayed cutaneous hypersensitivity. In a separate study Detsky et al[9] confirmed the relationship between malnutrition and the risk of major surgical complications. Those patients who were severely malnourished preoperatively had a complication rate of 67% compared with 10% for the group at large.

Table 15-2. Frequency of Weight Loss in Cancer Patients

		Weight loss in the previous 6 months (%)*			
Tumor type	N	0	0–5	5–10	>10
Favorable non-Hodgkin's lymphoma	290	69	14	8	10
Breast	289	64	22	8	6
Acute nonlymphocyte leukemia	129	61	27	8	4
Sarcoma	189	60	21	11	7
Unfavorable non-Hodgkin's lymphoma	311	52	20	13	15
Colon	307	46	26	14	14
Prostate	78	44	28	18	10
Lung, small cell	436	43	23	20	14
Lung, non small cell	590	39	25	21	15
Pancreas*	111	17	29	28	26
Nonmeasurable gastric	179	17	21	32	30
Measurable gastric	138	13	20	29	38
Total	3047	46[a]	22[a]	17[a]	15[a]

*Data for pancreatic cancer are weight loss in 2 months.
[a] Average for values listed for individual diseases. From DeWys WD, Begg D, Lavin PT, et al: Prognostic effect of weight loss prior to chemotherapy in cancer patients. Am J Med 1980;69:491.

Table 15-3. Effect of Weight Loss on Survival in Humans

	Median survival (weeks)		
Tumor Type	No Weight Loss	Weight Loss[a] (TCH)	P value[b]
Favorable non-Hodgkin's lymphoma	—[c]	138	<0.01
Breast	70	45	<0.01
Acute nonlymphocytic leukemia	8	4	NS
Sarcoma	46	25	<0.01
Unfavorable non-Hodgkin's lymphoma	107	55	<0.01
Colon	43	21	<0.01
Prostate	46	24	<0.05
Lung, small cell	34	27	<0.05
Lung, non small cell	20	14	<0.01
Pancreas	14	12	NS
Nonmeasurable gastric	41	27	<0.05
Measurable gastric	18	16	NS

[a] All categories of weight loss combined.
[b] The P value refers to a test of hypothesis that the entire survival curves are identical, not merely a test of the medians.
[c] Only 20 of 199 died, so median survival cannot be estimated.
From DeWys WD, Begg D, Lavin PT, et al: Prognostic effect of weight loss prior to chemotherapy in cancer patients. Am J Med 1980;69:491.

■

SUMMARY: PREVALENCE OF MALNUTRITION IN CANCER PATIENTS

1. Malnutrition is a common finding in cancer patients. Studies have shown that weight loss correlates significantly with decreased patient survival compared with no weight loss and a similar site and stage of disease (see Tables 15-2 and 15-3).

■

CAUSES OF MALNUTRITION IN CANCER PATIENTS

Anorexia

Anorexia is the inability to ingest adequate calories to meet energy expenditure and maintain lean body mass and body weight. Poor food intake in patients with cancer cachexia is nearly a universal finding and, according to some investigators, may be an adaptive response to having cancer.[10] There are many causes for anorexia in cancer patients but the most common is a loss of appetite. Poor appetite probably is due to the effects of circulating factors on the central nervous system. These factors include tumor necrosis factor, which when infused into the central nervous system causes profound anorexia in laboratory animals.[11] Other central nervous system alterations that have been found in tumor-bearing animals include increased serotonin production by the hypothalamus, which may activate the satiety center.[12] Feeding behavior is controlled by the ventromedial and ventrolateral nuclei of the hypothalamus. Selective destruction of the ventromedial hypothalamus forces rats to become hyperphagic, but cachexia still occurs with advanced malignant growth.[13]

Alterations of taste perception are another important reason why cancer patients fail to eat normally. Most commonly, patients have an elevated threshold for recognizing sweet. The normal excitatory stimuli from taste and smell sensation are blunted in cancer patients. In addition, cancer patients may have an aversion to meat. Typically, cancer patients have a lower threshold of urea-testing (the level of plasma urea that will produce the sensation of meat aversion) than controls.[14] The changes of taste sensation usually have been correlated to the level of tumor burden.

Compensatory mechanisms in feeding behavior also are affected by cancer. Normal rats will increase their daily food intake if the caloric value of provisions are decreased. This compensation allows equivalence of energy intake. However, tumor-bearing animals fail to adjust food intake when caloric density of provisions is decreased.[15]

Other causes of anorexia include the secondary effects of cancer treatment. Surgery produces intestinal ileus, pain, and changes of gastrointestinal function, which lead to poor appetite and early satiety. Radiation therapy can cause diarrhea and fatigue. Chemotherapy also causes diarrhea, nausea, and poor appetite as well as mouth sores and esophagitis, which impair the ability to eat.

Psychologic causes of anorexia are important factors as well. Depression in patients with advanced cancer reduces motivation to eat. Similarly, fatigue, weakness, and the asthenia of cachexia reduce the ability to produce the motor activity necessary to ingest adequate calories.

Metabolic Disturbances

Although a multitude of factors suppress food intake in cancer patients, many metabolic disturbances occur which increase the demand for nutrients. These phenomena exaggerate the imbalance of energy intake to energy expenditure. Some of the metabolic changes found in association with cancers are shown in Table 15-4. In glucose metabolism the tumor-bearing state is known to increase Cori cycle activity whereby glucose is rapidly consumed in peripheral tissues (including tumor cells) and resynthesized from lactate in the liver.[16,17] Clearance of glucose

Table 15-4. Metabolic Changes in the Cancer Patient

CARBOHYDRATE METABOLISM
Insulin resistance
Glucose intolerance
Increased gluconeogenesis
Increased Cori cycle activity
Increased glucose turnover
Increased serum lactate

FAT METABOLISM
Increased fatty acid mobilization
Increased fatty acid turnover
Increased glycerol turnover
Hyperlipidemia
Decreased lipoprotein lipase

PROTEIN METABOLISM
Increased whole body protein turnover
Increased skeletal muscle catabolism
Decreased skeletal muscle anabolism
Impaired keto-adaptation

From Daly JM, Torosian MH. Nutritional support. In: DeVita VT Jr, Hellman S, Rosenberg SA, eds. Cancer: Principles and practice of oncology. 4th ed. Philadelphia: JB Lippincott, 1993:2480.

from peripheral circulation decreases during tumor progression, resembling a metabolic picture of insulin resistance. Poor glucose tolerance probably is caused by accelerated hepatic gluconeogenesis as well as insulin resistance in muscle and fat. Pancreatic islets from tumor-bearing rats have significantly reduced insulin secretion.[19] One study showed that over one third of cancer patients have a diabetic pattern of glucose tolerance test.[18]

Metabolism of lipids also is affected by cancer. Hyperlipidemia generally occurs secondary to decreased activity of lipoprotein lipase. Turnover of glycerol and free fatty acids is increased.[20] The mechanism for these alterations may relate to a lipolytic factor found in tumor extracts and in serum of tumor-bearing mice.[21] In normal metabolism lipolysis, the mobilization of lipid stores into free fatty acids and glycerol, should slow down in response to infusion of adequate amounts of glucose. Experiments in cancer-bearing animals and humans have shown an inability to suppress lipolysis despite glucose infusion.[22,23] Other studies have shown that the rate of loss of body fat in the cancer-bearing state is greater than can be explained by anorexia alone.[24] Failure to appropriately use and restore fat reserves is a major metabolic disturbance in cancer patients that contributes to the syndrome of cachexia.

The efficiency of protein metabolism also is deranged in cancer cachexia. Whole-body protein turnover increases while the net rate of new muscle protein synthesis decreases.[25] The presence of tumor induces skeletal muscle protein catabolism beyond what would be expected by simple anorexia.[26,27] The findings by Shaw et al[28] included elevations of whole-body protein catabolism and synthesis rates in weight-losing cancer patients compared with weight-losing noncancer patients. Compensatory mechanisms to convert to lipid utilization during periods of prolonged hypocaloric intake are lost in the cancer-bearing state. Although lipolysis does increase during cancer cachexia, the reward of muscle protein preservation does not occur; proteolysis continues despite mobilization of lipids for energy supply. During starvation without cancer, the host can adapt by depleting fat reserves for energy compared with protein reserves in nearly a 15:1 ratio. In cancer, the ratio of protein to fat depletion is 3:1.[29,56] A comparison of characteristics of cancer cachexia with starvation cachexia is shown in Table 15-5.

Protein catabolism may be the result of a circulating factor based on data that show increased proteolysis of skeletal muscle samples in vitro using plasma from tumor-bearing animals compared with non-tumor-bearing controls.[30]

Glutamine is an essential amino acid that is rapidly consumed by tumors. Glutamine metabolism in the liver, gut mucosa, and kidney is affected by tumor growth.[31,32] These alterations may be secondary to consumption of available glutamine by tumor tissue or to an undiscovered agent released by tumors that affects glutamine metabolism at remote sites.

Numerous studies have been conducted to measure the rate of energy expenditure in

Table 15-5. Characteristics of Cancer versus Starvation Cachexia[69]

Starvation	Cancer
Preferential mobilization of fat, sparing skeletal muscle	Equal mobilization of fat and skeletal muscle
Decreased basal metabolic rate	Normal or increased basal metabolic rate
Liver atrophy	Increased liver size and metabolic activity
Normal LPL	Reduced LPL; acute-phase protein reaction; increased Cori cycle activity
Reduced glucose turnover	Normal or increased glucose turnover
Decreased protein breakdown	Increased protein breakdown

From Nelson KA, Walsh D, Sheehan FA. The cancer anorexia-cachexia, Cancer Res 1991;51(1):415.

cancer patients.[33–35] These experiments are difficult to control for all the variables that affect resting energy expenditure and results have been conflicting. One study in non–weight-losing sarcoma patients showed increased energy expenditure when compared with healthy volunteers.[35] The results were especially divergent when energy expenditure was standardized as a function of body cell mass, the energy producing compartment.

The disturbances of lipid, carbohydrate, and protein turnover are evidence that the tumor-bearing state induces metabolic changes that are separate and additive to the sequelae of anorexia. In fact, many of these catabolic phenomena have been described in cancer patients or laboratory animals without changes in food intake and before the overt signs of cachexia appear. The causative factors that mediate these phenomena are not completely understood. Several cytokines have been described that appear to correlate with cachectic decline. These include tumor necrosis factor (TNF), interleukin 1 (IL-1), interleukin 6 (IL-6), and interferon gamma (IFN-γ). Infusion of pharmacologic and physiologic preparations of these bioactive molecules can reproduce many elements of cachexia.[36] Most of these bioactive molecules have been undetectable in the serum of cancer patients. IL-6 levels, however, correlate with tumor progression.[37] Investigators are unsure, however, whether the origin of such substances is from tumor cells or from host inflammatory cells. Considering that similar acute phase response occurs in situations of sepsis and inflammation; the source of these substances is likely to be host cells such as macrophages. A hypothetical mechanism of cytokines in the syndrome of cancer cachexia is schematically shown in Figure 15-1.[36]

The summation of catabolic pathways is an overall utilization and demand for available energy that does not meet energy supply. Several clinical investigations have documented the rise in energy expenditure in patients with cancer. An acceleration of energy expenditure might explain why patients become cachectic despite apparently adequate caloric intake.

Treatment-Related Causes of Malnutrition

Nearly every form of cancer therapy has some impact on nutritional status. Chemotherapy acutely causes nausea and emesis. Later effects of many chemotherapeutic drugs include diarrhea, stomatitis, mucositis, and poor appetite. Other consequences of chemotherapy that affect nutrition are neutropenic fever and infections, which raise energy expenditure and suppress food intake. Fungal infections of the oropharynx also impair oral intake. Radiation therapy impacts nutritional status by causing generalized fatigue and appetite suppression. Diarrhea, stomatitis, and esophagitis are side effects that can cause nutritional deterioration. Surgical intervention for cancer can have severe nutritional consequences. The demands for healing and recovery from major surgery add to the catabolic processes of tumor-bearing. Paralytic ileus following abdominal or pelvic surgery

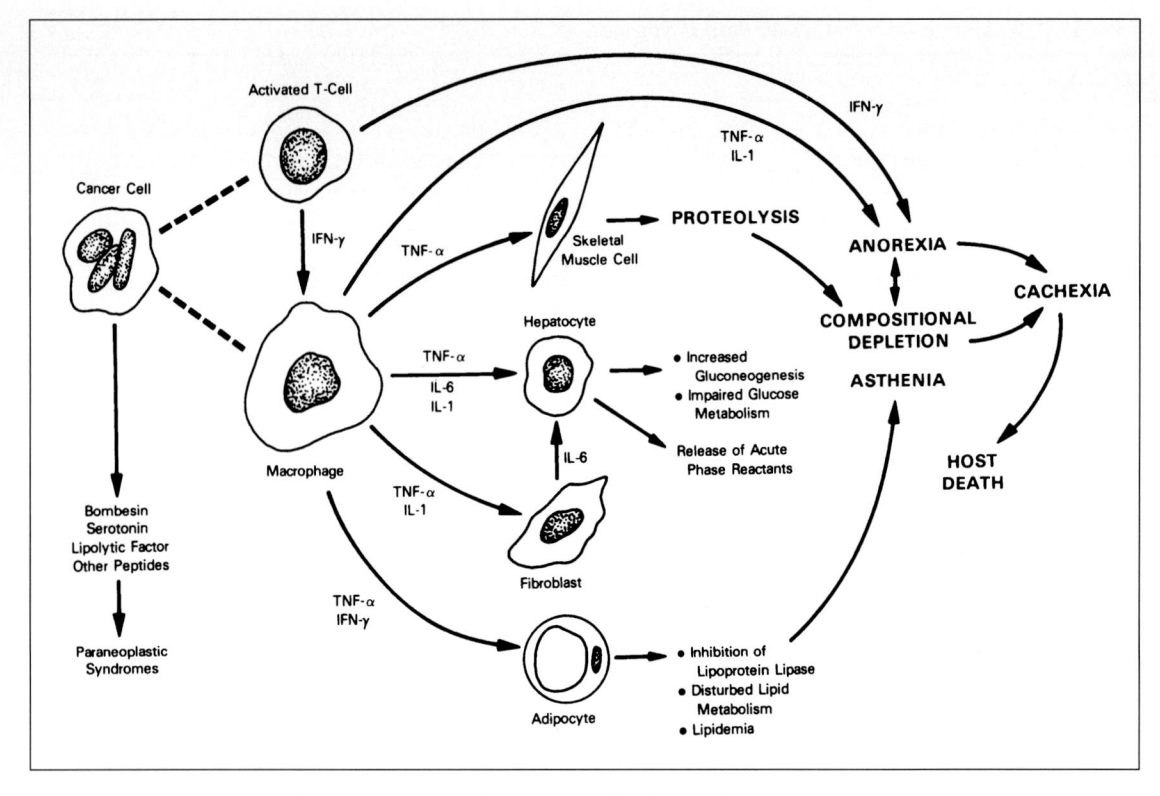

Figure 15-1. Cachexia in the tumor-bearing host is a result of complex interactions among numerous cytokines, some of which are illustrated here. From Langstein HN, Norton JA. Mechanisms of cancer cachexia. Hematol Oncol Clin North Am 1991;5(1):103; reprinted with permission.

as well as malabsorption due to major intestinal resection are contributors to malnutrition. Infection, fistulae, and obstruction are other potential sequelae of surgery that deprive the patient of nutritional intake.

SUMMARY: CAUSES OF MALNUTRITION IN CANCER PATIENTS

1. Cancer patients suffer a loss of appetite probably due to the effect of a number of circulating factors on the central nervous system. Taste perception also is altered, which leads to decreased appetite.
2. Food intake may also be decreased as a result of often complex therapies including surgery, radiation, and chemotherapy. Nearly every therapeutic intervention has some impact on nutritional status.
3. Metabolic alterations increase the demand for nutrients.
4. A number of cytokines probably are involved in the cachectic state, including TNF, IL-1, IL-6, and IFN-γ. Some of these interactions are shown in Figure 15-1.

TREATMENT OF MALNUTRITION IN CANCER PATIENTS

Replacement of Nutrients

Three decades ago Dudrick and associates proved that growth and development with positive nitrogen balance could be achieved exclusively by intravenous feeding solutions. Intravenous feeding has improved remarkably in the past two decades. Full replacement of carbohydrate, fat, and amino acids is achieved with total parenteral nutrition (TPN). In addition, essential fatty acids, trace minerals, and vitamins are provided. The benefits of TPN have dramatically changed the survival rates of patients with intestinal complications of surgery, particularly in the intensive care setting, inflammatory bowel disease, multiple trauma, sepsis, and even anorexia nervosa.

The benefit of TPN for the cancer patient is less certain. Patients with acute complications of cancer therapy who are unable to feed themselves are frequently given TPN although well-controlled trials that demonstrate efficacy are sparse. Tumors are known to be active consumers of glucose and amino acids, which raise the concern that aggressive nutritional support may accelerate tumor growth more than host weight. The methylcholantherene(MCA)-induced rat sarcoma model of cancer cachexia has shown increased tumor growth during hyperalimentation.[38] Other laboratory tumor models have not demonstrated acceleration of tumor growth out of proportion to host body weight. Human clinical studies in this regard have been largely retrospective; however, no convincing evidence exists that tumor growth rates accelerate in the presence of TPN. McGeer and co-workers[39] analyzed all published clinical trials testing TPN as an adjunct to systemic chemotherapy. Patients receiving TPN had overall survivals only 81% as long as patients who received no TPN. Klein et al[40] also pooled results from 28 prospective randomized clinical trials of TPN in cancer patients. No differences were found in survival, treatment tolerance, treatment toxicity, or tumor response in patients receiving chemotherapy or radiotherapy. Other studies, however, have shown metabolic benefits for patients with cancer receiving TPN. Burt et al[41] showed that esophageal cancer patients have improved protein synthesis and decreased excretion of urinary 3-methylhistidine, a parameter of skeletal muscle breakdown, when treated with TPN. Improvement of immune status (*i.e.*, reversal of skin anergy) has been demonstrated in cancer patients receiving nutritional support.

The specific circumstances in which nonsurgical patients might benefit from TPN include (1) inability to eat for a prolonged period of time; (2) the presence of cancer cachexia that can be demonstrated to be due to failure of nutrient intake rather than tumor-induced metabolic abnormalities; (3) a nutritional support team in place to decrease complications associated with nutritional support; and (4) the presence of a tumor that can be expected to respond to chemotherapy or radiotherapy.[42]

A meta-analysis of controlled trials in the literature has shown that short-term TPN during chemotherapy actually may be associated with decreased survival and increased complications.[39] Infection, glucose intolerance, and fluid overload are among the problems with TPN administration. Bone marrow transplant patients seem to be an exception. Randomized trials have shown an improved response to therapy and enhanced survival in patients receiving aggressive nutritional support.[44]

The role of nutritional support as an adjuvant for the cancer patient facing major surgery has been studied. Although most results have not justified routine use of preoperative TPN, one study by Muller et al[45] identified lower complication and mortality rates in patients with upper gastrointestinal cancer if TPN was given for 10 days before surgery. Other nonrandomized studies have supported the use of perioperative TPN in cancer patients. The largest prospectively randomized trial addressing the benefit of preoperative TPN was conducted by a US Department of Veterans Affairs (VA) multicenter group and published in 1991.[46] Malnourished patients facing major abdominal or thoracic procedures were randomly assigned to receive either TPN for 7 to 15 days before surgery and 3 days afterward or no perioperative TPN.

Differences in morbidity or mortality were noticed only in the most severely malnourished stratum. These patients had multiple or severe stigmata of malnutrition on history and physical examination. Routine use of preoperative TPN, therefore, was discouraged except for the subgroup of patients with severe weight loss (>25% total body weight). Interestingly, infectious complications were greater in the TPN-treated patients, an effect that had been noted in other studies and which suggests an immunosuppressive effect of intravenous hyperalimentation.[47,55] A summary of the findings from this important study are shown in Table 15-6.

TPN may also be necessary for nutritional support of radiation-related sequelae. Patients receiving radiation may develop mucositis, dysphagia nausea, vomiting, diarrhea, and anorexia. Indications for nutritional support intervention include (1) weight loss greater than 10%; (2) albumin less than 3.5 g/dL; and (3) presence of stomatitis or diarrhea. Usually patients with these side effects can be managed with oral supplements or intestinal feedings.

Intravenous hyperalimentation is not the only route for nutritional support. Use of the gastrointestinal tract is preferable if it is functional. Provision of nutrients through the gastrointestinal tract preserves mucosal barriers and enterocyte function. Atrophy of intestinal mucosal layers can allow bacterial translocation and potentiate sepsis in severely malnourished and immunosuppressed patients. Other physiologic benefits of enteral nutrition include liver function and avoidance of cholestasis. Enteral nutrition reduces glucose turnover and rates of gluconeogenesis more effectively than parenteral nutrition.

Enteral feeding can be accomplished with less morbidity than intravenous feeding and for lower cost. Daly et al[48] demonstrated the overall benefit of postoperative enteral feedings in patients with major abdominal surgery for cancer in a prospective, randomized trial. The results are summarized in Table 15-7 showing advantages in complication rate, recovery time, and immune status in patients receiving enteral nutrition supplemented with arginine, RNA, and omega-3 fatty acids.[48]

Parenteral Nutrition

Parenteral hyperalimentation may be administered by central or peripheral venous access. Central access is preferred in situations where parenteral nutrition is expected for longer than a few days. Access to the internal jugular or subclavian vein may be obtained by sterile cutdown techniques or percutaneous puncture. The tip of the catheter should be located in the superior vena cava. If nutri-

Table 15-6. Perioperative TPN in VA Cooperative Group Study: Cumulative Incidence of Complications 30 Days after Nutritional Stratification

	Degree of Malnutrition		
	Borderline	Mild	Severe
MAJOR INFECTIOUS COMPLICATIONS			
TPN group (%)	12.5	14.4	15.8
Control group (%)	9.1	3.7	21.4
P value (TPN vs. control)	0.75	0.004	1.00
MAJOR NONINFECTIOUS COMPLICATIONS			
TPN group (%)	12.5	20.0	5.3
Control group (%)	23.6	19.4	42.9
P value	0.20	1.00	0.03

From Buzby GP. The Veterans Affairs TPN Cooperative Study Group. Perioperative TPN in surgical patients. N Eng J Med 1991; 325:525, with permission.

Table 15-7. Enteral Nutrition with Supplemental Arginine, RNA, Omega-3 Fatty Acids: Cumulative incidence of complications

	Supplemented	Standard	P value
Infections	4/36	12/41	
Wound healing	0/36	4/41	
Total Infectious/healing complications	4/36	15/41	.02
Cardiopulmonary	30/36	34/41	
Urinary/other	4/36	5/41	
Total cardiopulmonary/urinary complications	30/36	35/41	NS
Mortality	1/36	0/41	NS

Adapted from Daly JM, et al[48]

tional support is expected for more than a few weeks a Hickman or Broviac catheter, which is tunneled subcutaneously is preferable. The use and complications of these devices is discussed at length in Chapter 9. Peripherally inserted central (PIC) lines are commercially available and provide an alternative to subclavian puncture for placement of a central line.

The solutions to be administered include a source of glucose, amino acids, and fat. Generally, these solutions contain 1.0 kcal/mL. Prevention of essential fatty acid deficiency requires administration of fat emulsion intravenously at least 2 days per week. Daily administration of fat is recommended to provide a higher proportion of calories as fat. Excessive fat administration can lead to protein depletion and hypertriglyceridemia.

Appropriate prescription of TPN solutions begins with an estimation of total caloric need. Precise measurement of caloric expenditure by indirect calorimetry requires patients to be on a mechanical ventilator or placed within a head canopy to capture exhaled air for CO_2 and O_2 analysis. A more practical method of predicting energy expenditure is the Harris-Benedict equation for basal energy expenditure:

Male: BEE (kcal) = 66 + 13.7 (weight, kg) + 5.0 (height, cm) − 6.8 (age, y)
Female: BEE (kcal) = 655 + 9.6 (weight, kg) + 1.7 (height, cm) − 4.7 (age, y)

Complete daily caloric requirements are met by adding 1000 kcal to the calculated basal energy expenditure or by multiplying the basal energy expenditure by 1.5. An even simpler method of estimating total energy expenditure is using the formula of 35 kcal/kg/d for maintenance and 45 kcal/kg/d for weight gain. A separate estimation of nitrogen requirements is needed to prescribe the appropriate amount of amino acids to administer. Generally 0.8 g nitrogen/kg/d will replace nitrogen losses in a nonstressed patient. Patients with postoperative stress or large tumor burden should have 1.0 to 1.2 g/kg/d.[49]

Formulas for carbohydrate and protein replacement should be used only as estimates for initiating parenteral nutrition. Monitoring nutritional status and adjustments of TPN solutions are critical for optimal nutritional support. The most sensitive parameters to monitor are serum pre-albumin and transferrin levels and total nitrogen balance. Pre-albumin and transferrin are serum proteins that have short half-lives and can accurately reflect current protein synthetic function. Total nitrogen balance is also a reliable indicator of successful nutritional support. This test requires, however, an accurate 24-hour urine collection. Evidence of weight gain is another simple but useful parameter for monitoring nutritional support. Short-term weight gain, however, is frequently secondary to fluid accumulation rather than replacement of lean body mass.

Complications of Parenteral Nutrition

Although parenteral nutrition has certainly made significant contributions to the care of critically ill patients, it is not without the potential for significant complications. These complications can be divided into mechanical, infectious, and metabolic complications. The mechanical and infectious complications associated with the central venous access necessary for TPN are extensively discussed in Chapter 9.

Patients receiving parenteral hyperalimentation also should be monitored for metabolic complications of therapy as well as for evidence of metabolic improvement. Such complications include hyperglycemia, hypertriglyceridemia, hypomagnesemia, and hypophosphatemia. These levels should be measured at least twice per week for timely corrections to be made.

The most frequent metabolic complication is hyperglycemia. This is defined as a glucose level greater than 200 mg/dL. It is important first to determine the cause of the hyperglycemia. Patients with new onset hyperglycemia must always be evaluated for an infection, particularly a line infection. Corticosteroids can cause hyperglycemia as well. Carbohydrate calories in excess of 30 to 35 kcal/kg should be decreased. Calories from fat can be adjusted to 30% of the nonprotein calories. Obviously, hyperglycemia is managed by both treating the underlying cause (*e.g.*, infection) as well as decreasing the serum glucose with insulin administration, using a sliding scale of regular insulin.

The refeeding syndrome can occur with parenteral or enteral nutrition and is mentioned below. The refeeding syndrome is a constellation of severe fluid and electrolyte shifts associated with initiating nutrition in the chronically malnourished individual. Typically, hypophosphatemia, hypomagnesemia, and hypokalemia are the electrolyte abnormalities that can result in cardiac and respiratory dysfunction and failure. Thiamine deficiency, hyperglycemia, and volume overload have also occurred. The best approach to the refeeding syndrome is prevention. TPN should be started at no more than 1000 kcals or 20 kcal/kg on the first day and titrated based on patient tolerance as defined by glucose monitoring and electrolyte values. Empiric replacement of vitamins, phosphorus, magnesium, and potassium is appropriate in the patient at risk.

In general, when electrolyte deficiencies are present in the patient prior to initiating TPN, it is best to correct the problems and delay intravenous feeding. Electrolyte deficiencies occurring once the patient is receiving parenteral nutrition should be corrected with runs outside of the parenteral nutrition. If the patient has increased maintenance requirements due to chronic gastrointestinal losses or other reasons, the maintenance requirements should be incorporated into the parenteral nutrition admixture. The use of inadequate or excessive amounts of any additive will result in the corresponding electrolyte abnormality. The amount of the corresponding electrolyte must be adjusted to correct the abnormality.

Hyperchloremic metabolic acidosis is fairly common in patients receiving TPN and may result from bicarbonate loss, such as that seen with severe diarrhea, pancreatic fistulas, or small bowel losses. The treatment is to administer more sodium and potassium as acetate salts (instead of the chloride salt) because the acetate covers the amino acids in the TPN.

Hepatic and biliary complications associated with parenteral nutrition generally are characterized by the duration of parenteral nutrition. Abnormal liver function tests are common in both short-term and long-term parenterally-fed patient populations. The most common hepatic complication associated with short-term TPN administration is hepatic steatosis. This fatty liver infiltration is thought to be due to overfeeding, especially of carbohydrate calories. The incidence of hepatic steatosis has decreased with the introduction of intravenous fat emulsion and the growing consideration of conservative caloric feeding. Biliary sludge formation and cholelithiasis with its associated complications have been noted in patients receiving TPN for 3 weeks or longer. Biliary stasis caused by lack of stimulation owing to bowel rest or short gut is thought to be the primary mechanism. Long-term TPN administration is associated with hepatic steatonecrosis. Its pathogenesis is unclear at this time.

The diagnosis of TPN-associated hepatotoxicity is a diagnosis of exclusion. Once other causes have been ruled out, management of hepatotoxicity includes reformulation of the caloric regimen, cyclic administration of TPN, and metronidazole.

Excessive amino acid infusion with inadequate calorie administration can result in prerenal azotemia. A rising blood urea nitrogen (BUN) should be monitored, but probably not treated until it is greater than 100 mg/dL, and then treated by reducing the amino acid intake and increasing calories administered as glucose. Prerenal azotemia due to intravascular volume depletion should be ruled out.

Bleeding abnormalities can be caused by inadequate amounts of vitamin K, iron, folate, or vitamin B_{12}. Adjust the nutrient administration to the required amount.

Overfeeding is always a potential problem in the nutritional support of the cancer patient. Once the decision is made to nutritionally support a patient, it is imperative to do so on a rational and quantitative basis. To do this, one must know the requirements for each nutritional component. Energy requirements are dependent on gender, weight, height, age, energy expenditure, and seriousness of the injury, as stated above. Overfeeding places patients at risk for hepatic complications, increased carbon dioxide production, and hyperglycemia.

TPN in Specific Disease States

Fluid administration must be carefully monitored and limited in patients with cardiac failure. Instead of the usual 1 mL water per calorie (as in tube feedings), water is given at 0.5 mL/cal. Alternatively, water can be given at a rate equal to 500 mL (insensible losses) plus measured losses. Protein can be limited to 0.8 to 1 g/kg, and sodium limited to 0.5 to 1.5 g/d.

Patients with diabetes receive increased calories from fat sources to limit the carbohydrate calories given while providing sufficient calories for protein anabolism. Insulin can be added to the feeding for a patient with stable insulin requirements. In general, fat should provide no more than 50% of total caloric intake, and no more than 2.5 g/kg/d.

Patients with hepatic dysfunction usually benefit from increased amounts of branched chain amino acids (leucine, valine, and isoleucine) and reduced amounts of aromatic amino acids, which are precursors to centrally active amines and thus contribute to hepatic encephalopathy. Specialized mixtures of amino acids are available and should be used only in patients with hepatic encephalopathy. Lipid emulsions should be limited in those with severe hepatic dysfunction.

Patients with renal disease have a number of specific restrictions that must be carefully accounted for in the administration of TPN including fluid, protein, potassium, magnesium, and sodium. Protein must be restricted to 0.6 to 0.8 g/kg/d in patients not undergoing dialysis. Patients receiving hemodialysis generally require 1.2 g/kg of protein per day and patients undergoing peritoneal dialysis need 1.5 g/kg. The latter patient also absorbs approximately 500 kcals/d of dextrose from the dialysate, which needs to be taken into account when designing the nutritional regimen. Patients on hemodialysis may receive the usual protein load of 1 to 1.5 g/kg/d. Specially formulated amino acid mixtures containing higher amounts of essential amino acids are used in these patients. In general, TPN should not contain potassium or magnesium in renal failure patients. Reduced sodium may also be necessary.

Patients with impaired ventilation, who already may retain CO_2, are further stressed if high carbohydrate loads are administered because carbohydrate metabolism results in the production of CO_2. This may be treated by increasing the percentage of calories provided by fat (up to 50%). Overall, calories should not exceed 30 to 35 kcal/kg. These patients also may be sensitive to phosphate depletion and should be monitored carefully for the development of hypophosphatemia. Once identified, this is treated with phosphate supplementation.

Enteral Nutrition

The intestinal tract is the preferred route for nutritional support in nearly all types of malnutrition, not just cancer cachexia. Absorption of nutrients throughout the intestinal tract improves visceral protein synthesis compared with nutrients given intravenously. Also, mucosal growth and function is improved by providing enteral nutrition.[50]

Interventional access to the intestinal tract frequently is required for patients who are recovering from surgery or who have other barriers to provision of food by oral routes. Also, patients who simply have severe cancer-related anorexia require mechanical access to the gastrointestinal tract.

Nasointestinal feeding tubes are an ideal method for nonsurgical access to the GI tract. These tubes are usually 5 to 7 mm in diameter and have a weighted tip to improve passage through the pylorus. Passage of the nasointestinal feeding tube is assisted by an intraluminal guide wire that can be withdrawn separately. Placement of the feeding tip beyond the pylorus is ideal to prevent reflux of feedings, especially in patients with depressed mental status who may not be able to prevent aspiration. Transpyloric intubation of the duodenum or jejunum is facilitated by placing the patient in a right lateral decubitus position following nasogastric placement. Administration of metoclopromide can increase gastric motility and improve the success rate of transpyloric placement. Confirmation of the feeding tube placement with an abdominal radiograph is necessary to assure proper location.

Gastrostomy tubes also can be used for feeding access. These tubes are generally larger in diameter and can accommodate less refined feeding formulas such as a blenderized diet. A gastrostomy for feeding would be selected for cancer patients who have esophageal obstruction and cannot have a nasointestinal tube or for patients who are going to require extended periods of nutritional support (i.e., greater than 6 weeks). Another advantage of nutritional support via gastrostomy tube is the convenience of bolus feeding. With a bolus feeding schedule, patients can take food three or four times per day in the form of meals. With a nasointestinal tube, the reservoir function of the stomach is not available and therefore feedings must be given as a continuous infusion.

Gastrostomy tubes can be placed surgically or percutaneously. Percutaneous placement requires endoscopic assistance, which may not be feasible in patients with esophageal or head and neck cancer. Techniques for direct percutaneous gastrostomy placement under fluoroscopic guidance have been reported.[51]

A third mechanism for access to the intestinal tract is a jejunostomy feeding tube. A jejunostomy can be created with a 12 F straight red rubber catheter placed through the antimesenteric border of the jejunum. Witzel's technique prevents leakage of jejunal contents or feedings into the peritoneal space. Another alternative is the needle catheter jejunostomy that tunnels a smaller catheter intramurally through the bowel wall. This device avoids the potential compromise of the small bowel lumen, which can be caused by the Witzel's technique. However, a smaller caliber catheter is used, which can be prone to clogging with fiber or high-protein diets.

Jejunostomy access is ideal for nutritional support following major upper abdominal surgery (i.e., esophagectomy, gastrectomy, or pancreatectomy). Feedings can begin within 48 hours of operation. Many references advocate feeding within 12 hours of surgery using dilute formulas.[48]

Formulas for feeding through the intestinal tract vary depending on intestinal function. Patients with intestinal ileus, malabsorption or pancreaticobiliary fistulas require chemically modulated diets. These diets are called elemental because they consist of simple sugars and amino acids which do not require enzymatic digestion for absorption. Most elemental diets are high in osmolarity, which can create diarrhea as a complication to their use. Patients who have better intestinal function can be fed a diet with complex sugars and polypeptides. These formulas are more iso-osmotic and contain fiber which helps prevent diarrhea. The most economical tube feeding is a blenderized diet. Any foods that can be blenderized are usable. These diets require more preparation time and a larger bore feeding tube.

The estimation of nutritional needs is the same for both enteral and parenteral support. Most enteral formulas contain 1.0 to 1.5 kcal/mL. The content of carbohydrate and fat is usually 150 nonprotein kcal/g of nitrogen. Generally an infusion of 75 to 100 mL/h provides adequate nutritional support by the enteral route. Supplementation of fats may be necessary. Many of the enteral formulas have only minimal amounts of fat. Patients with biliary fistulas or biliary obstruction usually require fat supplementation in the form of medium chain triglycerides which can be absorbed without bile salts and micelle formation.

Other important additives to enteral feedings include arginine, RNA, and omega-3 fatty acids. These compounds have immune regulatory function and have been shown in clinical studies to decrease infectious and wound complications after major abdominal surgery compared with standard enteral formulas.[48]

Complications of Enteral Nutrition

Complications from enteral nutrition are less common and less severe than those from parenteral nutrition. Nonetheless, some precautions are advised. Intestinal or gastric retention of feedings can lead to regurgitation and pulmonary aspiration. Gastric feedings especially should be monitored for residual volumes on a periodic basis. Diarrhea is the most common physiologic complication of enteral feeding. Diarrhea may occur secondary to a variety of reasons. High osmolarity of the feeding formula is a common cause of diarrhea. Hyperosmolar feedings, such as the elemental formulas, should be started at one half strength at 25 mL/h. The rate of feeding should be advanced to a target rate before increasing the concentration. Gastric feedings in patients whose pylorus is normal and the stomach can act as a reservoir for mixing do not require this precaution. Another cause of diarrhea is low serum albumin. Severely malnourished and stressed patients may have serum albumin levels less than 2.0 g/dL. This condition increases bowel wall edema and may have an impact on mucosal transport. Correction of serum hypoalbuminemia can improve tolerance of enteral feedings. Atrophy of the small bowel mucosa from lack of luminal nutrients is a major contributor to diarrhea with intestinal tube feedings. Therefore, enteral feeding is recommended early in the course of nutritional support.

Another complication of aggressive nutritional support in severely malnourished patients is the refeeding syndrome. Sudden replenishment of carbohydrates and fluid can cause severe hypophosphatemia, hypokalemia, and hypomagnesemia.[70] In addition, patients are likely to be more glucose- and fluid-intolerant. Anorexia nervosa patients are at highest risk for refeeding syndrome. The best method to prevent refeeding syndrome is careful monitoring of serum electrolytes over the first week of therapy and beginning hyperalimentation gradually (*i.e.*, by providing one third of total daily needs the first day and increase by one third each day).

Although less common than diarrhea, constipation can occur in the enterally fed patient. Check to be sure that adequate fluid volume is being given. Patients with additional requirements may benefit from water boluses or dilution of the enteral formulation. Fiber can be added to help regulate bowel function.

Aspiration is a serious complication of enteral feedings and is more likely to occur in the patient with impaired mental status. The best approach is prevention with elevation of the head of the bed and careful monitoring of residual fluid volume. Any patient suspected of possible aspiration or assessed to be at increased risk of aspiration prior to instituting enteral feedings should be further evaluated, and may not be a candidate for gastric feedings, necessitating small bowel feedings.

Patients who are suspected of aspiration should have the feedings stopped immediately, have a postero-anterior (PA) and lateral chest radiograph, and endotracheal intubation if indicated. Chest physiotherapy and antibiotics are useful adjuncts in the patient who has aspirated tube feedings.

The vitamin K content of various enteral products vary from 22 to 156 mcg/1000 kcal, which can significantly affect the anticoagulation profile of a patient receiving warfarin. Tetracycline products should not be administered 1 hour before or 2 hours after enteral feedings to avoid the inhibition of absorption. Similarly, enteral feedings should be stopped 2 hours before and after the administration of phenytoin.

Outpatient Supplements

Attention to nutritional status and attempts to intervene should not be confined to the hospital setting. Ambulatory patients or homebound patients with cancer may derive significant quality-of-life benefits from improvements in nutrition. Nutrients with calorie- and protein-rich liquid diets is a beginning. Most of these liquid supplements are not very palatable even with artificial flavoring. However, creative recipes can help the cancer patient consume adequate calories. Arrangements also can be made for continuous enteral and even parenteral nutritional support for outpatients. The use of home parenteral and enteral nutrition (HPEN) has increased markedly since 1985. The North American HPEN Patient Registry reported on nearly 3000 patients with active cancer receiving home nutrition support.[71] Mean survival time was 6 months. Twenty-five percent lived beyond a year and 20% resumed full oral nutrition. The appropriateness of home TPN for active cancer patients with prognosis less than 6 months is questionable.

Consumption of adequate calories and nitrogen is only the beginning of nutritional support for the cachectic cancer patient. The other objective is to improve the utilization of available nutrients toward synthesis of lean body mass and fat reserves. One maneuver to improve skeletal muscle mass is a program of exercise during nutritional support. Exercise increases uptake of amino acids as well as synthesis of new protein in skeletal muscle.[52] In addition, exercise can improve appetite and food intake. A study in tumor-bearing animals by Daneryd et al[53] demonstrated that forced exercise delayed the onset of anorexia and improved the body dry weight.

Various medications that have anabolic properties have been utilized to help improve nutritional status. Some of these drugs simply improve appetite whereas others have metabolic function. Megestrol acetate (Megace) is a progesterone derivative that has been used to treat metastatic breast cancer. A side effect of the drug, however, has been increased appetite and weight gain. Therefore, considerable interest has been directed toward clinical trials of megestrol to enhance weight gain in cachectic patients with cancer as well as AIDS. These studies indicate that megestrol in large doses can improve appetite and weight gain without acceleration of tumor proliferation.[54,57] A study from The Netherlands demonstrated that one third of patients experienced such an improvement in appetite and well-being after 10 days of treatment with megestrol acetate (160 mg three times daily) that they asked for continuation of therapy.[58]

The mechanism of megestrol toward appetite stimulation and anabolism is unknown. Further modifications of dosage and administration are needed for more practical clinical use.

SUMMARY: TREATMENT OF MALNUTRITION IN CANCER PATIENTS

1. An algorithm for the consideration of nutritional support in the cancer patient is shown in Figure 15-2.
2. Nutritional support is indicated in patients with greater than 10% weight loss or in patients expected not to be able to take adequate calories by mouth for 7 days due to therapeutic intervention.
3. Whenever possible, nutrition should be supplied by the enteral route. The amount of support should be estimated from formulas and adjustments made based on ongoing nutritional evaluation.
4. Complications of parenteral nutrition are categorized as mechanical (relating to the line used for administration), infectious, or metabolic. Common metabolic complications include hyperglycemia, hypertriglyceridemia, hypomagnesemia, and hypophosphatemia.
5. Enteral nutritional support may be administered by nasointestinal feeding tube, gastrostomy, or jejunostomy. Complications of enteral feeding include diarrhea, constipation, aspiration, and drug interactions.
6. Nutritional intervention includes the outpatient use of a variety of nutritional supplements. Megestrol may have a role in improving appetite.

FUTURE RESEARCH IN NUTRITIONAL SUPPORT

Advancements in nutritional support are needed in pathways of nutrient use as well as nutrient composition. As we learn more about the mechanisms that control both the inflammatory and the host response to tumor growth there will be an opportunity to modify nutritional support and to direct nutrients for the benefit of the host.

A potent anabolic agent under investigation is insulin. Insulin has been studied extensively in animal models of cancer cachexia but only to a limited degree in humans.[59] Insulin increases protein synthesis, promotes lipogenesis, and enhances hepatic glycogen storage. In addition, insulin stimulates appetite probably through induction of relative hypoglycemia. The benefit of insulin in tumor-bearing animals has improved food intake and body weight.[43,60] Other agents that improve overall metabolism include growth hormone and somatostatin. Recombinant growth hormone helps preserve protein stores in muscle tissue during periods of diminished nutrient availability.[61] Somatostatin theoretically blocks release of glucagon and thereby suppresses the catabolic sequelae of this endocrine hormone. Combinations of insulin, growth hormone, and somatostatin have been shown to have greater benefit in preserving host mass than insulin alone.[62]

Glutamine has emerged as a critical amino acid for metabolism especially in liver, gut, and tumor tissue. Enrichment of both parenteral and enteral feeding formulas with glutamine has been studied extensively. The advantages of added glutamine in the nutritional support of cancer patients include increased thickness and improved function of gut mucosa, resistance to radiation enteritis, and enhancement of liver protein synthesis.[63] The theoretical disadvantage of using excess glutamine is that tumor growth may accelerate because glutamine is a primary fuel of tumor cells. Experimental data have not supported this concern. In fact, increased glutamine levels may make some tumors more susceptible to chemotherapeutic destruction. Another strategy would be to use agents that antagonize entry of glutamine into the cancer cell. Acivicin is such an agent that has been tested by Chance et al in sarcoma-bearing rats[64]; tumor progression was retarded by treatment with TPN and acivicin compared with controls.

Arginine is another amino acid that has been studied as a supplement for nutritional support. Arginine is involved with nitric ox-

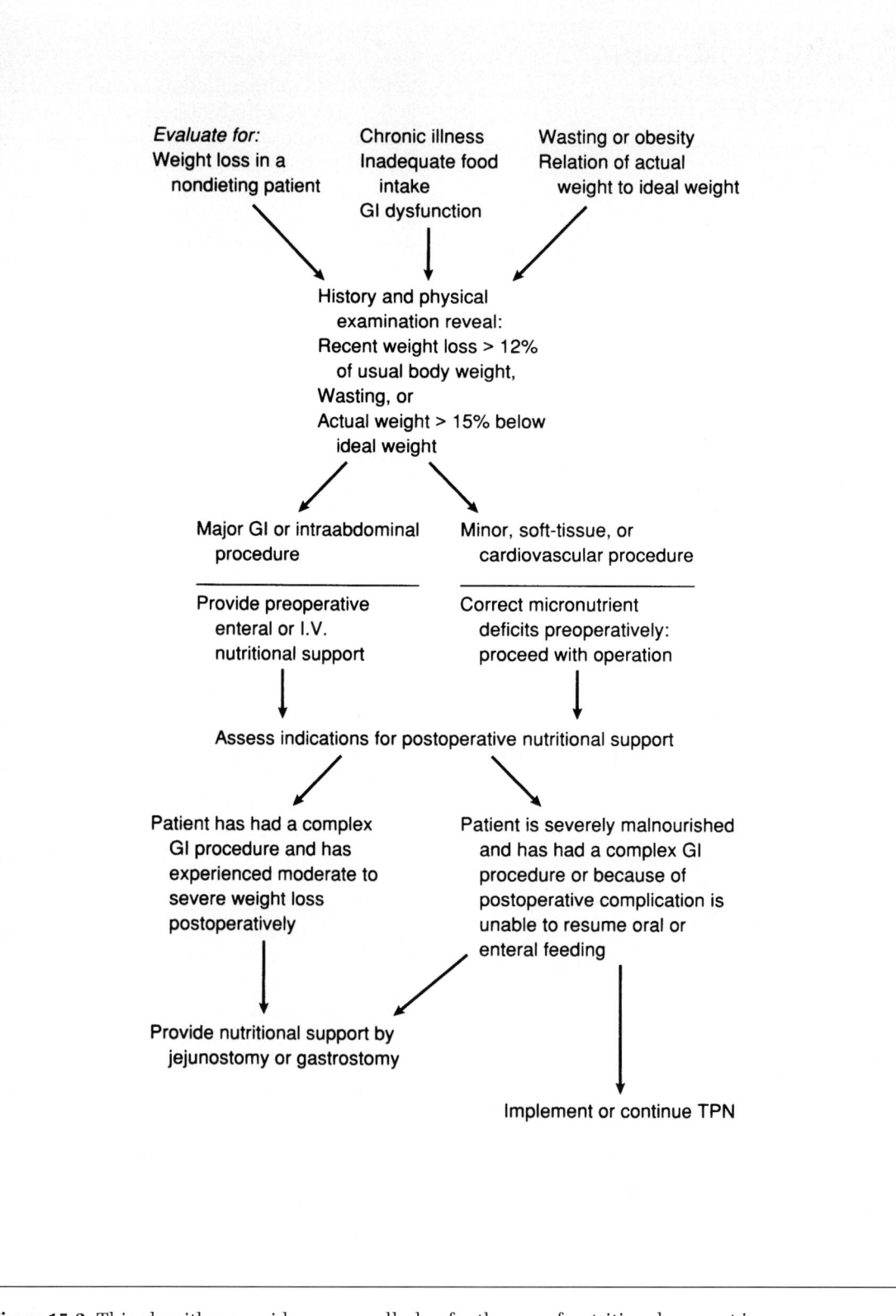

Figure 15-2. This algorithm provides an overall plan for the use of nutritional support in the cancer patient. From Daly JM, Torosian MH. Nutritional support. In: DeVita VT Jr, Hellman S, Rosenberg SA, eds. Cancer: principles and practice of oncology, 4th ed. Philadelphia: JB Lippincott, 1993;2480; reprinted with permission.

ide metabolism, which is an important factor in immune function. Arginine-enriched TPN solutions used in animal tumor models improved immune responses and retarded tumor growth in addition to preserving host weight.[65]

Control of nutrient intake through parenteral or enteral nutrition is an ideal strategy to test new compositions for efficacy in the cancer-bearing host. One approach has been to increase the number of tumor cells in active mitosis by providing specific nutrients. Tumors rapidly use glutamine and glucose. High concentrations of these nutrients may increase the proportion of tumor cells in the cycle of cell division and likewise increase their vulnerability to chemotherapy or radiation. In an animal tumor model, Torosian et al[66] showed that parenteral nutrition increases the S phase of tumor cell cycling and potentiates the antitumor efficacy of chemotherapy.

Administration of antibodies to the various cytokines that mediate cancer cachexia is another experimental approach. Anti-TNF and anti–interferon-γ have shown moderate capability to reverse anorexia and weight loss.[67] Antibodies to the IL-1 surface receptor also improve food intake and preserve body weight.[68] These effects, however, may be secondary to decreased tumor growth rather than improvements of host metabolism.

SUMMARY: FUTURE RESEARCH IN NUTRITION

1. Research in nutritional support may have direct benefits for the cancer patient. Combinations of insulin, growth hormone, and somatostatin may be beneficial.
2. Glutamine is a critical amino acid for gut metabolism. Glutamine results in increased thickness of gut mucosa, resistance to radiation enteritis, and enhancement of liver protein synthesis.
3. Antibodies to cytokines may be another fruitful intervention in nutritional support. It is unclear if this has clinical applications at this time.

SUMMARY

Anorexia and weight loss are ominous signs for the cancer patient. The advances of nutritional support invite the use of hyperalimentation to improve the length and quality of survival. A compendium of clinical studies and opinion articles conclude that surgeons and other oncologic clinicians must use discretion and selectivity in nutritional intervention. A representative schema for decision-making is shown in Figure 15-2. Guidelines issued by the American Society for Parenteral and Enteral Nutrition for cancer patients include:[72]

1. Enteral tube feeding and parenteral nutrition support may benefit some severely malnourished cancer patients or those in whom gastrointestinal or other toxicities are anticipated to preclude adequate oral nutritional intake for more than 1 week. Patients who are candidates for nutrition intervention under these circumstances should receive nutrition support, if possible, in conjunction with the initiation of oncologic therapy.
2. Specialized nutritional support is not routinely indicated for well-nourished or mildly malnourished patients undergoing surgery, chemotherapy, or radiation treatment and in whom adequate oral intake is anticipated.
3. TPN is unlikely to benefit patients with advanced cancer whose malignancy is documented as unresponsive to chemotherapy or radiation therapy.

The state of the art for nutritional support in the 1990s is use of the enteral route by whatever means possible. Each patient on venous hyperalimentation should have a solid contraindication for enteral feeding. More clinical studies with enteral feedings are needed to broaden the justification for nutritional support in cancer patients.

REFERENCES

1. Warren S: The immediate causes of death in cancer. Am J Med Sci 1932;184:610.
2. DeWys WD, Begg D, Lavin PT, et al: Prognostic effect of weight loss prior to chemotherapy in cancer patients. Am J Med 1908;69:491.
3. Hickman DM, Miller RA, Rombeau JL, et al: Serum albumin and body weight as predictors of postoperative course in colorectal cancer. JPEN J Parenter Enteral Nutr 1980;4:314.
4. DeWys WD: Abnormalities of taste as a remote effect of a neoplasm. Ann NY Acad Sci 1974; 230:427.
5. Buzby GP, Mullen JL, Matthews DC, et al. Prognostic nutritional index in gastrointestinal surgery. Am J Surg 1980;139:160.
6. Baker JP, Detsky AS, Wesson DE, et al. Nutritional assessment: comparison of clinical judgment and objective measurements. N Engl J Med 1982;306:969.
7. Nixon DW, Heymsfield SB, Cohen AE, et al. Protein-calorie undernutrition in hospitalized cancer patients. Am J Med 1980;68:684.
8. Smale BF, Mullen JL, Buzby GP, and Rosato EF. The efficacy of nutritional assessment and support in cancer surgery, Cancer 1981; 47:2375.
9. Detsky AS, Baker JP, O'Rourke. Predicting nutrition-associated complications for patients undergoing gastrointestinal surgery. JPEN J Parenter Enteral Nutr 1987;11(5):440.
10. Bernstein IL, Bernstein ID. Learned food aversions and cancer anorexia. Cancer Treatment Reports 1981;65(Suppl 5):43.
11. Tracey KJ, Morgello S, Koplin B, et al. Metabolic effects of cachectin/tumor necrosis factor are modified by site of production. Cachectin/tumor necrosis factor-secreting tumor in skeletal muscle induces chronic cachexia, while implantation in brain induces predominantly acute anorexia. J Clin Invest 1990;86(6):2014.
12. Krause R, James JH, Humphrey C, Fischer JE. Plasma and brain amino acids in Walker 256 carcinosarcoma-bearing rats. Cancer Res 1979; 39:3065.
13. Baille P, Miller FK, Pratt AW: Food and water intakes and Walker tumor growth in rats with hypothalamic lesions. Am J Physiol 1965;209: 293.
14. Kern KA, Norton JA. Cancer cachexia. JPEN J Parenter Enteral Nutr 1988;12:286.
15. Norton JA, Peacock JL, Morrison SD. Cancer cachexia. Crit Rev Oncol Hematol 1987;7:289.
16. Gold J. Proposed treatment of cancer by inhibition of gluconeogenesis. Oncology 1968;22: 185.
17. Holroyde CP, Reichard GA. Carbohydrate metabolism in cancer cachexia. Cancer Treatment Reports 1981;65(5):55.
18. Norton JA, Maher M, Wesley R, White D, Brennan MF. Glucose intolerance in sarcoma patients. Cancer 1984;54:302.
19. Fernandes lC, Machado UF, Nogueira R, Carpinelli AR, Curi R. Insulin secretion in Walker 256 tumor cachexia. Am J Physiol 1990;258: E1033.
20. Shaw JH, Wolfe RR. Fatty acid and glycerol kinetics in septic patients and in patients with gastrointestinal cancer. Ann Surg 1987;205: 368.
21. Beck SA, Tisdale MJ. Production of lipolytic and proteolytic factors by a murine tumor producing cachexia in the host. Cancer Res 1987; 47:5919.
22. Devereaux DF, Redgrave TG, Tilton B, et al. Intolerance to administered lipids in tumor bearing animals. Surg 1984;100:292.
23. Shaw JHF, Wolfe RR: Glucose and urea kinetics in patients with early and advanced gastrointestinal cancer: the response to glucose infusion, parenteral feeding, and surgical resection. Surgery 1986;101:181.
24. Costa G, Holland JF. Effects of Krebs-2 carcinoma on the lipid metabolism of male Swiss mice. Cancer Res 1962;22:1081.
25. Carmichael MJ, Clague MB, Keir MJ, et al: Whole body protein turnover synthesis and breakdown in patients with colorectal carcinoma. Br J Surg 1980;67:736.
26. Brennan MF. Total parenteral nutrition in the cancer patient. N Engl J Med 1981;305:375.
27. Kurzer M, Meguid MM. Cancer and protein metabolism. Surg Clin North Am 1986;66:969.
28. Shaw JH, Humberstone DA, Douglas RG, Koea J. Leucine kinetics in patients with benign disease, non–weight-losing cancer, and cancer cachexia: studies at the whole-body and tissue level and the response to nutritional support. Surgery 1991;109(1):37.
29. Radcliffe JD, Morrison SD. Histidine deficiency, food intake and growth in normal and Walker 256 carcinosarcoma-bearing rats. Nutr Cancer 1981;3:40.
30. Smith KL, Tisdale MJ. Mechanism of muscle protein degradation in cancer cachexia. Br J Cancer 1993;68(2):314.
31. Souba WW, Strebel FR, Bull JM, et al: Inter-

organ glutamine metabolism in the tumor-bearing rat. J Surg Res 1988;44:720.
32. Souba WW, Copeland EM: Hyperalimentation in cancer. CA 1989;39:5
33. Lundmark L, Bennegard K, Eden E, et al: Resting energy expenditure in malnourished patients with and without cancer. Gastroenterology 1984;87:407.
34. Merrick HW, Long CL, Grecos GP, et al: Energy requirements for cancer patients and the effect of total parenteral nutrition. JPEN J Parenter Enteral Nutr 1988;12:8.
35. Peacock JL, Inculet RI, Corsey R, et al. Resting energy expenditure and body cell mass alterations in noncachectic patients with sarcomas. Surgery 1987;102:465.
36. Langstein HN, Norton JA. Mechanisms of cancer cachexia. Hematol Oncol Clin North Am 1991;5(1):103.
37. Strassmann G, Fong M, Kenney JS, Jacob CO. Evidence for the involvement of interleukin 6 in experimental cancer cachexia. Journal of Clinical Investigation 1992;89(5):681.
38. Popp MB, Kirkemo AK, Morrison SD, et al: Tumor and host carcass changes during TPN in an anorectic rat-tumor system. Ann Surg 1984;199:205.
39. McGeer AJ, Detsky AS, O'Rourke K: Parenteral nutrition in cancer patients undergoing chemotherapy: a meta-analysis. Nutrition 1990;6:233.
40. Klein S, Simes J, Blackburn GL: Total parenteral nutrition and cancer clinical trials. Cancer 1986;58:1378.
41. Burt ME, Stein TP, Schwade JG, Brennan MF. Whole-body protein metabolism in cancer-bearing patients. Cancer 1984;53:1246.
42. Chlebowski RT. Nutritional support of the medical oncology patient. Hematol Oncol Clin North Am 1991;5(10:147.
43. Moley JF, Morrison SD, Norton JA. Insulin reversal of cancer cachexia in rats. Cancer Res 1985;45:4925.
44. Weisdorf SA, Lysne J, Wind D, et al. Positive effect of prophylactic total parenteral nutrition on long-term outcome of bone marrow transplantation. Transplantation 1987;43:833.
45. Muller JM, Dienst C, Brenner U, Pichlmaier H. Preoperative parenteral feeding in patients with gastrointestinal carcinoma. Lancet 1982;1:68.
46. Buzby GP. The Veterans Affairs TPN Cooperative Study Group. Perioperative TPN in surgical patients. N Engl J Med 1991;325:525.
47. Klein S, Koretz RL. Nutrition support in patients with cancer: what do the data really show? Nutrition in Clinical Practice 1994;9:91.
48. Daly JM, Lieberman MD, Goldfine J, et al. Enteral nutrition with supplemental arginine, RNA and omega-3 fatty acids in postoperative patients: immunologic, metabolic and clinical outcome. Surgery 1992;112:56.
49. Daly JM, Torosian MH. Nutritional support. In: DeVita VT Jr, Hellman S, Rosenberg SA, eds. *Cancer: principles and practice of oncology.* 4th ed. Philadelphia: JB Lippincott, 1993:2480.
50. Ng EH, Lowry SF. Nutritional support and cancer cachexia: evolving concepts of mechanisms and adjunctive therapies. Hematol Oncol Clin North Am 1991;5(1):161.
51. Deutsch LS, Kannegieter L, Vanson DT, Miller DP, Brandon JC. Simplified percutaneous gastrostomy. Radiology 1992;184(1):181.
52. Norton JA, Lowry SF, Brennan MF. Effect of work-induced hypertrophy on skeletal muscle of tumor- and nontumor-bearing rats, J Appl Physiol 1979;46:6540.
53. Daneryd PL, Hafstrom LR, Karlberg IH. Effects of spontaneous physical exercise on experimental cancer anorexia and cachexia. Eur J Cancer 1990;26(10):1083.
54. Loprinzi CL, Ellison NM, Schaid DJ, et al: A controlled trial of megestrol acetate in patients with cancer anorexia/cachexia. Proc Am Soc Clin Oncol 1990;9:321.
55. Szeluga DJ, Stuart RK, Brookmeyer R, et al. Nutritional support of bone marrow transplant recipients: a prospective randomized clinical trial comparing total parenteral nutrition to an enteral feeding program. Cancer Res 1987;47:3309.
56. Cahill GF. Starvation in man. N Engl J Med 1987;282:668.
57. Tchekmedyian NS, Tait N, Moody M, et al: High-dose megestrol acetate. A possible treatment for cachexia. JAMA 1987;257:1195.
58. Splinter TA. Cachexia and cancer: a clinician's view. Ann Oncol 1992;3(Suppl 3):25.
59. Moley JF, Morrison SD, Gorschboth CM, et al. Body composition changes in rats with experimental cachexia: improvements with exogenous insulin. Cancer Res 1988;48:2784.
60. Peacock JL, Norton JA. Impact of insulin on survival of cachectic tumor bearing rats. JPEN J Parenter Enteral Nutr 1988;12(3):260.
61. Ward HC, Holliday D, Sim AJW. Protein and energy metabolism with biosynthetic human growth hormone after gastrointestinal surgery. Ann Surg 1987;206:56.
62. Bartlett DL, Charland S, Torosian MH. Cancer 1994;73(5):1499.
63. Klimberg VS, Souba WW, Dolson DJ, et al. Prophylactic glutamine protects the intestinal mucosa from radiation injury. Cancer 1990;66:62.

64. Chance WT, Cao L, Fischer JE. Insulin and acivicin improve host nutrition and prevent tumor growth during total parenteral nutrition. Ann Surg 1988;208:524.
65. Tachibana K, Mukai K, Hiraoka I, et al. Evaluation of the effect of arginine enriched amino acid solution on tumor growth. JPEN J Parenter Enteral Nutr 1985;9:428.
66. Torosian MH, Tsou KC, Daly JM, et al. Alteration of tumor cell kinetics by total parenteral nutrition: potential therapeutic implications. Cancer 1984;53:1409.
67. Langstein JW, Fraker DL, Norton JA. Reversal of cancer cachexia by antibodies to interferon-gamma but not cachectin/tumor necrosis factor. Surgical Forum 1989;15:408.
68. Gelin J, Moldawer LL, Lonnroth C, Sherry B, Chizzonite R, Lundholm k. Role of endogenous tumor necrosis factor alpha and interleukin 1 for experimental tumor growth and the development of cancer cachexia. Cancer Res 1991;51(1):415.
69. Nelson KA, Walsh D, Sheehan FA. The cancer anorexia-cachexia syndrome. J Clin Oncol 1994;12:213.
70. Solomon SM, Kirby DF. The refeeding syndrome: a review. JPEN J Parenter Enteral Nutr 1990;14:90.
71. Howard L. Home parenteral and enteral nutrition in cancer patients. Cancer 1993;72:3531.
72. ASPEN Board of Directors. Guidelines for the use of parenteral and enteral nutrition in adult and pediatric patients. JPEN J Parenter Enteral Nutr 1993;17(Suppl):1SA.

16

Infections in the Immunocompromised Patient

CARL SHANHOLTZ

A variety of factors predispose the cancer patient to infection. These factors can be broadly categorized as:

- Disruption of barrier function
- Alterations in host flora
- Defects in humoral immunity
- Defects in cellular immunity
- Defects in phagocyte function

The patient with cancer is a host whose immune system is often in a state of flux with periods of altered immunity and periods of normal immune function. Multiple defects in immunity in the same patient are common.[1] For example, a patient with Hodgkin's disease has defective cellular immunity. This patient may undergo a splenectomy as part of a staging procedure, thus producing both a defect in immunity and a wound. The patient may subsequently receive chemotherapy with associated mucositis and neutropenia, producing another alteration in barrier function along with a loss in phagocytic function. Later, the patient may undergo bone marrow transplantation, which produces multiple alterations in immunity.[1] In addition, a specific defect in immunity may be difficult to isolate due to the interdependence of various aspects of the immune system. For example, defects in cell-mediated immunity owing to decreased helper thymus-derived (T) lymphocytes can alter the production of immunoglobulin by bone-marrow-derived, or bursa-equivalent, (B) lymphocytes.[2,3]

THE IMMUNOCOMPROMISED STATE

Disruption in Anatomic Barrier Function

The skin and mucosa form the primary barrier between the host and the environment. Treatment of malignancy frequently violates the integrity of these barriers. The integrity of the skin can be compromised by indwelling vascular access devices, surgical procedures, and infections such as herpes zoster. More importantly, mucosal damage, which frequently occurs as a consequence of cytotoxic chemotherapy, provides an important route for invasion by colonizing organisms in patients with concomitant pancytopenia. Patients with chronic neutropenia (*e.g.*, aplastic anemia) and no mucosal disruption have a much lower incidence of infection than patients with treatment-related neutropenia and mucositis. Mucositis often is complicated by viral infections, especially herpes simplex virus, which reactivate during periods of immunosuppression.[4]

Alterations in Host Flora

Environmental factors also place patients with cancer at increased risk for infection. A study of patients with acute leukemia at the

University of Maryland Cancer Center demonstrated that almost half of all bacteremias followed hospital acquisition of the organism.[5] Environmental surveillance cultures have revealed *Pseudomonas aeruginosa* and other gram-negative organisms growing in moist areas such as sink drains, water faucets, ice machines, and bath tubs. Water faucets are especially prone to contamination from the aerator, which traps sediment over time. Ice machines with storage bins are prone to contamination from the communal use of the scoop, or the direct handling of ice by hand, whereas ice dispensers are less prone to colonization.[6]

Certain organisms are also prone to nosocomial spread. Airborne transmission has been demonstrated with *Aspergillus* through hospital ventilation systems with life-threatening consequences.[7] *Clostridium difficile*, a common cause of diarrhea in cancer patients, can be transmitted by hospital personnel caring for these patients.[8] Antibiotic use may select for resistant organisms such as vancomycin-resistant *enterococcus*,[9] methicillin-resistant *Staphylococcus aureus*,[10] antibiotic resistant coagulase-negative *Staphylococcus* and *Enterobacter* organisms.[11] *Pseudomonas cepacia* has been associated with intravenous fluid bags used to mix heparin flush,[12] and also with contaminated ventilator nebulizers.[13]

Defects in Humoral Immunity

B lymphocytes secrete immunoglobulin or specific antibody after activation by a variety of stimuli.[2,3] The most specific activation of B cells occurs when the antigen, in association with a class II major histocompatibility complex (MHC) molecule on the monocyte-macrophage surface, is presented to an antigen-specific T helper cell. The monocyte secretes the lymphokine interleukin-1 (IL-1) which activates resting T cells and B cells. Once stimulated, the T cell produces a variety of lymphokines including IL-2, IL-4, and other B cell growth factors, which together promote B-cell proliferation, growth, differentiation, immunoglobulin synthesis, and antibody production, among other functions. Activated T cells also secrete gamma-interferon (IFN-γ), which increases expression of class I and class II MHC on T and B cells, in addition to increasing antibody production by B cells. The B cell, activated by processed antigen and lymphokines, proliferates and differentiates into an antibody-secreting plasma cell.[3,14–16] There are also nonspecific ways in which B cells can be triggered directly, either by the perturbation of surface membrane immunoglobulin or independently of surface immunoglobulin.[2]

Antibody secretion is essential in fighting infection, and defects in humoral immunity are associated with infections caused by encapsulated organisms, notably *Streptococcus pneumoniae, Hemophilus influenzae*, and *Neisseria meningitidis* (Table 16-1).[16] Defects in humoral immunity have been associated with B-cell malignancies such as chronic lymphocytic leukemia, multiple myeloma, and Waldenström's macroglobulinemia, as well as in patients with leukemia receiving intensive chemotherapy.[4,17] Patients with chronic lymphocytic leukemia often have low levels of measured immunoglobulin and are susceptible to recurrent bacterial and viral infections.[4] Similarly, patients with multiple myeloma and macroglobulinemia have an abnormal humoral response (because of impaired antibody response rather than abnormal immunoglobulin) and are also susceptible to recurrent infections.[17]

Splenectomy has been associated with alterations in humoral immunity because the spleen functions as a filter and a source for opsonization.[18] Splenectomy produces a deficiency in tuftsin, a phagocytosis-stimulating peptide, and cases of overwhelming infection caused by *S. pneumoniae, H. influenzae*, and *Neisseria meningitidis* have been reported.[19] Although the association is strong between splenectomy in childhood and subsequent infection with encapsulated organisms, the issue is controversial in individuals who have received splenectomy as adults. The experience at the University of

Table 16-1. Immune Defects, Commonly Associated Diseases, and Commonly Associated Pathogens

Immune Defect	Associated Diseases	Associated Pathogens			
		Bacteria	Fungi	Viruses	Parasites
Humoral immunity	Chronic lymphocytic leukemia, Multiple myeloma, splenectomy	S. pneumoniae, H. influenzae, N. meningitidis			
Cell-mediated immunity	Hodgkin's disease, Hairy cell leukemia, Transplant recipients, AIDS, adrenal corticosteroids	Listeria, Legionella, Salmonella, Nocardia, Typical and atypical mycobacteria	Candida Cryptococcus Histoplasmosis Coccidiodomycosis	Herpes simplex Varicella-zoster Cytomegalovirus Epstein-Barr virus	Protozoa: *Pneumocystis carinii*, *Toxoplasma gondii*, Helminths: *Strongyloides stercoralis*
Phagocytosis	Acute leukemia, Following cytotoxic chemotherapy	Enterobacteriaceae especially *E. coli*, *P. aeruginosa*, *K. pneumoniae*, Staphylococcus spp. Streptococcus spp. JK diphtheroids, Clostridium difficile	*Candida spp. Torulopsis glabrata, Aspergillus spp*, less commonly mucormycosis, trichosporon, *Pseudoallescheria boydii*	Herpes simplex, cytomegalovirus	

Maryland Cancer Center of the incidence of infection was reviewed in 92 previously untreated patients with Hodgkin's disease who underwent staging laparotomy and splenectomy. Severe infections were observed only in those patients with recurrent Hodgkin's disease who were profoundly granulocytopenic. Infections with *S. pneumoniae* and *Hemophilus* were uncommon during the remission period.[20] More recently, the incidence of fatal and nonfatal infections in adult patients with Hodgkin's disease who had undergone staging laparotomy with splenectomy was compared to nonsplenectomized patients over a period of 10 years, and no difference was found in frequency or death from infection.[21]

Defects in Cellular Immunity

The monocyte performs a crucial role in regulating the immune system, and is clearly necessary for specific T cell responses to antigen. T-cell receptors only recognize antigen in close physical association with an integral membrane protein called a *restriction element*. Restriction elements are glycoproteins closely resembling immunoglobulins and are coded for by the MHC.[2,3] Class I MHC molecules include human lymphocyte antigen (HLA) types A, B, and C, and serve as restriction elements for CD8 or T8 suppressor or cytotoxic T cells. Class II MHC molecules (HLA-DR) serve as restriction elements for CD4 or T4 helper or inducer T cells.[3] After antigen associated with a restriction element is presented to the resting T cell in the presence of monocyte secreted IL-1, the helper T cell becomes activated, producing the lymphokines IL-2, IL-3, IL-4, and IFN-γ. After activation, high-affinity receptors appear on the surface of T-cells. The binding of IL-2 to these receptors causes expansion of the activated clone. IL-2 may also have a role in T-cell maturation, activation and proliferation of cytotoxic lymphocytes, and the enhancement of natural killer (NK) cell activity.[14] IL-2 also transforms resting cytotoxic non-T cells into lymphokine-activated killer cells.[13] Thus, T-cell–mediated immunity is dependent on a complex interaction between monocytes, helper T cells, and suppressor T cells, and disruption of this interaction can lead to infection.

Defects in cell-mediated immunity are commonly encountered in the acquired immune deficiency syndrome (AIDS), Hodgkin's disease, transplant recipients, prolonged therapy with adrenocorticosteroids, and some chemotherapy agents such as fludarabine.[22] Commonly associated infections include intracellular pathogens including *Listeria monocytogenes*, *Nocardia asteroides*, salmonellosis, typical and atypical mycobacteria, most fungi, parasites such as *Pneumocystis carinii* (PCP), *Toxoplasma gondii*, *Strongyloides stercoralis*, and viruses, especially from the herpes family (herpes simplex, varicella-zoster, cytomegalovirus, and Epstein-Barr virus).[1,4,16,19] Although Hodgkin's disease is associated with defects in cell-mediated immunity, the study by Schimpff et al,[20] mentioned above, demonstrated no increase in infection, other than herpes zoster, during the remission period.

Defects in Phagocytic Function

Perhaps the most dramatic increase in the incidence of infection in cancer patients comes with the development of neutropenia. Even in Hodgkin's disease, with its associated defects in cell-mediated immunity, the most serious infections are associated with neutropenia occurring during therapy.[20,21] A study by Pizzo et al,[23] showed that nearly 80% of febrile episodes in children and young adults with cancer occurred while the patients were neutropenic. Bodey et al[24] examined the relationship between leukopenia and infection in patients with acute leukemia treated at the National Institutes of Health (USA). The incidence of severe infections was greatest in patients with less than 100 granulocytes/mm^3, and it dropped precipitously with increasing granulocyte levels, with a plateau in the incidence of infection occurring above 1000 granulocytes/mm^3 (Fig. 16-1**A**). A fal-

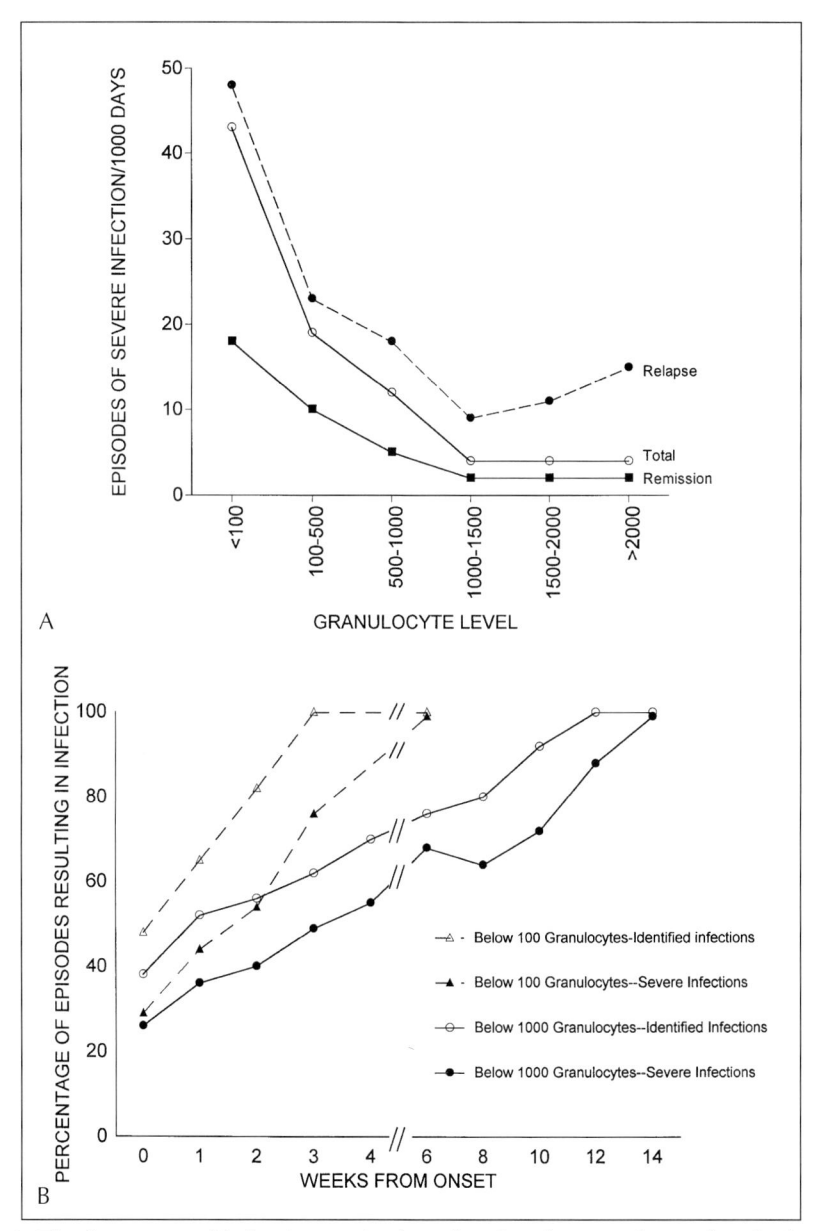

Figure 16-1. A. The frequency of infectious episodes related to the granulocyte level. The number of episodes of severe infection/1,000 days without severe infection is plotted for each granulocyte level. The risk of developing severe infection decreases with increasing granulocyte level. However, no further reduction occurs above a granulocyte level of 1,500/mm$_3$. The risk is greater in relapse than in remission for every granulocyte level. **B** The effect of duration of granulocytopenia on the frequency of infection. The duration of granulocytopenia is plotted against the percentage of episodes resulting in infection. Along the abscissa are recorded the number of episodes of granulocytopenia (<1,000/mm^3) and severe granulocytopenia (<100/mm^3) for each time interval. The curves illustrate the percentage of episodes at both granulocyte levels resulting in any infection and in severe infection. The risk of developing infection increases the longer granulocytopenia is present and this risk is consistently greater at the lower granulocyte level. (Adapted from Bodey GP, Buckley M, Sathe YS, Freireich EJ. Quantitative relationships between circulating leukocytes and infection in patients with acute leukemia. Ann Intern Med 1966;64:328; with permission.)

ling (as opposed to a stable or rising) granulocyte count was also associated with an increased risk of infection. In addition, the risk of infection increased with the duration of neutropenia (Fig. 16-1**B**).

The predominant organisms infecting the neutropenic host are the enterobacteriaceae and *Pseudomonas*, gram-positive bacteria including *Staphylococcus epidermidis*, and JK diphtheroids, fungi (especially *Candida* and *Aspergillus*), and the herpes family of viruses. Anaerobes are uncommon, occurring in less than 5% of patients. However, *C. difficile* is a notable exception.[25] Coagulase-negative staphylococcal species are now major pathogens, and the incidence of gram-positive organisms producing initial infections has grown, becoming the most frequent cause of initial infections in neutropenic patients in some centers.[26,27]

MANAGEMENT OF INFECTION IN THE CANCER PATIENT

Clinical Presentation of Infection in the Febrile Neutropenic Patient

The evaluation of febrile episodes in the neutropenic patient can be a confounding problem to the clinician. The clinical presentation of infection in the neutropenic patient can be subtle with few localizing signs. Because the defenseless host can rapidly deteriorate from sepsis, the consequences of delaying antibiotic therapy while awaiting positive cultures can be catastrophic. Nearly 85% of febrile episodes in neutropenic cancer patients are caused by infection.[28,29] A prospective study of consecutive patients with acute leukemia receiving induction chemotherapy at the University of Maryland Cancer Center demonstrated 306 febrile episodes in 130 patients. These episodes comprised 14% bacteremias, 2% fungemias, and 35% microbiologically proved infections without bacteremia. The remaining episodes comprised 36% clinically documented infections and 14% fever of unknown cause.[29]

The most frequent sites of infection in the neutropenic patient are natural anatomic barriers, which are vulnerable to damage from cytotoxic chemotherapy or a change in colonizing flora. They can be broadly divided into the alimentary tract, the respiratory tract, the skin, and the urinary tract.[5,25] Bacteremias may be associated with infections at some sites (anorectum and lungs) more than others (skin or urinary tract), although microbiologic documentation may be more difficult to achieve in the lungs than other sites. Anorectal infections occur in nearly 30% of neutropenic patients with acute leukemia, making a careful rectal examination an essential part of the fever work-up.[5] Acute periodontitis occurs as a result of a flare of chronic periodontal disease, and has been associated with up to 20% of febrile neutropenic episodes.[25]

Neutropenic patients have an altered clinical presentation of infection because localizing signs and symptoms of infection depend on the presence of granulocytes. Sickles et al,[30] reported the associated physical findings, symptoms, and pathologic features of the five most common localized infections (pharyngitis, skin infection, pneumonia, anorectal infection, and urinary tract infection) occurring in cancer patients. Erythema and local pain or tenderness occurred in all patients regardless of granulocyte count or site of infection. However, neutropenic patients had a greater prevalence of fever, and a lower prevalence of exudate, fluctuance, ulceration or fissure, local heat, swelling, and regional adenopathy. Therefore, fever, erythemia, and pain or tenderness should be considered evidence of infection in these patients.

The majority of pathogens responsible for initial infections in patients with neutropenia are bacterial.[6,18,28] Classically, the most common presenting organisms are gram-negative aerobic bacteria, particularly *Escherichia coli, Klebsiella pneumoniae,* and *Pseudomonas aeruginosa,* as well as gram-positive species such as *Staphylococcus aureus* and streptococcal species. Empiric antibiotic therapy directed at these pathogens has been essential in the initial management of febrile neutropenic patients. The advantages of combination therapy are: the contribution of additive or synergistic effects, the prevention of the emergence of resistant organisms, and the prevention of treatment failures.[28,29] Because prolonged, severe neutropenia (granulocyte counts <100/mm^3 for more than 14 days) is a risk factor for poor outcome in the neutropenic cancer patient with gram-negative bacteremia, the choice of initial antibiotic therapy is critical.[31] Studies have shown a poorer response if the recovered organism was resistant to one of the antibiotics administered than if it was sensitive to both.[6,31] A retrospective review of 410 episodes of *Pseudomonas* bacteremia in cancer patients showed cure rates diminished significantly (from 67% to 14%) if inappropriate antibiotics were used. A 1- to 2-day delay in appropriate antibiotic therapy was associated with a reduction in cure rate from 74% to 46%.[32]

Antibiotic strategies targeted at gram-negative bacteria have typically combined an aminoglycoside (gentamicin, tobramycin, or amikacin) with either an antipseudomonal penicillin (ticarcillin, piperacillin, azlocillin, or mezlocillin) or an antipseudomonal third-generation cephalosporin (cefoperazone, ceftazidime).[28,29] The advantages of this combination include synergy and a low emergence of resistant organisms. The disadvantages of combined therapy include ototoxicity, hypokalemia, and nephrotoxicity. Since so many cancer patients receive multiple nephrotoxic insults during therapy, an alternative strategy combining two antipseudomonal β-lactam antibiotics has been used in some centers. The combination of a third-generation cephalosporin (ceftazidime or cefoperazone) and an antipseudomonal penicillin (piperacillin, mezlocillin) has been found to be as effective as the combination of a penicillin and an aminoglycoside, with very low toxicity.[33] The disadvantages, however, include the occasional emergence of resistant organisms, possible antagonism of the combinations, and little effect of third-generation cephalosporins against anaerobic bacteria.[34] Different drugs and dosing schedules have been tried. Although no particular combination has been shown to be superior, cefotaxime and aztreonam seem to have less efficacy than most other combinations.[29]

Monotherapy as an alternative to combination antibiotic therapy is attractive because of reduced toxicity, cost, and ease of administration. The two most promising single-agent drugs are ceftazidime and imipenem. A prospective, randomized trial at the National Cancer Institute (USA) compared monotherapy using ceftazidime to combination therapy using cephalothin, carbenicillin, and gentamicin for initial empiric therapy in 550 episodes of febrile neutropenia.[35] Patients were evaluated at 72 hours to assess the efficacy of the antibiotics during the period of empiric use (before microbiologic data) and at the resolution of neutropenia. Endpoints were: successful resolution of febrile neutropenia without modification of the initial antibiotics, failure (death during neutropenia), and an intermediate endpoint of survival, but with modification of the initial regimen. There was no difference in terms of survival, but the monotherapy required significantly more modifications (58 of 282 compared with 29 of 268) at 72 hours because of anaerobic infections (necrotizing gingivitis and perirectal cellulitis), and a greater need for vancomycin in patients with gram-positive infections.[18,35]

A major criticism of the single-agent ceftazidime study has been targeted at the intermediate endpoint of survival with the modification of the initial empiric antibiotic regimen. Traditionally, the endpoint of failure includes the need for modification of the initial antibiotic regimen. Had this endpoint been used, success rates in this study would have been lower than in other trials reported. In addition, there were few documented infections, and few gram-negative infections, suggesting the study had a low power.[29] Nevertheless, a consensus conference has since adopted endpoints of success with modification if the primary infection was eradicated with initial empiric therapy, but a secondary infection arises that falls outside the initial spectrum of activity.[36]

Imipenem also has shown much promise for use as empiric monotherapy. A randomized controlled trial by Winston et al,[37] found imipenem to be as effective as the combinations of cefoperazone and piperacillin, or ceftazidime and piperacillin, with an 82% response rate to imipenem. This study used the traditional definition of failure (any modification of the initial antibiotics). The major drawback to single agent imipenem was a more frequent occurrence of superinfection with *Xanthomas maltophilia* (3 of 135 patients compared with 0 of 268 patients). In a large prospective, randomized, double-blinded trial at the University of Maryland Cancer Center, imipenem was found to be as effective as the synergistic antibiotic combination of amikacin and piperacillin.[29] Recently, a four-arm trial comparing ceftazidime alone, imipenem alone, ceftazidime plus amikacin, and imipenem plus amikacin, found single agent ceftazidime to be less effective than the other regimens using the classic endpoint of response without modification.[38] The spectrum of infections in the neutropenic patient population has shifted to include an increased number of gram-positive infections, especially with *S. epidermidis*. Although this organism is usually considered to be usual skin flora, a molecular epidemiologic study at the University of Maryland Cancer Center has found the respiratory tract and alimentary canal to be the predominant sites of origin.[27] The increased incidence of infection was not related to nosocomial transmission or the presence of indwelling catheters.[27] Because of the increased incidence of gram-positive infections in the neutropenic population, empiric use of vancomycin has been suggested. A randomized, controlled trial showed vancomycin decreased the median number of days of fever and the frequency of subsequent gram-positive infections.[39] A large multicenter trial by the European Organization for Research and Treatment of Cancer (EORTC) and the National Cancer Institute of Canada, however, demonstrated no difference in the proportion of febrile patients each trial day, or in the duration of fever in patients receiving, or not receiving, vancomycin. However, nephrotoxicity was more frequent in the vancomycin arm.[40]

Outpatient empiric antibiotic therapy can potentially reduce hospitalizations and reduce costs. In a prospective clinical trial by Rubenstein et al,[41] febrile neutropenic patients at low risk for complications were randomized to receive either oral ciprofloxacin and clindamycin, or intravenous aztreonam and clindamycin. Although the oral regimen was effective, it was associated with significantly more nephrotoxicity, necessitating early termination of the study.[41] More trials are needed to define a role for outpatient antibiotic therapy.

While initial infections usually are caused by bacteria and usually respond well to initial empiric antibiotic coverage, subsequent infections occur in patients with protracted neutropenia and are caused by resistant bacteria, fungi, viruses, and parasites. These pathogens are more difficult to diagnose, are resistant to treatment, and carry high rates of morbidity and mortality.[29] A review of the National Cancer Institute (USA) experience categorized neutropenic patients with fever of unknown origin into three groups based on their risk of infection. The low risk group had neutropenia for less than 7 days. The two high-risk subgroups included those with neutropenia for 7 to 14 days, and neutropenia for greater than 2 weeks. Low-risk patients had the lowest rate of recurrence of fever (0.6%) after defervescence following the initiation of antibiotic therapy. Recurrent fevers occurred in 4% of high-risk patients who remained neutropenic for 7 to 14 days, and in 38% of high-risk patients who remained neutropenic for greater than 2 weeks.[42] Therefore, patients with prolonged neutropenia frequently require modifications of antibiotics. Fever persisting more than 3 days implies: 1) infection with, or emergence of, resistant organisms, 2) infection with non-bacterial pathogens, 3) infection at an avascular site such as an abscess or catheter, or 4) a noninfectious cause of fever such as drug fever, or "tumor fever."[34] Options for modifying the initial empiric antibiotic therapy in persistently or recurrently febrile neutropenic patients is shown in Table 16-2.[28] During the first 4 to 5 days, initial antibiotics should be continued if the patient's clinical condition remains unchanged and reevaluation provides no new information. Consideration should be given to changing antibiotics for microbiologic documentation of resistant gram-negative organisms, isolation of gram-negative organisms while on therapy, drug fever, or clinical progression of disease. Vancomycin should be added if there is suspicion of infection with methicillin-resistant *S. aureus, S. epidermidis, Streptococcus viridans,* or *Corynebacterium* species.[34]

Evaluation and Treatment of Fungal Infections

Fungal infection, rarely seen prior to the 1960s, is a major problem in the immunocompromised patient population.[10,19] The most common fungal pathogens seen in neutropenic patients are *Candida* spp and *Aspergillus* spp,[43] although more exotic fungal species have been reported in cancer patients with increasing frequency. These include *Trichosporon beigelii, Fusarium* spp, *Geotrichum candidum, Curvularia* spp, *Drechslera* spp, *Penicillium* spp, *Rhodotorula rubra, Pseudoallescheria boydii, Pichia farinosa, Torulopsis pintolopesii, Saccharomyces cerevisiae, Cunninghamella bertholletiae, Scopulariopsis,* and *Kluveromyces.*[44,45] Invasive rhinocerebral fungal infections have been reported with the phycomycetes.[46] Cryptococcus, although a common pathogen in the AIDS population, is rarely encountered in neutropenic cancer patients.[43]

Predisposing factors to fungal infection include the underlying diagnosis of a hematologic malignancy, diabetes, prolonged neutropenia, and the breakdown of natural barriers.[47] Adrenal corticosteroids, frequently administered during therapy for leukemia and other hematologic malignancies, also increase the risk for fungal infections.[47] Subcutaneous catheters for parenteral nutrition, the administration of long-term antibiotics, phlebotomy, and repeated transfusions have been associated with an increased risk of fungemia.[10] Transient fungemia with *Candida* spp and *Torulopsis glabrata* is common in patients with indwelling catheters receiving parenteral nutrition and necessitates removal of the catheter. Although removal of the catheter may be all that is required to treat the infection, immunocompromised patients are at risk for persistent fungemia. Amphotericin in this patient population has been shown to reduce the incidence of disseminated fungal infection and persistent fungemia, and decrease the mortality rate related to fungemia.[45,47]

Candida *Infections*

Candida albicans is the major cause of disseminated candida infection, although *C. tropicalis* causes fungemia as frequently as *C. albicans.* A chemotherapy treated animal model has demonstrated *C. tropicalis* to be more pathogenic than *C. albicans.* This has been confirmed through isolates from patients' blood.[43] Other species of yeast that have been known to cause systemic fungal infections in immunocompromised patients include *C. parapsilosis, C. guillermondii, C. lusitaniae,* and *Torulopsis glabrata.*[43] *C. krusei* is emerging as a significant pathogen, especially with the prophylactic use of fluconazole.[48,49]

The average time interval for documented *Candida* sepsis to appear is 9 to 11 days after the onset of neutropenia. Diagnosis can be difficult because symptoms are nonspecific. Disseminated *Candida* infection is suggested by refractory fever, recurrence of fever after defervescence on antibacterial therapy, sepsis with hypotension, and embolic skin lesions. *C. tropicalis* is the most likely *Candida* species to cause embolic skin lesions.

Table 16-2. Common Modifications or Additions to Initial Empirical Antibiotic Therapy in Febrile Neutropenic Patients

Status or Symptoms	Modifications of Primary Regimen
FEVER	
Persistent for >1 week	Add empirical antifungal therapy with amphotericin B.
Recurrence after 1 week or later in patient with persistent neutropenia	Add empirical antifungal therapy.
Persistent or recurrent fever at time of recovery from neutropenia	Evaluate liver and spleen by CT, ultrasonography, or MRI for hepatosplenic candidiasis, and evaluate need for antifungal therapy.
BLOOD STREAM	
Cultures before antibiotic therapy	
Gram-positive organism	Add vancomycin pending further identification
Gram-negative organism	Maintain regimen if patient is stable and isolate is sensitive. If *P. aeruginosa,* enterobacter, or citrobacter is isolated, add an aminoglycoside or an additional β-lactam antibiotic.
Organism isolated during antibiotic therapy	
Gram-positive organism	Add vancomycin.
Gram-negative organism	Change to new combination regimen (e.g., imipenem plus gentamicin or vancomycin, or gentamicin plus piperacillin).
HEAD, EYES, EARS, NOSE, THROAT	
Necrotizing or marginal gingivitis	Add specific antianaerobic agent (clindamycin or metronidazole) to empirical therapy.
Vesicular or ulcerative lesions	Suspect herpes simplex infection. Culture and begin acyclovir therapy.
Sinus tenderness or nasal ulcerative lesions	Suspect fungal infection with aspergillus or mucor.
GASTROINTESTINAL TRACT	
Retrosternal burning pain	Suspect candida, herpes, simplex, or both. Add antifungal therapy and, if no response, acyclovir. Bacterial esophagitis also a possibility. For patients who do not respond within 48 hours, endoscopy should be considered.
Acute abdominal pain	Suspect typhlitis, as well as appendicitis, if pain in right lower quadrant. Add specific antianaerobic coverage to empirical regimen and monitor closely for need for surgical intervention.
Perianal tenderness	Add specific antianaerobic drug to empirical regimen and monitor closely for need for surgical intervention, especially when patient is recovering from neutropenia.
RESPIRATORY TRACT	
New focal lesion in patient recovering from neutropenia	Observe carefully, since this may be a consequence of inflammatory response in concert with neutrophil recovery.
New focal lesion in patient with continuing neutropenia	Aspergillus is the chief concern. Perform appropriate cultures and consider biopsy. If patient is not a candidate for procedure, administer high-dose amphotericin B (1.5 mg/kg/day).
New interstitial pneumonitis	Attempt diagnosis by examination of induced sputum or bronchoalveolar lavage. If not feasible, begin empirical treatment with trimethoprim-sulfamethoxazole or pentamidine. Consider noninfectious causes and the need for open-lung biopsy if condition has not improved after 4 days of therapy.

(continued)

Table 16-2. *(Continued)*

Status or Symptoms	Modifications of Primary Regimen
CENTRAL VENOUS CATHETERS	
Positive culture for organisms other than bacillus species or candida	Attempt to treat. Rotate antibiotic administration in patients with multiple-lumen catheters.
Positive culture for bacillus species or candida	Remove catheter and treat appropriately.
Exit-site infection with mycobacterium or aspergillus	Remove catheter and treat appropriately.
Tunnel infection	Remove catheter and treat appropriately.

(Adapted from Pizzo, PA, N Engl J Med 1993:328:1323; with permission.)

Myalgias can occur from muscle invasion by candida, and organisms can be recovered by biopsy. Renal dysfunction can be related to antifungal therapy, or invasion of the kidney by fungus.[43]

Hepatosplenic candidiasis has been seen with increasing frequency in patients with leukemia and other hematologic malignancies. Thaler et al,[50] reviewed eight cases at the National Institutes of Health (USA) and 60 immunocompromised patients reported in the world literature with hepatosplenic candidiasis. All patients had a documented antemortem diagnosis, and candida was proved by biopsy or on postmortem examination. Manifestations usually became apparent after recovery of the granulocyte count. None of the patients were diagnosed while neutropenic. Fever occurred in 85% and abdominal pain in 57% of these patients. The most consistently abnormal laboratory value was a persistently elevated alkaline phosphatase, for a median duration of 130 days. Total bilirubin and transaminase levels usually returned to normal in a few days. Computed tomographic (CT) scans were usually positive, with less than 10% of CT scans in this review being negative. Ultrasound, however, was normal in nearly a third of patients. Computed tomography was more sensitive, and ultrasound more specific, although falsely negative studies occurred with each. Typical ultrasound findings of early hepatosplenic candidiasis were the presence of "target" or "bull's eye" lesions: a hypoechoic lesion or hypoechoic ring around a central hyperechoic nidus. As the lesions shrank they became hyperechoic with occasional calcification. They may disappear completely. Computed tomography findings appeared as areas of decreased attenuation, with the target appearance only an occasional finding.[50] Target lesions have been demonstrated by magnetic resonance imaging scans (Fig. 16-2). Radionuclide imaging was found to be insensitive and nonspecific. Grossly, the liver and spleen were studded with white to yellow nodules ranging in size from 1 mm to 2 cm. The early histologic appearance showed abscess formation, with a necrotic center surrounded by inflammatory infiltrate and fibrosis, making needle biopsy difficult. Yeast forms and pseudohyphae were found only in the center of the lesions. Therefore, serial sections needed to be performed and stained with methenamine silver or periodic-acid Schiff (PAS). There was a large variation in therapy in this series of patients with cumulative doses of amphotericin B ranging from 0.7 to 9 g. Many patients receiving 2 g or less of amphotericin B had residual disease at autopsy, implying that large doses are needed to eradicate disease.[50]

Primary *Candida* pneumonia, defined invasive infection limited to the lungs, has also been reported. A review of autopsy records at the University of Texas MD Anderson Cancer Center (Houston, TX) revealed a 9% inci-

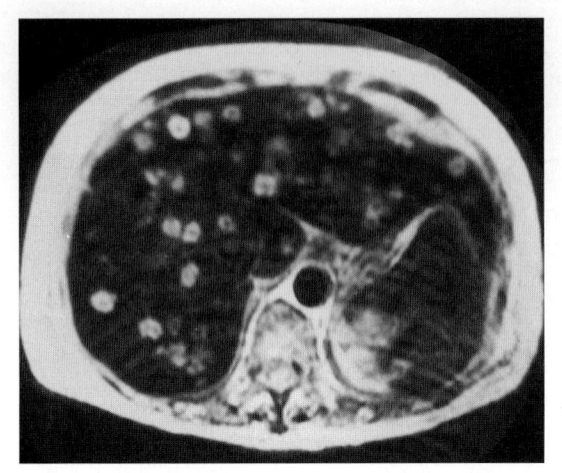

Figure 16-2. Hepatosplenic Candidiasis. This 27-year-old woman with acute leukemia was transferred to the University of Maryland Medical Center with candidemia. This magnetic resonance T$_2$-weighted image demonstrates decreased signal intensity of the liver and spleen consistent with iron deposition from hemosiderosis related to multiple transfusions. There are multifocal, round, hyperintense "target" lesions appearing within the liver and spleen consistent with hepatosplenic candidiasis.

dence of primary *Candida* pneumonia out of all invasive *Candida* pulmonary infections.[51] Unlike hepatosplenic candidiasis, there was an equal distribution among patients with solid tumors and hematologic malignancies. Factors associated with primary *Candida* pneumonia include prior antibiotic use (90%), steroids, central venous catheters, and esophagitis. Dyspnea was the most frequent symptom, occurring in 97% of patients, and fever occurred in 87%. Hypoxemia was found in 90% of patients. Chest radiographic appearance had diffuse bilateral infiltrates in roughly half of patients, and infiltrates limited to one or more lobes in others. Antemortem sputum cultures yielded *Candida* spp in most of the patients in which they were obtained; however bronchoscopies and transbronchial biopsies were negative in the two patients from whom they were obtained. Bronchopneumonia and intra-alveolar hemorrhage were the most common histopathologic finding. Microabscesses were seen with limited areas of hemorrhage in adjacent lung, unlike the large areas of infarction and hemorrhage seen in *Aspergillus* infections. Primary *Candida* pneumonia was a contributing cause of death in 84% of patients.[51]

Aspergillus *Infections*

Aspergillus has emerged as a frequent fungal pathogen in patients with cancer, having life-threatening implications. *Aspergillus* is ubiquitous in the environment, and the portal of entry is usually the respiratory tract.[43,47] Primary cutaneous *Aspergillus* infection has been seen in the setting of indwelling vascular catheter infections, and has been linked to the exposure to aspergillus spores in the air of the operating room.[43] Outbreaks of nosocomial transmission have been reported.[7,52] The most common species associated with infection are *A. fumigatus* and *A. flavus*, although other species, such as *A. niger* have also been known to cause infection.

Protracted neutropenia is the most significant risk factor for developing invasive aspergillosis, with the risk rising dramatically after 3 weeks of neutropenia. In addition to environmental exposure of exogenous organisms, reactivation of endogenous organisms may also produce infection. Patients with acute leukemia who have had fungal pneumonia while neutropenic have a significant risk of developing another episode of fungal pneumonia during subsequent courses of treatment and periods of neutropenia.[43]

Infection with *Aspergillus* is primarily pulmonary, and patients frequently present with pleuritic chest pain, fever, hemoptysis, adventitious breath sounds, and hypoxemia.[53] Radiographic findings include infiltrates and nodules, with serial radiographs demonstrating cavitary lesions as the granulocyte count recovers. Computed tomographic scans may demonstrate a characteristic zone of low attenuation surrounding a mass-like infiltrate ("halo" sign), nodular infiltrates, or cavitary lesions[53] (Fig. 16-3). *Aspergillus* invades the walls of blood vessels,

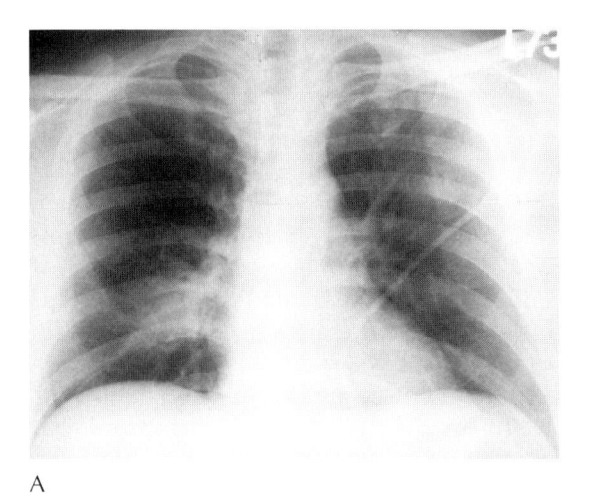

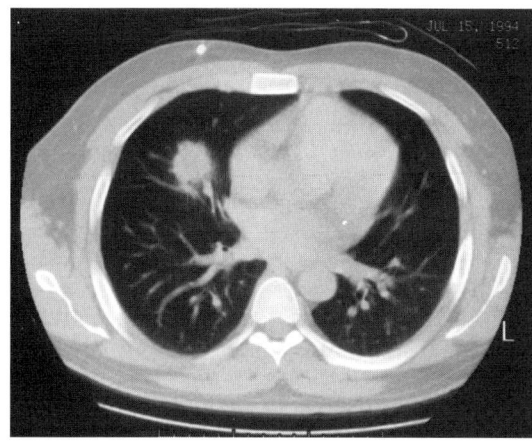

Figure 16-3. A. Pulmonary Aspergillosis. This 42-year-old man with acute myeloid leukemia developed a pulmonary infiltrate during a period of chemotherapy-induced neutropenia with fever. This chest radiograph demonstrates a right middle lobe infiltrate. **B.** Computed tomographic scan of the lungs demonstrates a large right middle lobe nodule with surrounding area of decreased attenuation, known as the CT "halo" sign. **C.** Computed tomographic scan of the patient's lungs performed 24 days later demonstrates cavitation of the nodule. The lesion was later resected and shown to be *Aspergillus*.

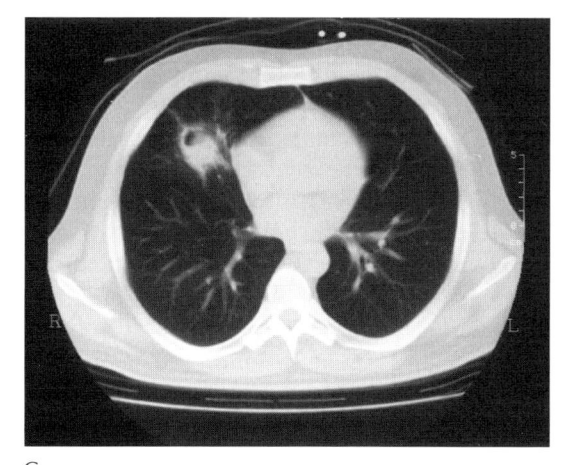

usually causing necrotizing bronchopneumonia or hemorrhagic pulmonary infarction[47] and can lead to massive hemoptysis.[54] Disseminated *Aspergillus* infections can occur with invasion of multiple organs producing embolization, infarction, and hemorrhage.[47] Invasive pulmonary aspergillosis may be difficult to diagnose. Although routine surveillance cultures have not been shown to be predictive or cost effective in general,[55] recovery of aspergillus from the nose or respiratory secretions has been shown to be very highly predictive of invasive pulmonary aspergillosis.[56,57]

Survival rates from invasive pulmonary aspergillosis traditionally ranged from 0% to 35%. A series from the Johns Hopkins Oncology Center, however, reported survival in 13 of 14 patients who received high-dose (1.0 to 1.5 mg/kg/d) amphotericin B with, or without, flucytosine (5-FC). Therapy was initiated a mean of 2 days after the first clinical findings, often prior to the establishment of a definitive diagnosis.[53]

In addition to pulmonary infection, *Aspergillus* also can produce rhinocerebral infection. This infection originates in the sinuses and invades through the soft tissues, cartilage, and bone, leading to destructive lesions of the nose and palate.[47] Patients may present with unusual forms of sinusitis associated with periorbital cellulitis, conjunctivitis, and eschar formation in the nasal passages or on the palate.[7] Cerebral involvement can occur if the infection invades through the base of the skull.[47]

Phycomycetes Infections

An increased incidence of infections with phycomycetes (*Rhizopus, Mucor,* and *Absidia*) has been recognized in cancer patients between the 1960s and 1970s.[46] In this report of the experience at the Memorial Sloan-Kettering Cancer Center (New York, NY), these infections occurred only in patients with hematologic malignancies. Vascular invasion and infarction were typical. The respiratory tract was the most common site of involvement. Radiographic changes included patchy infiltrates, bronchopneumonia, consolidation, cavitation, and cavitation with fungus-ball formation. Presenting symptoms and signs included pleuritic chest pain, hemoptysis, and a pleural friction rub. Cerebral infection was the second most common site of involvement. Most of these infections arose from rhinocerebral infection with invasion of the nasal sinus, penetration of the cribriform plate, and extension into the meninges. Brain lesions also occurred from systemic involvement.[46] Invasive sinus infections have been successfully treated with amphotericin B and surgical resection.[58]

Empiric Treatment of Fungal Infections

Delayed treatment of fungal infections negatively affects survival.[52] In children with neutropenia and fever of unknown origin, broad-spectrum antibiotics reduced the incidence of bacterial infections, but were associated with an increased incidence of infections caused by *Candida* and *Aspergillus*. The empiric addition of amphotericin B, 0.5 mg/kg/d, after 7 days of antibacterial therapy in persistently febrile patients resulted in a trend toward a reduction in fungal infections. There was also a reduction in the number of disseminated fungal infections found as the cause of death at autopsy.[59] In a large controlled trial by the EORTC, 132 patients remaining febrile after 4 days of broad-spectrum antibacterial antibiotics were randomized to receive either empiric amphotericin B or no antifungal therapy. There was a trend toward improved response (resolution of fever) in the amphotericin arm (69%) over the no antifungal therapy arm (53%), but there was no difference in 30-day mortality between the two arms. However, there were six documented fungal infections and four deaths among the 64 patients in the control group compared with only one case of fungemia and no deaths among the 68 patients randomized to receive amphotericin B.[60]

Of the drugs used to treat fungal infections in immunocompromised patients, amphotericin B is the most reliable agent.[61] Amphotericin B, a polyene antibiotic, binds irreversibly to ergosterol, an essential component of fungal cell membranes.[62] This results in increased membrane permeability and diminishes membrane-associated enzyme activity, thus inhibiting fungal cell growth and reproduction.[63] Most empiric regimens have used doses of 0.5 mg/kg daily, but breakthrough infections of *Aspergillus* have been reported. As mentioned above, successful therapy for *Aspergillus* infection has been reported with high-dose amphotericin therapy. Potential adverse reactions include fevers, chills, nausea, vomiting, bronchospasm, hypotension, and even anaphylaxis with drug administration. Many of these effects can be reduced or avoided through pretreatment with acetaminophen, diphenhydramine, and hydrocortisone. Meperidine has been useful in lysing chills.[61] Other side effects of amphotericin B include renal failure, renal tubular acidosis, and renal wasting of potassium and magnesium. The glomerular filtration rate falls 40% in most patients given amphotericin B for more than 2 weeks. The postulated mechanism is tubuloglomerular feedback defined as the reflex vasoconstriction of the afferent arteriole in response to an increased delivery of sodium chloride ions to the distal tubule. Sodium loading has been shown to reduce tubuloglomerular feedback, and saline loading (150 mEq/d) has been shown to have a protective effect in patients administered amphotericin B.[64] Liposomal preparations also hold promise in delivering effective doses with reduced toxicity.[61]

Flucytosine is a fluorinated pyrimidine,[62] which may have activity against invasive pulmonary aspergillosis in combination with amphotericin B.[53] The usual dose is 50 to 150 mg/kg daily in four divided doses. The major toxicity is bone marrow suppression, but this can be attenuated by monitoring blood levels of the drug and maintaining peak serum concentrations of 30 to 60 µg/ml.[53]

Interest has grown in the new triazole drugs. Azoles are inhibitors of ergosterol synthesis and include the imidazoles (miconazole and ketoconazole) and triazoles (fluconazole and itraconazole).[63] Fluconazole is available in both oral and intravenous preparations, whereas itraconazole is available only for oral use. Itraconazole, in contrast to fluconazole, requires an acidic environment for absorption, and absorption is increased when taken with food. The azoles are active against *Candida albicans, Cryptococcus neoformans, Coccidioides immitis, Histoplasma capsulatum, Blastomyces dermatitidis, Paracoccidioides brasiliensis,* and *Sporothrix schenckii.* However, these drugs are less active against nonalbicans *Candida* species and yeast such as *C. krusei* and *Torulopsis glabrata.* Itraconazole, but not fluconazole, is active against *Aspergillus* species. Fluconazole has been shown to be effective for the treatment of cryptococcal meningitis of mild severity in patients with AIDS, and candidemia in patients without neutropenia. The role of azoles in the treatment of disseminated fungal infections in neutropenic patients has not been well defined.[64]

Management of Viral Infections

Viral infections in the immunocompromised oncology patient have recently been recognized to be a major cause of morbidity and mortality. The overwhelming majority of these viruses are members of the herpes family. These viruses are a group consisting of a large envelope of DNA containing viruses which establish latent states within the cells that they infect.[65]

HERPES SIMPLEX VIRUS

Infections with herpes simplex virus (HSV) are being seen with increasing frequency in oncology patients. A study of 130 consecutive patients with acute leukemia at the University of Maryland Cancer Center showed that 48% developed reactivation of herpes simplex virus a median of 17 days into induction chemotherapy.[65] Seropositivity was highly predictive with 66% of seropositive patients experiencing reactivation of infection, and no reactivation in seronegative patients. Recurrent infections with herpes simplex virus in immunocompromised patients tend to be more severe than in the normal host with patients experiencing multiple mucocutaneous ulcers which often persist. These infections occur primarily from the reactivation of latent virus. Primary sites are the nasal, labial, and genital mucocutaneous areas, especially at sites of disruption caused by chemotherapy-induced oral mucositis, periodontitis, and dental appliance or nasogastric tube irritation. Oropharyngeal herpes simplex virus infection usually presents as multiple vesicles that rupture and cause confluent ulceration and can involve the labia, gums, oropharynx and hard and soft palates. Oropharyngeal infections are frequently polymicrobial due to co-infection with bacterial and fungal pathogens.

Herpes simplex virus infections of the respiratory tract can present as nasal mucositis, and can be complicated by cellulitis and epistaxis. Involvement of the tracheobronchial tree can occur, and may be responsible for 5% of nonbacterial pneumonias, occurring mostly in recipients of allogeneic bone marrow transplants. Esophageal HSV infection is a common problem in immunocompromised cancer patients and is mostly likely related to chemotherapy, radiation, graft-versus-host disease, and mechanical trauma from nasogastric intubation. Patients may present with odynophagia, dysphagia, chest pain, nausea and vomiting, fever, and gastrointestinal bleeding. These infections are often polymicrobial in origin with bacteria, fungi (usually *Candida* spp), and occasionally cytomegalovirus. In a study (unpublished) from the University of Maryland Cancer Center, 76 patients were examined endoscopically for symptoms of esophagitis. Sixty-seven of these patients had esophageal inflammation, 39 had an infectious cause, and 7 of these cases had HSV infection, either as a single pathogen, or as part of a polymicrobial infection. Pharyngeal cultures showed low sensitivity, but high specificity, for HSV infection with a positive predictive value of 60%. Disseminated infection involving the liver, lungs, adrenal glands, gastrointestinal tract, central nervous system, and skin can occur in patients without circulating antibodies, or with defects in cellular immunity.

Management of HSV infection is primarily with acyclovir. Acyclovir is an acyclic purine nucleotide which is converted by viral thymidine kinase from acyclovir monophosphate to acyclovir triphosphate. Acyclovir triphosphate acts as a potent inhibitor of viral DNA polymerase. Oral acyclovir is poorly absorbed with a bioavailability of approximately 20%. Nausea is common and generally resolves with continued use. Renal dysfunction has been seen in 5% of patients treated with intravenous acyclovir and has been attributed to crystallization within the renal tubules. Acyclovir has also been associated with neurotoxicity including lethargy, tremor, delirium, and seizures. Neurotoxicity is often preceded by a resting or intention tremor. Toxicities may be avoided with adequate hydration.[65]

Herpes simplex virus infection is associated with a high incidence of antibiotic fever in neutropenic patients, which may be an incentive for the initiation of antiviral therapy. Double-blind, placebo-controlled studies have shown acyclovir to be effective. The usual dosage for HSV infection in immunocompromised patients is 250 mg/m^2 of acyclovir intravenously every 8 hours for 7 days, or oral acyclovir 400 mg five times daily for 10 days. Acyclovir is a virustatic drug and so lack of immediate response does not automatically imply resistance. Resistant HSV infections have been reported, but the incidence is extremely low in patients who have not previously been exposed to acyclovir. Resistant infections may respond to foscarnet.[65]

CYTOMEGALOVIRUS

Cytomegalovirus (CMV) is a ubiquitous virus in the general population with potentially catastrophic consequences for immunosuppressed patients with cancer, particularly patients who have undergone allogeneic bone marrow transplantation. Perinatal infections occur in 1% of newborns in the United States, and adolescents and young adults get infected at a rate of 2% to 10% per year with primary CMV infections usually producing a mononucleosis-like syndrome.[66] Infection in immunocompromised patients is usually from the reactivation of latent virus. In patients undergoing bone marrow transplantation the incidence of cytomegalovirus pneumonitis is 15% to 20% and carries a high mortality rate.[67]

An epidemiologic study at the University of Maryland Cancer Center confirmed the importance of cytomegalovirus as a pathogen in patients undergoing treatment for acute leukemia. A total of 130 consecutive adult patients with acute leukemia undergoing therapy were evaluated for CMV disease. Thirty-one of 97 patients who were seropositive for cytomegalovirus prior to therapy developed disease. Of these, 14 had biopsy-proven infections, 16 had CMV excretion, and 1 had seroconversion alone. Of 33 patients who were seronegative prior to the initiation of therapy, 19 had developed evidence of cytomegalovirus disease, including 5 with biopsy-proven infections, 5 with CMV excretion, and 9 with seroconversion without recovery of virus. In 14 of these 19 patients, CMV infections developed during the period of profound neutropenia, and 8 of these 19 patients died of their cytomegalovirus infection.[29]

The spectrum of disease caused by CMV in cancer patients usually includes pneumonitis, hepatitis, esophagitis, enteritis, and colitis. Cytomegalovirus disease also can lead to prolonged bone marrow suppression. In the University of Maryland Cancer Center study, cytomegalovirus infection occurred at a median of 39 days after beginning induction chemotherapy in seropositive patients and a median of 49 days in seronegative patients.[29]

In the bone marrow transplant population, the seropositivity of the donor and the presence of graft-versus-host disease are important risk factors for the subsequent development of CMV pneumonitis. The incidence of cytomegalovirus pneumonitis is much higher in patients receiving allogeneic bone marrow transplantation than in patients receiving syngeneic or autologous transplantation even though the incidence of CMV infections is similar between these groups. This suggests immune activation in the pathogenesis of interstitial pneumonia.[66]

An accurate diagnosis of cytomegalovirus infection is made by recovering cytomegalovirus in the diseased organ. However, bronchoalveolar lavage, with a sensitivity of 95% to 100% and a specificity of 80% to 100% in diagnosing CMV pneumonitis, is a successful and less invasive diagnostic method. The identification of large cytomegalic cells in tissue establishes a histopathologic diagnosis. Immunocytochemistry with labelled antibody can also yield rapid results. Other molecular techniques have been useful in establishing a diagnosis including *in situ* hybridization with RNA or DNA probes and polymerase chain reaction. However, the definitive test remains the culture of virus on human fibroblasts with the production of typical cytopathic effects resulting in a characteristic plaque formation. The culture technique is prolonged, however, and can take several days or weeks before a diagnosis can be made. A modification of this, the shell vial centrifugation technique, was developed, which allows the diagnosis to be made in 16 to 18 hours by centrifuging the specimen onto fibroblast shell vials and detecting cytomegalovirus with monoclonal antibodies.[68]

Until recently, the outcome from the treatment of cytomegalovirus infections was dismal, with survival rates of only 15% in patients with CMV pneumonitis.[69] The most active agent against cytomegalovirus is the acyclic nucleoside analogue ganciclovir.[67] Although ganciclovir has been demonstrated to eliminate viral excretion and decrease the titer of CMV in lung tissue, the efficacy of ganciclovir, either alone or in combination with corticosteroids in the treatment of CMV pneumonia, has been poor. However, the combination of ganciclovir and intravenous high-dose immunoglobulin has produced significantly better results with survival rates increasing to 50% to 70%. These regimens have been combined in an induction phase of ganciclovir (either 2.5 mg/kg three times a day, or 5 mg/kg twice a day for 14 to 21 days) with intravenous immunoglobulin (400–500 mg/kg every other day for 14 to 21 days, or on days 1, 2, and 7). The induction phase of treatment has been followed by a maintenance treatment with ganciclovir (5 mg/kg once a day for 14 days or 3–5 times weekly for 21 doses) and immunoglobulin (200 mg/kg on days 14 and 21 or 500 mg/kg twice weekly for 8 doses).[69,70] The major toxicity of ganciclovir in these studies was bone marrow suppression.

Foscarnet, a pyrophosphate analogue which does not require viral enzymes to phosphorylate the drug to its active form, directly inhibits DNA polymerase of the herpes viruses, and is the treatment of choice for acyclovir-resistant herpes simplex virus and varicella-zoster virus, and ganciclovir-resistant cytomegalovirus. Renal toxicity is the major side effect of treatment of foscarnet, and it occurs in most patients.[61]

Several strategies have been employed in the prophylaxis of cytomegalovirus infections. These include vaccination with Towne live attenuated virus in high-risk patients prior to receiving kidney transplantation,[71] cytomegalovirus immunoglobulin,[72] and high-dose acyclovir (500 mg/m^2 every 8 hours) in bone marrow transplant patients.[73] Evidence has grown that ganciclovir is also effective for cytomegalovirus prophylaxis. In a study by Goodrich et al,[74] early treatment with ganciclovir in allogeneic bone marrow transplant patients with positive surveillance cultures was shown to reduce the incidence of CMV disease and improve survival. Patients who were seropositive for CMV, or who received marrow from a CMV seropositive donor, underwent surveillance screening for cytomegalovirus excretion from the throat, blood, urine and with surveillance bronchoalveolar lavage. Seventy-two patients with marrow engraftment who were excreting virus were randomly assigned to receive either placebo or ganciclovir (5 mg/kg twice daily for 1 week followed by 5 mg/kg/day for the first 100 days after transplantation). Cytomegalovirus developed in only 3% of the patients randomized to the ganciclovir arm and 43% of the patients assigned to receive placebo. Significant benefit and improved survival was seen in the ganciclovir group at 100 days and 180 days after transplantation. Two recent studies have reported efficacy in ganciclovir prophylaxis in reducing cytomegalovirus infection and disease in recipients of bone marrow transplants, with neutropenia being the most important side effect.[75,76]

SPECIFIC INFECTIOUS PROBLEMS IN IMMUNOCOMPROMISED PATIENTS

Vascular Access Catheter Infections

The use of long-term tunneled intravenous catheters has provided great comfort to cancer patients requiring frequent blood sampling and the administration of blood products and chemotherapy, particularly vesicants (extensively discussed in Chapter 9). However, this practice can be complicated by catheter-related infection. It has been postulated that the incidence of intravenous catheter-related infection may be related to the type of device used. Several strategies have been employed to counter this problem. The mechanism of catheter infection is through the migration of skin flora through the subcutaneous tract with subsequent colonization of the catheter.[77] Infections can also occur through colonization of the hub or by the administration of contaminated fluids.[78] Once established in the lumen of the catheter, microorganisms can adhere to the wall and encase themselves in a glycocalyx making antibiotic penetration more difficult.[79]

Several strategies to combat the infectious complications with the use of central venous access catheters have been developed allowing long-term use. Smooth surface silastic catheters, rather than the rough surface polyvinylchloride catheters, have been used to prevent adherence of bacteria. In addition, catheters are tunneled in a long (at least 10 cm) subcutaneous tunnel to prevent migration of organisms. The addition of a Dacron cuff extends the infection-free survival of the catheter. Catheter infections still occur, however. Attempts to further reduce the incidence of infection have been tried, including the use of the silver-impregnated cuff. However, in a prospective randomized controlled trial of tunneled silastic catheters in cancer patients, the use of the silver-impregnated cuff had no effect in decreasing the incidence of catheter-related infections.[80] Groeger et al,[81] prospectively observed the incidence of infection in long-term intravenous access devices.[81] They found a 43% incidence of catheter-related infection in tunneled catheters compared with an 8% incidence of infection in subcutaneous infusion ports. There were 2.77 infections per 1000 device days for catheters compared with 0.21 infections per 1000 device days for ports. Gram-negative bacilli infections predominated in tunnel catheters (55%) whereas gram-positive cocci predominated in subcutaneous infusion port-related infections (65.5%). The underlying diagnoses of the patients receiving these devices were different, however. Subcutaneous infusion ports were inserted primarily in patients with solid tumors, whereas patients with hematologic malignancies and patients receiving bone marrow transplants had catheters implanted. The patients who had a catheter implanted tended to have more aggressive chemotherapy. Other contributing factors to the decreased incidence of infections in subcutaneous infusion ports include: the need for less frequent irrigation, the lack of requirement for home care, and decreased exposure to environmental contamination. Twenty-five of 26 subcutaneous infusion port-associated bacteremias and fungemias as a first infection were treated successfully without device removal. However, 73 of 264 catheter-related bacteremias and fungemia first infections required removal, with many catheters also developing second, third and fourth bacteremias. The organism responsible for the first infection in catheters was often non-predictive of subsequent infections. Almost all tunnel and port pocket infections, however, required removal.[81] Sterilization of catheter-related fungemias is controversial. In a review of 155 episodes of catheter-associated fungemia at the National Cancer Institute (USA), Lecciones et al[82] found a negative outcome in 82% of the cases managed with antifungal therapy alone. Disseminated fungal infection also occurred in 35% of less severe cases treated with catheter removal. These data suggest that intravascular catheters should be removed in cases of catheter-associated fungemia, and that patients be treated with amphotericin B.[82] Infectious complications of catheters and subcutaneous infusion ports are also discussed extensively in Chapter 9.

In the case of temporary central venous and pulmonary artery catheters, the conventional wisdom was to either routinely replace the catheter, or exchange the catheter over a guidewire to prevent infection. Data from the University of Virginia reported by Cobb et al,[83] showed no benefit from routine replacement of central vascular catheters and an actual increased of risk of infection from the use of guidewire exchanges. These data suggest that temporary vascular catheters should be changed when clinically indicated rather than routinely.

Evaluation of Pulmonary Infiltrates in the Immunocompromised Host

Pulmonary disease is the most common complication in the immunocompromised host and a leading cause of mortality in patients undergoing bone marrow transplantation. The differential diagnosis of pulmonary infiltrates is rather broad, but the diagnoses can be narrowed somewhat by recognition of the patient's underlying condition, the type of impairment of host defense, the timing of the infiltrates and the radiographic appearance. Infiltrates in immunocompromised cancer patients can be caused by extension of the basic underlying disease process to involve the lungs (as in the case of metastatic disease), infection (community acquired and opportunistic), pulmonary reaction to drugs (from cytotoxic chemotherapy, biologic response modifiers, and radiation), or a new process (pulmonary embolism, hemorrhage or pulmonary edema). Frequently, pulmonary infiltrates are caused by a combination of the above. The timing of infection gives some insight as to the differential diagnosis of the pathogens. In patients undergoing bone marrow transplantation, bacterial pneumonias, HSV infections, and *candida* infections tend to occur early, whereas interstitial pneumonia, cytomegalovirus, adenovirus varicella-zoster virus infections, *Aspergillus*, infections with encapsulated organisms, and graft-versus-host disease tend to occur later in the course of therapy.[84] Pulmonary infiltrates can be localized or diffuse. Localized infiltrates include pulmonary infarction, lymphoma, a new bronchocarcinogenic carcinoma, hemorrhage, and infection (usually bacterial, nocardia, fungal, microbacterial, or parasitic). The cause of diffuse infiltrates includes drug reaction, pneumocystis pneumonia, cytomegalovirus, miliary tuberculosis, leukemic infiltrate, bacteremic infection, pulmonary edema, adult respiratory distress syndrome (ARDS), lymphangitic spread of carcinoma, viral pneumonia, fungal infection, or interstitial pneumonitis in bone marrow transplant patients.[85]

The approach to the diagnosis of pulmonary infiltrates in cancer patients has evolved over the last decade (see Chapter 12). Traditionally, open lung biopsy has been the standard for the antemortem diagnosis of pulmonary infiltrates in the immunocompromised cancer patient, with the ability to make a specific diagnosis in over 60% of cases of diffuse pneumonia, as opposed to only a third of cases in which no procedure was performed.[86] Open lung biopsy, however, is associated with significant morbidity. Warner et al[87] reviewed the experience of 11 years at the Mayo Clinic (Rochester, MN) of all patients who had diffuse infiltrates on chest x-ray film and respiratory failure and underwent open lung biopsy. Although open lung biopsy provided a specific diagnosis in 66% and influenced therapy in 70% of patients, only 30% of these patients survived for hospital discharge, and only 11% survived 1 year or more. Nineteen percent had complications, possibly related to the procedure, such as pneumothorax, air leak, subcutaneous emphysema, and myocardial infarction.[87] In general, the highest diagnostic yield for open lung biopsy is in patients with discrete nodules, masses, or cavities. It is less useful in patients with diffuse infiltrates.[88] In view of the relatively high morbidity that has been associated with open lung biopsy, the use of thoracoscopy has expanded to obtaining tissue for pathologic diagnosis. This is extensively discussed in Chapter 12. Thoracic surgeons at the University of Maryland and elsewhere have had excellent results with thoracoscopic lung biopsy.

Fiberoptic bronchoscopy provides the ability to sample the lower respiratory tract through the technique of bronchoalveolar lavage, bronchial washings, bronchial brushings, and transbronchial biopsy.[88,89] Data reported by Stover et al, on the usefulness of bronchoalveolar lavage in the diagnosis of diffuse pulmonary infiltrates in immunocompromised cancer patients demonstrated a sensitivity of at least 80% in the diagnosis of *Pneumocystis carinii* pneumonia, viral pneumonia, fungal pneumonia, bacterial pneumonia and mycobacterial disease.[90] Transbronchial biopsy and bronchial washings or brushings were complementary in increasing the yield.[90] Springmeyer et al[91] demonstrated an 89% sensitivity of diagnosing CMV pneumonia by bronchoscopy in bone marrow transplant recipients with diffuse pulmonary infiltrates. The specificity of bronchoalveolar lavage in diagnosing the cause of diffuse infiltrates remains controversial. *Pneumocystis* and *mycobacterium tuberculosis* as well as *legionella, histoplasma, coccidioides,* and *blastomyces* are usually pathogens whenever isolated.[92] However, the positive predictive value of isolating *Aspergillus, Candida,* or CMV as the cause of the infiltrates is dependent on the immune defect of the host. For instance, CMV isolated from a patient who received an allogeneic bone marrow transplant is more likely to represent disease than if it were isolated from a patient with AIDS, although these patients also die from CMV pneumonitis.[89] The specificity of recovering *Aspergillus* by bronchoalveolar lavage is also controversial. Studies in a heterogeneous group of immunocompromised patients have shown that the recovery of *Aspergillus* by bronchoalveolar lavage may signify either pathogenicity or colonization.[92,93] Therefore, the detection of invasive organisms by transbronchial biopsy is often considered necessary to confirm infection with *Aspergillus*.[89] However, it is worth noting that in the patients reported by Stover et al,[90] most of whom had a hematologic malignancy as their underlying disease, there were no cases in which the lavage fluid cultures gave false–positive results for *Aspergillus* or cryptococcus. Bronchial washings were less specific, however, with half of the positive washings being associated with negative lavage fluid cultures, and no confirmation of invasive pulmonary aspergillosis.[90] The cause of bacterial pneumonia can be difficult to assess because of the contamination of a bronchoscopy specimen by flora colonizing the upper airway. Sensitivity and specificity can be increased, however, to greater than 70%, by the use of a protected catheter brush to obtain uncontaminated specimens and semi-quantitative cultures.[94-96]

Pulmonary surveillance using serial examinations by bronchoscopy or high-resolution CT of the chest, has been used for the early detection of pulmonary complications in high risk immunocompromised patients. Vaughan et al,[97] performed bronchoscopy with bronchoalveolar lavage in patients undergoing high-dose chemotherapy for leukemia or bone marrow transplantation prior to therapy and at the onset of granulocytopenia. Of the 57 patients managed in this program, 40 patients had significant abnormalities noted by bronchoscopy prior to treatment including 12 of 19 patients with no clinically suspected pulmonary disease. Twenty-seven patients had significantly abnormal findings by bronchoscopy or bronchoalveolar lavage at the onset of granulocytopenia, and 13 patients required additional bronchoscopy during aplasia due to new or progressive pul-monary findings. Patients with abnormal pretreatment bronchoscopy had a higher incidence of pulmonary complications than patients with normal pretreatment bronchoscopy, and patients with persistent or new findings on bronchoscopy at the onset of aplasia had a significantly higher incidence of pulmonary complications than patients whose bronchoscopic findings became or remained normal. Twelve patients died during aplasia and all underwent autopsy. In no case was an etiology of pulmonary failure found that had not been documented antemortem.[97] Surveillance CT scans also have promise in reducing complications of pulmonary disease. In patients receiving bone marrow transplantation, a serial high-resolution CT scan of the chest has resulted in a change in clinical management or added confidence to the diagnosis in the presence of normal or nonspecific chest radiographs.[98]

Intra-abdominal Infections

Typhlitis, a necrotizing enterocolitis that typically involves the cecum, is found primarily in children and adults with acute leukemia.[99-101] This disease has been found in association with chemotherapy-related neutropenia and prolonged treatment with broad spectrum antibiotics. The incidence in autopsy series ranges from 10% to 24%. Patients almost universally have fever, and most have abdominal pain and distention. The problem of right lower quadrant pain in the neutropenic cancer patient is extensively discussed in Chapter 1 in which an algorithm for the management of this complicated problem is shown in Figure 1-3.

Other common presentations include peritoneal signs, lower gastrointestinal bleeding, a right lower quadrant mass, vomiting, diarrhea, and respiratory distress. Radiographic findings include a dilated cecum with air fluid levels and dilated small bowel and decreased large bowel gas. Ultrasound and computed tomographic may demonstrate cecal wall thickening or ascites. Perforation can occur with the appearance of intraperitoneal free air. Nonspecific gas patterns are also commonly seen, as well as *pneumatosis intestinalis*. Premortem blood cultures are primarily bacterial with the most common pathogen being *Pseudomonas*, but *E. coli*, *Klebsiella*, *S. aureus*, and alpha streptococci were also prevalent. Postmortem blood cultures may show a predominance of fungal pathogens, primarily *Candida* and *Aspergillus*, suggesting progressive disease is fungal in nature. Patterns of involvement found include cecal involvement alone; cecal and appendicial involvement; cecal and ileal involvement; cecal, ileal and ascending colon involvement; and cecal involvement with sporatic ulcers throughout the intestines.[99] Successful medical and surgical management has been reported.[99-101] Nonoperative management includes antibiotics, fluid and electrolyte replacement, nasogastric suction, and blood product support. Although these patients have been typically considered poor operative risks, a review by Skibber et al of right lower quadrant complications in young patients with leukemia showed a postoperative mortality rate of 8% and a median postoperative duration of survival of 7 months, concluding that these patients could be operated on safely (refer to Chapter 1).[100]

Clostridium Difficile *Colitis*

Clostridium difficile colitis is a significant cause of morbidity in cancer patients. The pathogenesis is related to the inhibition of normal colonic flora by the use of antibiotics, particularly broad-spectrum antibiotics, frequently used in treating infections in cancer patients. *C. difficile* forms spores which can persist in the environment and colonization occurs through the ingestion of these spores.[102] Evidence exists for nosocomial acquisition of *C. difficile*. Transmission occurs through contact with infected patients, contaminated rooms, and hospital personnel with hand carriage of *C. difficile* due to caring for patients who carry the organism.[8] Pathogenic strains of *C. difficile* produce toxins that cause fluid secretion and mucosal damage in the colon. The clinical spectrum of *C. difficile* colitis ranges from mild to moderate diarrhea with abdominal cramping, to severe colitis with fever, nausea, anorexia, malaise and dehydration and, occasionally, colonic bleeding. The more severe form of *C. difficile* disease, pseudomembranous colitis, is associated with more profound diarrhea, abdominal tenderness and systemic manifestations. Endoscopy reveals adherent yellow plaques which range in diameter from 2 to 10 mm or coalesce to cover larger areas of the mucosa. More extreme forms of the disease include acute abdomen, toxic megacolon, colonic perforation, and peritonitis. Radiographic findings include free air associated with colonic perforation, mucosal edema appearing as thumb-printing on an abdominal plain film, or colonic thickening on computed tomography scan of the abdomen. The diagnosis of *C. difficile* colitis is made by the detection of *C. difficile* toxins in the stool. The most accurate test is the tissue culture assay for stool cytotoxin which has a sensitivity and specificity nearing 100%. Cultures for *C. difficile* are less specific because there are nontoxigenic strains of the organism. Latex agglutination tests, although rapid, are poorly sensitive and nonspecific. Other enzyme immunoassays to detect *C. difficile* toxins may have better sensitivity and specificity. The first line treatment for *C. difficile* colitis is oral metronidazole 250 mg four times daily. For patients who do not tolerate or do not respond to oral metronidazole, oral vancomycin 125 mg four times daily is equally effective. Patients who are unable to tolerate oral medication can be treated with parenteral metronidazole. Relapse can occur in 10% to 20% of patients due to the organisms ability to form resistant spores. Patients who receive multiple cycles of chemotherapy with associated neutropenia are particularly susceptible.[102]

PREVENTION OF INFECTION IN THE IMMUNOCOMPROMISED PATIENT

It is clear from the preceding sections that certain patterns of infection can be somewhat predictable. Therefore, strategies to prevent infection have been attempted using this knowledge about typical pathogens, colonization, and portals of entry, but success has been variable. These strategies have been directed at the protection of the host from the environment, the use of prophylactic antimicrobials to suppress colonizing flora, and the restoration of normal host immunity.

Environmental Protection

Because patients are often infected with hospital-acquired flora[5] a logical strategy to prevent infection would be to isolate the patient from the surrounding hospital environment while susceptible to infection. The strictest form of this reverse isolation technique is the total protected environment. This practice includes the use of laminar air flow rooms in which air is passed through high-efficiency particulate air (HEPA) filters, the daily cleaning of all surfaces with antiseptics, the use of sterile supplies, sterile water, and cooked food, the decontamination of the patient's skin and gastrointestinal tract. Visitors stand downstream from the patient wearing sterile caps, masks, gloves, and shoe covers.[103–105] The protected environment is effective in reducing the risk of serious infection in patients with protracted neutropenia,[103] and it has been shown to reduce the incidence and severity of graft-versus-host disease and improve survival in patients receiving bone marrow transplants.[106] Infections by airborne pathogens such as *Aspergillus* species are likely to be prevented by using laminar air flow rooms.

Limitations exist with this technique. Protected environments will not prevent complications from the reactivation of viruses such as HSV and CMV, and therefore they will not reduce deaths caused by CMV pneumonitis. Constant decontamination of the gastrointestinal tract is essential, and compliance with oral nonabsorbable antibiotics can be a problem. A study at the National Cancer Institute (USA) found that less than half the patients in protected environments were compliant with taking oral nonabsorbable antibiotics throughout the study period because of the bad taste, nausea, and diarrhea.[103] In addition, the added benefit of the laminar air flow room has not been observed in all studies. In a controlled trial performed at the University of Maryland Cancer Center, adult patients with acute myeloid leukemia were randomized to receive care in a protected environment including the use of oral nonabsorbable antibiotics, on the ward with oral nonabsorbable antibiotics, or on the ward without oral nonabsorbable antibiotics. No advantage was seen in the group of patients randomized to receive care in the protected environment over the patients randomized to receive care on the ward along with nonabsorbable antibiotics. Patients receiving nonabsorbable antibiotics had a reduced rate of infection and longer median survival than the patients receiving routine care on the ward alone, and patients who stopped taking their prophylactic antibiotics also had an incidence of infection similar to that observed in patients randomized to receive care on the ward alone.[104]

The expense of protected environments is high due to the costs of construction of laminar air flow rooms, sterile supplies, food, water, consumables, and added professional support from dietary, housekeeping, and nursing.[105] Recently the Bone Marrow Transplant Committee of the Eastern Cooperative Oncology Group recommended protective isolation for patients receiving bone marrow transplantation where there is a high institutional prevalence of *Aspergillus* species and for recipients of allogeneic bone marrow transplants.[107]

Oral Antimicrobial Prophylaxis

The gastrointestinal tract is a significant reservoir of potential pathogens. Therefore, the use of antibiotics to suppress colonizing organisms in the gastrointestinal tract to lower the risk of infection is intuitive. Consistent benefits have not been seen, however, with the use of oral nonabsorbable antibiotics to suppress endogenous flora. These agents do not prevent infection by organisms colonizing sites other than the gastrointestinal tract, are poorly tolerated, and can only suppress, not eliminate, gastrointestinal flora.[105] Noncompliance can lead to rapid recolonization with subsequent infection.[104] Furthermore, the emergence of antibiotic-resistant organisms, especially resistance to aminoglycosides, has been seen with the use of oral nonabsorbable antibiotics.[105]

A different prophylactic antibiotic strategy employs the use of absorbable antibiotics. The benefits of this approach were first reported by Hughes et al[108] in 1977. In a trial using trimethoprim-sulfamethoxazole to prevent *Pneumocystis carinii* pneumonia in children treated for acute lymphoblastic leukemia, the incidence of bacterial infections was reduced as well.[108] There may be an added benefit of this approach from selective gut decontamination: the suppression of aerobic flora while leaving anaerobic flora intact. This has also been called "colonization resistance," because a higher bacterial load is needed to colonize the gastrointestinal tract when competing with anaerobic bacteria.[103] Although studies with trimethoprim-sulfamethoxazole prophylaxis appeared promising in reducing the incidence of microbiologically documented infections in neutropenic patients, the need for parenteral antibiotics was unchanged.[105] The importance of compliance with the use of prophylactic absorbable antibiotics was also demonstrated by Pizzo et al,[109] in a randomized, double-blinded, placebo-controlled trial of trimethoprim-sulfamethoxazole plus erythromycin in cancer patients at risk for chemotherapy-related neutropenia. The benefits of prophylactic antibiotics were seen only in the group of patients with excellent compliance and were lost if even occasional doses were missed. The most interesting finding of this study was the significant decrease in the infection rate of patients compliant with placebo. Compliance with medication may reflect compliance with other infection control measures such as hygiene or diet, or it may be an indirect marker of general health (ill patients being less likely to be compliant). Other drawbacks to the use of trimethoprim-sulfamethoxazole prophylaxis include bone marrow suppression and an increased risk of fungal infections.[29]

The quinolones (*e.g.*, norfloxacin and ciprofloxacin) are a class of antibiotics that inhibit DNA gyrase and have had some promise in their use as oral absorbable antibiotic prophylaxis against bacterial infections. Selective gut decontamination is possible with these drugs because they are effective against gram-negative bacteria but not anaerobes. They lack activity, however, against streptococci and coagulase-negative staphylococci that are being found with increasing frequency as causes of infection in neutropenic cancer patients.[29] The emergence of resistant organisms is another disadvantage.[28,29] Because the quinolones are absorbed systemically, it is unclear how much of the prophylaxis is due to systemic antimicrobial activity rather than colonization resistance. It is possible that these drugs prevent microbiologic documentation of infection, thereby causing them to be classified as "fevers of unknown origin."[105] Prophylactic use of the quinolones has not been shown to decrease the incidence of febrile episodes, reduce the need for systemic antibiotic therapy, or improve survival in neutropenic cancer patients.[29] Attempts at prophylaxis against fungal infections have been made using nystatin, clotrimazole, ketoconazole, and miconazole with disappointing results.[29] More recently, trials of antifungal prophylaxis have been performed with fluconazole in neutropenic cancer patients. An early report of its use in patients undergoing bone marrow transplantation was promising, with fewer systemic fungal infections occurring in patients receiving fluconazole.[110] However, a recent study in patients with acute leukemia reported no reduction in invasive fungal infections or use of amphotericin B with prophylactic use of fluconazole.[111] In addition, prophylactic use of fluconazole has not been associated with an increase in survival.[110,111] A disadvantage of antifungal prophylaxis is the emergence of resistant organisms. Wingard et al,[48] reported an increased incidence of infection with *Candida krusei* after fluconazole was adopted for routine use as antifungal prophylaxis. Consequently, the incidence of disseminated candida or other yeast infections was not reduced by fluconazole in this review.

Antiviral prophylaxis is more successful. The administration of intravenous acyclovir 250 mg/m^2 every 8 hours to bone marrow transplant recipients who were seropositive for HSV prevented the appearance of culture-positive HSV lesions in a randomized, double-blinded, placebo-controlled study.[111] Oral acyclovir (800 mg twice daily) also has proven efficacy in preventing infections with HSV.[29]

Restoration of Host Immunity

Restoration of normal host immunity has been attempted in a variety of ways, depending on the immune defect. Specifically, these methods entail the administration of immune globulin to hypogammaglobulinemic patients, the transfusion of leukocytes to neutropenic patients, and the use of growth factors to promote bone marrow recovery.

Hypogammaglobulinemia is a common complication of chronic lymphocytic leukemia. A multicenter randomized, double-blinded, placebo-controlled trial of intravenous immune globulin demonstrated a significant decrease in the incidence of bacterial infections in these patients, although no increase in survival was seen. This practice, however, is expensive, inconvenient for the patient, and produces very little improvement in the quality of life.[112] Early approaches at restoring the granulocyte count have included leukocyte transfusions and lithium administration.[105] These practices had technical limitations (the collection of adequate numbers of functional granulocytes) and toxicity (leukocyte reactions, alloimmunization, lithium toxicity). The use of hematopoietic growth factors for the restoration of normal bone marrow function is more encouraging.

The cytokines granulocyte colony-stimulating factor (G-CSF) and granulocyte-macrophage colony-stimulating factor (GM-CSF) are regulatory glycoproteins that influence myeloid proliferation, differentiation, survival, and function.[113] G-CSF and GM-CSF are commercially available through the use of recombinant DNA technology. The administration of growth factors after cytotoxic chemotherapy does not prevent neutropenia, but it does shorten its duration.[113,114] Studies in patients receiving standard cytotoxic chemotherapy, and some studies in patients receiving bone marrow transplants, have demonstrated a decrease in neutropenia or its duration with the use of G-CSF or GM-CSF. Decreases in the incidence of documented infections, days of fever, days on antibiotics, and hospital days, however, were not universally seen (refer to Chapter 17 for further discussions of the use of growth factors).[114]

There are also drawbacks to the use of growth factors. Adverse effects range from bone pain (with either drug) to myalgias, flushing, rash, venous thrombosis, and a capillary-leak syndrome with fluid retention, pleural and pericardial inflammation and effusions, and arterial oxygen desaturations (with GM-CSF).[113] Fever, occurring as a side-effect of GM-CSF, can potentially defeat the desired benefit of the drug.[113,114]

SUMMARY

Infections are a major source of morbidity and mortality in the cancer patient. It is incumbent upon the treating surgeon to understand the interactions between infections and surgical therapy in these complex patients. The cancer patient is predisposed to the development of infection as a result of disruption of barrier function (*e.g.*, the surgical wound), defects in cellular immunity, defects in humoral immunity, alterations in host flora and defective phagocytosis. Environmental factors also increase the risk of infection, particularly by alterations in host flora.

The evaluation of febrile episodes in the neutropenic patient remains a clinical challenge. The clinical presentation of infection can be subtle, yet delay in initiating therapy can lead to disastrous results. The usual sites of infection remain the natural barriers that are vulnerable to damage by cytotoxic therapy. Most of the pathogens responsible for clinically significant infection are bacterial. Antibiotic strategies usually combine an aminoglycoside with an antipseudomonal penicillin. Single agent strategies also have been used. Although a majority of the responsible organisms have been gram-negative, there has been a recent shift to include an increased number of gram-positive organisms. Fungal pathogens, most commonly *Candida* and *Aspergillus*, are seen with increasing frequency. Amphotericin B is the standard therapy. Viral infections are also a significant cause of morbidity and mortality in the immunocompromised host.

Long-term intravenous catheters are complicated by infections, despite the fact that they have a Dacron cuff and are tunneled in the subcutaneous tissue (refer also to Chapter 9). Although bacterial infections can occasionally be treated without removal of the device, catheter-associated fungemia usually necessitates removal of the device. Pulmonary infiltrates are a common problem in cancer patients and require specific diagnostic tests to maximize therapeutic results (refer also to Chapter 12). Although open lung biopsy has been the traditional method of obtaining tissue, newer techniques, most notably thoracoscopic biopsy, has more recently been used with excellent results. Fiberoptic bronchoscopy may also be of use. Intra-abdominal infections, especially in the neutropenic patient are a clinical and diagnostic challenge (refer also to Chapter 1). Therapy may be nonoperative or surgical, depending on the specific clinical presentation.

Resistance to infection requires the integrity of a variety of host defenses that have a complex interaction. Knowledge of the specific defect in host defenses, as well as the nature of the hostile environment, can provide clues to particular patterns of infection. Frequently, the difficulty in establishing a microbiologically documented diagnosis, combined with the prognosis of an infected, defenseless host, creates the need for empiric antimicrobial coverage. Methods of preventing infection have been met with variable success, but the use of cytokines to restore immunity is promising.

REFERENCES

1. Rubin RH, Ferraro MJ. Understanding and diagnosing infectious complications in the immunocompromised host. Current issues and trends. Hematol Oncol Clin North Am 1993; 7:795.
2. Fauci AS. Basic mechanisms of activation and immunoregulation of human B-lymphocyte responses. In: Fauci AS, moderator. Activation and regulation of human immune responses: implications in normal and disease states. Ann Intern Med 1983;99:61.
3. Nossal GJV. Current concepts: Immunology: The basic components of the immune system. N Engl J Med 1987;316:1320.
4. Chanock S. Evolving risk factors for infectious complications of cancer therapy. Hematol Oncol Clin North Am. 1993;7:771.
5. Schimpff SC, Young VM, Greene WH, et al. Origin of infection in acute nonlymphocytic leukemia. Significance of hospital acquisition of potential pathogens. 1972;77:707.
6. Schimpff SC. Gram-negative bacteremia. Support Care Cancer 1993;1:5.
7. Mahoney DH, Steuber CP, Starling KA, et al. An outbreak of aspergillosis in children with acute leukemia. J Pediatr 1979;95:70.
8. McFarland LV, Mulligan ME, Kwok RYY, Stamm WE. Nosocomial acquisition of *clostridium difficile* infection. N Engl J Med 1989;320:204.
9. Nosocomial enterococci resistant to vancomycin—United States 1989–1993. MMWR 1993;42:597.
10. McGowan JE Jr. Changing etiology of nosocomial bacteremia and fungemia and other hospital-acquired infections. Rev Infect Dis 1985;7:S371.
11. Chow JW, Fine MJ, Shlaes DM, et al. *Enterobacter* bacterium: clinical features and emergence of antibiotic resistance during therapy. Ann Intern Med 1991;115:585.
12. Pegues DA, Carson LA, Anderson RL, et al. Outbreak of *Pseudomonas cepacia* bacteremia in oncology patients. Clin Infect Dis 1993;16:407.
13. Yamagishi Y, Fujita J, Takigawa K. Clinical features of *Pseudomonas cepacia* pneumonia in an epidemic among immunocompromised patients. Chest 1993;103:1706.
14. Fauci AS. The human immunoregulatory network. In: Fauci AS, moderator. Immunomodulators in clinical medicine. Ann Intern Med 1987;106:421.
15. Dinarello CA, Mier JW. Lymphokines. N Engl J Med 1987;317:940.
16. Robinson BE, Donowitz GR. Infections in patients with cancer: host defenses and the immune-compromised state. In: Moossa AR, Schimpff SC, Robson MC, eds. Comprehensive textbook of oncology. 2nd ed. Baltimore: Williams and Wilkens, 1991:1733.
17. Fahey JL. Scoggins R, Utz JP, et al. Infection, antibody response and gamma globulin components in multiple myeloma and macroglobulinemia. Am J Med 1973;35:698.

18. Pizzo PA, Meyers J, Freifeld AG, Walsh T. Infections in the Cancer Patient. In: DeVita VT Jr, Hellman S, Rosenberg SA, eds. Cancer: principles and practice of oncology. 4th ed. Philadelphia: J.B. Lippincott, 1993:2292.
19. Bodey GP. Infection in cancer patients. A continuing association. Am J Med 1986;81(Suppl 1)A:11.
20. Schimpff SC, O'Connell MJ, Greene WH, Wiernik PH. Infections in 92 splenectomized patients with Hodgkin's Disease. A clinical review. Am J Med 1975;59:695.
21. Abrahamsen AF, Borge L, Holte H. Infection after splenectomy for Hodgkin's disease. Acta Oncologica 1990;29:167.
22. Anaissie E, Kontoyiannis DP, Kantarjian H, et al. Listeriosis in patients with chronic lymphocytic leukemia who were treated with fludarabine and prednisone. Ann Intern Med 1992;117:466.
23. Pizzo PA, Robichaud RN, Wesley R, Commers JR. Fever in the pediatric and young adult patient with cancer. Medicine 1982;61:153.
24. Bodey GP, Buckley M, Sathe YS, Freireich EJ. Quantitative relationships between circulating leukocytes and infection in patients with acute leukemia. Ann Intern Med 1966;64:328.
25. Schimpff SC. Infections in patients with cancer: overview and epidemiology. In: Moossa AR, Schimpff SC, Robson MC, eds. Comprehensive textbook of oncology. 2nd ed. Baltimore: Williams and Wilkens, 1991:1720.
26. Carlisle PS, Gucalp R, Wiernik PH. Nosocomial infections in neutropenic cancer patients. Infect Control Hosp Epidemiol 1993; 14:320.
27. Wade JC, Schimpff SC, Newman KA, Wiernik PH. *Staphylococcus epidermidis*: an increasing cause of infection in patients with granulocytopenia. Ann Intern Med 1982;97:503.
28. Pizzo PA. Management of fever in patients with cancer and treatment-induced neutropenia. N Engl J Med 1993;328:1323.
29. Wade JC. Management of infection in patients with acute leukemia. Hematol Oncol Clin North Am 1993;7:293.
30. Sickles EA, Greene WH, Wiernik PH. Clinical presentation of infection in granulocytopenic patients. Arch Intern Med 1975;135:715.
31. Love LI, Schimpff SC, Schiffer CA, Wiernik PH. Improved prognosis for granulocytopenic patients with gram-negative bacteremia. Am J Med 1980;68:643.
32. Bodey GP, Jadeja L, Elting L. *Pseudomonas* bacteremia. Retrospective analysis of 410 episodes. Arch Intern Med 1985;145:1621.
33. DeJongh CA, Joshi JH, Thompson BW, et al. A double beta-lactam combination versus an aminoglycoside-containing regimen as empiric antibiotic therapy for febrile granulocytopenic cancer patients. Am J Med 1986;80:101.
34. Hughes WT, Armstrong D, Bodey GP, et al. Guidelines for the use of antimicrobial agents in neutropenic patients with unexplained fever. J Infect Dis 1990;161:381.
35. Pizzo PA, Hathorn JW, Hiemenz J, et al. A randomized trial comparing ceftazidime alone with combination antibiotic therapy in cancer patients with fever and neutropenia. N Engl J Med 1986;315:552.
36. Anonymous. The design, analysis, and reporting of clinical trials on the empirical antibiotic management of the neutropenic patient. Report of a consensus panel. J Infect Dis 1990;161:397.
37. Winston DJ, Ho WG, Bruckner DA, Champlin RE. Beta-lactam antibiotic therapy in febrile granulocytopenic patients: a randomized trial comparing cefoperazone plus piperacillin, ceftazidime plus pipercillin, and imipenem alone. Ann Intern Med 1991;115:849.
38. Rolston KVI, Berkley P, Bodey GP, et al. A comparison of imipenem to ceftazidime with or without amikacin as empiric therapy in febrile neutropenic patients. Arch Intern Med 1992;152:283.
39. Karp JE, Dick JD, Angelopulos C, et al. Empiric use of vancomycin during prolonged treatment induced granulocytopenia. Am J Med 1986;81:237.
40. EORTC International Antimicrobial Therapy Cooperative Group and the NCI of Canada-Clinical Trials Group: Vancomycin added to empirical combination antibiotic therapy for fever in granulocytopenic cancer patients. J Infect Dis 1991;163:951.
41. Rubenstein EB, Rolston K, Benjamin RS, et al. Outpatient treatment of febrile episodes in low-risk neutropenic patients with cancer. Cancer 1993;71:3640.
42. Pizzo PA. After empiric therapy: what to do until the granulocyte comes back. Rev Infect Dis 1987;9:214.
43. Saral R. *Candida* and *aspergillus* infections in immunocompromised patients: an overview. Rev Infect Dis 1991;13:487.
44. Anaissie E, Bodey GP, Kantarjian H. New spectrum of fungal infections in patients with cancer. Rev Infect Dis 1989;11:369.
45. Walsh TJ, Lee J, Lecciones J. Empiric therapy with amphotericin B in febrile granulocytopenic patients. Rev Infect Dis 1991;13:496.
46. Meyer RD, Rosen P, Armstrong D. Phycomycosis complicating leukemia and lymphoma. Ann Intern Med 1972;77:871.

47. Bodey GP. Fungal infections and fever of unknown origin in neutropenic patients. Am J Med 1986;80:(Suppl 5C):112.
48. Wingard JR, Merz WG, Rinaldi MG, et al. Increase in *Candida krusei* infection among patients with bone marrow transplantation and neutropenia treated prophylactically with fluconazole. N Engl J Med 1991;325:1274.
49. Goldman M, Pottage JC, Weaver DC. *Candida krusei* fungemia: report of 4 cases and review of the literature. Medicine 1993;72:143.
50. Thaler M, Pastakia B, Shawker TH, O'Leary T, Pizzo PA. Hepatic candidiasis in cancer patients: the evolving picture of the syndrome. Ann Intern Med 1988;108:88.
51. Haron E, Vartivarian S, Anaissie E, Dekmezian R, Bodey GP. Primary *Candida* pneumonia. Experience at a large cancer center and review of the literature. Medicine 1993;72:137.
52. Aisner J, Schimpff SC, Wiernik PH. Treatment of invasive aspergillosis: relation of early diagnosis and treatment to response. Ann Intern Med 1977;86:539.
53. Burch PA, Karp JE, Merz WG, Kuhlman JE, Fishman EK. Favorable outcome of invasive aspergillosis in patients with acute leukemia. J Clin Oncol 1987;5:1985.
54. Panos RJ, Barr LF, Walsh TJ, Silverman HJ. Factors associated with fatal hemoptysis in cancer patients. Chest 1988;94:1008.
55. Kramer BS, Pizzo PA, Robichaud KJ, Witebsky F, Wesley R. Role of serial microbiologic surveillance and clinical evaluation in the management of cancer patients with fever and granulocytopenia. Am J Med 1982;72:561.
56. Aisner J, Murillo J, Schimpff SC, Steere AC. Invasive aspergillosis in acute leukemia: correlation with nose cultures and antibiotic use. Ann Intern Med 1979;90:4.
57. Yu VL, Muder RR, Poorsattar A. Significance of isolation of aspergillus from the respiratory tract in diagnosis of invasive pulmonary aspergillosis: results from a three-year prospective study. Am J Med 1986;81:249.
58. Eden OB, Santos J. Effective treatment for rhinopulmonary mucormycosis in a boy with leukaemia. Arch Dis Childhood 1979;54:557.
59. Pizzo PA, Robichaud KJ, Gill FA, Witebsky FG. Empiric antibiotic and antifungal therapy for cancer patients with prolonged fever and granulocytopenia. Am J Med 1982;72:101.
60. EORTC International Antimicrobial Therapy Cooperative Group. Empiric antifungal therapy in febrile granulocytopenic patients. Am J Med. 1989;86:668.
61. Freifeld AG. The antimicrobial armamentarium. Hematol Oncol Clin North Am 1993;7(4):813.
62. Sande MA, Mandell GL. Antimicrobial agents. In: Goodman LS, Gilman A, eds. Goodman and Gilman's the pharmacological basis of therapeutics. 6th ed. New York: Macmillan, 1980:1222.
63. Como JA, Dismukes WE. Oral azole drugs as systemic antifungal therapy. N Engl J Med 1994;330:263.
64. Branch RA. Prevention of amphotericin B-induced renal impairment: a review on the use of sodium supplementation. Arch Intern Med 1988;148:2389.
65. Bustamante CI and Wade JC. Herpes simplex virus infection in the immunocompromised cancer patient. J Clin Oncol 1991;9:1903.
66. Zaia JA. Epidemiology and pathogenesis of cytomegalovirus disease. Semin Hematol 1990;27:(Suppl 1):5.
67. Emanuel D. Treatment of cytomegalovirus disease. Semin Hematol 1990;27(2)(Suppl 1):22.
68. Spector SA. Diagnosis of cytomegalovirus infection. Semin Hematol 1990;27:(Suppl 1):11.
69. Reed EC, Bowden RA, Dandliker PS, et al. Treatment of cytomegalovirus pneumonia with ganciclovir and intravenous cytomegalovirus immunoglobulin in patients with bone marrow transplants. Ann Intern Med 1988;15:783.
70. Emanuel D, Cunningham I, Jules-Elysee K, et al. Cytomegalovirus pneumonia after bone marrow transplantation successfully treated with the combination of canciclovir and high-dose intravenous immune globulin. Ann Intern Med 1988;109:777.
71. Plotkin SA, Starr SE, Friedman HM, et al. Effect of towne live virus vaccine on cytomegalovirus disease after renal transplant. A controlled trial. Ann Intern Med 1991;114:525.
72. Balfour HH Jr. Options for prevention of cytomegalovirus disease. Ann Intern Med 1991;114:598.
73. Meyers JD, Reed EC, Shepp DH, et al. Acyclovir for prevention of cytomegalovirus infection and disease after allogeneic marrow transplantation. N Engl J Med 1988;318:70.
74. Goodrich JM, Mori M, Gleaves CA, et al. Early treatment with ganciclovir to prevent cytomegalovirus disease after allogeneic bone marrow transplantation. N Engl J Med 1991;325:1601.
75. Winston DJ, Ho WG, Bartoni K. Ganciclovir prophylaxis of cytomegalovirus infection and disease in allogeneic bone marrow trans-

75. (continued) plant recipients: results of a placebo-controlled, double-blind trial. Ann Intern Med 1993;118:179.
76. Goodrich JM, Bowden RA, Fisher L, et al. Ganciclovir prophylaxis to prevent cytomegalovirus disease after allogeneic marrow transplant. Ann Intern Med 1993;118:173.
77. Maki DG, Weise CE, Sarafin HW. A semiquantitive culture method for indentifying intravenous-catheter-related infection. N Engl J Med 1977;296:1305.
78. Linares J, Sitges-Serra A, Garau J, Perez JL, Martin R. Pathogenesis of catheter sepsis: a prospective study with quantitative and semiquantitative cultures of catheter hub and segments. J Clin Microbiol 1985;21:357.
79. Cheesbrough JS, Elliott TSJ, Finch RG. A morphological study of bacterial colonisation of intravenous cannulae. J Med Microbiol 1985; 19:149.
80. Groeger JS, Lucas AB, Coit D, et al. A prospective, randomized evaluation of the effect of silver impregnated subcutaneous cuffs for preventing tunneled chronic venous access catheter infections in cancer patients. Ann Surg 1993;218(2):206.
81. Groeger JS, Lucas AB, Thaler HT, et al. Infectious morbidity associated with long-term use of venous access devices in patients with cancer. Ann Intern Med 1993;119:1168.
82. Lecciones JA, Lee JW, Navarro EE, et al. Vascular catheter-associated fungemia in patients with cancer: analysis of 155 episodes. Clin Infect Dis 1992;14:875.
83. Cobb DK, High KP, Sawyer RG, et al. A controlled trial of scheduled replacement of central venous and pulmonary-artery catheters. N Engl J Med 1992;327:1062.
84. Masur H. The differential diagnosis of respiratory disease in patient subgroups. In: Shelhamer JH, moderator. Respiratory disease in the immunosuppressed patient. Ann Intern Med 1992;117:415.
85. Rosenow EC III, Wilson WR, Cockerill FR III. Pulmonary disease in the immunocompromised host (first of two parts). Mayo Clin Proc 1985;60:473.
86. Singer C, Armstrong D, Rosen PP, Walzer PD, Yu B. Diffuse pulmonary infiltrates in immunosuppressed patients: prospective study of 80 cases. Am J Med 1979;66:110.
87. Warner DO, Warner MA, Divertie MB. Open lung biopsy in patients with diffuse pulmonary infiltrates and acute respiratory failure. Am Rev Respir Dis 1988;137:90.
88. Suffredini A. Diagnosis of infection: noninvasive and invasive procedures. In: Shelhamer JH, moderator. Respiratory disease in the immunosuppressed patient. Ann Intern Med 1992;117:415.
89. Baughman RP. Use of bronchoscopy in the diagnosis of infection in the immunocompromised host. Thorax 1994;49:3.
90. Stover DE, Zaman MB, Hajdu SI, et al. Bronchoalveolar lavage in the diagnosis of diffuse pulmonary infiltrates in the immunosuppressed host. Ann Intern Med 1984; 101:1.
91. Springmeyer SC, Hackman RC, Holle R, et al. Use of bronchoalveolar lavage to diagnose acute diffuse pneumonia in the immunocompromised host. J Infect Dis 1986;4:604.
92. Pisani RJ, Wright AJ. Clinical utility of bronchoalveolar lavage in immunocompromised hosts. Mayo Clin Proc 1992;67:221.
93. Martin WJ II, Smith TF, Sanderson DR, et al. Role of bronchoalveolar lavage in the assessment of opportunistic pulmonary infections: utility and complications. Mayo Clin Proc 1987;62:549.
94. Wimberley NW, Bass JB Jr., Boyd BW, et al. Use of a bronchoscopic protected catheter brush for the diagnosis of pulmonary infections. Chest 1982;81:556.
95. Xaubet A, Torres A, Marco F, et al. Pulmonary infiltrates in immunocompromised patients: diagnostic value of telescoping plugged catheter and bronchoalveolar lavage. Chest 1989; 95:130.
96. Thorpe JE, Baughman RP, Frame PT, Wesseler TA, Staneck JL. Bronchoalveolar lavage for diagnosing acute bacterial pneumonia. J Infect Dis 1987;155:855.
97. Vaughan WP, Linder J, Robbins R, Arneson M, Rennard SI. Pulmonary surveillance using bronchoscopy and bronchoalveolar lavage during high-dose antineoplastic therapy. Chest 1991;99:105.
98. Barloon TJ, Galvin JR, Mori M, Stanford W, Gingrich RD. High-resolution ultrafast chest CT in the clinical management of febrile bone marrow transplant patients with normal or nonspecific chest roentgenograms. Chest 1991;99:928.
99. Katz JA, Wagner ML, Gresik MV, Mahoney DH, Fernbach DJ. Typhlitis: an 18-year experience and postmortem review. Cancer 1990; 65:1041.
100. Skibber JM, Matter GJ, Pizzo PA, Lotze MT. Right lower quadrant pain in young patients with leukemia: a surgical perspective. Ann Surg 1987;206:711.
101. Varki AP, Armitage JO, Feagler JR. Typhlitis in acute leukemia. Successful treatment by early surgical intervention. Cancer 1979;43: 695.

102. Kelly CP. Pothoulakis C, LaMont JT. *Clostridium difficile* colitis. N Engl J Med 1994;330:257.
103. Pizzo PA. Antimicrobial prophylaxis in the immunosuppressed cancer patient. In: Remington JS, Swartz MN, eds. Current clinical topics in infectious diseases. Vol. 4. New York: McGraw Hill, 1983:153.
104. Schimpff SC, Greene WH, Young VM, et al. Infection prevention in acute nonlymphocytic leukemia. Laminar air flow room reverse isolation with oral, nonabsorbable antibiotic prophylaxis. Ann Intern Med 1975;82:351.
105. Pizzo PA. Considerations for the prevention of infectious complications in patients with cancer. Rev Infect Dis 1989;11:S1551.
106. Meyers JD. Infection in bone marrow transplant recipients. Am J Med 1986;81:suppl 1A:27.
107. Rowe JM, Lazarus HM. Are protected environments necessary for recipients of bone marrow transplants? Ann Intern Med 1994;121:76.
108. Hughes WT, Kuhn S, Chaudhary S, et al. Successful chemoprophylaxis for *Pneumocystis carinii* pneumonitis. N Engl J Med 1977;297:1419.
109. Pizzo PA, Robichaud KJ, Edwards BK, et al. Oral antibiotic prophylaxis in patients with cancer: a double-blind randomized placebo-controlled trial. J Pediatr 1983;102:125.
110. Goodman JL, Winston DJ, Greenfield RA. A controlled trial of fluconazole to prevent fungal infections in patients undergoing bone marrow transplantation. N Engl J Med 1992;326:845.
111. Saral R, Burns WH, Laskin OL, Santos GW, Lietman PS. Acyclovir prophylaxis of herpes-simplex-virus infections: a randomized, double-blind, controlled trial in bone-marrow-transplant recipients. N Engl J Med 1981;305:63.
112. Weeks JC, Tierney MR, Weinstein MC. Cost effectiveness of prophylactic intravenous immune globulin in chronic lymphocytic leukemia. N Engl J Med 1991;325:81.
113. Lieschke GJ, Burgess AW. Granulocyte colony-stimulating factor and granulocyte-macrophage colony-stimulating factor. Part I. A review article. N Engl J Med 1992;327:285.
114. Lieschke GJ, Burgess AW. Granulocyte colony-stimulating factor and granulocyte-macrophage colony-stimulating factor. Part II. A review article. N Engl J Med 1992;327:99.

17

Cancer and Therapy-Related Hematologic Abnormalities

MEYER R. HEYMAN

Bone marrow function may be disturbed in cancer patients as a result of primary bone marrow disorders (*e.g.*, leukemia and myeloma), metastases (*e.g.*, breast and lung cancer) as well as myelosuppressive chemotherapy and radiation therapy. The production of all elements including red cells, neutrophils, and platelets may be impaired, although often to different degrees depending on the type of underlying malignancy and the therapy administered.

Similarly, the coagulation (and fibrinolytic) mechanisms may be dysfunctional in cancer patients as a result of impaired production of coagulation factors (*i.e.*, drug- or tumor-induced hepatic injury) or abnormal consumption of coagulation factors such as occurs in tumor-driven, disseminated intravascular coagulation (DIC). Such abnormalities may result in an abnormal predisposition for hemorrhage and thrombosis.

It is incumbent on the surgeon to be aware of both bone marrow and coagulation abnormalities in order to provide safe and appropriate pre-, intra-, and postoperative management. Hematologic and coagulation abnormalities may dictate both the timing and extent of surgical intervention. Close cooperation among the surgeon, hematologist–oncologist, anesthesiologist, and the blood bank is imperative in guiding complicated patients through surgical interventions. This chapter provides both general and practical guidelines to familiarize surgeons with the hematologic complications of malignancy and to aid in their recognition and management.

CHEMOTHERAPY-INDUCED MYELOSUPPRESSION

The effect of a particular chemotherapeutic agent on bone marrow function depends on its mechanisms of action, dose, and schedule of administration. The surgeon should be aware when myelosuppression is likely to be maximal as well as its duration so that elective surgery can be performed when bone marrow recovery has occurred. In emergent situations it is important for the surgeon to know the extent and duration of myelosuppression to be certain that adequate amounts of blood products will be available. A further discussion of the preoperative considerations in patients who have received chemotherapy is found in Chapter 13.

In general, drugs that interfere with DNA synthesis and repair (*i.e.*, antimetabolites—cytosine arabinoside, methotrexate; topoisomerase inhibitors; and anthracyclines—adriamycin, mitoxantrone, etoposide) and which are given in large pulse doses produce rapidly developing (7 to 14 days) variably severe neutropenia and thrombocytopenia often resulting in the need for platelet transfusion as well as neutropenic fever (see

Chapter 16) requiring empiric antibiotic therapy. These agents also are the most likely to produce severe mucositis given their predominant effect on rapidly dividing cells which requires continual DNA synthesis. Such mucositis compounds the risk of neutropenia-related infection and thrombocytopenic bleeding because of interruption of normal mucosal barriers. Mucositis is further discussed in Chapter 4. Myelosuppression often lasts for 7 to 14 days but can be prolonged in patients who have been previously treated with multiple doses of the same or other chemotherapeutic agents. In many instances, the period of severe neutropenia may be shortened by the administration of recombinant hematopoietic growth factors such as granulocyte or granulocyte-macrophage colony stimulating factors (G-CSF, GM-CSF),[1,2] but only if they are given shortly after the completion of chemotherapy.

The duration and severity of myelosuppression caused by the various alkylating agents (*i.e.*, cyclophosphamide, melphalan, chlorambucil, busulfan) are variable and depend on the specific agent, the dose and schedule of administration, and the degree of toxicity directed toward hematopoietic stem cells. Although many alkylating agents have enhanced toxicity for dividing as compared to resting cells, as a group they cause considerably less mucosal disruption than the drugs discussed previously. Those alkylating agents that have the greatest toxicity to hematopoietic stem cells (*i.e.*, melphalan, chlorambucil) may have considerable cumulative toxicity and result in prolonged neutropenia and thrombocytopenia. The nitrosoureas (*i.e.*, Carmustine (BCNU), Lomustine (CCNU)) are examples of such drugs. Of the alkylating agents, cyclophosphamide is associated with less marked and less prolonged thrombocytopenia.

To take advantage of steep dose-response curves for particular drugs against various malignancies, myeloablative doses of chemotherapy followed by autologous bone marrow transplantation is an increasingly used modality of therapy. This is particularly true for some of the more common solid tumors such as breast cancer.[3] The use of growth factors (*e.g.*, G-CSF and GM-CSF) to shorten the duration of neutropenia and more recently the use of mobilized autologous peripheral blood stem cells to shorten the period of thrombocytopenia has become standard practice in many centers.[4,5]

ANEMIA IN THE CANCER PATIENT

Anemia is present in almost all cancer patients at sometime during the course and treatment of their disease. Anemia in the cancer patient may be caused by bone marrow metastases, primary bone marrow disorders (leukemia, lymphoma), blood loss (colon, gastric, uterine cancer), chemotherapy and radiation-induced myelosuppression, immune destruction (chronic lymphatic leukemia, drug induced), and non-immune hemolysis as may occur in DIC and in cancer-related thrombotic microangiopathy (Table 17-1).

Anemia is the most easily managed of the blood cytopenias due to the immediate availability of packed red cells in all centers and their long shelf life (42 days). This may not always be the case, however, because patients may be sensitized to multiple red cell antigens due to previous transfusion or multiple pregnancies and may be extremely difficult if not impossible to crossmatch. In such instances it may require hours or even days before compatible blood can be obtained from rare donor pools maintained by the American Red Cross in the United States. A sample of red cells and serum should be sent to the blood bank promptly for typing and antibody screening in anticipation of the need for transfusion. A sufficient number of compatible units should be available in the local hospital blood bank to cover any unexpected intra- or postoperative bleeding.

Autologous Blood Donation

The transfusion of pre-donated autologous blood during surgical procedures is unequiv-

Table 17-1. Cause of Cancer-Related Anemia

IMPAIRED RBC PRODUCTION		
	• Marrow invasion	Leukemia, myeloma, breast, and lung cancer
	• Marrow fibrosis	Myeloproliferative disorder, radiation
	• Myelosuppression	Chemotherapy, radiotherapy
	• Vitamin deficiency	B_{12} (postgastrectomy, ileal resection, blind loop)
		Folate (alcoholism, malabsorption, poor dietary intake increased need—hemolysis)
		Iron (blood loss—GI and uterine malignancies)
	• Impaired erythropoietin secretion	Anemia of chronic disease, cancer, malnutrition, infection, chronic inflammation
RBC SEQUESTRATION		
	• Hypersplenism	Splenomegaly - myeloproliferative disorders, portal hypertension with cirrhosis, hairy cell leukemia, lymphoma
INCREASED RBC DESTRUCTION		
	• Immune hemolysis	CLL and other lymphoproliferative disorders
		Drug induced—penicillin, *cis*-platinum
	• Microangiopathic (mechanical destruction)	Cancer-related DIC, cancer-related thrombotic microangiopathy (colon cancer-nitrosoureas)
RBC LOSS		
	• Bleeding	Gastrointestinal malignancies
		Uterine malignancies
		Gastritis, peptic ulcer

ocally the safest for the patient as it absolutely avoids the risk of all transfusion-related infections and the risk of alloimmunization to nonself red cell antigens.

Autologous blood donation has been shown to be a practical, effective method of conserving homologous blood resources in both elective cardiovascular and orthopedic surgery.[6,7] Goodnough[8] was able to demonstrate a decrease in homologous blood exposure from 41% to 17% in patients undergoing orthopedic surgery.

Unfortunately, autologous donation is not possible for many if not most cancer patients because they often are anemic with chemotherapy-induced myelosuppression and surgical intervention is often of an emergent nature. Also, many patients require much greater amounts of red cells as well as other blood products (plasma, platelets), which preclude autologous donation. Nonetheless, autologous blood should be collected if possible for elective surgical procedures. Adequate lead time prior to planned surgery should be allowed to collect a sufficient volume of autologous blood because the American Association of Blood Banks guidelines require a minimum hematocrit of 33 for donation and that blood be collected no more than every 3 days and not within 72 hours of surgery.[9] It is important that the collection of autologous blood be restricted to those instances in which there is a significant risk for major intraoperative blood loss requiring replacement. Recent data have suggested that autologous blood transfusion is unnecessarily expensive and in many instances autologous blood is collected needlessly resulting in unnecessary costs and waste of blood bank time and resources.[10]

Many physicians minimize the risks of standard transfusions in cancer patients because of their often limited life expectancy. There are, however, a number of reports of transfusion-related AIDS in leukemic patients, some of whom died in long-term remission and were possibly cured of their leukemia.[11] Therefore, autologous donations should certainly be considered for patients with clinically localized malignancies in whom curative surgery is contemplated. Although in some studies a relationship between perioperative homologous transfusion and an increased risk of tumor recurrence has been suggested,[12] it is not at all clear that homologous transfusion-related immunosuppression (and presumably decreased tumor surveillance) is of clinical relevance. One cannot support the use of autologous transfusion to reduce these unproved risks.

Recombinant Human Erythropoietin (rhEPO)

Erythropoietin (EPO), a glycoprotein hormone produced primarily in the kidney, is essential for bone marrow production of red blood cells (RBC). Sensors in the kidney cause release of EPO in response to decreased renal oxygen tension. Thus, a fall in red cell mass leading to decreased O_2 delivery to the kidney results in an increase in EPO production and an appropriate increase in RBC production. Recently the cloning of the gene for EPO and other recombinant genetic techniques have allowed for the *in vitro* synthesis of recombinant human EPO (rhEPO) in large quantities for clinical use. Recombinant human EPO administration has resulted in dramatic increases in hematocrit and improved quality of life for patients undergoing hemodialysis. A large number of clinical trials using rhEPO have been completed or are presently ongoing including the use of rhEPO in cancer-related anemia.

The EPO response to the mild anemia induced by serial phlebotomies has been shown to be a limiting factor in the donation of multiple autologous units.[13,14] The administration of rhEPO has been shown to allow for increased preoperative autologous donation in patients undergoing elective orthopedic surgery.[15] This finding cannot necessarily be extrapolated to the patient with cancer; however, it does suggest that in selected patients such an approach might be considered. The Food and Drug Administration (FDA) has not yet approved the use of rhEPO to support preoperative autologous donation and therefore many insurers may refuse reimbursement for the use of this very expensive agent for this purpose.

Endogenous EPO levels have been demonstrated to be inappropriately low in cancer-related anemia,[16] indicating that decreased red blood cell production has an important role in causing the anemia of cancer. Not surprisingly, a number of trials of rhEPO in patients with various malignancies have shown an improvement in hematocrit.[17-19] A recent three-arm double-blind randomized trial of rhEPO versus placebo in patients with advanced cancer receiving no therapy, cisplatin-containing and non–cisplatin-containing combination chemotherapy showed an increased hematocrit, decreased blood transfusion requirement, and improved quality of life in EPO responders when compared with placebo.[20] This trial recently resulted in the FDA approval of rhEPO for cancer patients receiving chemotherapy. Because a response to erythropoietin occurs only after weeks of therapy, rhEPO is of little use in cancer patients with the need for semi-elective or urgent surgical intervention. It is as yet unclear whether prolonged postoperative EPO administration will significantly decrease the need for RBC transfusion in patients with prolonged and complicated postoperative courses.

SPECIAL TRANSFUSION CONSIDERATIONS IN BONE MARROW TRANSPLANT RECIPIENTS

Surgical intervention is often necessary in patients who are future bone marrow transplant candidates or who already have undergone bone marrow transplantation (BMT). It is imperative that the surgeon be aware of the special transfusion requirements of these individuals to avoid potentially catastrophic complications.

Cytomegalovirus (CMV) Prophylaxis

Cytomegalovirus may cause life-threatening infection in heavily immunosuppressed autologous and allogeneic BMT recipients (see Chapter 16). CMV infection is known to be transmitted by leukocytes in transfused blood products. For this reason, all CMV seronegative BMT recipients should receive blood products (RBC and platelets) prepared from CMV seronegative donors. Those BMT patients who are seropositive for CMV antibodies need not receive CMV seronegative blood products because they are already at risk for reactivation of endogenous latent CMV infection. It is important that the blood bank be immediately notified of the expected need for CMV-negative blood products because significant time may be necessary for procurement.

Transfusion-Associated Graft-Versus-Host Disease

Immunocompetent cytotoxic T lymphocytes transfused along with donor red cells and platelets may produce transfusion-associated graft-versus-host disease (GVHD) in severely immunosuppressed allogeneic and autologous bone marrow transplant recipients. Transfusion associated-GVHD, as with the GVHD of allogeneic bone marrow transplantation, is characterized by skin rash, liver dysfunction, and diarrhea. Unlike bone marrow transplant-related GVHD, however, transfusion-associated GVHD is associated with pancytopenia most likely a result of attack on recipient marrow by immunocompetent donor lymphocytes. The onset of transfusion-associated GVHD occurs more rapidly than bone marrow transplant-related GVHD (within 3 to 30 days of infusion) and is associated with a much higher mortality rate (>80%) than bone marrow transplant-related GVHD (10% to 20%). Moreover, the efficacy of immunosuppressive agents such as methotrexate, steroids, cyclosporine, and antilymphocyte globulin is unproved in transfusion-associated GVHD. To avoid transfusion-associated GVHD in bone marrow transplant recipients, all transfused blood products should be gamma irradiated with a minimum dose of 2500 cGY. It is mandatory that this not be forgotten during emergent procedures. Gamma irradiation of blood components using Cesium-137 irradiation devices specifically designed for this purpose takes only a few minutes.[21,22]

LEVELS OF PERIOPERATIVE RBC TRANSFUSION SUPPORT

Despite the lack of clinical or physiologic data to support the practice, for many years it was customary for surgeons and anesthesiologists to maintain a perioperative hematocrit of 30% (Hgb 10 gm/dL) to provide adequate tissue oxygen delivery. Considerable clinical and physiologic evidence indicates that the use of this trigger (the 10/30 rule) is unjustified in most individuals and that in otherwise healthy normovolemic individuals, a hemoglobin as low as 7 g/dL may be well tolerated and unassociated with any dramatic increase in cardiac output.[23,24] Moreover, there is no evidence that maintaining the hematocrit at 30 or above improves wound healing or decreases the incidence of postoperative infection. Obviously, the level of transfusion support should be individualized in each patient, taking into account factors such as patient age, underlying cardiac and pulmonary dysfunction, as well as the probability and extent of intraoperative blood loss.[23–25] These factors are thoroughly discussed with reference to the preoperative evaluation of the cancer patient in Chapter 13.

MANAGEMENT OF THROMBOCYTOPENIA IN THE PERIOPERATIVE SETTING

Sources and Storage of Platelets for Transfusion

Unlike RBCs, the shelf life of platelets is only 5 days, making procurement and maintenance of adequate blood bank inventories a more difficult task. Platelets are stored at room temperature (22°C) with gentle horizontal agitation. Platelets can be obtained by simple centrifugation of a unit of fresh whole blood. The supernatant platelet-rich plasma is expressed sterilely into a polyolefin bag. Platelets processed in this fashion are referred to as *random donor units*.[26] For convenience, multiple (6 to 10) random donor platelet units are often pooled into a single larger bag immediately before transfusion.

An equivalent number of platelets can be obtained from a single donor by automated pheresis. Although this is more expensive and time consuming, the use of completely or partially Human Leukocyte Antigen (HLA)-matched platelets from a single donor may often be the only source of platelet support for recipients who are alloimmunized against multiple HLA antigens.[27] It remains unproved whether the use of single donor units obtained by apheresis *in lieu* of multiple random donor platelets delays HLA alloimmunization in a given recipient by decreasing the number of HLA types to which the recipient is exposed.[28] A large multi-group national trial (TRAP study [Trial To Reduce Alloimmunization To Platelets]) is presently underway to answer this question.

Prophylactic Platelet Transfusion

Considerable controversy still exists regarding the level of platelet count below which patients should receive transfusion to avoid serious spontaneous hemorrhage. Based on early studies in acute leukemia, a platelet count of 20,000 µL often is used as the level below which platelets are administered.[29] To date, there are no well-controlled randomized trials that establish a specific threshold below which platelets should be transfused prophylactically. Indeed, a recent National Institutes of Health Consensus Conference statement acknowledged that, although it was "common practice" to give patients a transfusion prophylactically below a predetermined level of platelet count (such as 20,000/µL), even lower levels might be safely tolerated "based on clinical judgement and close observation."[30]

Clinical experience clearly indicates that the decision to administer prophylactic platelet transfusions should be individualized for each patient. For example, sepsis, chemotherapy-induced emesis and mucositis, and coexistent coagulation abnormalities such as hepatic failure and disseminated intravascular coagulation (DIC) may be associated with serious hemorrhage at levels of platelet count at which one does not usually expect bleeding. In such patients it is prudent to be more vigorous with platelet transfusion. At the University of Maryland Cancer Center, platelet counts are often maintained in the 40,000 to 50,000 µL range for patients with a particularly high risk of bleeding such as those with acute promyelocytic leukemia accompanied by DIC and acute myeloid leukemia with high blast counts (>100,000/µL) who are at risk for cerebral infarction and hemorrhage.

Two large retrospective reviews of patients with solid tumor with thrombocytopenia have indicated that even severe thrombocytopenia (<10,000/µL) can be tolerated in stable patients whereas those with sepsis, coexistent coagulation abnormalities, and direct tumor invasion were liable for hemorrhage even at platelet counts not ordinarily associated with bleeding.[31,32] Thus, the need for assessing additional risk factors for hemorrhage in each patient cannot be overemphasized in deciding at what level of platelet count prophylactic platelet transfusion should be administered.

Perioperative Platelet Support

Patients with thrombocytopenia secondary to bone marrow failure and chemotherapy often require surgical intervention for diagnostic and therapeutic purposes. There are no prospective trials to date that elucidate the minimal level of platelet count necessary to prevent bleeding with specific procedures. Because there are many factors other than thrombocytopenia that may increase the risk for perioperative hemorrhage, the minimal platelet count sufficient to prevent bleeding for a particular procedure may vary among individual patients.

In a retrospective review of 167 surgical procedures among 95 patients with acute leukemia at the University of Maryland Cancer Center, platelet transfusions were given to achieve a minimal level of 50,000/µL. No hemorrhage-related deaths were noted within 1 month of surgery with a median 1-hour posttransfusion or immediate postoperative platelet count of 56,000/μL. Moreover, intraoperative blood loss greater than 500 mL and perioperative transfusion requirements greater than 4 U of packed red blood cells occurred in only 7% of procedures. Not surprisingly, patients with preoperative fever, those with other coagulation abnormalities, and those undergoing more extensive surgical procedure had more bleeding and required greater amounts of transfusion.[33]

Based on these data, investigators at the University of Maryland Cancer Center have maintained a minimal level of 50,000 platelets/μL in the intra- and immediate postoperative period. Certainly higher levels may be considered in patients with other coexisting coagulation disturbances and in those procedures (e.g., neurosurgery) where even a small amount of bleeding is likely to be catastrophic. With some procedures such as endoscopic esophageal biopsy, lumbar puncture, and bronchoalveolar lavage, a platelet count of 40,000/μL has been adequate to prevent serious bleeding. Whether or not such procedures could be safely carried out at lower platelet counts is uncertain. Minor procedures, such as radial artery puncture and bone marrow aspiration, where direct pressure can be applied to the operative site may be done safely even with platelet counts below 20,000 μL. Whenever possible, other coagulation disturbances should be corrected before undertaking surgical intervention in the thrombocytopenic patient.

Assessment of Response to Platelet Transfusion

Before operative intervention begins, it is imperative that the surgeon verify that the target platelet count has been reached following platelet transfusion. This is best done with a 10-minute posttransfusion platelet count.[34] The absence of any increment in platelet count following transfusion is indicative of the presence of alloantibodies against HLA antigens (and less frequently platelet-specific antigens) found on platelets. The demonstration of lymphocytotoxic antibody in the recipient's serum is confirmation that alloantibodies are present, precluding the use of random donor platelets.[35] In the presence of alloimmunization, surgery must be delayed until adequate amounts of platelets matched to the recipient's HLA type are obtained. In those patients with uncommon HLA types, procurement of matched platelets can be difficult if not impossible.[36] Recently, the use of in vitro platelet crossmatching techniques has shown promise in selecting potentially matched donors without the need for HLA typing.[37,38] Even with the use of HLA-matched platelets, a 10-minute postinfusion count is necessary because transfusion with platelets matched for major HLA types are not always successful. In the event that HLA-matched platelets are not available for an alloimmunized recipient and surgery is deemed absolutely emergent, large amounts of random donor platelets given during the procedure may sometimes provide hemostasis even in the absence of a measurable increase in platelet count.[28] Operating under such conditions should be considered a measure of last resort.

Massive bleeding, sepsis, DIC, and splenomegaly may markedly reduce the survival of transfused platelets, necessitating frequent intraoperative platelet counts with further transfusion when necessary. The surgeon must be certain that adequate amounts of platelets are available before proceeding.

Treatment of Immune Thrombocytopenic Purpura

Although immune thrombocytopenic purpura (ITP) is most often idiopathic, it also frequently complicates AIDS and lymphoproliferative disorders, particularly chronic lymphatic leukemia and Hodgkin's Disease. Less often, ITP may be seen in patients with non-Hodgkin's lymphoma and occasionally with solid tumors. With chronic lymphatic leukemia and Hodgkin's Disease, ITP may occur even in the absence of active disease.

Patients with ITP having platelet counts in excess of 50,000 μL rarely need platelet transfusion support to maintain hemostasis in the intra- and perioperative setting. Because the circulating platelets are younger and more hemostatically effective in patients with ITP, patients may tolerate surgery at surprisingly low platelet counts (<20,000/μL) without serious hemorrhage. Nonetheless it seems prudent to increase the platelet count perioperatively whenever possible. Although prednisone remains the mainstay of initial therapy for ITP, response sometimes is obtained only after days of treatment. When surgery becomes emergent in patients with ITP not yet in remission, high dose intravenous gammaglobulin (1 gm/kg daily × 2 days) often results in a prompt increase in platelet count, usually within the first 24 to 48 hours.[39] Surgery can then be carried out with little or no risk of excessive bleeding. When ITP is refractory to all therapy and emergent surgery is required, platelet transfusion can be given intraoperatively if serious bleeding ensues. There is often a measurable increment in platelet count in the presence of autoantibody, although platelet survival is short. Hemostasis may also be obtained even in the absence of a measurable increase in platelet count following transfusion. Splenectomy should be strongly considered in cancer patients where ITP persists following steroids, high-dose intravenous IgG, and treatment for their primary malignancy. This is particularly the case in chronic lymphatic leukemia and lymphomas where treatment may result in years of survival and sometimes cure.

DISTURBANCES OF THE COAGULATION SYSTEM IN THE CANCER PATIENT

Disseminated Intravascular Coagulation (DIC)

Disseminated intravascular coagulation (DIC) is characterized as a pathologic, often diffuse activation of the coagulation system as a result of wide-spread endothelial cell or tissue injury. Such activation can occur via the intrinsic coagulation system (factor XII) as is often seen in gram-negative endotoxemia or via the extrinsic system (direct factor X activation) as may occur with massive trauma or metastatic carcinoma.[40] Central to the development of DIC is the generation of thrombin resulting in fibrinogen consumption (hypofibrinogenemia), fibrin deposition, platelet consumption, and consumption of factors V and VIII that results in tissue ischemia and a hemorrhagic diathesis. Invariably there is a concomitant activation of the fibrinolytic mechanism resulting in plasmin generation. Although plasmin will degrade fibrin and will restore vascular patency in DIC, plasmin is a nonspecific protease and will degrade other plasma coagulation factors including native fibrinogen, factors V and VIII, and further aggravate the hemorrhagic tendency.[40]

Depending on the extent and rapidity of activation of the coagulation system, the ability of the liver to compensate with increased coagulation factor synthesis, and the ability of the natural anticoagulants and fibrinolytic inhibitors (i.e., antithrombin III, antiplasmin) to contain the process, DIC may be an acute overwhelming process or a chronic subacute one.

Acute DIC

The patient with acute DIC often exhibits hypotension and acidosis related to overwhelming sepsis or trauma. Cyanosis and gangrene often involves the acral parts including fingers, toes, nose, and ear lobes. Continuous oozing from surgical wounds, sites of trauma, central venous catheter sites, Foley catheters, and endotracheal tubes reflect hypocoagulability and secondary fibrinolysis. Impaired mentation and respiratory failure often coexist with acute DIC.

The prothrombin time (PT) is often markedly prolonged. Hypofibrinogenemia is usually severe (<50 mgm/dL) and fibrin split products (FSPs) usually are markedly elevated (>40 μgm/dL).

The most important modality of treatment in acute DIC is the correction of the precipitating cause. For example, volume resuscitation with correction of hypoxia and acidosis along with immediate administration of antibiotics is critical in patients whose DIC is precipitated by sepsis.[41] There are no properly controlled clinical trials demonstrating the efficacy of heparin in acute DIC and its use is rarely justified. Although heparin may antagonize the action of thrombin, it may also produce worsening hemorrhage. Some have advocated the use of subcutaneous heparin (80 U/kg every 4 to 6 hours) in acute DIC;[41] however, there appears to be no corroborating evidence that this approach is either safe or efficacious. Reversal of the precipitating cause of DIC (and thus the continued generation of thrombin) followed by correction of the hypocoagulable state by transfusion with platelets, and cryoprecipitate (as a source of fibrinogen) is the cornerstone of appropriate management.[42] It should be remembered that approximately 450 to 700 mL of relatively fresh plasma (≤ 5 days old) is administered when 6 to 10 U of platelets are transfused. Correction of the hypofibrinogenemia with cryoprecipitate along with platelet transfusion is most often adequate to promote hemostasis without the administration of additional fresh frozen plasma. The use of fibrinolytic inhibitors, such as epsilon aminocaproic acid (AMICAR), must be avoided in the patient with active DIC because it will allow for the unopposed deposition of fibrin in the microcirculation, which can result in severe organ ischemia and failure.[42] Although some have claimed that administration of platelets and plasma products without the "cover" of heparin only adds "fuel to the fire" and worsens the coagulopathic state,[41] there is no clinical evidence that this is so. Failure to correct the precipitating cause of acute DIC usually leads to the patient's demise regardless of the therapy employed to correct the coagulopathy.

Chronic DIC of Malignancy

Chronic DIC associated with malignancy is most often manifested clinically by episodes of thrombosis. Bleeding often ensues as a result of surgical intervention when a preexisting coagulopathy has gone unrecognized.

Chronic DIC can be manifested by migratory and recurrent superficial and deep vein thrombosis (Trousseau's syndrome, see Chapter 11), arterial occlusion such as stroke, and nonbacterial thrombotic endocarditis (marantic endocarditis) involving the aortic and mitral valves.[40] The latter may be associated with arterial emboli particularly to the cerebral circulation, the onset of a new heart murmur, and occasionally demonstrable valvular vegetations by cardiac echocardiography. Chronic DIC may also manifest itself as a microangiopathic hemolytic anemia (MAHA) resulting from fragmentation of red blood cells on fibrin thrombi in the microcirculation. Microangiopathic hemolytic anemia is manifested by transfusion dependency, reticulocytosis, fragmented RBCs on smear (helmet cells or schistocytes), and chemical evidence of hemolysis (hyperbilirubinemia and increased serum lactate dehydrogenase [LD]).

Chronic DIC is most often associated with adenocarcinomas involving the stomach, pancreas, colon, breast, lung, and prostate. Tumor-associated mucin, proteases, and tissue factor have been implicated in activation of the coagulation system.[40,43]

Although both acute and chronic myeloid leukemias may be associated with chronic DIC, it occurs invariably in patients with acute promyelocytic leukemia (APL). Constituents of the large promyelocytic granules are responsible for activation of the coagulation system with resultant thrombin generation.[44] Prolonged PT, partial thromboplastin time (PTT), hypofibrinogenemia, increased FSPs, and thrombocytopenia of variable severity are present. These patients often have considerable bleeding even in the face of moderate thrombocytopenia. Thrombosis is uncommon but does occur. We have recently seen a patient with APL who presented with aortic thrombosis and bilateral lower extremity ischemia. Characteristically, the DIC and bleeding worsen with induction chemotherapy, resulting in lysis of the leukemic promyelocytes and release of their granular contents. When inappropriately treated, severe and often fatal (particularly intracranial) hemorrhage may result.

Laboratory evidence of chronic DIC is often subtle and often difficult to interpret. The usual screening tests for coagulopathy including the PT and activated PTT are often normal or minimally prolonged until prominent hypofibrinogenemia ensues (<100). Normal fibrinogen level (150 to 250 mgm/dL) are often inappropriately low in patients with metastatic malignancy, where in the absence of chronic DIC or hepatic failure, fibrinogen level usually are increased (400 to 500 mgm/dL). Although the platelet count may be normal, mild to moderately severe thrombocytopenia often is present even in the absence of other coagulation test abnormalities. Coexistent bone marrow invasion by tumor and myelosuppressive chemotherapy often are significant contributing factors to thrombocytopenia. Fibrin split products are usually elevated (>40 μgm/dL).

Treatment of Chronic DIC

Many patients with metastatic adenocarcinoma may have laboratory evidence of DIC in the absence of clinical bleeding or thrombosis. Such patients are often best served by observation without specific therapeutic intervention. Chemotherapy-induced tumor lysis, however, may be associated with sudden worsening of the coagulopathy with resultant hemorrhage or thrombosis. Patients with clinical evidence of thrombosis deserve immediate anticoagulation with heparin and if markedly thrombocytopenic (<50,000/μL) or hypofibrinogenemia (<100 mgm/dL), platelets, and cryoprecipitate should be given concomitantly. In those patients with a markedly increased risk of potentially cataclysmic bleeding (i.e., in the presence of vascular brain metastases and mucosal tumor invasion) the risk of bleeding must be weighed against any potential benefit of anticoagulation. The use of platelet function inhibitors (i.e., aspirin, sulfinpyrozone, and dipyridamole) has been advocated to antagonize the platelet-aggregating activity attributed to various tumors.[41,43] The efficacy of this approach has been reported only anecdotally and certainly cannot be considered proved therapy in chronic DIC.[41]

Most patients with chronic DIC and widespread adenocarcinoma succumb to the progression of disease in spite of appropriate management of their coagulopathy. This is not surprising due to the relative ineffectiveness of currently available chemotherapeutic regimens in these malignancies. Still, some patients with responsive tumors (i.e., breast or prostate cancer) may benefit from anticoagulation with or without coagulation factor replacement. Coumadin anticoagulation is ineffective in the DIC of malignancy and may contribute to severe bleeding without protection from thrombosis. If chronic anticoagulation is necessary, adjusted-dose heparin can be administered subcutaneously on an outpatient basis.[45,46]

All patients with acute promyelocytic leukemia should be vigorously supported with fresh frozen plasma, cryoprecipitate, and platelet transfusions. In our institution platelets are maintained in excess of 50,000/μL and fibrinogen (≥100 mgm/dL) with the concomitant administration of heparin to block thrombin activity.[47] Although excellent results have been obtained, equally good outcomes have been reported with replacement of platelet and coagulation factors without concurrent heparinization.[42,48] Semi-elective procedures, such as Hickman catheter insertion, are best delayed in acute promyelocytic leukemia until adequate leukemic cytoreduction has been accomplished with chemotherapy and the coagulopathy has resolved.

Surgical Intervention and DIC

Surgical intervention is best delayed whenever possible in patients with both acute and chronic DIC until the coagulopathy is corrected.

In some instances, however, surgical intervention plays an important role in gaining control of the coagulopathy, such as in septic patients with a perforated viscus or typhlitis. Obviously, surgery should be carried out only with meticulous attention to adequate antibiotic administration, vigorous volume replacement, and prompt correction of hypoxia and acidosis in addition to platelet and coagulation factor replacement. Immediate establishment of central venous access is therefore sometimes necessary even in the presence of a severe hemorrhagic diathesis if the coagulopathy is to be reversed.

The first evidence of impaired hemostasis with chronic DIC may be precipitated by surgical intervention, such as central line insertion. Thus, it is important to obtain preoperative screening studies of coagulation (particularly fibrin split products and plasma fibrinogen) in patients with metastatic carcinomas likely to be associated with chronic DIC. The surgeon must be prepared to correct the coagulopathy with the transfusion of appropriate blood products perioperatively should bleeding ensue. Following the establishment of intraoperative hemostasis, postoperative anticoagulation with heparin may be necessary to interfere with continual thrombin generation and postoperative deep venous thrombosis. Fibrinolytic inhibitors, such as epsilon aminocaproic acid (AMICAR), should be used only when all other measures to control bleeding have failed and *only* when adequate heparinization has been ensured. In situations where bleeding persists following the correction of appropriate laboratory parameters, a surgical bleeding site must be ruled out.

Use of Fibrinolytic Agents in Cancer Patients

The procoagulant activation accompanying many metastatic malignancies, even in the absence of chronic DIC, predispose the cancer patient to an increased risk of *spontaneous* as well as postoperative deep vein thrombosis and resultant pulmonary emboli.

The frequent coexistence of severe thrombocytopenia and other coagulation abnormalities as well as the frequent need for invasive diagnostic and therapeutic surgical procedures precludes the use of thrombolytic (fibrinolytic therapy) in many cancer patients owing to the disproportionate bleeding risk. Active bleeding and intracranial lesions (infectious, vascular, and neoplastic) represent absolute contraindications to the use of fibrinolytic agents. The use of systemic fibrinolytic therapy to treat lower extremity deep vein thrombosis, submassive pulmonary emboli, and arterial occlusion should be considered only in carefully selected patients with malignancies likely to be associated with a prolongation of quality survival.[49]

Local instillation of urokinase in central venous catheters has been shown to be safe and associated with significant restoration of catheter patency without systemic fibrinolysis and its attendant bleeding risks.[50] Systemic fibrinolytic agents also have been used safely in patients with subclavian vein thrombosis related to indwelling venous catheters. A high rate of thrombus resolution without the need for catheter removal has been obtained only when the fibrinolytic agents have been introduced directly into the thrombus.[51]

SURGICAL COMPLICATIONS OF MYELOPROLIFERATIVE DISORDERS

The myeloproliferative disorders (MPD), which include chronic myeloid leukemia, myeloid metaplasia and myelofibrosis, polycythemia vera, and essential thrombocythemia, are clonal disorders of hematopoietic stem cells. All of these disorders are associated paradoxically with a variable degree of increased risk of thrombosis as well as hemorrhage.[52] The pathogenesis of this increased risk of thrombosis and hemorrhage is complex and likely related to increased platelet count, defective platelet function and, in the case of polycythemia vera, increased whole blood viscosity due to increased hematocrit.

Amongst the myeloproliferative disorders, bleeding and thrombosis are infrequent in chronic myeloid leukemia with an incidence of less than 5%. Hemorrhage seems to be particularly common in myeloid metaplasia and myelofibrosis, whereas thrombosis is more typical of polycythemia vera.[52] Essential thrombocythemia is characterized by an increased risk of both hemorrhage and thrombosis, although the latter seems to be more common. Bleeding in the myeloproliferative disorders is typically mucocutaneous in nature, whereas soft tissue and deep visceral bleeding is rare. Thrombosis in myeloproliferative disorders may present with ordinary deep vein thrombosis of the lower extremities with or without pulmonary embolism. However, unusual sites of venous thrombosis, including the hepatic veins (Budd-Chiari syndrome, refer to Chapter 5), portal vein, and mesenteric veins, also are typical of myeloproliferative disorders. Arterial occlusion including stroke, myocardial infarction, and peripheral arterial thrombosis also occur. Acral ischemia and occasionally gangrene are seen particularly in association with polycythemia vera and essential thrombocythemia. Unfortunately, neither the bleeding time, platelet function studies, nor height of the platelet count are predictive of the risk for bleeding or thrombosis in the myeloproliferative disorders.[52-54] There is, however, a close correlation between packed cell volume (hematocrit) and the risk for thrombosis in polycythemia vera.

The patient with myeloproliferative disorders is at significantly increased risk of hemorrhage or thrombosis when undergoing surgical procedures. There are many reports in the older literature of severe and often fatal thrombohemorrhagic complications in patients with uncontrolled myeloproliferative disorders undergoing surgery, particularly among patients with polycythemia vera.[55-57] Although there are no definitive guidelines for operative management of patients with myeloproliferative disorders, certain maneuvers appear to lessen the risk of perioperative thrombosis or hemorrhage. It is mandatory that patients with polycythemia vera be adequately phlebotomized (<45%) prior to surgical intervention. Following phlebotomy, normal red cell mass should be confirmed, when possible, using chromium 51 methods. When the need for operative intervention is urgent in a newly diagnosed patient with polycythemia vera, reduction of red cell mass can be performed quickly and safely by automated pheresis devices. Whether or not lowering the platelet count to normal in patients with polycythemia vera by the use of myelosuppressive chemotherapy will decrease the incidence of perioperative hemorrhage or thrombosis is unknown.

Keeping in mind the reports of major thrombotic and hemorrhagic events in patients with essential thrombocythemia undergoing surgery,[57] normalization of the platelet count with myelosuppressive agents should be considered prior to elective surgery. This can be done safely (and temporarily if desired) by the use of hydroxyurea with little risk of protracted bone marrow suppression. In urgently symptomatic essential thrombocythemia patients, such as those with mesenteric venous thrombosis or peripheral arterial occlusion who require immediate surgical intervention, rapid lowering of the platelet count can be accomplished by automated pheresis. All such patients will require concomitant hydroxyurea therapy to prevent rebound thrombocytosis.

Most hematologists will discontinue aspirin (which may have been given therapeutically or prophylactically to myeloproliferative disorder patients) at least a week before surgery to reduce the risk of perioperative hemorrhage. The wisdom of this approach is unproven but certainly is reasonable especially in patients who have demonstrated previous perioperative bleeding.

The potential benefits of perioperative prophylactic anticoagulation in patients with myeloproliferative disorders to prevent postoperative thrombotic events have not been studied in a controlled fashion. The decision for prophylactic perioperative anticoagulation should be made for an individual patient based on the type of surgery, the risks for both perioperative hemorrhage or thrombosis, and when possible the patient's prior history of thrombohemorrhagic complications with surgical interventions.

CHEMO-HORMONAL THERAPY-RELATED THROMBOSIS

Patients with cancer often have multiple factors putting them at increased risk for thrombosis. These factors include age, premorbid cardiovascular disease, the thrombogenicity of the particular tumor type, extent and sites of metastases, and performance status. Thrombosis is a major cause of morbidity and mortality in the cancer patient. Major pulmonary embolism has been observed in up to 35% of patients with advanced cancer. The problem of deep venous thrombosis in the cancer patient is thoroughly discussed in Chapter 11. More recently, it has been noted that thrombosis can occur as a complication of cancer therapy. Specifically, this section addresses the risk of thrombosis caused by chemo-hormonal therapy.

The heterogeneity of the risk factors for thrombosis among individual patients has made it difficult to sort out a specific role for chemotherapeutic agents in producing thrombosis. The recent and numerous trials of adjuvant chemo- and hormonal therapy in early stage breast cancer has provided a unique opportunity to evaluate the relationship between chemotherapy and thrombotic risk because the patients in these trials are a more homogeneous group without overt evidence of persistent tumor.

Weiss et al[58] described a 5% incidence of venous thrombosis among 433 stage II breast cancer patients undergoing 2 years of adjuvant chemotherapy with cytoxan, methotrexate and 5-fluorouracil (CMF), CMF with vincristine (V) and prednisone (P), or CMF and immunotherapy with the methanol extraction residue of bacillus Calmette-Guerin (MER). All episodes of venous thrombosis occurred during the 2 years while the patients were on therapy and none occurred in any patient after completion of the 2-year course of treatment. This suggested a causal role for chemotherapy in the genesis of these thrombotic events.

Levine et al[59] from the Ontario Cancer Treatment and Research Foundation reported a 6.8% incidence of thrombosis among 205 patients receiving adjuvant chemotherapy with CMFVP or CMFVP plus adriamycin (A). In this trial, no thrombotic events were noted during 2413 patient-months without therapy. Saphner et al[60] reported an incidence of thrombotic events (venous and arterial) among 5.4% of 2673 patients who received adjuvant chemo-hormonal therapy or hormonal therapy alone in seven consecutive Eastern Cooperative Oncology Group (ECOG) studies. In these trials, the incidence of venous thrombosis was 2.8% in premenopausal patients who received both chemotherapy and tamoxifen compared with those who received chemotherapy alone (0.8%). Similarly, among postmenopausal patients who received chemotherapy and tamoxifen there was an 8% incidence of venous thrombosis compared with 2.3% in those receiving tamoxifen alone. These differences were statistically significant ($p = 0.03$). Also, there was a highly statistically significant ($p = 0.004$) increase in arterial thrombosis among premenopausal patients receiving chemotherapy and tamoxifen when compared with those patients receiving chemotherapy alone (1.6% vs. 0.0%). Wall et al[61] reported seven (0.8%) arterial thromboses among 901 patients with stage II breast cancer who received adjuvant chemotherapy without tamoxifen in two Cancer and Leukemia Group B (CALGB) trials.

The National Surgical Adjuvant Breast and Bowel Project (NSABBP) reported a considerably lower incidence of venous thromboembolic events (0.7% [5 of 696]) in patients with stage II breast cancer receiving adjuvant chemotherapy with phenylalanine mustard (P) plus 5-fluorouracil (F) and PAF.[62] In contrast, there was a 3.6% incidence (37 of 1082) of venous thromboses in patients receiving the same drugs plus tamoxifen. The corresponding rates for arterial emboli were 0.3% and 0.0% respectively, none of which occurred while patients were receiving tamoxifen alone. In a later NSABP adjuvant trial in which stage II breast cancer patients received chemotherapy alone, venous thrombotic events occurred in only 0.2 to 1.7% among the three treatment arms.[63]

Two recent large studies, including 2644[64] and 2365[65] patients with early stage breast cancer in which patients were randomized to either tamoxifen alone or no therapy, demonstrated rates of thrombosis among the tamoxifen arms of 0.9% and 4.1% versus rates of 0.15% and 3.8% respectively in the no-therapy arms.

In summary, the above data suggest that chemotherapy alone is associated with an increased risk of both venous and arterial thrombosis, at least in patients with early stage breast cancer. The reported rates for venous thrombosis range from as low as 0.7% to as high as 6.8% with considerably lower rates for arterial thrombosis (0.3% to 0.8%). The fact that both venous and arterial thrombosis occur while patients are on chemotherapy and that further events are infrequent after the completion of chemotherapy suggest a causal role for chemotherapy in the development of these thromboses. The addition of tamoxifen to chemotherapy appears to increase the risk of thrombotic events when compared with chemotherapy alone. There may be a small increase in the risk of thrombosis related to hormonal therapy (tamoxifen) alone but this effect is less clear.

The mechanism by which chemotherapy produces thrombotic disease remains unclear but could be related to alteration in levels of prothrombotic and anticoagulant proteins as well as direct vascular toxicity.[66,67] For example, deficiencies of proteins C and S have been reported in breast cancer patients receiving CMF chemotherapy.[67] Chemotherapy-associated thrombosis has not been restricted only to patients with breast cancer. Veno-occlusive disease of the liver often is seen in bone marrow transplant patients who have received high doses of chemotherapy as part of their primary treatment or their pre-transplant conditioning regimen. Both myocardial infarction and stroke have been associated with *cis*-platinum–based chemotherapy.[66,68] A thrombotic microangiopathy clinically indistinguishable from hemolytic uremic syndrome has been well described in patients receiving mitomycin chemotherapy.[66] Injury to vessels, by a number of mechanisms including endothelial cell injury, vasospasm, and fibroblast stimulation also has been implicated as a mechanism for chemotherapy-induced hypercoagulability.[69]

The surgeon must remain alert to the possibility of chemotherapy-related thrombotic events in their patients because these events may seriously complicate both pre- and postoperative management.

SUMMARY

The use of multimodality therapy in the modern treatment of the cancer patient makes it incumbent on each person involved in the care of the patient to be familiar with the myriad effects of treatment. One of the most dramatic and far-reaching effects of chemotherapy is the occurrence of hematologic abnormalities that can have a direct impact on the planning and execution of surgical therapy.

A number of chemotherapeutic agents have a myelosuppressive effect. Those drugs that interfere with DNA synthesis and repair and those that are given in large pulse doses produce neutropenia and thrombocytopenia within 7 to 14 days of administration. This period of neutropenia may be shortened by the administration of recombinant growth factors.

Anemia is a common finding in cancer patients and can have many causes including metastatic disease, primary bone marrow disorders, blood loss, myelosuppression, immune destruction, and hemolysis. Although red blood cells are usually available for transfusion, crossmatch may be difficult due to antigen sensitization. Autologous blood donation may be difficult or impossible in many cancer patients. The level of transfusion support must be individualized, taking into account physiologic factors rather than a *trigger point* for transfusion at a hematocrit less than 30%.

Bone marrow transplantation patients have several special considerations that must be taken into account in their care. All CMV-seronegative bone marrow transplant recipients should receive blood products from seronegative donors. To avoid transfusion-associated graft-versus-host disease in marrow transplant recipients, all transfused blood products should be gamma irradiated with a minimal dose of 2500 cGy.

Platelet transfusions are often administered for counts less than 20,000/μL to prevent spontaneous bleeding, although it is unclear at the present time whether transfusion at lower levels is as safe in many instances. Again, the decision to administer platelets must be made on an individual basis. There are no prospective trials that elucidate the minimal platelet count necessary to prevent bleeding from a specific invasive procedure. It is important to correct other coagulation disturbances prior to the conduct of such procedures. At the University of Maryland Cancer Center, a minimal platelet count of 50,000/mL is used for intraoperative and postoperative management. Whether or not these procedures could be carried out safely at lower counts is uncertain.

DIC is a result of diffuse activation of the coagulation system as a result of widespread endothelial cell or tissue injury. Acute DIC is often characterized by cyanosis and gangrene affecting the acral parts, with continuous oozing from surgical wounds, venous access sites, Foley catheters, and endotracheal tubes. The most important modality in treating this condition is to correct the underlying cause. Chronic DIC of malignancy is most often manifest by episodes of thrombosis and is most commonly associated with adenocarcinomas involving the stomach, pancreas, colon, breast, lung, and prostate. Surgical intervention should be delayed if possible in patients with acute and chronic DIC until the coagulopathy is corrected.

It has been recently noted that patients receiving chemo-hormonal therapy are at increased risk for the development of thrombotic complications. Thus, not only can the underlying malignancy predispose a patient to thromboses, but the therapy can also increase the incidence of this potentially fatal complication.

A thorough knowledge of the effects of a malignancy and its treatment on the hematologic system is essential for surgeons involved in the care of cancer patients.

REFERENCES

1. Demetri GD, Antman KHS. Granulocyte-macrophage colony stimulating factor (GM-CSF): preclinical and clinical investigations. Semin Oncol 1992;19:362.
2. Glaspy JA, Golde DW. Granulocyte colony stimulating factor (G-CSF): preclinical and clinical studies. Semin Oncol 1992;19:386.
3. Myers SE, Williams SF. Role of high dose chemotherapy and Autologous Stem cell support in the treatment of breast cancer. Hematol Oncol Clin North Am 1993;7:631.
4. Kessinger A. Utilization of peripheral blood stem cells in autotransplantation. Hematol Oncol Clin North Am 1993;7:535.
5. Peters WP, Ross M, Vredenburgh J, et al. Role of cytokines in autologous bone marrow transplantation. Hematol Oncol Clin North Am 1993;7:737.
6. Goodnough LT, Shaffron D, Marcus RE. Impact of preoperative autologous blood donation in elective orthopaedic surgery. Vox Sang 1990;59:65.
7. Owings DV, Kruskall MS, Thurner RL, et al. Autologous blood donations prior to elective cardiac surgery. Safety and effect on subsequent blood use. JAMA 1989;262:1963.
8. Goodnough LT. Toward bloodless surgery: erythropoietin therapy in the surgical setting. Semin Oncol 1992;19:19.
9. American Association of Blood Banks. Standards for blood banks and transfusion services. 13th ed. Arlington, VA 1989:40.
10. Krusuall MS, Yomtovian WH, Dzik KD, et al. On improving the cost-effectiveness of autologous blood transfusion practices. Transfusion 1994;34:259.
11. Minamoto GY, Scheinberg DA, Dietz K, et al.

Human immunodeficiency virus infection in patients with leukemia. Blood 1988;71: 1147.
12. Henry DH. Changing patterns of care in the management of anemia. Semin Oncol 1992;19 (8):3.
13. Kickler TS, Spivak JL. Effect of repeated whole blood donations on serum immunoreactive erythropoietin levels in autologous donors. JAMA 1988;260:65.
14. Goodnough LT, Brittenham G. Limitations of the erythropoietic response to serial phlebotomy: implications for autologous blood donor programs. J Lab Clin Med 1990;115:28.
15. Goodnough LT, Rudnick S, Price TH, Ballas SK, Collins ML, et al. Increased preoperative collection of autologous blood with recombinant human erythropoietin therapy. N Engl J Med 1989;321(17):1163.
16. Miller CB, Jones RJ, Piantadosi S, Abeloff MD, Spivak JL. Decreased erythropoietin response in patients with the anemia of cancer. N Engl J Med 1990;322(24):1689.
17. Platanias LC, Miller CB, Mick R, Hart RD, Ozer H, et al. Treatment of chemotherapy-induced anemia with recombinant human erythropoietin in cancer patients. J Clin Oncol 1991;9(11):2021.
18. Oster W, Herrmann F, Gamm H, Zeile G, Lindemann A, et al. Erythropoietin for the treatment of anemia of malignancy associated with neoplastic bone marrow infiltration. J Clin Oncol 1990;8(6):956.
19. Ludwig H, Fritz E, Kotzmann H, Höcker P, Gisslinger H, et al. Erythropoietin treatment of anemia associated with multiple myeloma. N Engl J Med 1990;322(24):1693.
20. Abels RI. Use of recombinant human erythropoietin in the treatment of anemia in patients who have cancer. Semin Oncol 1992;19(3):29.
21. Linden JV, Pisciotto PT. Transfusion-associated graft-versus-host disease and blood irradiation. Transfus Med Rev 1992;6(2):116.
22. Rowe JM, Ciobanu N, Ascensao J, et al. Recommended guidelines for the management of autologous and allogeneic bone marrow transplantation. Ann Intern Med 1994;120:143.
23. Perioperative red cell transfusion. National Institutes of Health Consensus Development Conference Statement. Transfusion Medicine Reviews 1989;3:63.
24. Welch HG, Meehan KR, Goodnough LT. Prudent strategies for elective red blood cell transfusion. Ann Intern Med 1992;116(5):393.
25. American College of Physicians. Practice strategies for elective red blood cell transfusion. Ann Intern Med 1992;116(5):403.
26. Schiffer CA, Lee EJ, Ness PM, Reilly J. Clinical evaluation of platelet concentrates stored for one to five days. Blood 1986;67:1591.
27. Lohmann HP, Bull MI, Decter JA et al. Platelet transfusions from HLA compatible unrelated donors to alloimmunized patients. Ann Intern Med 1974;80:9.
28. Heyman MR, Schiffer CA. Platelet transfusion therapy for the cancer patient. Semin Oncol 1990;17:198.
29. Gaydos LA, Freireich EJ, Mantel N. The quantitative relation between platelet count and hemorrhage in patients with acute leukemia. N Engl J Med 1962;13:283.
30. NIH Consensus Development Conference Statement. Platelet transfusion therapy. In: NIH consensus development conference on platelet transfusion therapy. Bethesda, National Institutes of Health, 1986;(Suppl 7):6.
31. Belt RJ, Leite C, Haas CD, Stephens RL. Incidence of hemorrhagic complications in patients with cancer. N Engl J Med 1978;239:2571.
32. Dutcher JP, Schiffer CA, Aisner J, et al. Incidence of thrombocytopenia and serious hemorrhage among patients with solid tumors. Cancer 1984;53:557.
33. Bishop JF, Schiffer CA, Aisner J, et al. Surgery in leukemia: a review of 167 operations in thrombocytopenic patients. Am J Hematol 1987;26:147.
34. O'Connell B, Lee EJ, Schiffer CA. The value of 10-minute posttransfusion platelet counts. Transfusion 1988;28:66.
35. Lee EJ, Schiffer CA. Serial measurement of lymphocytotoxic antibody and response to nonmatched platelet transfusions in alloimmunized patients. Blood 1987;70:1727.
36. Schiffer CA, Keller C, Dutcher JP, et al. Potential HLA-matched platelet donor availability for alloimmunized patients. Transfusion 1983;23:286.
37. O'Connell B, Schiffer CA. Donor selection for alloimmunized patients by platelet crossmatching of random donor platelet concentrates. Transfusion 1990;30:314.
38. Kickler TS, Braine H, Ness PM. The predictive value of crossmatching platelet transfusion for alloimmunized patients. Transfusion 1985;25:385.
39. Heyman MR, Schiffer CA. Clinical use of high dose intravenous gamma globulin In: Dutcher JP, ed. Modern Transfusion Therapy. Vol 1. Boca Raton, Florida, CRC Press;1990.
40. Colman RW, Rubin RN. Disseminated intravascular coagulation due to malignancy. Semin Oncol 1990;17:172.
41. Bick RL. Disseminated intravascular coagulation and related syndromes: a clinical review. Semin Thromb Hemost 1988;14:299.

42. Feinstein DI. Treatment of disseminated intravascular coagulation. Semin Thromb Hemost 1988;14:351.
43. Rickles FR, Edwards RL. Activation of blood coagulation in cancer: Trousseau's syndrome revisited. Blood 1983;62:14.
44. Sterrenberg L, Haak HL, Brommer EJP, Nieuwenhuizen W. Evidence of fibrinogen breakdown by leukocyte enzymes in a patient with acute promyelocytic leukemia. Haemostasis 1985;15:126.
45. Bell WR, Starksen NF, Tong S, Porterfield JK. Trousseau's syndrome. Am J Med 1985;79:423.
46. Sack GH, Levin J, Bell WR. Trousseau's syndrome and other manifestations of chronic disseminated coagulopathy in patients with neoplasm: clinical, pathophysiologic, and therapeutic features. Medicine (Baltimore MD) 1977;56:1.
47. Daly PA, Schiffer CA, Wiernik PH. Acute promyelocytic leukemia—clinical management of 15 patients. Am J Hematol 1980;8:347.
48. Goldberg MA, Ginsburg D, Mayer RJ, Stone RM, Maguire M, Rosenthal DS, Antin JH. Is heparin administration necessary during induction chemotherapy for patients with acute promyelocytic leukemia? Blood 1987;69:187.
49. Gray WJ, Bell WR. Fibrinolytic agents in the treatment of thrombotic disorders. Semin Oncol 1990;17:228.
50. Hurtubise MR, Bottino JC, Lawson M, et al. Restoring patency of occluded venous catheters. Arch Surg 1980;115:212.
51. Fraschini G, Jadeja J, Lawson M, et al. Local infusion of urokinase for the lysis of thrombosis associated with permanent central venous catheters in cancer patients. J Clin Oncol 1987;5:672.
52. Schafer AI. Bleeding and thrombosis in the myeloproliferative disorders. Blood 1984;64:1.
53. Murphy S, Davis JL, Walsh PN, Gardner FH. Template bleeding time and clinical hemorrhage in myeloproliferative disease. Arch Intern Med 1978;138:1251.
54. Barbui T, Cortelazzo S, Viero P, Bassan R, Dini E, Semderaros N. Thrombohaemorrhagic complications in 101 cases of myeloproliferative disorders: relationship to platelet number and function. Eur J Cancer Clin Oncol 1983;19:1593.
55. Fitts WT, Erde A, Peskin GW, Frost JW. Surgical implications of polycythemia vera. Ann Surg 1960;152:548.
56. Rigby PG, Leavell BS. Polycythemia vera. Arch Intern Med 1960;106:622.
57. Ravocj RBM, Gunz FW, Reed CS, Thompson IL. The dangers of surgery in uncontrolled haemorrhagic thrombocythaemia. Med J Aust 1970;704.
58. Weiss RB, Tormey DC, Holland JF, Weinberg VE. Venous thrombosis during multimodal treatment of primary breast carcinoma. Cancer Treatment Reports 1981;65:677.
59. Levine MN, Gent M, Hirsh J, Arnold A, Goodyear MD, Hryniuk W, DePauw S. The thrombogenic effect of anticancer drug therapy in women with stage II breast cancer. N Engl J Med 1988;318:404.
60. Saphner T, Tormey DC, Gray R. Venous and arterial thrombosis in patients who received adjuvant therapy for breast cancer. J Clin Oncol 1991;9:286.
61. Wall JG, Weiss RB, Norton L, Perloff M, Rice MA, Korzun AH, Wood WC. Arterial thrombosis associated with adjuvant chemotherapy for breast carcinoma: a cancer and leukemia group B study. Am J Med 1989;87:501.
62. Fisher B, Redmond C, Wickerham DL, et al. Doxorubicin-containing regimens for the treatment of stage II breast cancer: the national surgical adjuvant breast and bowel project experience. J Clin Oncol 1989;7:572.
63. Fisher B, Brown AM, Dimitrov NV, et al. Two months of doxorubicin-cyclophosphamide with and without interval reinduction therapy compared with 6 months of cyclophosphamide, methotrexate, and fluorouracil in positive-node breast cancer patients with tamoxifen-nonresponsive tumors: Results from the national surgical adjuvant breast and bowel project B-15. J Clin Oncol 1990;8:1483.
64. Fisher B, Costantino J, Redmond C, et al. A randomized clinical trial evaluating tamoxifen in the treatment of patients with node-negative breast cancer who have estrogen-receptor-positive tumors. N Engl J Med 1989;320:479.
65. Rutqvist LE, Mattsson A. Cardiac and thromboembolic morbidity among postmenopausal women with early stage breast cancer in a randomized trial of adjuvant tamoxifen. J Natl Cancer Inst 1993;85:1398.
66. Doll DC, Ringenberg QS, Yarbro JW. Vascular toxicity associated with antineoplastic agents. J Clin Oncol 1986;4:1405.
67. Rogers JS, Murgo AJ, Fontana JA, Raich PC. Chemotherapy for breast cancer decreases plasma protein C and protein S. J Clin Oncol 1988;6:276.
68. Doll DC, List AF, Greco FA, Hainsworth JD, Hande KR, Johnson DH. Acute vascular ischemic events after cisplatin-based combination chemotherapy for germ-cell tumors of the testis. Ann Intern Med 1986;105:48.
69. Myhand RC and Weiss RB. Causes and management of treatment-related thrombosis. Contempory Oncology 1994;37.

Index

Abdominal aortic aneurysm, 241, 242
Abdominal distention
  in *Clostridium difficile* colitis, 105
  in constipation, 162
  in pancreatitis, 117
Abdominal pain, 3–23
  in bone marrow transplantation, 17–20
  in cholangitis, 116
  in *Clostridium difficile* colitis, 105
  in disseminated infection, 13–15
  following colonoscopy, 89
  in gastrointestinal obstruction, 15–16
  initial empirical antibiotic therapy in, 352
  in neutropenic enterocolitis, 5–10
  in pancreatitis, 10–11, 117
  in radiation enteritis, 103, 145
  in spontaneous rupture of hepatic tumor, 120
  in vascular and ischemic events, 16–17
Abdominal wall hernia, 128
Absidia, 356
Acalculous cholecystitis, 114–115
Acidosis, disseminated intravascular coagulation and, 382
Acivicin, 337
Acquired immunodeficiency syndrome, 315
Actinomycin D, 171, 311, 314
Acute promyelocytic leukemia, 383–384
Acute tubular necrosis, 289–290
Acyclovir
  in herpes simplex virus infection, 99, 358–359
  prophylactic, 367
Adenocarcinoma, small bowel, 34
Adrenal insufficiency, 297–299
Adrenocorticotropic hormone stimulation test, 297–298
Adriamycin; *See* Doxorubicin
Airway management, 273–274
Alkylating agents
  extravasation injury and, 212, 218–219
  myelosuppression caused by, 376
  and preoperative evaluation, 295–296
Allopurinol, 309
Alpha blockade drugs, 282
Alpha-fetoprotein, 257

5-Aminosalicylic acid, 151
Amitriptyline, 164
Amphotericin B
  in candidiasis, 14
    esophageal, 100
    hepatosplenic, 354
  in fungal infection, 357
  in pulmonary aspergillosis, 355
Anal cancer and obstruction, 47–48
Anastomotic leak, colonic, 40, 41
Anemia, 376–378
  microangiopathic hemolytic, 383
  preoperative evaluation of, 283–285
Anesthesia
  for central venous access, 188
  mediastinal mass and, 276
Aneurysm, abdominal aortic, 241, 242
Angiodysplasia and gastrointestinal bleeding, 73
Angiography, pulmonary, 233
Animal model
  in chemotherapy effects on wound healing, 314
  in malignant ascites, 126
Anorectal infection, 349
Anorexia
  in malignant ascites, 128
  malnutrition and, 325
  refeeding syndrome and, 335
Antacids, 65
Anterior mediastinal mass, 257, 276–279
Anthracycline
  cardiac toxicity of, 293–294
  extravasation injury and, 212
Anthraquinone glycosides, 166–167
Antibiotics
  in acalculous cholecystitis, 115
  in cholangitis, 116
  in device-related bacteremia, 203
  neutropenia and, 349–350, 351, 352
  in perforated duodenal ulcer, 83
  and preoperative evaluation, 293–294
Antibody alterations in humoral immunity, 344
Anticipatory emesis, 171
Anticoagulation
  in deep venous thrombosis, 234

Anticoagulation *Continued*
  in disseminated intravascular coagulation, 384
  perioperative prophylactic, 386–387
Antidepressants and constipation, 164–165
Antiemetic agents, 176
Antihistamines, 281
Antioxidants and radiation induced bowel injury, 146
Antithrombin-III, 228
Antrectomy
  for malignant duodenal obstruction, 33
  in perforated gastric ulcer, 67, 82
Anxiolytics, 171
Aortic sarcoma, 224
Appendicitis, 88, 91
Appetite loss, 325
Ara-C; *See* Cytosine arabinoside
Arginine, 335, 337–339
Arterial rupture, 240
Arteriography
  in carotid body tumor, 225, 226
  in erosive gastritis, 66
  in hemobilia, 68
  in lower gastrointestinal bleeding, 70, 72
Arteriovenous fistula and vascular access devices, 204
Ascites, 125–142
  chemotherapy in, 137–138
  diagnosis of, 126–128
  etiology of, 125–126
  immunotherapy and biologic response modifiers in, 138–140
  LeVeen and Denver shunt results, 131–137
  in malnutrition, 322
  natural history and complications of, 128
  need for intervention, 128–129
  paracentesis in, 129–131
Ascitic fluid chemistry determinations, 127
L-Asparaginase
  emetic potential of, 171
  pancreatitis and, 10
  preoperative evaluation of, 297, 298
Aspergillus infection, 13
  in neutropenic patient, 355–356
  nosocomial spread of, 344
Aspiration during enteral feeding, 336
Aspirin, preoperative discontinuation of, 386
Atherosclerosis
  accelerated, 242
  radiation-induced, 230
  secondary effects of tumor on, 229
ATN; *See* Acute tubular necrosis
Atrial myxoma, 226–227
Atrium, direct access to, 195
Autologous blood donation, 284, 376–378
Awake intubation, 274
Azacitidine, 171
Azole, 357–358
Azygous vein access, 195

B cell activation, 344
Bacteria, immune defects and, 345
Bacteroides, 116
Balloon dilatation of obstructing colonic lesions, 40
Balloon pericardiostomy, 254
Balloon tamponade of esophageal varix, 64
Basal energy expenditure, 331
Bile salts and radiation injury, 152

Biliary tract
  candidiasis of, 14
  infections of, 114–117
  malignant obstruction of, 111–114
  stasis of, 333
Biologic response modifiers, 138–140
Biopsy
  in candidiasis, 14, 100
  lung, 265, 266–267
  in malignant pericardial effusion, 253
  in malignant pleural effusion, 250
  in mediastinal mass, 258, 259
Bisacodyl, 167
Bladder distention, 145, 146
Bleeding, 232
  anticoagulation and, 234–235
  cancer-related anemia and, 377
  during central venous access, 196–197
  in myeloproliferative disorders, 386
  in spontaneous rupture of hepatic tumor, 120
Bleomycin
  effects on wound healing, 309, 314
  emetic potential of, 171
  in malignant pleural effusion, 251
  preoperative evaluation of, 294–295
Blood, withdrawal through catheter, 203
Blood transfusion
  autologous, 284, 376–378
  cancer recurrence and, 284
  graft-*versus*-host disease and, 379
Blue toe syndrome, 239
Boerhaave's syndrome
  esophageal perforation in, 75
  Mallory-Weiss syndrome *versus,* 65
Bone marrow dysfunction, 375–391
  anemia in, 376–378
  bone marrow transplant transfusion considerations in, 378–379
  chemotherapy-induced myelosuppression in, 375–376
  chemotherapy-related thrombosis in, 387–388
  disseminated intravascular coagulation in, 382–385
  myeloproliferative disorders in, 385–387
  red blood cell transfusion support in, 379
  thrombocytopenia in, 379–382
Bone marrow transplantation
  abdominal pain following, 17–20
  Budd-Chiari syndrome following, 118
  cytomegalovirus and, 359–360
  herpes simplex virus hepatitis following, 14
  myeloablative doses of chemotherapy and, 376
  nutritional support in, 329
  pancreatitis following, 11
  transfusion considerations in, 378–379
  varicella-zoster virus infections following, 15
Bone tumor, thoracic spine, 259
Brachytherapy and internal complications, 144
Breast cancer
  malignant ascites in, 137
  pulmonary metastasis from, 263
Bronchoalveolar lavage, 363
Bronchoscopy
  in immunocompromised patient, 363–364
  in interstitial lung disease, 266
Budd-Chiari syndrome, 118–120

Index

deep venous thrombosis and, 237
upper gastrointestinal bleeding and, 63–64
Bulk-forming agents, 166
Busulfan, 296
Bypass
  in bowel obstruction after pelvic irradiation, 151
  in bowel obstruction caused by carcinomatosis, 52
  carotid, 240
  esophageal, 80
  in gastric cancer, 30
  in pancreatic cancer, 32
  in radiation enteritis, 155
  in radiation-related carotid atherosclerosis, 230
  in rectovaginal fistula, 156

Calcitonin, 288
Caloric requirements, 331
Cancer; *See* Malignancy; specific cancer
Cancer cachexia, 321–342
  assessment for, 321–323
  causes of, 325–328
  enteral nutrition in, 334–336
  future research in, 337–339
  nutrient replacement in, 328–330, 331
  outpatient supplements in, 336
  parenteral nutrition in, 330–334
  prevalence of, 323–325
Cancer procoagulant, 228
Candida infection, 13
  esophageal, 100, 101
  in neutropenic enterocolitis, 6
  in neutropenic patient, 353–355
Carbohydrate metabolism, 326
Carbon dioxide partial pressure, 274–275
Carboplatin, 171
Carcinoid syndrome, 34–35
  preoperative evaluation of, 280–283
  upper gastrointestinal bleeding in, 67
Cardiac tamponade, 279–280
Carmustine
  emetic potential of, 171
  pulmonary toxicity of, 296
Carotid body tumor, 224–226
Carotid bypass, 240
Carotid rupture, 240
Cascara, 167
Catheter, venous access
  fungal infection and, 353
  removal of, 198–199
  shearing of, 203–204
Cecum, neutropenic enterocolitis and, 6
Ceftazidime, 350
Cell-mediated immunity, 345, 346
Cell-saver blood, 284–285
Central venous access, 183–209
  catheter shear and, 203–204
  cutdown venotomy for, 193, 194, 195
  extravasation injury prevention and, 219
  failure to place device, 197
  fluoroscopy and radiography in, 195–196
  hemorrhage during, 196–197
  Hickman catheter in, 184–185
  indications for, 183–184
  infection and, 202–203, 361–362
  intra-abdominal, 193–194
  intraoperative preparation in, 188

intrathoracic, 194–195
operative approach for, 189, 191
parenteral hyperalimentation by, 330–331
P.A.S. Port in, 186
patient positioning for, 188, 190
percutaneous, 190–193
peripherally inserted central catheter in, 184
pneumothorax and hemothorax during, 197
postoperative care in, 198–199
preoperative care in, 187–188
subclavian catheter in, 184
subcutaneous infusion port in, 185–186
thrombosis following, 200–202
withdrawal occlusion and, 203
Cephalic vein cutdown, 189, 193
Cerebral infarction, 239
Cervical esophageal perforation, 76
Charcot's triad, 116
Chemoreceptor trigger zone, 169–170
Chemotherapy
  colitis and, 74
  constipation and, 164
  deep venous thrombosis and, 237–238
  emesis and, 168–177
    combination therapy for, 175–176
    general guidelines in, 171–172
    harmful effects of, 168–169
    neurophysiology of, 169–170
    single agent therapy for, 172–175
    temporal patterns of, 170–171
  in esophageal cancer, 26
  extravasation during, 211–222
    algorithm for treatment, 220
    initial nonoperative care of, 214–215
    of non-nucleic acid-binding agents, 218–219
    of nucleic acid-binding agents, 212–214
    operative management of, 215–218
    prevention of, 219
    risk factors for, 211
  in gastric cancer, 30
  gastrointestinal obstruction and, 48–51
  in malignant ascites, 137–138
  malnutrition and, 327–328
  myelosuppression and, 375–376
  obstructive symptoms and, 15–16
  pancreatitis and, 10, 11
  stomatitis and, 98–99
  vascular effects of, 231
  wound healing and, 307–315
    actinomycin D in, 311
    animal models in, 314
    bleomycin in, 309
    cisplatin in, 309–310
    corticosteroids in, 310–311
    cyclophosphamide in, 311
    dacarbazine in, 311
    doxorubicin in, 308–309
    etoposide in, 311–312
    5-fluorouracil in, 312
    6-mercaptopurine in, 312
    methotrexate in, 312–313
    mitomycin in, 313
    mitoxantrone in, 313
    systemic effects, 307–308
    vinblastine in, 313
    vincristine in, 313

Chest pain
  in malignant pericardial effusion, 253
  in malignant pleural effusion, 250
Chest roentgenogram
  in esophageal perforation, 75–76
  in gastric or duodenal perforation, 81
  in malignant pericardial effusion, 253
  in mediastinal tumor, 257
Chlorambucil, 296
Cholangiocarcinoma, 111–114
Cholangitis, 115–117
Cholecystectomy, 115
Cholecystitis
  acalculous, 114–115
  after bone marrow transplant, 19
Cholelithiasis and TPN, 333
Cholesterol determination, of ascitic fluid, 127
Cholestyramine
  in enteritis, 103
  in radiation-induced diarrhea, 106
Chronic myeloid leukemia, 386
Chronic venous access; *See* Central venous access
Cisplatin
  effects on wound healing, 309–310, 314
  emetic potential of, 171
  in malignant ascites, 138
  preoperative evaluation of, 296–297
Clam-shell incision, 264
Clonidine, 281
Clostridium difficile colitis, 105, 354–365
  colonic perforation in, 88–89
  in neutropenic patient, 6
  nosocomial spread of, 344
  rectal bleeding in, 74
Clotrimazole, 100
Clotting factors
  disseminated intravascular coagulation and, 382
  tumor growth and, 228–229
CMV; *See* Cytomegalovirus
Coagulation, growth of tumors and, 227–229
Coagulopathy
  after peritoneovenous shunt, 136
  preoperative evaluation of, 285–286
Colace; *See* Docusate sodium
Cold therapy for doxorubicin extravasation, 214
Colitis, 105–107
  chemotherapy-induced, 74
  Clostridium difficile, 105, 354–365
    colonic perforation in, 88–89
    in neutropenic patient, 6
    nosocomial spread of, 344
    rectal bleeding in, 74
  diversion, 105–106
Collagen, wound repair and, 306–307
Colon
  fistula of, 91
  lower gastrointestinal bleeding and, 73–74
  neutropenic enterocolitis and, 6
  perforation of, 88–91
  physiology of, 162
  radiation effects on, 106
Colon cancer
  colonic perforation in, 88, 90–91
  gastrointestinal obstruction in, 36–47
    electrocautery fulguration in, 46–47

laser ablation in, 45–46
  left-sided, 39–41
  radiation therapy in, 43–45
  rectosigmoid, 42–43
  surgical resection or diversion in, 43, 44
lung metastasis and, 262
radiation-induced, 154
small bowel obstruction after cancer surgery and, 49
Colonoscopy, 70
Colostomy
  in anal squamous cell carcinoma, 48
  in colon cancer, 38, 39
  in diverticular perforation, 90
Colyte, 167
Complete blood count, preoperative, 286
Computed tomography
  in abdominal pain, 7, 8
  of carotid body tumor, 225
  in hepatosplenic candidiasis, 354
  in interstitial lung disease, 266
  in malignant pericardial effusion, 253
  of mediastinal mass, 257, 277
  in pancreatitis, 117
  in pulmonary aspergillosis, 355, 356
Congestive heart failure
  adriamycin-induced, 293
  in atrial myxoma, 226
Constipation, 161–168
  adverse effects of, 165
  causes of, 162–165
  in colonic or rectal perforation, 89
  enteral feedings and, 335
  hemorrhoids and, 161
  physiology of, 162
  treatment of, 166–168
  vincristine and, 16
Constipation Assessment Scale, 165
Contraction of wound, 307
Contrast phlebography, 232–233
Contrast venography, 187
Corticosteroids
  in doxorubicin extravasation, 215
  effects on wound healing, 310–311
Cortisol, 297–299
Cortisone acetate, 310
Corynebacterium parvum, 138
Cosyntropin, 297
Cough
  in malignant pericardial effusion, 253
  in malignant pleural effusion, 250
Creatinine-height index, 322
Crohn's disease, 84–85
Culture
  of *Clostridium difficile,* 365
  of cytomegalovirus, 360
Cushing's ulcer, 65
Cutaneous vasculitis, 238
Cutdown, 193, 194, 195
Cyclophosphamide
  effects on wound healing, 311, 314
  emetic potential of, 171
  preoperative evaluation of, 295
Cytokines
  antibodies to, 339
  cachexia and, 327, 328

Cytology
    in ascites, 127
    in pericardial effusion, 253
    in pleural effusion, 250
Cytomegalovirus infection
    after bone marrow transplant, 15, 378–379
    biopsy in, 101
    in colitis, 105
    in gastritis, 103
    in neutropenic patient, 359–360
Cytosine arabinoside
    neutropenic enterocolitis and, 5–6
    pancreatitis and, 10
    toxicity of, 296
Cytoxan, 387

Dacarbazine
    effects on wound healing, 311, 314
    emetic potential of, 171
Dactinomycin; See Actinomycin D
Daily caloric requirements, 331
Daunomycin, 293
Daunorubicin, 212
Debridement in doxorubicin extravasation, 215, 216–217
Debulking of mediastinal mass, 259
Decompressing colostomy, 38
Decompression of esophageal varix, 64
Deep venous thrombosis, 232–239
    disseminated intravascular coagulation and, 383
    late complications of, 237–238
    prophylaxis and surveillance against, 238–239
    treatment of, 234–237
    tumor mass and, 229
Dehydration
    constipation and, 163
    vomiting and, 168
Delayed gastric emptying, 32
Delta 9 tetra hydrocannabinol, 174–175
Dentition, constipation and, 163
Denver shunt, 131–135, 252
Depression, vomiting and, 169
Dermatitis, therapeutic radiation and, 143–144
Desipramine, 164
Dexamethasone, 174
Diabetes mellitus and TPN, 333
Diarrhea
    after bone marrow transplant, 17
    antiemetic agents and, 176
    enteral feeding and, 335
    in enteritis, 103
    malnutrition and, 327
    in neutropenic enterocolitis, 6
    in pancreatitis, 117
    radiation therapy and, 144, 145
Dietary fiber, constipation and, 162–163, 166
Digital artery occlusion, 238
Dimethyl sulfoxide, 214–215
Diphenoxylate, 103
Disseminated intravascular coagulation, 382–385
    malignancy and, 228
    peritoneovenous shunting and, 133, 135–136
    preoperative evaluation for, 285–286
Distal common bile duct cholangiocarcinoma, 111
Distal splenorenal shunt, 64

Diuretics
    constipation and, 163
    in hypercalcemia, 288
    in malignant ascites, 129
Diversion
    in bowel obstruction after pelvic irradiation, 151
    esophageal, 79
Diversion colitis, 105–106
Diverticular disease
    colonic perforation in, 88, 89–91
    lower gastrointestinal bleeding in, 73
Diverting colostomy
    in anal squamous cell carcinoma, 48
    in colorectal cancer, 38–39
Docusate sodium, 166
Double-lumen catheter, 185
Doxepin, 164
Doxorubicin
    cardiotoxicity of, 293
    effects on wound healing, 308–309, 314
    emetic potential of, 171
    extravasation injury and, 212
Doxycycline
    in pericardial effusion, 254
    in pleural effusion, 251
Drainage procedures
    in acalculous cholecystitis, 115
    in malignant ascites, 129
Dressings
    in central venous access, 198
    for doxorubicin infiltration injury, 217
Dronabinol; See Marinol
Drug-induced disorder
    colitis as, 74
    constipation as, 163–165
    deep venous thrombosis as, 237–238
    pancreatitis as, 10, 11
    stomatitis as, 98–99
Duodenal ulcer perforation, 83
Duodenitis, 69
Duodenum
    perforation of, 81–84
    upper gastrointestinal bleeding and, 68–69
Duplex scan
    in deep venous thrombosis, 233
    in thrombus-associated catheter malfunction, 201
DVT; See Deep venous thrombosis
Dyspnea
    in ascites, 128
    in candidal pneumonia, 355
    in esophageal perforation, 75
    in pericardial effusion, 253
    in pleural effusion, 250

Early Postoperative Intraperitoneal Chemotherapy, 48–49
Echocardiography, 253, 280
Edema
    after peritoneovenous shunt, 136
    of airway structures, 273
    in malnutrition, 322
Effusion
    pericardial, 253–256, 279–280
    pleural, 249–252
Electrocardiography, 253

Electrocautery fulguration, 46–47
Electrolyte deficiencies
　parenteral nutrition and, 332
　preoperative evaluation of, 286–291
Embolic arterial occlusion, 239–240
Embolism
　in atrial myxoma, 226
　pulmonary
　　chemotherapy-related, 387
　　deep venous thrombosis and, 232
　　diagnosis of, 233–234
Embolization in hemobilia, 68
Emesis; *See* Vomiting
Emollient laxatives, 166
Endocarditis, nonbacterial thrombotic, 239
Endoscopic laser tumor ablation, 27–29
Endoscopic retrograde cholangiopancreatography, 111
Endoscopy
　in bleeding gastric ulcer, 67
　in esophageal candidiasis, 100
　in esophageal varices, 64
　gastric perforation and, 83
　in lower gastrointestinal bleeding, 72
　in Mallory-Weiss syndrome, 65
　in upper gastrointestinal bleeding, 63
Enema, 167
Enteral feeding, 330, 331, 334–336
Enteritis, 103–105
　following bone marrow transplant, 17
　radiation-induced, 143–160
　　acute and subacute, 145
　　bowel obstruction and, 150–152
　　chronic, 147–150
　　prevention of, 152–153
　　risk of recurrent obstruction and, 50
　　treatment of, 145–147, 153–156
Enterobacter
　in cholangitis, 116
　in neutropenic enterocolitis, 6
　nosocomial spread of, 344
　in oral infection, 99
Enterococcus, 344
Enterocutaneous fistula, 85, 86–87
Enteroenteric fistula, 85, 87
Enterovaginal fistula, 85, 87
Enterovesical fistula, 85, 87
Epirubicin, 212
Epsilon aminocaproic acid, 383
Erosive gastritis, 65–66
Erythema
　in device-related bacteremia, 203
　in extravasation injury, 212
Erythropoietin, 377, 378
Escherichia coli
　in cholangitis, 116
　in neutropenic enterocolitis, 6
　neutropenic patient and, 349
　in oral infection, 99
Esmolol, 283
Esophageal varix, 63–64
Esophagitis, 99–102, 327
Esophagus
　bypass of, 80
　cancer of, 25–29
　herpes simplex virus infection of, 358

　perforation of, 27, 75–80
　tracheoesophageal fistula and, 80
　upper gastrointestinal bleeding and, 63–65
Etoposide
　effects on wound healing, 311–312, 314
　emetic potential of, 171
　toxicity of, 296
Evacuation of clot
　in erosive gastritis, 66
　in upper gastrointestinal bleeding, 62
Excision in doxorubicin extravasation, 215–216
Exit site infection and central venous access devices, 203
External beam irradiation, 144, 253–254
Extrapyramidal reaction, 176
Extravasation, 211–222
　algorithm for treatment, 220
　device fracture and, 203
　initial nonoperative care of, 214–215
　of non-nucleic acid-binding agents, 218–219
　of nucleic acid-binding agents, 212–214
　operative management of, 215–218
　prevention of, 219
　risk factors for, 211
Extrinsic compression by malignancy, 54–56
Exudate effusion, 250

Facial purpura, 169
Failure to place device, 197
Fat metabolism, 326
Fatigue, vomiting and, 169
Fecal impaction, 161, 167–168
Femoral vein
　venous cutdown and, 193
Fever
　in cholangitis, 116
　in disseminated fungal infection, 14
　in esophageal perforation, 75
　in fecal impaction, 161
　granulocyte-macrophage colony stimulating factor and, 368
　initial empirical antibiotic therapy in, 352
　in neutropenic enterocolitis, 6
　in neutropenic patient, 348–351, 352–353
　in pancreatitis, 117
Fiberoptic bronchoscopy, 363
Fiberoptic esophagogastroduodenoscopy, 63
Fiberoptic intubation, 274
Fibrin, 228
Fibrin split products
　disseminated intravascular coagulation and, 382, 384
　tumor growth and, 229
Fibrinogen, 384
Fibrinolytic therapy, 385
　in deep venous thrombosis, 236
　disseminated intravascular coagulation and, 383
　in thrombus-associated catheter malfunction, 201–202
Fibroblast, 306
Fibronectin, ascitic fluid, 127
Fistula
　arteriovenous, 204
　colonic, 89, 91
　enterocutaneous, 86–87
　enteroenteric, 85, 87
　enterovaginal, 85, 87

enterovesical, 85, 87
perforation of small intestine and, 84–85
radiation-induced, 155–156
rectovaginal, 156
tracheoesophageal, 79–80
Flap
in esophageal perforation repair, 78
in extravasation injury, 218
Flipped port, 204
Flow cytometry, 128
Flow volume loop, 276, 277
Fluconazole, 357–358
in esophageal candidiasis, 100
prophylactic, 367
Flucytosine, 355, 357
Fluid overload after peritoneovenous shunt, 136
Fluoroscopy
to ascertain guidewire position, 191
in central venous access, 195–196
in malignant pericardial effusion, 253
5-Fluorouracil
in cholangiocarcinoma, 113
effects on wound healing, 312, 314
emetic potential of, 171
radiation injury to bowel and, 150–151
in recurrent rectal cancer, 44
toxicity of, 296
venous thrombosis and, 387
Focal hepatic candidiasis, 14
Forced expiratory volume in 1 second, 274–275
Formula
enteral, 335
parenteral, 331
Foscarnet, 360
Fractional excretion of sodium (FEN$_a$), 291
Fracture, vomiting and, 169
Free flap, 218
Free water deficit, 287
Fresh frozen plasma, 63
Fulguration, 46–47
Fungal infection, 351–358
abdominal pain in, 13–15
catheter-associated, 361
immune defects and, 345
oral, 99
prophylaxis for, 367

Gallbladder cancer, 113, 114
Ganciclovir, 360
Gangrene, 382
Gastrectomy, 29
in erosive gastritis, 66
gastritis following, 102
in perforated gastric neoplasm, 82
Gastric outlet obstruction
malignant causes of, 29
in periampullary malignancy, 32
Gastric sarcoma perforation, 82
Gastric ulcer
perforation of, 13, 82
upper gastrointestinal hemorrhage in, 66–67
Gastritis, 102–103
Gastrointestinal bleeding, 61–74
anticoagulation therapy and, 235
lower, 69–75

colon and rectum and, 73–74
initial management of, 69–71
jejunum and ileum and, 71–73
upper, 61–69
duodenum and, 68–69
esophageal, 63–65
hemobilia and, 67–68
initial management of, 61–63
stomach and, 65–67
Gastrointestinal obstruction, 25–60
abdominal pain in, 15–16
anal region cancer and, 47–48
cancer therapy and, 48–51
colon and rectum cancer and, 36–43
constipation and, 163
esophageal cancer including gastric cardia in, 25–29
extrinsic compression by malignancy and, 54–56
gastric cancer and, 29–31
mesenteric small bowel malignancy and, 34–36
palliative management of recurrent colorectal cancer and, 43–47
periampullary region cancer and, 31–34
peritoneal carcinomatosis and, 51–54
Gastrointestinal perforation, 74–91
abdominal pain in, 12–13
colonic, 88–91
esophageal, 75–80
small intestine and, 84–88
stomach and duodenum and, 81–84
Gastrointestinal tract
graft-*versus*-host disease and, 18
inflammatory lesions of, 97–109
colitis in, 105–107
enteritis in, 103–105
esophagitis in, 99–102
gastritis in, 102–103
stomatitis in, 98–99
radiation-induced injury to, 143–160
acute and subacute, 145
bowel obstruction and, 150–152
chronic, 147–150
prevention of, 152–153
treatment of, 145–147, 153–156
Gastrojejunostomy, 30, 32
Gastrostomy tube
for feeding, 334
in gastric cancer, 30–31
in ovarian cancer, 52
Gauze dressing at catheter exit site, 198
Germ cell tumor, mediastinal, 257
Glucocorticoids
in hypercalcemia, 288
preoperative evaluation and, 297
Glutamine, 326
in preserving host mass, 337
in radiation enteritis, 146–147
Goiter, retrosternal, 257
Golytely (Colyte), 167
Graft-*versus*-host disease
abdominal pain in, 17–18
transfusion-associated, 379
Graham patch, 83
Granisetron, 173–174
Granulation tissue, 306
Granulocyte colony stimulating factor, 367–368

Granulocyte level, infection and, 347
Granulocyte-macrophage colony stimulating factor, 367–368
Granulocytopenia
    chemotherapy and, 231
    frequency of infection and, 348
Gray (Gy), defined, 143
Greenfield filter, 235–236
Grillo flap, 77, 78
Growth factors
    doxorubicin toxicity and, 309
    for restoration of host immunity, 367–368
Growth hormone, 337
Guidewire, fluoroscopic positioning of, 191

Harris-Benedict equation, 331
Hartmann's procedure in colonic obstruction, 38, 39
Head and neck tumor
    airway considerations in, 273–274
    pulmonary metastasis from, 263
    resection of, 240
Heart
    chemotherapy toxicity and, 292
    disease of
        association with cancer, 229
        embolic arterial occlusion and, 239
        total parenteral nutrition in, 333
    tumor of, 226
Helper T cell, 346
Hemangiopericytoma, 223
Hemangiosarcoma, 223
Hematemesis, 61
Hematochezia
    in lower gastrointestinal bleeding, 69
    in upper gastrointestinal bleeding, 61
Hematocrit, perioperative, 379
Hematologic abnormalities, 375–391
    anemia in, 376–378
    bone marrow transplant transfusion considerations in, 378–379
    chemotherapy-induced myelosuppression in, 375–376
    chemotherapy-related thrombosis in, 387–388
    disseminated intravascular coagulation in, 382–385
    myeloproliferative disorders in, 385–387
    preoperative evaluation of, 283–286
    red blood cell transfusion support in, 379
    thrombocytopenia in, 379–382
Hemicolectomy, 38, 39
Hemigastrectomy, 82
Hemobilia, 67–68
Hemodialysis and TPN, 333
Hemolytic anemia, microangiopathic, 383
Hemorrhage, 232
    anticoagulation and, 234–235
    cancer-related anemia and, 377
    during central venous access, 196–197
    in myeloproliferative disorders, 386
    in spontaneous rupture of hepatic tumor, 120
Hemorrhoids, 161
Hemothorax during central venous access, 197
Heparin
    in catheter thrombosis, 198, 201
    in deep venous thrombosis, 234
    in disseminated intravascular coagulation, 383, 384
    low molecular weight, 236
    prophylactic, 238
    tumor growth and, 228
Hepatic artery chemotherapy, 103
Hepatic candidiasis, 14
Hepatic steatosis, 332
Hepatic tumor rupture, 120–121
Hepatic vein occlusion, 18–19, 118
Hepatitis
    herpes simplex virus, 14
    varicella-zoster virus, 15
Hepatobiliary disease, 111–123
    acalculous cholecystitis in, 115–117
    Budd-Chiari syndrome in, 118–120
    cholangiocarcinoma in, 111–114
    cholangitis in, 115–117
    pancreatitis in, 117–118
    portal vein occlusion in, 118–120
    rupture of hepatic tumor in, 120–121
Hepatoma and Budd-Chiari Syndrome, 118
Hepatosplenic candidiasis, 14, 354
Hernia, abdominal wall, 128
Herpes simplex infection
    in neutropenic patient, 14, 358–359
    oral, 99
Hickman catheter, 184–185
High-affinity receptor, 346
High-efficiency particulate air filter, 365
High-resolution computed tomography, 266
Histamine$_2$ blockers
    in erosive stress gastritis, 65
    in perforated duodenal ulcer, 83
Histiocytoma, malignant fibrous of the great vessels, 224
Hodgkin's disease
    infections during, 346
    mediastinal lymph nodes and, 256
Home parenteral and enteral nutrition, 52–54, 336
Host flora alterations, 343–344
Human leukocyte antigen, 346
Human leukocyte antigen-matched platelets, 380, 381
Humoral immunity defects, 344–346
Hydrocortisone, 298–299
Hydrothorax, venous access devices and, 204
5-Hydroxytryptamine receptor, 164
Hydroxyurea in thrombocytopenia, 386
Hypercalcemia
    constipation and, 163
    preoperative evaluation of, 288
Hyperchloremic metabolic acidosis, 332
Hyperglycemia, 332
Hyperkalemia, 287–288
Hyperlipidemia, 326
Hypernatremia, 287
Hyperosmolar feedings, 335
Hypersplenism, 377
Hypertension, portal venous, 63
Hypertriglyceridemia, 332
Hypoalbuminemia, 249
Hypocalcemia, 288–289
Hypofibrinogenemia, 382, 384
Hypogammaglobulinemia, 367
Hypokalemia
    constipation and, 163

Index

preoperative evaluation of, 287
vomiting and, 168
Hypomagnesemia
   parenteral nutrition and, 332
   preoperative evaluation of, 289
Hyponatremia, 286–287
Hypophosphatemia, 332
Hypotension
   in disseminated intravascular coagulation, 382
   in spontaneous rupture of hepatic tumor, 120

Idiopathic thrombocytopenic purpura, 381–382
Ifosfamide, 295–296
Ileocecal syndrome, 5
Ileostomy, 86
Ileum
   adenocarcinoma of, 34
   lower gastrointestinal bleeding and, 71–73
Ileus
   from chemotherapeutic agent, 16
   neutropenic enterocolitis and, 6
Iliofemoral deep venous thrombosis, 237
Imipenem, 350
Imipramine, 164
Immune hemolysis, 377
Immunity
   defects in, 344–346
   restoration of, 367–368
Immunocompromised host infection, 343–373
   cellular immunity defects in, 346
   central venous catheter-associated, 361–362
   Clostridium difficile, 364–365
   disruption of anatomic barrier function in, 343
   fever in, 348–351, 352–353
   fungal, 351–358
   host flora alterations in, 343–344
   humoral immunity defects in, 344–346
   intra-abdominal, 364
   phagocytic function defects in, 346–348
   prevention of, 365–368
   pulmonary infiltrates and, 362–364
   viral, 358–360
Immunoglobulin therapy, 360
Immunotherapy, 138–140
Impedance plethysmography, 232–233
Incision
   clam shell, 264
   in cutdown venotomy, 193
   for peritoneovenous shunt, 130
   in pulmonary metastasis resection, 264
   for subcutaneous port, 192
   thoracoabdominal, 260
Indomethacin, 146
Indwelling venous access device, 183–184
Infection
   abdominal pain in, 5–15
      in disseminated infection, 13–15
      in gastrointestinal perforation, 12–13
      in neutropenic enterocolitis, 5–10
      in pancreatitis, 10–11
   biliary tree, 114–117
   in bone marrow transplant patient, 17
   in immunocompromised host, 343–373
      cellular immunity defects in, 346
      central venous catheter-associated, 361–362

Clostridium difficile, 364–365
disruption of anatomic barrier function in, 343
fever in, 348–351, 352–353
fungal, 351–358
host flora alterations in, 343–344
humoral immunity defects in, 344–346
intra-abdominal, 364
phagocytic function defects in, 346–348
prevention of, 365–368
pulmonary infiltrates and, 362–364
viral, 358–360
indwelling central venous access device and, 202–203
shunt, 136–137
Inferior vena cava
   accessing, 188
   chronic thrombus, 237
   Greenfield filter in, 235–236
   leiomyosarcoma of, 224
Infiltration injury; See Extravasation
Inflammatory disease
   abdominal pain in, 5–15
      in disseminated infection, 13–15
      in gastrointestinal perforation, 12–13
      in neutropenic enterocolitis, 5–10
      in pancreatitis, 10–11
   pulmonary, 265
Inflammatory lesion, gastrointestinal, 97–109
   colitis as, 105–107
   enteritis as, 103–105
   esophagitis as, 99–102
   gastritis as, 102–103
   stomatitis as, 98–99
Inflammatory phase of wound healing, 305–306
Insulin
   in cancer cachexia, 337
   resistance to, 326
Interferons
   cachexia and, 327, 328
   major histocompatibility complex and, 344
   in malignant ascites, 138–139
Interleukin-1
   cachexia and, 327, 328
   in T cell activation, 344
Interleukin-2
   in therapy of malignant ascites, 139
   prior to metastasectomy, 263
   T cell and, 346
Interleukin-6, 327, 328
Internal jugular vein
   accessing, 190
   cutdown of, 193, 194
Interstitial lung disease, 266
Interstitial pneumonitis, 352
Intra-abdominal infection, 364
Intra-abdominal venous access, 193–194
Intraoperative port accession, 198
Intraperitoneal chemotherapy
   bowel obstruction following, 48–49
   in malignant ascites, 138
Intrathoracic venous access, 194–195
Intravena caval devices, 236
Intravenous feeding, 329
Intravenous immunoglobulin, 360
Intrinsic renal failure, 289–290

Ischemic venous thrombosis, 237
Itraconazole, 357–358

Jaundice
　in cholangiocarcinoma, 111
　in cholangitis, 116
　in hemobilia, 67
Jejunostomy
　for feeding, 334
　in gastric outlet obstruction, 31
Jejunum
　adenocarcinoma of, 34
　lower gastrointestinal bleeding and, 71–73

Kaposi's sarcoma, 223–224
Ketanserin, 281
Ketoconazole, 100
Klatskin tumor, 112
Klebsiella, 349
　in cholangitis, 116
　in neutropenic enterocolitis, 6
　in oral infection, 99

Lactulose, 167
Laminar air flow room, 365–366
Large intestine; *See* Colon
Large vessel
　thrombosis of, 238–239
　tumor of, 224–227
Laser therapy
　in colon cancer, 40, 45–46
　in esophageal cancer, 27–29
　lung biopsy and, 267
　in rectal cancer, 42–43
Lavage
　bronchoalveolar, 363
　peritoneal, 7
Laxatives, 164, 166
Lean body mass, 322
Leiomyoma, 67, 71
Leiomyosarcoma, 67, 224
Leucovorin, 44
Leukemia
　disseminated intravascular coagulation in, 383–384
　neutropenic enterocolitis in, 5
Leukocytosis
　in acalculous cholecystitis, 114
　in cholangitis, 116
LeVeen shunt, 131–135
Ligation of esophageal varix, 64
Linitis plastica, 30
Liver disease, 111–123
　acalculous cholecystitis in, 115–117
　Budd-Chiari syndrome in, 118–120
　cholangiocarcinoma in, 111–114
　cholangitis in, 115–117
　fungal, 14
　pancreatitis in, 117–118
　parenteral nutrition and, 332, 333
　portal vein occlusion in, 118–120
　rupture of hepatic tumor in, 120–121
Lomustine, 296
Loperamide, 103
Lorazepam, 175
Loss of appetite, 325

Low molecular weight heparin, 236
Lower gastrointestinal bleeding, 69–75
　colon and rectum and, 73–74
　initial management of, 69–71
　jejunum and ileum and, 71–73
Lung
　chemotherapy toxicity and, 292
　disease of
　　biopsy in, 265, 266–267
　　total parenteral nutrition in, 333–334
　infiltrates in, 362
　metastasis to, 262–265
　resection of, 274–276
Lymphokine-activated killer cell, 139
Lymphoma
　gastrointestinal perforation and, 12–13
　of small bowel, 35
　upper gastrointestinal bleeding in, 67
Lymphoproliferative disease of mediastinum, 256–259
Lytic therapy, 236

Macrophage, 305
Magnesium citrate, 167
Major histocompatibility complex, 344
Malabsorption, 154
Malignancy
　extrinsic compression by, 54–56
　hematologic complications of, 375–391
　　anemia in, 376–378
　　bone marrow transplant transfusion considerations in, 378–379
　　chemotherapy-induced myelosuppression in, 375–376
　　chemotherapy-related thrombosis in, 387–388
　　disseminated intravascular coagulation in, 382–385
　　myeloproliferative disorders in, 385–387
　　red blood cell transfusion support in, 379
　　thrombocytopenia in, 379–382
　immunocompromised state and, 343–348
　　cellular immunity defects in, 346
　　disruption of anatomic barrier function in, 343
　　host flora alterations in, 343–344
　　humoral immunity defects in, 344–346
　　phagocytic function defects in, 346–348
　thoracic complications of, 249–270
　　lymphoproliferative disease of mediastinum in, 256–259
　　parenchymal lung disease in, 265–267
　　pericardial effusion in, 253–256
　　pleural effusion in, 249–252
　　pulmonary metastases in, 262–265
　　surgical approach to thoracic spine in, 259–261
　vascular complications of, 223–248
　　accelerated chronic arterial occlusive disease in, 242
　　concomitant conditions and, 241–242
　　embolic arterial occlusive disease in, 239–240
　　hemorrhage in, 232
　　large vessel primary vascular tumors in, 224–227
　　small vessel primary vascular tumors in, 223–224
　　tumor effects in, 227–231
　　vascular reconstruction associated with resection in, 240–241
　　venous thromboembolism in, 232–239

Malignant ascites, 125–142
  chemotherapy in, 137–138
  diagnosis of, 126–128
  etiology of, 125–126
  immunotherapy and biologic response modifiers in, 138–140
  LeVeen and Denver shunt results, 131–137
  natural history and complications of, 128
  need for intervention, 128–129
  paracentesis in, 129–131
Malignant fibrous histiocytoma of the great vessels, 224
Malignant obstruction
  biliary, 111–114
  gastrointestinal, 25–60
    anal region cancer and, 47–48
    cancer therapy and, 48–51
    colon and rectum cancer and, 36–43
    constipation and, 163
    esophageal cancer including gastric cardia in, 25–29
    extrinsic compression by malignancy and, 54–56
    gastric cancer and, 29–31
    mesenteric small bowel malignancy and, 34–36
    palliative management of recurrent colorectal cancer and, 43–47
    periampullary region cancer and, 31–34
    peritoneal carcinomatosis and, 51–54
Malignant pericardial effusion, 253–256
Malignant pleural effusion, 249–252
Mallory-Weiss tear, 64–65
Malnutrition, 321–342
  assessment for, 321–323
  causes of, 325–328
  enteral nutrition in, 334–336
  future research in, 337–339
  in malignant ascites, 128
  nutrient replacement in, 328–330, 331
  outpatient supplements in, 336
  parenteral nutrition in, 330–334
  prevalence of, 323–325
  secondary to radiation-induced malabsorption, 154
  vomiting and, 168–169
Marinol, 174–175
Maturation phase of wound repair, 307
Maximal oxygen consumption, 275
Maximal tolerance dose (TD 50/5), 144
Maximal volume ventilation, 274–275
McCorkle and Young Symptom Distress Scale, 165
Mechlorethamine, 212, 218–219
Median sternotomy
  in mediastinal tumor, 257
  in pulmonary metastasis resection, 264
  in thoracic spine tumor, 260
Mediastinal lymphoproliferative disease, 256–259
Mediastinal mass, 256
Megestrol acetate and appetite stimulation, 336
Melanoma, pulmonary metastases, 262–263
Melena
  in lower gastrointestinal bleeding, 69
  in upper gastrointestinal bleeding, 61
Melphalan, 296
6-Mercaptopurine
  effects on wound healing, 312, 314
  emetic potential of, 171
  toxicity of, 296
Mesh sling to prevent pelvic radiation injury, 151

Metabolic acidosis, hyperchloremic, 332
Metabolic disturbances, 325–327
Metastasis
  pancreatitis and, 11
  pulmonary, 262–265
  small bowel, 36
Metastasectomy, 262, 264
Methotrexate
  effects on wound healing, 312–313, 314
  emetic potential of, 171
  toxicity of, 296
  venous thrombosis and, 387
Methylcellulose fiber, 166
Metoclopramide, 172–173
Metopimazine, 164
Metronidazole, 105, 365
Miconazole, 100
Microangiopathic hemolytic anemia, 383
Microvascular thrombosis, 238
Middle mediastinal mass, 276–279
Milk of Magnesia, 167
Minimal tolerance dose, (TD 5/5), 144
Mini-thoracotomy, 264
Misoprostol, 151
Mithramycin
  extravasation injury and, 212
  in hypercalcemia, 288
  preoperative evaluation of, 295
Mitomycin C
  effects on wound healing, 313, 314
  emetic potential of, 171
  extravasation injury and, 212
  preoperative evaluation of, 295
Mitotic inhibitors, 296
Mitoxantrone
  cardiotoxicity of, 294
  effects on wound healing, 313, 314
Mucor, 13, 356
Mucositis
  myelosuppression and, 376
  viral infections and, 343
Myeloproliferative disorders, 385–387
Myelosuppression, chemotherapy-induced, 375–376
Myxoma, atrial, 226–227

Narcotics, constipation and, 163–164, 167
Nasogastric tube in gastrointestinal bleeding, 62
Nasointestinal feeding tube, 334
Nausea
  in bowel obstruction caused by carcinomatosis, 52
  harmful effects of, 168–169
  neurophysiology of, 169–170
  in neutropenic enterocolitis, 6
  in pancreatitis, 117
  in radiation enteritis, 145
Navelbine, 164
Necrosis
  in doxorubicin extravasation, 212–214
  in neutropenic enterocolitis, 6
Needle biopsy, percutaneous, 266
Needle catheter jejunostomy, 334
Neodymium:yttrium aluminum garnet laser (Nd:YAg)
  in colon cancer, 40
  in esophageal cancer, 27–29
  in rectal cancer, 42

Neurotensin, 147
Neutropenia
  febrile, 348–351, 352–353
  infections and, 346–348
  myelosuppression and, 376
  wound healing and, 307
Neutropenic enterocolitis, 5–10
Neutropenic enteropathy, 5
Nevin classification of gallbladder carcinoma, 114
Nitrogen mustard
  emetic potential of, 171
  extravasation injury and, 212, 218–219
  in malignant pleural effusion, 251
Nitroprusside, 283
Nitrosourea, 296
Nonbacterial thrombotic endocarditis, 239
Non-Hodgkin's lymphoma
  gastrointestinal perforation and, 12
  mediastinal lymph nodes and, 256
Nonsteroidal anti-inflammatory drugs, 102
Nortriptyline, 164
Nosocomial infection, 344
Nutrient replacement, 328–330, 331
Nutritional defects, tumor mass and, 230
Nutritional support, 321–342
  assessment for, 321–323
  in chronic radiation enteritis, 154
  future research in, 337–339
  malnutrition and
    causes of, 325–328
    enteral nutrition in, 334–336
    nutrient replacement in, 328–330, 331
    outpatient supplements in, 336
    parenteral nutrition in, 330–334
    prevalence of, 323–325
Nystatin, 100

Obstruction
  biliary, 111–114
  gastrointestinal, 25–60
    abdominal pain in, 15–16
    anal region cancer and, 47–48
    cancer therapy and, 48–51
    colon and rectum cancer and, 36–43
    constipation and, 163
    esophageal cancer including gastric cardia in, 25–29
    extrinsic compression by malignancy and, 54–56
    gastric cancer and, 29–31
    mesenteric small bowel malignancy and, 34–36
    palliative management of recurrent colorectal cancer and, 43–47
    periampullary region cancer and, 31–34
    peritoneal carcinomatosis and, 51–54
  small bowel
    after cancer surgery, 49–51
    after intraperitoneal chemotherapy, 48–49
    after pelvic irradiation, 150–152
    chronic radiation enteritis and, 149, 150
    perforation and, 84
Occlusion of peritoneovenous shunt, 136
Octreotide, 281
OK-432 in malignant ascites, 139
Omega-3 fatty acids, 335
Oncovin; See Vincristine

Ondansetron
  for chemotherapy-induced emesis, 172–173
  constipation and, 164
Open lung biopsy
  in diagnosis of pulmonary infiltrates, 362
  in interstitial lung disease, 266
Opioids, constipation and, 163–164
Oral intake in constipation, 166
Oral mucosa, stomatitis and, 98
Oropharyngeal herpes simplex virus infection, 358
Osmotic diuresis, 287
Osmotic laxatives, 167
Ovarian cancer
  gastrointestinal obstruction in, 51–54
  malignant ascites in, 128–129
Overfeeding, 333
Oxyphenisatin, 167

Pain; See also Abdominal pain
  in bowel obstruction caused by carcinomatosis, 52
  in constipation, 161
  in esophageal perforation, 75
  in extravasation injury, 212
  in hemobilia, 67
  in pericardial effusion, 253
  in pleural effusion, 250
  in small bowel malignancy, 34
  in thrombus-associated catheter malfunction, 201
Palliative procedures
  in esophageal cancer, 25–27
  in gastric cancer, 30–31
  in tracheoesophageal fistula, 80
Pancreatic cancer, 31–34
Pancreatitis, 10–11, 117–118
Paracentesis, 129–131
Paraganglioma of carotid bifurcation, 224–226
Parasite, immune defects and, 345
Parenchymal lung disease, 265–267
Parenteral nutrition, 154, 330–334
Partial thromboplastin time, 286
P.A.S. Port, 186
Patient positioning for central venous access, 188, 190
Peel-away introducer, 193
Pelvic irradiation, bowel obstruction after, 150–152
Percutaneous needle biopsy, 266
Percutaneous venous access, 190–193
Perforation
  fecal impaction and, 165
  gastrointestinal, 74–91
    abdominal pain in, 12–13
    abscess and, 85
    colonic, 88–91
    esophageal, 75–80
    small intestine and, 84–88
    stomach and duodenum and, 81–84
Perfusion scan and pulmonary embolism, 233–234
Periampullary region cancer, 31–34
Pericardial biopsy, 253
Pericardial effusion, 253–256, 279–280
Pericardial window, 254
Pericardialperitoneal shunt, 255–256
Pericardiectomy, 255
Pericardioscopy, 255
Peripheral bile duct cholangiocarcinoma, 113
Peripheral venous access, 183

Peripherally inserted central catheter (PIC catheter), 184
Peripherally inserted subcutaneous port, 186
Peritoneal carcinomatosis, 51–54
Peritoneal lavage, 7
Peritoneovenous shunt
  complications of, 135–137
  in malignant ascites, 129–131
Phagocytic defects, 346–348
Phagocytosis, associated diseases, 345
Phenolphthalein, 167
Phenoxybenzamine, 282
Phentolamine, 283
Phenylalanine mustard, 387–388
Phenytoin, 336
Pheochromocytoma, 281–283
Phlebography, 232–233
Phlebotomy, 386
Phlegmasia cerulea dolens, 237
Phycomycetes, 13, 356
Physical examination
  in colonic or rectal perforation, 89
  in gastric or duodenal perforation, 81
  in malnutrition, 322
  in mediastinal tumor, 257
  in upper gastrointestinal bleeding, 63
Pitressin, 64
Platelet count
  posttransfusion, 381
  preoperative, 285
Platelet transfusion, 379–381
  in disseminated intravascular coagulation, 384
  prior to venous access, 187, 196
Pleural biopsy, 250
Pleural effusion, 249–252
Pleural fluid, 249
Pleural symphysis, 251
Pleurectomy, 252
Pleuropericardial window, 254
Pleuroperitoneal shunt, 252
Pneumatosis intestinalis, 364
Pneumonia, candidal, 354–355
Pneumonitis, interstitial, 352
Pneumoperitoneum, 13
Pneumothorax during central venous access, 197
Polycythemia vera, 386
Polyglycolic acid mesh to suspend small bowel, 153
Popliteal vein scan, 234
Port pocket infection, 203
Portal vein occlusion, 118–120
Portal venous hypertension, 63
Posterolateral thoracotomy, 259
Postrenal failure, 289
Pre-albumin and nutritional status, 322
Prednisone, 382
Preoperative evaluation, 273–304
  airway considerations in, 273–274
  of carcinoid syndrome, 280–283
  of cardiac tamponade, 279–280
  in central venous access, 187–188
  of chemotherapy patient, 291–297
  hematologic considerations in, 283–286
  in lung resection, 274–276
  of mediastinal mass, 276–279
  of pericardial effusion, 279–280

  of pheochromocytoma, 281–283
  in renal and electrolyte disorders, 286–291
Prerenal azotemia, 333
Prerenal failure, 289
Primary anastomosis without bowel preparation, 40–41
Procarbazine
  emetic potential of, 171
  preoperative evaluation of, 297
Prochlorperazine, 175
Proctitis, radiation, 106, 156
Prognostic nutritional index, 322
Proliferation phase of wound repair, 306–307
Prophylaxis
  bone marrow transplantation, 378–379
  carcinoid syndrome, 281
  deep venous thrombosis, 238–239
  for immunocompromised patient, 366–367
  platelet transfusion as, 380
  radiation-induced injury, 152
Prostaglandin inhibitors, 145–146
Prosthetic mesh to suspend small bowel, 152–153
Protein catabolism, 326
Protein metabolism, 326
Proteus, 99
Prothrombin time, 286
Proximal biliary duct cholangiocarcinoma, 112
Pseudomembranous colitis, 74
Pseudomonas
  in cholangitis, 116
  in neutropenic enterocolitis, 6
  neutropenic patient and, 349
  nosocomial spread of, 344
  in oral infection, 99
Psychologic factors
  in anorexia, 325
  in vomiting, 169
Psyllium derivatives, 166
Pulmonary angiography, 233
Pulmonary artery catheterization, 279–280
Pulmonary artery malignancy, 224
Pulmonary edema, 136
Pulmonary embolism
  chemotherapy-related, 387
  deep venous thrombosis and, 232
  diagnosis of, 233–234
Pulmonary fibrosis, bleomycin-induced, 294–295
Pulmonary function tests
  chemotherapy and, 291
  preoperative, 274–275
Pulmonary infiltrates, 362–364
Pulmonary vascular resistance, 275
Purpura
  facial, 169
  idiopathic thrombocytopenic, 381–382

Quinacrine, 251
Quinolone, 367

Radiation enteritis, 143–160
  acute and subacute, 145
  bowel obstruction and, 150–152
  chronic, 147–150
  prevention of, 152–153
  risk of recurrent obstruction and, 50
  treatment of, 145–147, 153–156

Radiation esophagitis, 99–100
Radiation proctitis, 106, 156
Radiation stomatitis, 98
Radiation therapy
  airway complications in, 273–274
  in cholangiocarcinoma, 112, 113
  in colorectal cancer, 43–45
  in esophageal cancer, 26, 29
  in gastric cancer, 30
  in mediastinal mass, 258
  in rectal cancer, 42
  vascular effects of, 230
  wound healing and, 315
Radiography
  in central venous access, 195–196
  in esophageal perforation, 75–76
  in gastric or duodenal perforation, 81
  in malignant pericardial effusion, 253
  in mediastinal tumor, 257
  in neutropenic enterocolitis, 6–7
Random donor units, 379–380
Recall enteritis, term, 147
Recombinant human erythropoietin (Rh EPO), 378
Rectal cancer
  gastrointestinal obstruction in, 36–47
    electrocautery fulguration in, 46–47
    laser ablation in, 45–46
    left-sided, 39–41
    radiation therapy in, 43–45
    rectosigmoid, 42–43
    surgical resection or diversion in, 43, 44
  radiation-induced, 154
Rectovaginal fistula, 156
Rectum
  extrinsic compression of, 54–55
  lower gastrointestinal bleeding and, 73–74
  radiation effects on, 106
Red blood cell
  cancer-related anemia and, 377
  erythropoietin and, 378
Refeeding syndrome, 332, 335
Remodeling stage of wound repair, 307
Renal cell carcinoma, 263
Renal disease
  preoperative evaluation of, 286–291
  total parenteral nutrition in, 333
Renal potassium wasting, 287
Resection
  in bowel obstruction after pelvic irradiation, 151
  in colon cancer, 38, 39
  in esophageal cancer, 25–26
  in gallbladder cancer, 113
  in gastric cancer, 30
  lung, 262, 274–276
  in mediastinal mass, 258, 259
  of periampullary cancer, 31
  in radiation enteritis, 155–156
  of radiation-damaged colon, 106
  of soft tissue sarcoma, 263
  vascular reconstruction associated with, 240–241
Residual volume, 274–275
Resuscitation
  in lower gastrointestinal bleeding, 70
  in upper gastrointestinal bleeding, 61–62

Retrocolic loop gastrojejunostomy, 32
Retrosternal goiter, 257
rhEPO; *See* Recombinant human erythropoietin
Rhinocerebral infection, 355–356
Rhizopus, 356
Rupture of hepatic tumor, 120–121

Saphenous vein cutdown, 193, 195
Sarcoma
  aortic, 224
  gastric, 82
  Kaposi's, 223–224
  soft tissue, metastatic to lungs, 263
Sclerotherapy
  in esophageal varices, 64
  in malignant pleural effusion, 250–252
Selective gut decontamination, 367
Semustine, 296
Senna, 166–167
Serratia, 99
Serum-ascites albumin difference, 127
Shunt
  Denver, 131–135, 252
  LeVeen, 131–137
  pericardialperitoneal, 255–256
  peritoneovenous, 133, 135–136
  pleuroperitoneal, 252
  splenorenal, 64
  transjugular intrahepatic portosystemic (TIPS), 64, 119–120
Sigmoid colon cancer and obstruction, 42
Sigmoidoscopy
  in lower gastrointestinal bleeding, 70
  in recurrent rectal cancer, 45
Single-lumen catheter, 185
Skin disruption, 343
Skin graft and extravasation injuries, 216, 217–218
Small bowel
  cancer of
    gastrointestinal obstruction in, 34–36
    lower gastrointestinal bleeding in, 71
  chronic radiation enteritis involving, 148, 149
  lymphoma of, 35
  obstruction of
    after cancer surgery, 49–51
    after intraperitoneal chemotherapy, 48–49
    after pelvic irradiation, 150–152
  perforation of, 84–88
Small vessel tumor, 223–224
Soft tissue sarcoma metastatic to lungs, 263
Somatostatin
  in carcinoid syndrome, 281
  in preserving host mass, 337
Spine, thoracic, 259–261
Spironolactone and ascites management, 129
Splanchnic outflow obstruction, 118
Spleen, disseminated fungal infection and, 14
Splenectomy
  alterations in humoral immunity and, 344–346
  in idiopathic thrombocytopenic purpura, 382
Splenic vein thrombosis, 63
Split-thickness skin graft, 216, 217–218
Spontaneous perforation, term, 12
Spontaneous rupture of hepatic tumor, 120
Squamous cell carcinoma of anal canal, 47–48

Staphylococcus aureus
    neutropenic patient and, 349
    nosocomial spread of, 344
Staphylococcus epidermidis, 351
Starvation cachexia, 327
Steatosis, hepatic, 332
Stent
    in cholangiocarcinoma, 113
    in cholangitis, 116
    in gastrointestinal obstruction
        esophageal cancer and, 27–29
        stomach cancer and, 31
    in pancreatic cancer, 33
Steroid-induced cell death, 310
Steroids
    in carcinoid syndrome, 281
    in radiation-induced injury, 152
    stress steroids, 297–299
Stomach
    cancer of
        gastrointestinal obstruction in, 29–31
        upper gastrointestinal bleeding in, 67
    perforation of, 81–84
Stomatitis, 98–99, 327
Stool evaluation, 7
Streptococci, 349
Streptozocin
    emetic potential of, 171
    pulmonary toxicity of, 296
Stress gastritis, 65–66, 102
Stress steroids, 297–300
Stricture, radiation-induced bowel, 149, 150
Subclavian catheter, 184
Subclavian vein access, 190–193
Subcutaneous infusion port, 185–186, 192
    infection and, 203, 361
    removal of, 198–199
Subxiphoid pericardiectomy, 255
Subxiphoid pericardiocentesis, 254
Sulfasalazine, 151
Superior vena cava access, 188
Superior vena cava syndrome
    deep venous thrombosis and, 237
    lymphoma and, 256
Supraclavicular needle entry, 190
Syndrome of inappropriate antidiuretic hormone, 287
Synthetic polyphenolics, 167

T cell
    activation of, 344
    in wound repair, 306
Tagged red blood cell scan, 70
Tamoxifen
    in malignant ascites, 137
    venous thrombosis and, 387–388
Taste alterations, 321
Tenckhoff catheter
    in malignant ascites, 129
    in pleural effusion, 252
Tetracycline
    enteral feedings and, 336
    in malignant pleural effusion, 251
Thoracentesis, 250
Thoracic disorders, 249–270
    lymphoproliferative disease of mediastinum in, 256–259
    malignant pericardial effusion in, 253–256
    malignant pleural effusion in, 249–252
    parenchymal lung disease in, 265–267
    pulmonary metastases in, 262–265
    surgical approach to thoracic spine in, 259–261
Thoracic esophageal perforation, 76–79
Thoracoscopy
    in malignant pleural effusion, 250
    in mediastinal tumor, 257
    in metastatectomy, 264
Thoracostomy
    in interstitial lung disease, 266–267
    in malignant pleural effusion, 250
Thoracotomy
    in esophageal perforation, 78
    in malignant pleural effusion, 251
    in pulmonary metastasis resection, 264
    in thoracic spine tumor, 259
Thrombocythemia, 386
Thrombocytopenia, 379–382
    after peritoneovenous shunt, 136
    chemotherapy and, 231
    disseminated intravascular coagulation and, 384
    heparin anticoagulation and, 235
    perioperative platelet support in, 380–381
    preoperative evaluation of, 285
    venous access and, 187
Thrombocytopenic purpura, idiopathic, 381–382
Thrombocytosis, 285
Thrombolytic therapy, 19
Thrombosis, 232–239
    chemotherapy-related, 387–388
    deep venous, 232–239
        disseminated intravascular coagulation and, 383
        late complications of, 237–238
        prophylaxis and surveillance against, 238–239
        treatment of, 234–237
        tumor mass and, 229
    indwelling central venous access device and, 200–202
    large vessel, 238–239
    microvascular, 238
    in myeloproliferative disorders, 386
    preoperative evaluation for, 285–286
    splenic vein, 63
    tumor mass and, 230
Thymoma, 257
TIPS; *See* Transjugular intrahepatic portosystemic shunt
Tissue, radiation effects on, 143
Tissue factor, tumor growth and, 228
Tissue plasminogen activator, 236
Total nitrogen balance, 331
Total parenteral nutrition, 146, 329–334
Towne live attenuated virus, 360
Toxicity of radiation, 144
Tracheoesophageal fistula, 79–80
Transfusion; *See* Blood transfusion
Transhiatal esophagectomy, 26
Transjugular intrahepatic portosystemic shunt, 64, 119–120
Transudative effusion, 250
Trazodone, 164

Trendelenburg position for central venous access, 188
Triazole, 357–358
Triceps skin fold, 322
Trimethoprim-sulfamethoxazole, 366
Trimipramine, 164
Triple-lumen catheter, 185
Trypsin, 152
Tube decompression in recurrent small bowel cancer, 49
Tuftsin, 344
Tumor, vascular effects of, 227–231
Tumor markers, 257
Tumor necrosis factor
　cachexia and, 327, 328
　in malignant ascites, 139
Tunnel infection in central venous access devices, 203
Typhlitis, 5, 88–89, 364

Ulcer
　Cushing's, 65
　skin in doxorubicin extravasation, 212–214
　duodenal
　　perforation of, 83
　　upper gastrointestinal bleeding in, 68–69
　gastric
　　perforation of, 13, 82
　　upper gastrointestinal hemorrhage in, 66–67
　in neutropenic enterocolitis, 6
Ultrasound
　in acalculous cholecystitis, 114
　in deep venous thrombosis, 233
　in malignant ascites, 127–128
Upper gastrointestinal bleeding, 61–69
　duodenum and, 68–69
　esophageal, 63–65
　hemobilia and, 67–68
　initial management of, 61–63
　stomach and, 65–67
Urokinase, 385
　in deep venous thrombosis, 236
　in thrombus-associated catheter malfunction, 201–202
　in withdrawal occlusion, 203

Vagotomy
　in duodenal ulcer, 69, 83
　in gastric ulcer, 82
Vancomycin, 105
Varicella-zoster virus, 14–15
Vascular access devices, 184–187
Vascular permeability factor, 126
Vascular problems, 223–248
　arterial occlusive disease in
　　accelerated chronic, 242
　　embolic, 239–240
　in chronic radiation enteritis, 149–150
　concomitant conditions and, 241–242
　hemorrhage in, 232
　primary vascular tumors in, 223–227
　　large vessel, 224–227
　　small vessel, 223–224
　small vessel injury caused by radiation and, 104
　tumor effects in, 227–231
　vascular reconstruction associated with resection in, 240–241
　venous thromboembolism in, 232–239

Vascular system
　cellular effects of tumors on, 227–229
　central venous access and, 189
　chemotherapy effects on, 231
　effects of surgery on, 230–231
　radiation therapy effects on, 230
Vascular tumor, 223–227
　large vessel, 224–227
　small vessel, 223–224
Vasopressin, 64
Venography, 201, 202
Venotomy, 193, 194, 195
Venous access; *See* Central venous access
Venous cutdown, 189, 193, 194, 195
Venous duplex scan, 187
Venous gangrene, 237
Venous thromboembolism, 232–239
VePesid; *See* Etoposide
Verapamil, 164
Vertebral column tumor, 259
Vinblastine
　constipation and, 164
　effects on wound healing, 313, 314
　extravasation injury and, 212, 218–219
　toxicity of, 296
Vinca alkaloids
　constipation and, 164
　extravasation injury and, 212, 218–219
Vincristine
　constipation and, 164
　effects on wound healing, 313, 314
　emetic potential of, 171
　extravasation injury and, 212, 218–219
　ileus and, 16
　toxicity of, 296
Vindesine, 212, 218–219
Viral infection
　immune defects and, 345
　in neutropenic patient, 14, 358–360
Vitamin deficiency, 377
Vitamin E
　to prevent pelvic radiation injury, 151
　in radiation enteritis, 146
Vitamin K, 336
Vomiting
　in bowel obstruction caused by carcinomatosis, 52
　chemotherapy-induced, 168–177
　　combination therapy for, 175–176
　　general guidelines in, 171–172
　　harmful effects of, 168–169
　　neurophysiology of, 169–170
　　single agent therapy for, 172–175
　　temporal patterns of, 170–171
　in neutropenic enterocolitis, 6
　in pancreatitis, 117
　radiation therapy and, 144, 145
von Willebrand factor, 228–229
VP-16; *See* Etoposide

Warfarin, 234
Wedge resection of lung, 262, 264
Weight loss
　in cachexia syndrome, 321–322
　in colonic or rectal perforation, 89
　frequency and survival, 324

Index

White blood cell count, 114
Withdrawal occlusion, 203
Wound healing, 305–319
   basic principles of, 305–307
   cancer effects on, 230
   chemotherapy effects on, 307–315
      actinomycin D in, 311
      animal models in, 314
      bleomycin in, 309
      cisplatin in, 309–310
      corticosteroids in, 310–311
      cyclophosphamide in, 311
      dacarbazine in, 311
      doxorubicin in, 308–309
      etoposide in, 311–312
      5-fluorouracil in, 312
      6-mercaptopurine in, 312
      methotrexate in, 312–313
      mitomycin in, 313
      mitoxantrone in, 313
      systemic, 307–308
      vinblastine in, 313
      vincristine in, 313

Xanthomas maltophilia, 350

DELAWARE ACADEMY OF MEDICINE
LEWIS B. FLINN LIBRARY
1925 LOVERING AVE.
WILMINGTON, DEL. 19806